The British Horse Society

THE BHS COMPLETE MANUAL OF
HORSE AND STABLE MANAGEMENT

Revised and expanded by

Josephine Batty-Smith BHSI, CERT. ED

KENILWORTH PRESS

This revised and expanded edition, with the new title *The BHS Complete Manual of Horse and Stable Management,* was published in 2008 in the UK by Kenilworth Press, an imprint of Quiller Publishing Ltd

Reprinted 2010, 2011

First edition published in the UK in 1998 under the title *The BHS Complete Manual of Stable Management* by Kenilworth Press, an imprint of Quiller Publishing Ltd

Reprinted 1998, 1999, 2000 (twice), 2001, 2002, 2003 (twice), 2004, 2005, 2006 (twice), 2007

British Library Cataloguing-in-Publication Data
A catalogue record for this book
is available from the British Library

ISBN 978 1 905693 18 4

Cover and prelim design by Sharyn Troughton

Printed by Bell & Bain Ltd, Glasgow

Kenilworth Press

An imprint of Quiller Publishing Ltd
Wykey House, Wykey, Shrewsbury, SY4 1JA
Tel: 01939 261616 Fax: 01939 261606
E-mail: info@quillerbooks.com
Website: www.kenilworthpress.co.uk

THE BHS COMPLETE MANUAL OF
HORSE
AND
STABLE
MANAGEMENT

CONTENTS

Preface 8
Acknowledgements 9

Section 1 THE HORSE
1 Conformation and How to Assess it 13
2 Action 29
3 The Psychology of the Horse 32
4 The Teeth and Ageing 34
5 Breeds 39
6 Breeding 45
7 Identification 55
8 Buying and Selling a Horse 61

Section 2 CARE OF THE HORSE
9 Management Methods 67
10 Handling the Horse 71
11 Grooming 81
12 Clipping, Trimming, Pulling and Plaiting 88
13 The Foot and Shoeing 101
14 Bedding 116
15 Signs of Good and Ill-Health, and Sick Nursing 123
16 Basic Systems of the Horse and How to Get a Horse Fit 133
17 Internal Parasites 138
18 Stable Vices and Problem Behaviour 144

Section 3 WATERING AND FEEDING
19 Watering 153
20 Food and Digestion 159
21 The Rules of Feeding 166
22 Food – Composition and Types 169
23 Deciding on a Ration 186
24 Feeding Problems and Non-routine Feeding 200
25 Managing Forage 205
26 The Feed Shed and Storing Food 208

Section 4 SADDLERY AND TACK
27 The Saddle 215
28 Bridles 226
29 Other Saddlery 231
30 Bits 243
31 Boots and Bandages 254
32 Clothing 265
33 Care and Cleaning 271
34 Saddling up and Unsaddling 280

Section 5 SPECIALIST CARE OF THE COMPETITION HORSE
35 Guidelines for Competition Horses 287
36 The Event Horse 291
37 The Dressage Horse 298
38 The Show Jumper 300
39 The Endurance Horse 302
40 The Driving Horse or Pony 307
41 The Hunter 309
42 The Point-to-Pointer 314
43 The Show Horse or Pony 319
44 The Polo Pony 326
45 Transportation 330

Section 6 THE HORSE AT GRASS
46 Grassland Management 347
47 Management of Horses and Ponies at Grass 357
48 Working the Grass-kept Horse or Pony 371
49 Bringing a Horse up From Grass 376

Section 7 THE STABLE YARD
50 Construction of Stables 381
51 Design of Stables 387
52 Riding Areas 410
53 Buying Fodder and Bedding 417
54 Organising and Running a Yard 422
55 The Law 448

Appendices

1 Measurements 471

2 The British Horse Society 472

3 Equine Passports 477

4 Vaccinations 479

5 Government Publications and Codes of Practice 481

6 The National Equine Database 486

7 Animal Transport Certificate and Route Plan 487

8 Stable Fires 490

Further Reading 492
Index 494

PREFACE

The aim of this volume is to provide a reliable source of information and advice on all practical aspects of horse and stable management. Throughout the book emphasis is placed on the adoption of correct and safe procedures for the welfare of all who come into contact with horses, as well as for the animals themselves. The book has been compiled by a panel of experts, each drawing on considerable experience and contributing specialised knowledge on his or her chosen subject.

There is no one 'BHS method' or procedure for doing any task. Any procedure that is safe for both handler and equine, is practical and efficient and achieves the right outcome is acceptable practice.

ACKNOWLEDGEMENTS

The British Horse Society would like to acknowledge the contribution made by the late Pat Smallwood FBHS, who undertook much of the initial work on this project.

The British Horse Society is also grateful to the following individuals for their invaluable assistance:

Joan Allen; Islay Auty FBHS; Goran Breisner FBHS; Carole Broad FBHS; Jo Claridge; Dr James L. Duncan; Eric Ellis; Sidney Free; Judy Harvey FBHS; Stewart Hastie MRCVS; Jeremy Houghton-Brown BPhilEd; Jane Kidd; Elizabeth Launder MSc; James Lord; Deborah Lucas MSc; Gillian McCarthy BSc; Jane McHugh; Dr David Marlin; Tessa Martin-Bird FBHS; Stella Hore; Clive Scott; Richard Shepherd; the late Michael Simons MRCVS; Barbara Slane Fleming FBHS; Sue Tanzer; Claire Tomlinson; Gillian Watson FBHS; Helen Webber FBHS; and members of the 1997 BHS Training Committee.

Illustrations
The line drawings are all by Dianne Breeze, except for the foot detail diagrams on pages 15 and 102 (left), which are by Christine Bousfield.

NOTE: Throughout the book the term 'horses' is used and it will often include ponies.

THE HORSE

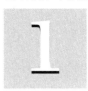

CONFORMATION AND HOW TO ASSESS IT

The conformation of a horse or pony affects his soundness, ability to perform and comfort as a ride. If the horse is in good condition, the following features should be sought:

General Impression

The general impression should be that he is built in proportion, with all sectors matching and his outlook is alert, bold and confident.

The 'top line' – the neck, withers, back, loins and dock – should form a succession of well-developed outlines, each of which blends smoothly into the next. He should have a good sloping shoulder, a relatively short back and a long croup, i.e. length from hip to point of buttock, giving an appearance of 'standing over a lot of ground', whilst being well balanced over his legs, which are four square underneath him.

If the horse is in poor condition, only an experienced person with a 'good eye' can assess his potential. It takes skill to recognise whether he has the right make and shape; and to see that when given suitable care, food and work, he will make up into a worthwhile or even top-class animal.

Similarly, too much fat can disguise a horse's outline, and can make it difficult to visualise what he will be like when the excess weight is lost and he is fit.

A horse with good skeletal structure, but poor muscle development, can be transformed by being given suitable work and the opportunity to use and develop his muscles in the correct way.

Feet

The much-quoted saying 'no foot, no horse' is very true. The make and shape of feet are vital to the soundness and functioning of the horse.

Front feet and hind feet should be matching pairs. Any obvious difference in outline, angle of foot to the ground, or size of frog, should be viewed with suspicion. The only exception is the horse whose foot has been worn down through losing a shoe.

- The front feet should slope at an angle of 45–50° from the ground.

- The hoof wall should continue at the same angle as the pastern when viewed from the side.

- The hind feet should have a slightly steeper slope, and should be longer and narrower than the front feet.

- All feet should point straight forwards. Any deviation from this is usually caused by poor conformation of the leg, and will result in faulty action.

The heels should be wide, with a well-developed frog to help absorb concussion. The sole should be slightly concave. Contracted heels and poorly developed frogs restrict the blood supply to the foot, and increase the vulnerability to navicular disease.

Large, flat feet can cause problems, particularly on stony ground. They are liable to develop corns and are easily bruised.

Small feet are a disadvantage, as they give a smaller weight-bearing surface, and there is a greater tendency

The points of the horse

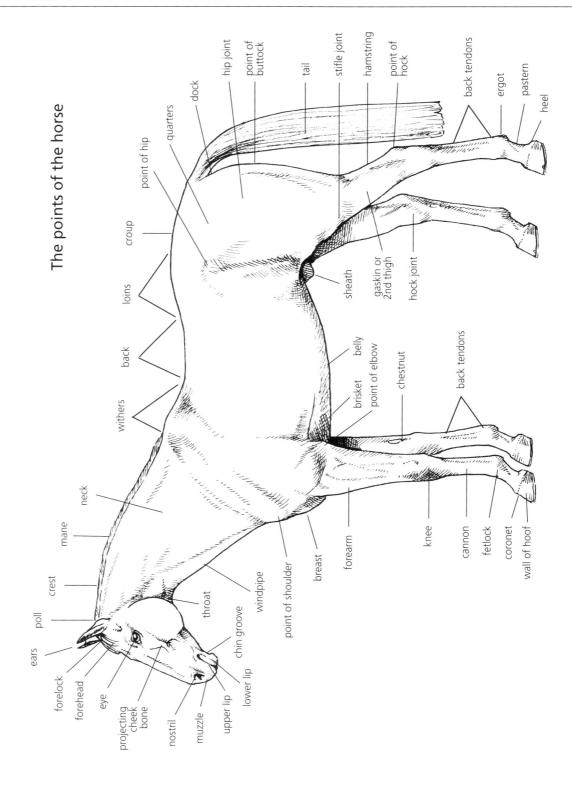

The skeleton

Bones of the foot

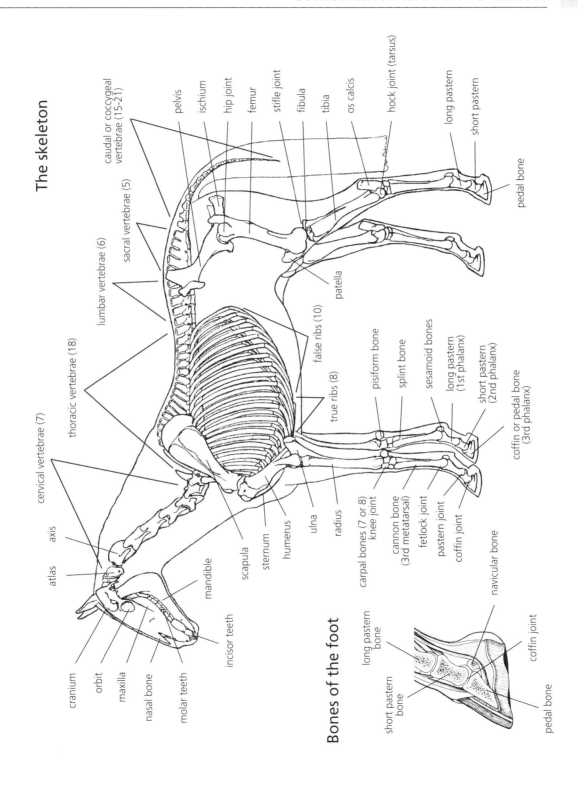

The skeleton labels:
cranium, orbit, maxilla, nasal bone, molar teeth, incisor teeth, mandible, atlas, axis, cervical vertebrae (7), thoracic vertebrae (18), lumbar vertebrae (6), sacral vertebrae (5), caudal or coccygeal vertebrae (15-21), pelvis, ischium, hip joint, femur, stifle joint, fibula, tibia, os calcis, hock joint (tarsus), long pastern, short pastern, pedal bone, patella, false ribs (10), true ribs (8), pisiform bone, splint bone, sesamoid bones, long pastern (1st phalanx), short pastern (2nd phalanx), coffin or pedal bone (3rd phalanx), scapula, sternum, humerus, ulna, radius, carpal bones (7 or 8) knee joint, cannon bone (3rd metatarsal), fetlock joint, pastern joint, coffin joint, navicular bone

Bones of the foot labels:
long pastern bone, short pastern bone, pedal bone, coffin joint, navicular bone

The main superficial external muscles

semitendinosus

biceps femoris

deep digital flexor

gluteal fascia or
superficial gluteal

intercostal

latissimus dorsi

digital extensor

deep pectoral

lateral carpal flexor

trapezius

splenius

rhomboideus

masseter

sternocephalicus

brachiocephalicus

deltoid

triceps

superficial pectoral

radial carpal extensor

common digital extensor

Simple Facts About the Superficial Muscles

Body muscles are responsible for maintaining posture and preserving the overall shape of the horse when he is standing still.

Some muscles limit movement and provide joint stability by preventing too much movement or preventing unwanted movement.

Muscles can only work in contraction, so are always arranged in opposing groups performing opposing actions.

Muscles must be attached at each end in order to produce their required action. They are attached at either end by tendons which are formed from dense white fibrous tissue. Each tendon is continuous with the belly of the muscle at one end and attaches seamlessly to the periosteum of the bone at the other.

There are different types of muscles to perform different tasks.

Muscles that cause a joint to bend are called *flexors*.

Muscles that cause a joint to straighten are called *extensors*.

A muscle which carries a limb further away from the body than it was previously is called an *abductor*.

The opposite action is produced by an *adductor* muscle.

Some of the Major Superficial Muscles and Their Actions

Brachiocephalic: extending from the front of the upper arm to the head. When the horse is standing still this muscle helps to swing the head and neck to the side. During movement it draws the forelimb forwards when the foot is raised from the ground at the end of the stride.

Trapezius: the muscle on either side of the withers, over the top of the *Rhomboideus* and *Splenius* muscles. It draws the scapula up and back.

Rhomboideus: draws the scapula upwards and forwards; it elevates the shoulder.

Splenius: elevates the head and turns the head and neck to one side.

Latissimus dorsi: runs from shoulder blade to back. It draws the scapula down and back. It draws the humerus up and back and supports the dorsal part of the thorax.

Longissimus dorsi: runs along the back. The muscle the rider sits upon. It supports the rider's weight.

Sternocephalicus: flexes the head and neck forwards and downwards.

Serratus ventralis: the cervical and thoracic part acts as a sling for the trunk.

Triceps: extensor muscle of the elbow.

Biceps: flexor muscle of the elbow.

Semitendinosus: extends hip and flexes the stifle.

Biceps femoris: extends the hip joint, flexes the stifle joint. The main belly flexes the hock, the anterior part extends the stifle.

Gluteus medius: extends the hip joint.

towards unsoundness in the foot.

The wall of the foot should be smooth and free from cracks. Rings and grooves are a sign of change of management or diet; pronounced rings can signify laminitis (see Shoeing, page 101 onwards).

The texture of the horn is of importance. Some breeds of horses have naturally hard feet, especially native ponies, Arabs and Hackneys. Poor horn texture can be improved by careful feeding, particularly the use of the additive biotin, and by the use of horn stimulants.

A skilled farrier can greatly improve a horse's feet through regular attention. Equally, lack of care or an inexperienced farrier can spoil good feet.

Head

The head should be lean, well set on to the neck and of a size and style to suit the type of horse. There should be sufficient width between the branches of the lower jaw to allow ample room for the top of the windpipe. The jaw bone itself should not be too large. There must be room between the lower edge of the jaw bone and the jugular furrow, to allow the horse to flex.

The set of the head on the neck is very important, as it affects respiration, and ease of flexion, which in its turn affects the control and balance of the horse.

Eyes

The eyes should be of a good size and expression, and widely set to give broad vision. Their expression is a key to temperament and reliability, and should be bold and generous, not mean and sharp, if the horse is to work well.

Muzzle

The muzzle should be fine with a well-defined nostril. The jaws should be of equal length. If overshot (parrot-mouthed) or undershot, the horse may have problems when biting grass, although his ability to chew will not be affected. This is an hereditary fault which could be passed on through breeding. Horses with this conformational fault should not be used for breeding.

If the jaw is too narrow in width or short in length it will make choosing the right bit more difficult.

Ears

The ears should be relaxed, mobile and of a good size. When pricked, they should be carried forward. Lop ears droop forwards and down, or to the side and down, but they have no ill effects other than to give an impression of dejection; some people say they are the sign of a generous nature.

Neck

The neck should be muscular and of a length and substance proportional to the body. The top line should be convex, with a definite arch between the withers and poll. A heavy crest, expected in a stallion, is to be regretted in a mare or gelding. The muscle under the neck should appear to slip into the shoulder without any definite division. The neck should not be set into the shoulder so low that there is a big dip between it and the withers.

Neck muscles, and thus outline, can be improved by correct training.

Shoulder

The shoulder should be deep with a definite slope forward from the withers to its point. This shape gives a better ride, and longer, more flowing strides. The top of the shoulder blades should be close together; if wide apart they make a lumpy or 'loaded' shoulder, which gives an uncomfortable ride and poor movement. When looked at from in front, they should appear as a flat, widening V from the withers downwards, not rounded or bulging.

Upright shoulders allow the saddle to slip forward, make the rider feel that he has little in front of him, and restrict the freedom of movement of the horse. This type of shoulder is more suitable for the harness horse.

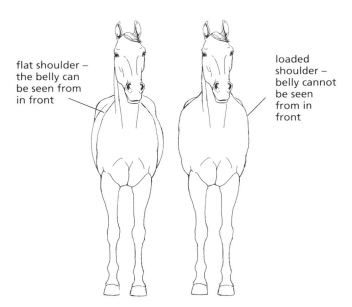

flat shoulder – the belly can be seen from in front

loaded shoulder – belly cannot be seen from in front

Flat (good) and loaded (poor) shoulders.

Withers

The withers should be clearly defined and of a sufficient height to provide room for the attachment of the covering muscles of the shoulders. If too high, this will make it difficult to fit a saddle; if too low the saddle tends to work forward – which may result in girth galls.

In a mature horse, the withers and croup should be of a similar height. If the croup is higher, known as 'croup high', the horse appears to be standing downhill and tends to be on his forehand when ridden. There are, however, some good jumpers and racehorses with this conformation.

Chest

The chest should be of medium width, giving plenty of heart room. If too narrow, the horse moves very close in front with the likelihood of brushing. If too wide, he tends to roll in canter and have limited ability to gallop.

Forelegs

The forelegs' positioning will depend on the length and angle of the humerus bone, lying between the elbow and the point of shoulder. If this is too long, the legs are too far under the body, and the elbow is likely to be tied in, with a consequent lack of freedom of movement. The elbow should stand well away from the ribs.

The forelegs should be straight from the top of the leg to the foot when looked at from the front, and straight from the top of the leg to the front of the fetlock when looked at from the side. Any deviation from a straight line when looked at from the front is a serious fault, which affects the straightness of the action and gives extra strain on the tendons, ligaments and joints.

The forearm should be well developed, and longer than the leg below the knee, which should be relatively short so as to minimise strain on the ligaments and tendons.

Good column of support through centre of limb.

'Out of one hole.'

Splayed feet.

Pigeon-toed.

good column of support through limb   over at the knee   back at the knee

Good knees.   Bad knees.

Knees

The knees should be broad, flat and deep to give room for the tendons which are attached over the top of the knee, and also to give room for the attachment of tendons and ligaments at the back of the knee.

A horse '**back at the knee**' (concave when viewed from the side) or 'calf kneed' will be suitable for slower work, but is more likely to strain tendons when galloping and jumping.

A horse a little '**over at the knee**' (convex when viewed from the side) is less likely to sprain tendons. This conformation, in many people's opinion, is no drawback. It sometimes becomes more noticeable with age, especially in Thoroughbred horses.

Swollen knees caused by injury are always suspect, and the cause should be investigated.

Cannon Bones

The cannon bones should be short and straight. If narrower below the knee than at the fetlock, the horse is said to be 'tied in below the knee'. There is less room for tendons and ligaments, and therefore a greater risk of strain.

'Bone' is measured immediately below the knee and is the circumference of the leg at that point. By placing the thumb and first finger round the leg an approximate measurement can be taken: 20cm (8ins) is sufficient bone for a riding horse or lightweight hunter, although this will depend on breeding; 21.5cm (8½ins) for a mediumweight hunter and 23–23.8cm (9–9½ins) for a heavyweight hunter.

A well-known saying is that 'blood carries weight'. Thoroughbred and Arab horses have much denser bone structure than a horse of common breeding, i.e. of cart-horse blood. Horses with this denser bone are capable of carrying more weight, relative to their size, than the commoner breeds.

Fetlock

The fetlock joint should give an appearance of flatness rather than roundness. Lumps on the front or back of the joint are a sign of work and age; on the inside they indicate that the horse moves close and brushes.

Pasterns

Pasterns should be of medium length. Long, sloping pasterns make for a springy ride, but are liable to strain. Short, upright pasterns are strong, but give a bumpy ride, and tend to cause lameness through the extra jar and concussion.

The angle of the pastern and hoof should match that of the shoulder (see page 103, hoof/pastern axis).

When looking at the horse's legs as a whole, it is best if they are two matching pairs. If one leg is twisted or bent it may put some strain on the tendons and ligaments, and the joints. This may result in the leg not moving straight. The straighter the horse's action the less likelihood there is of lameness.

Body

The body should be deep through the heart, with well-sprung ribs and plenty of room for the lungs. This gives a natural girth line.

A horse who is shallow through the heart is described

A herring-gutted horse.

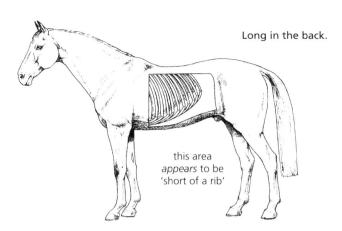

Long in the back.

this area *appears* to be 'short of a rib'

A short-coupled horse.

Roach back.

as 'showing a lot of daylight' or 'on the leg'. The measurement from the lowest part of the girth to the withers should approximately equal that from the girth to the ground. Many young horses have a 'leggy' appearance, but lose this look as they mature.

By taking a piece of string and measuring from the elbow to the ground and then reversing it and taking it up from the elbow towards the withers, an approximate indication of the height at maturity can be made.

Ribs

There are eight true ribs attached to both the vertebrae and the sternum, and ten false ribs attached to the vertebrae at the top and interconnected by cartilage at the bottom. The first rib is only slightly curved, the curvature of each succeeding rib gradually increasing to give a well-rounded appearance and internal space for many of the main organs of the body.

A 'well sprung' rib cage will support the saddle more easily.

An animal who is flat-sided, who runs up light, and who is 'herring-gutted', is usually a 'poor doer', lacking in stamina. There should be only a short gap between the last rib and the point of hip, i.e. 5–8cm (2–3ins). When looked at from the side, the flank should have depth.

Back

The back, having to carry the weight, should be of medium length and almost level.

- LONG BACKS give a comfortable ride but are liable to strain. It is usual for mares to be longer in the back than stallions or geldings.

- SHORT BACKS are strong, but give a less comfortable ride.

- HOLLOW BACKS are a sign of weakness in young horses, but are also a sign of age in an older horse. Weak- or dip-backed horses are often suffering from progressive arthritis.

- ROACH BACKS – i.e. arched upwards – are strong but give an uncomfortable ride. This outline can develop with age, and may then signify arthritis. It can be difficult to fit a saddle.

The correct muscular development of the back and loin area is essential if the horse is to perform well under the weight of the rider.

Loins

The loins are immediately behind the saddle and on either side of the spinal processes. They should be broad and well developed. Their strength and correct muscular development play a major part in the horse's balance and ability to perform. A slack loin goes with a weak back and should be avoided.

Quarters

The quarters provide power and should be muscular, the hips broad, rounded and a pair.

'**Hip down**' (a fracture of the point of the hip caused by a fall or hitting a door post) is shown by the flatter outline of the injured hip. It can be unsightly but often goes unobserved, and once the initial bruising has subsided, it rarely causes lameness. It can sometimes cause problems in pregnancy.

A '**goose-rumped**' horse has quarters which slope sharply from croup to dock, and this often accompanies jumping ability. A prominence on the croup is called a 'jumping bump'.

The dock should not be set on too low. There should be plenty of length between the hip and the point of buttock and the point of the hip and point of hock.

Viewed from behind, the impression should be one of strength, with rounded quarters and upper or first thighs sloping down to a well-developed second thigh or gaskin. 'Split up behind' means a poorly developed upper thigh.

'Split up behind'.

Cow hocks.

Wide behind.

Good hocks.

Hocks out behind.　　Straight hocks.　　Good hocks well supported under the body.　　Sickle-shaped hocks.　　Hocks too high.

Hind Legs

When the horse is standing naturally and the hind leg is viewed both from the side and from immediately behind, there should be a straight line from the point of buttock through the point of hock down to the fetlock and so to the ground. Any deviation from this shows a weakness, and places greater strain both on the stifle joint, or the patella above, and the hock joint below it. When viewed from the side, the angles from point to hip to point of buttock, from point of buttock to stifle and from stifle to hock need to be similar and sufficient to be able to close to allow for engagement and open to allow for extension. These three joints work in harmony, and provide the main propelling force for galloping and jumping. When in movement, the stifle joint should not be thrown outwards, but should stay in line with the body. The stifle joint is the equivalent of the human knee.

Hocks

The hocks should be large, and the outline should be clean and flat with a prominent point at the back. There should be plenty of bone below the hock. There should be length from hip to hock. The hock should be 'well let down', i.e. the section of the limb from hock to fetlock should appear short.

There are various weak shapes of hock:

- BENT OR SICKLE HOCKS If viewed from the side, there is a more acute angle to the hocks, which are too much under the horse, usually with a poor second thigh and cut-in above the hock.

- COW HOCKS If viewed from the rear, the points of the hocks come together and the toes turn out. Such a horse is liable to brush but is often able to jump.

- BOWED HOCKS If viewed from behind, the points of the hocks are wide apart, the toes turn in and the foot is likely to screw as it comes to the ground.

- STRAIGHT HOCKS These are good for galloping, but have less leverage for jumping. There is more concussion unless compensated for by a long pastern. They are liable to strain, and young horses with straight hocks may suffer from a slipped stifle joint. This is usually rectified as the horse matures and the muscles and ligaments strengthen.

- HOCKS OUT BEHIND Viewed from the side, such hocks are way out behind the horse. There is a big angle above the hock over the hamstring. Such horses often jump well, but rarely gallop and would have difficulty if asked to do dressage at any high level.

When viewed from behind when the horse is moving,

the hocks should move strongly forward with no visible 'wobble'. Hocks that deviate to the inside or outside when moving are more prone to strain or damage.

DEVELOPING AN EYE FOR A HORSE

It takes considerable experience and constant practice to 'develop an eye' for a horse and to be able to assess a horse's conformation correctly. It can only be achieved by looking at many different types and sizes of horses and learning to compare and evaluate mentally what has been seen.

Assessing Conformation

First look at the horse at rest in the stable. Then ask the attendant to bring him out and stand him up for inspection.

General Impression

- Is the first impression good? If so, why? If not, why not?

- Is he true to type?

- Is he the right size, weight, etc. for the job required?

- If the first impression is good, look further. Remember, few horses within the budget of the average buyer are perfect. If the faults are minor or irrelevant to the job the horse is required to do, they do not necessarily preclude purchase.

- Does everything match?

- Assess the size of head in relation to body, and parts of the body in relation to each other.

- Consider the size of body in relation to the amount of 'bone' and to the length or shortness of legs.

- Assess structure and size of forehand in relation to hindquarters.

- Look at the size and shape of the feet.

Head, Neck, Forehand, Legs and Feet

- Check teeth for age, wolf teeth, and bit injuries.

- Check shape of the upper and lower jaw, and width between the branches of the lower jaw.

- Check the set of the head on the neck.

Stand in front of the horse and check:

- Width of the chest.

- Straightness of the legs – are they a pair?

- Size and shape of the knees.

Stand on the left or near side and:

- Check the shape and feel of the withers.

- View the angle and length of the shoulders.

- Check by eye and right hand the position and set of the elbow joint.

Face towards the tail and:

- Run the left hand down the back of the forearm, knees, tendons and fetlock joint of the left leg.

- Move to the right or off-side and compare the look and feel of the right leg.

Face the horse and:

- View the size and shape of the knee, the cannon bone, fetlock joint and pastern.

- Crouch down and, using both hands, check the front and back of the knee and leg to the coronet.

Face towards the tail and:

- Run the left hand down the shoulder and leg and pick up the foot. If necessary, pick out the foot. Check the size and shape of the foot, sole and frog.

- If shod, check the shoes for fit, type and wear.

Repeat the above procedure with the right leg.

The Middle

Stand back and view:

- The general outline.
- Top line.
- Length of back.
- Depth of girth.
- Shape of ribs.
- Strength of loins.
- Run your left hand over the withers and along the back. Then feel the ribs and loin area.
- Feel for muscle development and condition.

As a rule of thumb, in a well-proportioned horse the length of the horse's head (A) is approximately equal to: the distance between the back of the shoulder blade and the point of hip; the depth of body at the girth; and the distance between the point of hock and the ground. The horse's body from shoulder to point of hip should roughly fit into an imaginary square whose sides are A x 2.5.

The Hindquarters, Legs and Feet

Stand back and view the outline, particularly:

- Length from hip joint to hock.
- Stifle to hock.
- Hock to fetlock.
- The size and shape of the hock, and the angle at which it is set on. The development of the muscles of the second thigh.

Run your hand along the body and over the quarters.

Take hold of the tail, and standing behind the horse check:

- The levelness of the points of the hips, and the width between the points of the hips.
- The muscular development of the buttocks and upper thighs.
- The straightness of the hind leg from point of buttock through the hock joint to the ground.
- The angle of the foot.

Standing to the side:

- Run your hand down the quarters and with both hands examine the hock joint for signs of strain or injury.

Feel down the hind leg in the same way as for the front leg, particularly the inside of the fetlock joint.

Check the hind feet in the same way as the front feet.

Repeat the last three procedures with the other leg.

Standing in front of the horse:

- Look through the front legs and, diagonally, at the inner outline of the hock. Compare the outline of each hock joint.

Consider:

- The **general impression**, from expression of eyes and appearance of skin, coat and colour of gums. A running nose or eyes should be noted and mentioned.

- The feel of the **coat and skin**: staring coat and tight skin may imply worms or other illness and lack of condition.

- The feel of the horse's **body**.

- **Neck**. The crest should feel tough and strong. Poor crest means no reserves of fat.

- **Back and ribs**. These should be well covered. In old age or pregnancy the weight of belly may give an impression of poorness above it. A second feel along the backbone should verify condition.

- **Quarters**. Their shape varies according to breed and type. A fit horse has firm, well-developed muscles. A fat horse will show a round outline. A poor horse shows poverty lines down the back of the quarters, and the muscles will feel underdeveloped and soft.

- **The feet**. These reflect general condition and management. The outward evidence of changes – either for the better or worse – may take nine to eighteen months to show.

Assessing Condition

Developing 'an eye for a horse' will include both conformation and condition. An unscrupulous seller may try to hide poor conformation with too much condition. The inexperienced handler may think that the very lean fit horse is in poor condition. Assessing the horse's condition is called '**Condition Scoring**' and is an important skill to learn. It is as harmful to the horse to be too fat as to be too thin.

If the horse is too fat he will be unable to work satisfactorily. He will be more prone to laminitis and joint problems. His heart and lungs will be put under extra strain and he may also be difficult to fit a saddle to.

SCORE 0

SCORE 1

SCORE 2

SCORE 3

SCORE 4

SCORE 5

CONDITION SCORING

SCORE	DESCRIPTION	PELVIS	BACK AND RIBS	NECK
0	**Very Poor**	Angular, skin tight. Very sunken rump. Deep cavity under tail.	Skin tight over ribs. Very prominent and sharp backbone.	Marked ewe neck. Narrow and slack at base.
1	**Poor**	Prominent pelvis and croup. Sunken rump but skin supple. Deep cavity under tail.	Ribs easily visible. Prominent backbone with sunken skin on either side.	Ewe neck, narrow and slack base.
2	**Moderate**	Rump flat either side of back bone. Croup well defined, some fat. Slight cavity under tail.	Ribs just visible. Backbone covered but spines can be felt.	Narrow but firm.
3	**Good**	Covered by fat and rounded. No gutter. Pelvis easily felt.	Ribs just covered and easily felt. No gutter along the back. Backbone well covered but spines can be felt.	No crest (except for stallions), firm neck.
4	**Fat**	Gutter to root of tail. Pelvis covered by fat. Need firm pressure.	Ribs well covered – need pressure to feel. Slight crest to feel.	Wide and firm.
5	**Very Fat**	Deep gutter to root of tail. Skin distended. Pelvis buried, cannot be felt.	Ribs buried, cannot be felt. Deep gutter along back. Back broad and flat.	Marked crest very wide and firm. Fold of fat.

(Based on the Carroll and Huntington Method)

To obtain a body condition score, score the pelvis first, then adjust by half a point if it differs by one point or more from the back or neck.

The horse who is too thin may well be subject to worms and lice. He will have difficulty finding the energy to work and may be prone to more sprains and strains because of tiredness. It may also be difficult to fit a saddle on him.

The Fit Horse

The backbone is not visible, and the flesh on either side is level. The ribs are barely distinguished, though they can just be felt. The shoulders and neck blend smoothly into the body. The neck, when felt, is hard and has substance. The skin over the ribs is loose and easily moved. The muscles are well developed and firm to the touch.

Four categories of fitness may be recognised:

- **The ridden show animal**. Fairly well muscled up, but often overfat. Ribs not visible and can only just be felt.

- **The show jumper/dressage horse**. Well muscled, but may carry some fat. Ribs cannot be seen, but can be felt.

- **The event horse**. Very well muscled, but should not be carrying much excess weight. Ribs can be seen and felt. A three-day event horse will be much leaner than a one-day event horse.

- **The racehorse**. Very well muscled but with no surplus fat. Muscles are rounded and can be clearly seen and felt, including above the bony points, especially over the loins and croup. There is little fat in the spaces between muscles. This horse, to an uneducated eye, may appear thin.

Assessing Temperament

Whilst moving around the animal and handling him, be aware of his reaction. Note whether he is calm and confident when handled or nervous, pushy or stiff. Remember that age and experience will have a bearing but if you have doubts repeat the procedure and note the reaction.

Breeding Conformation

If a mare is going to be used for breeding note the shape and size of the udder. If she has already had a foal, the teats will usually be more prominent and she will not mind being touched in that area.

Examine the vulva; it should be perpendicular and firmly closed. If the mare has bred there may be some wrinkling but it should be closed. If the vulva slopes backwards towards the rectum there is more risk of infection.

Final Assessment

Once you have examined the whole horse in detail, take another step back and look at the whole again. If you still like what you see you will want to assess the action, see Chapter 2.

CHAPTER

2 ACTION

The ability of a horse to move well greatly depends on his conformation, breeding and type. A good mover uses himself equally well in front and behind.

To move well in front, a horse must actively use his shoulders as well as his knees and fetlock joints. He should move straight, with a length of stride suitable to his make and shape. He should flow, giving an impression of moving with ease, which will be more likely if the elbow is well positioned, allowing plenty of room between elbow and ribs. There should be slight knee elevation, but if this is exaggerated the horse may be better suited to driving rather than riding.

A horse with an upright shoulder rarely moves well: he has a short stride and is a moderate ride. A show horse should always move straight. Horses destined for most competitive disciplines will usually be less susceptible to strains and injury if their action is 'straight'.

The movement of the hind leg is equally important. Good movement comes from well-developed loins, quarters and thighs, and from active hocks. The appearance should be of strength and power. The action should again be straight, with the hocks brought well forward underneath the body.

In trot, if as the horse moves away from you he is sound and has full use of his joints, it should be possible to see briefly the whole sole of each foot when the foot is at its highest point.

Some allowance should be made for young horses, particularly when trotted in-hand, and for four-year-olds when ridden. Lack of balance and muscular development may affect their action. As the horse matures and comes off his forehand, small defects in his action often disappear. A skilled farrier can do much to improve a horse's movement.

DEFECTIVE ACTION

Dishing

The front foot is thrown outwards, particularly in trot, and although this action appears to come from below the knee it is related to the flexion of the elbow. When still, the horse will often stand with toes turned in – 'pigeon-toed'. The movement can occur in one or both front legs. As long as it is only moderate dishing it is of little detriment to the horse, except for showing. An exaggerated movement puts great strain on the fetlock joints, and this may eventually cause unsoundness.

Plaiting or Lacing

At walk and trot the horse places one of the hind or front pairs of feet in front of the other. Narrow-chested horses are prone to this. Excessive plaiting is likely to make the horse stumble and even fall. A slight deviation can be acceptable. The knee should be carefully checked for any scarring or bruising.

Toes Turned Out

Horses who stand with either front or hind feet pointing outwards usually brush their legs, knocking the inside of their fetlock joint with the opposite foot. Evidence of this is an enlarged joint from constant bruising and/or rubbing off of the hair over the joint. It is a serious fault, as it necessitates always using protective boots when the horse is ridden, which can cause other problems.

Going Wide Behind

This often relates to stiffness in the back, and the hind legs are frequently bowed outwards. It is unsightly.

It can put extra strain on the hocks. When viewed from behind if the hocks appear to 'wobble' when the horse moves it sometimes means he will have difficulty when asked to do dressage or jump beyond novice level. In the young horse, judicious work may strengthen the hock joints.

Forging

Forging is not considered to be a defect, as it can usually be corrected. It occurs in trot when the toe of the hind shoe strikes the underneath surface of the front shoe on the same side. The front foot lingers and is caught by the back shoe.

It is sometimes found in free-moving young horses, not yet sufficiently balanced and strong under the weight of the rider, and thus not able to bring the weight off the forehand. The problem ceases when the horse is stronger and better balanced. Another cause is trotting too fast. This is usually the rider's fault – if the trot is slowed down, the forging ceases.

Poor conformation can sometimes lead to forging. The remedy is schooling to improve and build up muscles. If the feet are too long at the toe this can also cause forging, but this can be corrected by a farrier.

Over-reaching

Over-reaching occurs when the hind limb over-extends and the toe of the hind shoe interferes with or strikes into the forelimb between the knee and the bulbs of the heel. Usually the lower part of the limb is most affected,

Forging.　　　　Over-reaching.

particularly the bulbs of the heels. A high over-reach can cause severe damage to the tendons in the back of the leg. Over-reaching usually occurs when galloping or jumping, or through loss of balance, or when overworking a tired horse.

Pigeon-toed – weight not evenly distributed down the centre of the limb.

Plaiting.　　　　Dishing.

ASSESSING ACTION AND SOUNDNESS

- Ask the attendant to walk the horse away, turn and walk back. Check on evenness and length of stride, and head movement. Always ensure the attendant allows free movement of the head and neck whilst walking and trotting up the horse.

- Ask the attendant to trot the horse away, turn and trot back, keeping to as straight a line as possible. Check on the straightness of movement, the activity and levelness of the trot, and the evenness of the movement of the horse's head.

- Ask for the horse to be trotted up again, and view from the side. Observe the general attitude of the horse.

- When assessing the walk from the side, the front and hind leg should appear to form a V underneath the belly. If both legs on the same side appear to be going forward at the same time, the walk will not be a regular 4:4 rhythm and this can be difficult to correct with training.

- In trot when viewed from the side, the feet should be raised a similar amount behind and in front. When viewed from behind, the hips should appear even and the hocks both active to the same degree. The head and neck should be carried straight. Sometimes, if the tail is carried to one side, it can indicate back problems. The area the horse is trotted up on can make a considerable difference to his action, as can whether he is shod or unshod. A smooth, level surface will give the horse the best chance of showing good action. If it is concrete or tarmac it will also enable the assessor to hear the rhythm of the footfalls, which can be very helpful when assessing soundness.

- In trot watching the movement of the head and neck can be a good indicator of soundness. In a sound horse the head and neck should remain fairly steady, with very little movement. If lame in front, the head is often raised above the norm when the lame leg hits the ground, and if lame behind it drops below the norm when the lame leg hits the ground.

CHAPTER 3

THE PSYCHOLOGY OF THE HORSE

Understanding the psychology of the horse is key to managing him successfully. At any time when there is a 'problem' with a horse, consider how it has arisen. It is almost certainly due to some mistake or error in his handling.

Stable management might better be called horse management. In order to manage horses and ponies efficiently it is important to understand their natural lifestyle.

HORSE PSYCHOLOGY

Horses are herd animals. In the wild they live in family groups and roam over a wide area grazing for up to eighteen hours a day. They are flight animals, running away from perceived danger but when cornered will bite, kick, strike out and buck or rear in an attempt to rid themselves of the danger.

When kept in a group, they quickly establish a 'pecking order'. When a new animal is introduced into the group this order may change. It may also change if an animal is removed. This may result in the group biting and squealing and attempting to kick each other. Unless stallions are involved, if the animals are unshod behind, they seldom inflict much damage on each other.

Horses are large, flighty and unpredictable. They are also sensitive, have excellent memory and are creatures of habit. All these natural attributes need to be used to our advantage when caring for them.

Successfully balancing the horse's natural lifestyle against the practicalities of caring for and riding him is the key to good management.

Horses do not know the difference between good and bad but they are quick to learn and react to the way they are handled.

For many centuries they were nomadic, grass-eating, herd animals, and speed was their greatest protection against enemies. Even a newly born foal was soon on his feet, ready to keep up with his mother and, if the necessity arose, to join the rest of the herd in flight. Bucking was an instinctive defence reaction to dislodge a predator leaping on the back. Thus, if a horse is frightened, his first thought is to gallop off, bucking as he goes.

If a frightened horse is cornered, his instinct is to kick his way out. He may also stamp and strike out with his front feet. Allied with this protective behaviour is very acute hearing, good eyesight both forwards and to the side – and a nose sensitive to any strange or foreign smell. Horses therefore react very quickly when anything disturbs or alarms them. Their first thought is flight; if this is made impossible they resist and fight. It is essential that on these occasions any person dealing with the horse is of a calm temperament and unafraid.

Horses have little reasoning power but excellent memories. Their training from the earliest age must establish confidence, trust and good habits, which in time become instinctive. Their memory can, however, also work against them. If startled or frightened by circumstances or people, a horse never forgets. Given the same situation he will always be likely to think back and react in a similar way.

Most bad behaviour by horses, both in and out of the stable, is caused by incorrect handling, particularly when the horse is young. The horse is a creature of habit, and appreciates a regular routine. He can be easily upset by sudden and unexpected change.

THE HERD INSTINCT

This is exhibited in the following ways:

- Young horses often show unwillingness to leave others or reluctance to work alone.

- Horses left on their own when others are taken away will often gallop about, and may even jump over a fence or gate.

- A group of horses or ponies in a field will usually have a herd leader and a very distinctive pecking order. This is very obvious when hay is fed loose on the ground in winter.

As the herd instinct is very strong it can be used to help control and manage horses in such instances as:

- When horses are stabled they are always happier and more settled if other horses are within sight and hearing.

- When travelling, a young or nervous horse often settles if allowed a quiet older pony as a travelling companion.

- Horses at grass are happier when in company. Ponies who are difficult to catch will often give in if encouraged to follow others to the gate.

- A horse who gets loose when away from his stable or field feels insecure and worried and tends to return to familiar surroundings. He usually goes back to either the stable or outside the field gate.

PROBLEMS AND POSSIBLE CAUSES

Pulling back when tied up
Cause: Tying up before the horse is calm. Tying up too short, so that the horse feels restricted. Typing up when horse is standing on an unsuitable surface.

Kicking or biting when being groomed
Cause: Nervous groom, sensitive skin, rough handling. Poor choice of grooming equipment. Brushing hair against the lie of the coat. A build-up of static electricity in the coat cause by synthetic rugs and/or grooming tools.

Bad to shoe
Cause: Insufficient handling of feet when young. Hasty or rough farrier. If in older horses, they may be suffering from arthritis or joint problems and finding it difficult to stand on three legs.

Bad to box
Cause: Hasty or rough handling, insufficient time taken to box. Frightening the horse by driving too fast, particularly on corners. Poorly positioned lorry or trailer with the ramp too steep or not firm when stepped on. Leading the horse incorrectly.

Kicking when travelling
Cause: Insufficient room to balance, resulting in restriction and fear. Poor driving, especially cornering too fast or accelerating or decelerating too quickly.

Pulling back when in trailer
Cause: Tying up before back strap and back are put up. Tying up too short or too high.

Resisting examination and treatment
Cause: Fear, pain, nervous handler.

THE TEETH AND AGEING

The horse has three types of teeth. These are:

(1) the molars or grinding teeth;
(2) the incisors or biting teeth; and
(3) the tushes.

The **molars** are situated to the rear of the mouth, on either side of the face and in the upper and lower jaws. The **incisors** are in the upper and lower jaws in the front of the mouth. The **tushes** are found in the space between the other two groups of teeth. To open the mouth safely the fingers may be inserted into this space, which is where the bit lies.

The horse grows two sets of teeth during his lifetime: temporary milk or deciduous teeth, and permanent teeth. The temporary teeth are small and white, with a distinct neck. Permanent teeth are larger, stronger, pale fawn or yellow in colour, with no distinct neck.

TYPES AND NUMBER OF TEETH

Molars or Grinding Teeth

These are in the long head bones and jaw bones. Their function is to grind food. There are twelve temporary molars (also called premolars): three in each side of the upper and lower jaws; these are eventually replaced by permanent teeth. There are twelve permanent molars (also called true molars): three in each side of the upper and lower jaws. In addition, there are twelve true molars, which are permanent from the outset. By the time the horse is three-and-a-half to four years old, he

has a total of twenty-four permanent cheek teeth.

The upper jaw is wider than the lower jaw and this, in conjunction with the criss-cross movement of the jaws as the horse eats, causes the teeth to wear unevenly and require regular rasping to maintain a level surface. It is the outside of the upper teeth and the inside of the lower teeth which will need attention. If the sharp edges are left, mastication is affected, and the horse may also cut the inside of his mouth. All horses' teeth should be checked every six months right through their lives and not just when they become older or there are obvious signs of problems.

Incisors or Biting Teeth

These form a rather flat arch in the front of the top jaw or maxilla, and in the front of the lower jaw, the mandible. Their function is to bite through growing herbage and to collect food.

There are twelve temporary incisors and twelve permanent incisors, six in each jaw. The centre teeth are called 'centrals', on either side of them are the 'laterals' and the remaining ones are called 'corner' teeth.

Tushes

These are found in the mouths of adult male horses and very occasionally in mares. They appear between the incisor and molar teeth, one in each jaw, four in all. They appear at the age of three-and-a-half to four years, and are fully developed twelve months later. They were originally 'weapons', but now serve no purpose in the mouth of the domesticated horse.

If awkwardly placed, they can sometimes cause discomfort when a bit is in the mouth. As the horse grows older they often become encrusted with tartar, which should be removed to prevent the gum from becoming inflamed.

Wolf Teeth

These small extra teeth which may erupt between the ages of two and five years old are usually found more commonly in the upper jaw, close up against the first molar tooth. They may vary in size and root depth, but are always smaller than the true molar. They are usually discarded with the milk teeth. There are occasions when they remain in the jaw and cause the horse considerable discomfort when bitted. Their presence often goes unnoticed, and they can be the cause of mouth problems.

It is almost always advisable to have wolf teeth removed by your veterinary surgeon. This should be a simple task, but occasionally may require surgery if deep roots are encountered.

Before starting to train young horses or retrain older horses their mouths should be inspected in case of tooth problems. When inspecting the mouth, always untie the horse. Most horses will show some resentment when having their mouths looked at, so a tactful approach is needed and this should be carried out by an experienced person.

THE PARTS OF THE TEETH

The surface of the tooth which bites and/or grinds the food is called the **table**, also known as the tabular surface, masticating surface or occlusal surface; it is this which gets worn down.

The **crown** of the tooth is that part which is above the gum. In milk teeth, the point where gum and tooth meet is the **neck**.

The **root** part of the tooth lies within the jaw. It is hollow and its cavity contains the nerves and the blood vessels which nourish the tooth.

As the incisor tooth grows older, this cavity, the **fang hole**, fills up with a substance of a lighter colour. As the table of the tooth wears down, this will eventually appear as a small white area on the centre of the tooth in front of the **mark**.

The **mark** or **infundibulum** is the blackened depression seen on the table of the permanent incisors. It is lined by a ring of enamel. In the young tooth the mark is broad and deep, but as the table of the tooth wears down, the mark becomes shallower and eventually disappears. The blackening of the mark is due to discoloration from food and is not present in the new tooth.

TEETHING

When new teeth are coming through, the horse's gums become inflamed and painful, and if the animal is on feed other than grass they may make eating uncomfortable. Such animals should be put on a soft diet and meadow hay. Ridden horses can become more sensitive in their mouths, and if the problem is not recognised this 'mouthiness' can turn into a permanent habit.

Horses should not have a bit in their mouths until the teeth are through and the gum healed, so the mouths of all young horses should be checked regularly, particularly when they are likely to be cutting teeth. Should there be any unusual tooth formation or wolf teeth present, veterinary advice should be sought.

AGEING THE HORSE

The official age of Thoroughbred and warmblood horses is taken from 1 January.

Ageing the horse by looking at his teeth is not an exact science and with the introduction of passports it is very easy to verify the horse's age. However, it is still a requirement in BHS exams and is a useful aid when buying horses or assessing their potential. It is done by

2 years

all baby teeth

2½ years

through, but
not yet in wear

central
adult teeth

3 years

baby teeth

adult teeth

3½ years

adult lateral
teeth come
through
towards four
years old

4 years

baby teeth

adult teeth

4½ years

baby teeth will
be replaced by
adult teeth

adult corners
just through, as are tushes

5 years

corners not in wear

oval teeth;
well-defined
infundibulum

young teeth;
corners not in wear

6 years

full mouth in
wear;
infundibulum
still visible in all
incisors

tooth in wear

7 years

infundibulum
well defined in
corners, fading
in centrals

hook on corner tooth

8 years

remains of infundibulum

fang hole

9 years

slightly longer teeth

10 years

infundibulum almost gone   fang hole

10–12 years

angle becoming greater   less oval; infundibulum gone

15 years

increasingly angular   more triangular in shape; pulp cavity or fang hole shows alone

Milk Teeth

Birth or shortly after	Two central incisors appear in each jaw
4–6 weeks	Lateral incisors appear
9–10 months	Corner incisors appear
12 months	All incisor teeth are in full wear
2 years	Incisor teeth show signs of wear

Permanent Teeth

2½ years	The central milk teeth are gradually replaced by the permanent incisors which at 3 years are in full wear
3½ years	The lateral permanent incisors appear and at 4 years are in full wear
4½ years	The corner incisors appear and in the male, the tush
5 years	The corner incisors are well up but smaller than their neighbours. The tables are not quite level or in full wear. The tush is well grown
6 years	The corner incisors are in full wear but the infundibulum or 'mark' is less distinct
7 years	The mark on the central incisors may have gone, and that on the lateral incisors may be less obvious. A distinct hook shows on the edge of the upper corner incisor: the 'seven-year hook'
8 years	The mark may have disappeared from the lateral incisor and is less distinct on the corner incisors. The seven-year hook has been worn level. The fang hole or 'dental star' is seen in the central incisors as a line in front of the mark
9 years	The mark has all but gone from all the incisors. The dental star appears on the lateral incisors
10–12 years	The dental star gradually becomes a spot rather than a line and is present in all incisors

examining the incisors.

Ageing the horse by looking at his teeth should be done in conjunction with looking at the animal as a whole. Take into account make, shape and condition when coming to a conclusion. The way in which the horse has been managed, whether he lives out and has grazed all his life and the diet he has been fed will also make a difference to the colour and length of the teeth. A pony is quite likely to have much shorter, whiter incisors than a Thoroughbred of the same age who has always been stabled.

Horses who have a malformation of the jaw, undershot or overshot, or horses who have suffered injuries that affect the jaw action will be more difficult to age accurately.

When ageing, always have the horse untied, stand at the side of the horse facing the front and place the arm nearer the horse, under the jaw and steady the muzzle with your hand. With your free hand it may be sufficient just to push the lips apart in the area of the corners.

Always look at both sides of the mouth before making a judgement, as they often differ.

It is easier to age if it is done in 'blocks'. Up until two years the horse will only have milk teeth and be obviously very young in his build.

- From 2–4 he will be changing his milk teeth for permanent teeth.

- 4½–6 The permanent teeth will be gradually more in wear.

- 7–10 Mature mouth, hooks come and go. Marks on the tables change shape and prominence.

- 10–15 Shape of tables changes. Galvayne's groove often present. Marks on tables fade. Teeth longer and more angled.

- 15+ Triangular tables. Long teeth. Galvayne's groove disappeared. Horse may show other signs of age.

By working within these 'blocks' you are working within a 3–4 year age range which is easier for the less experienced handler.

Galvayne's Groove

This is a depression on the outer side of the upper corner incisor. It is seen mainly in cold-blood heavy horses. It is often absent in warmblood light horses or ponies. It appears just below the gum at nine to ten years, has grown halfway down by fifteen years, and to the bottom by twenty years. Very often staining on the teeth due to diet is mistaken for Galvayne's groove.

Hooks

Hooks occur on the edge of the upper, corner teeth. A hook is usually obvious at seven and may recur at nine and eleven when it may persist for the rest of the horse's life.

Shape of the Table and Angle of the Teeth

From the age of seven years onward, the tables of the teeth will change from oval to round and then to triangular. The back of the tooth forms the apex of the triangle. As the horse ages, his gums recede, his teeth appear to be longer and they project more forward and at a more acute angle.

Bishoping

This is the practice of attempting to make an old mouth look young. The teeth are filed short, and a false mark is gouged out of the centre of the table. The practice can be recognised, as the teeth do not meet naturally, and there is no enamel lining to the false mark.

Crib Biting

When examining a horse for age it is easy to recognise signs of crib biting. The central, and possibly lateral, upper teeth are worn on their outer edges.

5 BREEDS

Breed societies keep a stud register. For a horse or pony to be recognised as belonging to a certain breed and to be recorded in the stud book of that breed society they must be qualified. Many breed societies are affiliated to the British Horse Society. An up-to-date list can be found in the current **BHS Year Book**.

The Rare Breeds Survival Trust (RBST) currently lists no fewer than eleven of Britain's breeds on their 'watchlist', categorised as critical, endangered, vulnerable or at risk.

THOROUGHBRED (TB)

The word Thoroughbred is used to describe horses registered in the **General Stud Book.** In 1791 **An Introduction to a General Stud Book** first appeared, followed by several more editions until, in 1808, Volume I of the **General Stud Book,** now usually referred to as the GSB, was published.

All Thoroughbred horses can trace their ancestry in the male line to three stallions imported into Britain in the late seventeenth and early eighteenth centuries: the Byerley Turk, the Darley Arabian and the Godolphin Arabian. On the female side, all horses in the GSB trace back to some thirty mares, mostly of Arab blood, originally bred or imported by King Charles II in the seventeenth century and known as the 'Royal Mares'.

The breed has become extremely successful in racing, and Thoroughbred blood has been introduced to improve and upgrade the quality of old-established breeds. Nowadays the Thoroughbred can be found in horse racing countries all over the world.

The **General Stud Book** is kept by Messrs Weatherby of Wellingborough, Northamptonshire, and TB types are registered by reference to them. Foals should be registered before they are four months old. The information required is sex, age, colour and markings, name of previous owner and/or breeder, and the sire and the dam.

Since 1974 Weatherbys have kept a **Non-Thoroughbred Register**, previously published by Miss F. M. Prior as the HB (half-bred) Stud Book. Up to 1987 this was for the produce of TB stallions out of mares who had been identified by Weatherbys. Entry has now been widened to include the produce of certain non-TB stallions registered with Weatherbys.

BRITISH SPORT HORSE

The Sport Horse Breeders of Great Britain (SHB) is now the name of what used to be called the National Light Horse Breeding Society or Hunters' Improvement Society (HIS). Its aim is to identify and promote breeding of the range and type of horse for the future, largely using Thoroughbred blood. It will also assist in the registration, promotion and marketing of horses bred in the UK and establish British-bred horses internationally.

BRITISH WARMBLOOD

This is a new breed group started in the 1970s. The foundation stock are the Continental warmbloods (Hanoverian, Danish, Dutch, etc.), many of which have been mated with the Thoroughbred in Britain. Mares and stallions are eligible for the stud book on the basis of pedigree, plus conformation, action and veterinary tests. The aim is to produce a British warmblood with correct conformation, athletic movement and a tractable temperament, particularly suitable for dressage, jumping and general riding.

ARAB

The Arab is a foundation breed, crossing with which has improved other breeds of horses. Many countries now have their own Arab breed societies and stud books. In the United Kingdom the Arab Horse Society produces three stud books:

- for pure-bred Arabs

- for Anglo Arabs – Arabs crossed with Thoroughbreds

- for part-bred Arabs

Anglo Arabs and part-bred Arabs must have a minimum of 12.5% Arab blood to be eligible for registration.

CLEVELAND BAY

This is a breed of great antiquity originating in north-east Yorkshire. In the 1960s there were only four Cleveland Bay stallions left, and although their numbers have increased, the breed remains on the RBST's critical list. This is an excellent carriage horse, and is also a good show jumper and eventer. When crossed with the Thoroughbred this breed produces some of the best hunters.

Cleveland Bays must be bay with black points, and have no white other than a small star. Their ideal height is 16–16.2hh (162–168cm).

IRISH DRAUGHT

This breed has been used in Ireland as a general farm horse. A stud book was started in 1917, and in the 1970s steps were taken to maintain the breed which, because of the popularity of its cross, was diminishing in numbers. When crossed with Thoroughbred or Arab blood they produce quality weight-carrying stock who have achieved great success in competitive sports and as hunters.

HACKNEY

The Hackney horse is descended from two regional types: the Yorkshire and the Norfolk Roadster. The Hackney Horse Society was founded in 1883. Today the two types have been fused to produce what we know as the Hackney Horse, standing 15–15.3hh (152–160cm); a harness horse with a spectacular trotting gait, good use of the shoulders and great flexion and thrust from the hock. While most people view the Hackney as a carriage horse, the breed is actually extremely versatile.

The Hackney Pony was developed in the 1870s by crossing a Hackney stallion called Sir George with pure-bred Fell ponies, the resultant offspring having quality, substance, extravagant action and great presence. Hackney ponies do not exceed 14hh (142cm) and are now seen mostly in the show ring in driving competitions.

Both the Hackney Horse and Pony are listed as endangered by the RBST.

Cross-breds

The pure-bred Hackneys do not fulfil all the demands of riders or drivers, and in Britain there has been considerable cross-breeding to produce cobs, hacks, hunters and show jumpers. The mountain and moorland breeds, particularly the Welsh Cob and Connemara, are popular for this purpose.

HEAVY HORSE BREEDS

These are also used for cross-breeding. Many good riding horses are produced by putting a Shire or Clydesdale mare to a TB horse. If Percheron or Suffolk Punch mares are used, the offspring grow less feather on the legs. The Percheron cross tends to have the better action. Though Suffolk Punch numbers are improving, the breed remains on the RBST's critical list, whilst the Clydesdale is classified as vulnerable and the Shire as at risk.

Some shows are now holding ridden classes for the heavies, and these are proving extremely popular.

EUROPEAN WARMBLOODS

There are a considerable number of Continental breeds, often referred to as warmbloods. They are descendants of the riding and carriage horses who used to be bred in the various areas, mixed with TB, Arab and each other to varying degrees. Although their lineage is mixed, they are tested for type, conformation, action, aptitude for performing, etc. and will only be branded and accepted into the relevant stud book if they conform to the breed specifications. They are in high demand for all types of competition. Many have British branches of their stud books.

MOUNTAIN AND MOORLAND BREEDS

Nine of these breeds are indigenous to the British Isles. Many of the smaller breeds have had some Arab blood in them, whereas the larger ponies such as the Dales were crossed with Clydesdales to give the offspring greater size and strength.

The severity of the native environment has made the breeds very hardy. For many centuries they have had to survive in winter with the minimum of food and shelter, which has ensured that only the toughest of them have been left to carry on the breed.

The growth of trekking holidays increased the demand for the larger ponies and cobs. They make admirable mounts for novice adults, and are capable of carrying heavy riders. All the native breeds have experienced a huge increase in popularity during the last decade, and today large numbers of them can be seen competing at major shows.

Nevertheless, six of our native mountain and moorland breeds remain on the RBST's 'Watchlist.'

Welsh

There are four types of ponies and cobs registered with the Welsh Pony and Cob Society:

Section A is the Welsh Mountain Pony, the foundation stock of all the other sections. The ponies make excellent mounts for children, and are very successful in the show ring in leading rein, first ridden, open ridden and working hunter classes. They have also been used to improve other breeds. They are well-made, pretty ponies with a small, clean-cut head, short, flat bone and free, straight movement. They should not exceed 12hh (121.9cm) and can be any colour except piebald and skewbald, though grey tends to be dominant.

Semi-feral Section A ponies are listed on the RBST's 'Watchlist' as vulnerable.

Section B is the Welsh Pony up to 13.2hh (137.2cm). The general description of ponies in Section A of the Stud Book is applicable to those in Section B, but more particularly the Section B pony shall be described as a riding pony, with quality, riding action, adequate bone and substance, hardiness and constitution and with a pony character.

Section C is the Welsh Pony of cob type over 12hh (121.9cm) but not exceeding 13.2hh (137.2cm).

Section D is the Welsh Cob. They exceed 13.2hh (121.9cm) but there is no upper height limit, though they must have pony character and as much substance as possible. When crossed with TB stock they have produced successful dressage horses, show jumpers and driving horses.

Both Section Cs and Ds make excellent riding or driving ponies, and are good jumpers. Their action is true and forceful, and in trot the whole foreleg should be extended straight from the shoulder and as far forward as possible, with hocks flexed under the body with straight and powerful leverage. Colour can be anything except piebald and skewbald.

Exmoor

The oldest of our British native pony breeds, the Exmoor pony traces back to Roman times. The RBST lists the Exmoor as endangered because of the low number of breeding animals. Recently Exmoors have found a new role in managing nature reserves for English Nature and the National Trust. Their willingness to eat various coarse plants makes them ideal for conservation grazing, and on the Purbecks in Dorset a small herd is successfully helping the rare orchid population to survive.

The preferred height range is stallions and geldings 11.3hh (119.4cm) to 12.3hh (129.5cm) and mares 11.2hh (116.8cm) to 12.2hh (127cm). Colour is bay, brown or dun, with black points, 'mealy' colour on the muzzle, round the eyes and inside the flanks. There should be no white markings anywhere. The ponies have short ears, a clean-cut face with a broad forehead, and large, prominent eyes with a well-defined fleshy hood ('toad eyes'). In winter, they have a double-layered dense coat with an under-insulating layer of fine, springy hair and an outer waterproofing layer of hard, greasy hair.

They make good riding ponies for older children and are capable of carrying an adult. They can always be identified by brand marks, which are given when the pony is examined as a foal by the Exmoor Pony Society inspectors. If of a suitable standard, the pony is allocated a number which is branded on the near flank; the Exmoor star and the herd number are then branded on the near shoulder.

Movement should be straight and smooth, without exaggerated action.

Connemara

These ponies, which originated in western Ireland, are now very popular in the United Kingdom. They make excellent mounts for teenagers and light adults, and are known for their good temperament and jumping ability. Crossed with a Thoroughbred they make good all-round competition horses. Pure-bred Connemaras range in height from 12.2hh (127cm) to 14.2hh (148cm).

Colours are grey, black, bay, brown and dun with occasional roan, chestnut, palomino and dark-eyed cream. They are a well-balanced riding type with depth, substance and good heart room, standing on short legs covering a lot of ground. Movement is free, easy and true, without undue knee action but active and covering the ground.

New Forest

These ponies have bred in the New Forest for many centuries. There are now many private studs, where selective breeding has improved the stock. They make good, versatile riding ponies, with an upper height limit of 14.2hh (148cm). There is no lower height limit.

They can be any colour except piebald, skewbald or blue-eyed cream. They have an equable temperament and are easy to train. Their action is free, active and straight, but not exaggerated. Crossed with TB or Arab blood they make excellent small riding horses of great versatility.

Dartmoor

These ponies are indigenous to Dartmoor, though they are also bred privately off the moor, and are currently listed as vulnerable by the RBST. They make good children's ponies, being quiet, kind and reliable. They are versatile in that they are used successfully for lead rein, first ridden, open ridden, working hunter and driving.

In height they should not exceed 12.2hh (127cm). They can be black, bay, brown, chestnut, grey or roan. Piebalds and skewbalds are not allowed, and excessive white markings are discouraged. Their movement is low and straight, with good shoulder and hock action but without exaggeration.

They make good foundation stock and, when crossed with breeds such as TB or Arab, have produced many successful show animals.

Dales

Dales ponies are native to north-eastern England, and are on the RBST's critical list. They are a well-built cob-type, with active paces, full of quality and spirit. The preferred height range is 14hh (142cm) to 14.2hh (148cm).

Their colours are black, brown, bay, grey and occasionally roan. Markings include a star and/or snip, with white to the fetlocks on the hind legs only.

They have 20–23cm (8–9ins) of flat, flinty bone with ample, silky feather, and a long, flowing tail and mane, traditionally 'a yard long'. Their movement is clean, high, straight and true, with tremendous energy, going forward on 'all fours.'

It is said that a Dales pony should be capable of pulling a plough, trotting a mile in 3 minutes and giving a good ride to hounds.

This pony is always referred to as a 'Dales,' and not a 'Dale.'

Fell

The Fell pony is native to the northern Pennines and Cumbria, and is currently classified as at risk by the RBST. Smaller than its close neighbour the Dales, it should not exceed 14hh (142cm). They are strongly built and can be black, brown, bay or grey. Chestnuts, piebalds and skewbalds are barred. A star and/or a little white on or below the hind fetlock is acceptable, although an excess of white markings is discouraged. They have a lively and alert appearance, and great bone, with plenty of fine hair at the heels. The mane and tail are left to grow long.

Their walk is smart and true, with a well-balanced trot with good knee and hock action, going well from the shoulder and flexing the hocks. They make excellent ride-and-drive ponies.

Highland

The Highland pony is one of the two native breeds of the Scottish Highlands and Islands. Their height is 13hh (132cm) to 14.2hh (148cm). They were used for work on the crofts, ploughing and carrying peat. Being sure-footed and placid, they were ideal for deer stalking and for carrying the carcases. They make good riding ponies, capable of carrying adults. The RBST list them as at risk.

Colours include a range of duns: mouse, yellow, grey and cream. They can also be grey, brown, black and occasionally bay and liver chestnut with silver mane and tail. Many ponies have a dorsal stripe and some show zebra markings on legs and shoulders. A small star is acceptable, but other white markings are discouraged.

Their action is straight and free-moving, without undue knee action.

Shetland

These ponies originated in the Shetland Isles, where many are still bred. They are a very ancient breed, exceptionally strong for their size. In former years they were employed as pit ponies. They are now very popular for riding and driving.

Registered stock must not exceed 42 inches (107cm) at four years old. Shetland ponies may be any colour known in horses except spotted. They have great presence and stamina. The head should be small, carried well and in proportion. Their action should be straight and free, using every joint and tracking up.

DESCRIPTIVE TERMS

HALF-BRED Denotes a horse of whom one parent is a Thoroughbred.

THREEQUARTER-BRED Denotes that one parent is a Thoroughbred and the other a half-bred.

TYPES These include hunters, hacks, polo ponies, cobs and vanners. They are usually cross-breds, and are distinguished from breeds as they are not registered in a stud book.

COLD-BLOOD Applies to heavy work-horses such as Shires, Clydesdales and Percherons.

HOT-BLOOD OR FULL-BLOOD Applies to Thoroughbreds and to Eastern breeds such as Arabs, Barbs, etc.

WARMBLOOD Applies to horses with a mixture of 'hot' and 'cold' blood in their foundation stock.

HORSE Technically anything standing over 14.2hh (148cm) can be deemed a horse. However Arabs, whatever their size, are always referred to as horses, as are minute Falabellas, which do not exceed 30 inches (76cm).

PONY Traditionally, a pony does not exceed 14.2hh (148cm). However, the difference between a horse and a pony lies more in type, build and movement than in exact height. Polo ponies have no upper height limit, with the average being about 15hh (153cm). Today there are show classes for working hunter ponies and show hunter ponies not exceeding 15hh (153cm).

HACK A lightweight horse of TB type. Show hacks range from 'small', not exceeding 14.3hh (150cm), to 'large', not exceeding 15.3hh (160cm).

COB A sturdy, weight-carrying type, not exceeding 15.3hh (160cm). Until recently, show cobs could not exceed 15.1hh (155 cm) but due to popular demand there are now classes for 'maxi-cobs' over 155cm.

HUNTER A type, usually a half- or threequarter-bred animal, ranging from 15.2hh (157cm) upwards.

POLO PONY A Thoroughbred type under 16hh (162cm) with weight-carrying ability and suitable for adult riders.

COLOUREDS Piebald and skewbald horses and ponies. They include hunters, sports horses, riding horses, cobs, vanners, traditionals, draughts, paints, natives, part-bred Arabs, Thoroughbreds, warmbloods, coldbloods, driving types, working horses and ponies.

MULE A cross between a donkey stallion and a pony mare.

HINNY A cross between a horse or pony stallion and a female donkey. The name 'Jennet' is also used to denote this cross.

CHAPTER

6 BREEDING

Breeding a foal is an expensive and labour-intensive business and should not be undertaken without considerable thought and planning. Unless either the stallion or the mare has a proven record, it is unlikely that the breeder will make a profit on the eventual progeny, whether it is a small pony or a racehorse.

Facilities

It is essential to provide safe facilities for rearing a foal. Good clean grazing of not less than 3 acres is required. 'Clean' means that it has not been grazed by horses with a worm burden; that is not 'horse sick' (see Grassland Management, page 347 onwards). Ideally, it should have been cross-grazed by cattle or sheep during the previous twelve months. Fertilisers, if used, should be organic. The grazing should have very safe fencing, as foals have little sense of self-preservation, and shelter should be available from the prevailing winds.

A loosebox or barn large enough to hold the mare and foal is another requirement: 4.25 x 4.25m (14 x 14ft) is the minimum size for Thoroughbreds, but 4.6 x 4.6m (15 x 15ft) is more suitable. A smaller size is adequate for ponies.

Selection of Mare and Stallion

It is important to breed from tough, strong mares of good conformation, who are free from known hereditary disease, and who, if possible, have stood up to work and have a proven performance record. Do not consider breeding from a mare just because she is an old friend

and can no longer work!

Consideration must be given to the type of young horse required and, if he is to be sold, whether there is a market for him. It is pointless to breed a foal whom no one wants. Proven ability and soundness in both mare and stallion should be considered. The eligibility of the foal to obtain registration papers is becoming more important, so both parents should be registered or eligible to be registered with a society.

A stallion who complements the mare should be chosen. Breed societies have lists of the various stallions standing at stud. The British Warm-Blood Society has a list of their graded stallions. The stallion should be seen and the quality of the stable management at the stud taken into consideration.

In many cases it is sensible to delay sending the mare for service until late April or May. The foal will then be born in the warmer weather, and the fresh grass will encourage a good supply of milk from the mare. Foals destined to be shown in-hand are better born earlier, as they are more mature for the first shows.

Thoroughbreds bred for racing are born as early in the year as possible but that is a specialist occupation and outside the remit of this book.

MANAGEMENT OF THE MARE

Before Being Sent to the Stallion

- The mare should be in good condition but not fat or over-fit.

- She should have been wormed regularly, and been kept on very clean pasture.

- She should have been immunised against influenza within the last two months. Her tetanus vaccinations should be up to date.

- She should have had her hind shoes removed (some studs prefer the front shoes to be removed as well).

- Note should have been taken of the dates she came in season over the previous six weeks.

- Most studs insist that mares are swabbed by a veterinary surgeon, and passed clean before they are served. This can be carried out at home, but some studs insist that it is done at the stud.

The stallion owner/stud groom should be informed of all the above facts. In addition, they should be told if the mare is a maiden or barren and – if she has previously had a foal – whether there were difficulties getting her in foal. If she is due to foal at the stud, details of the last date of service and anything known about her previous breeding history should be supplied.

She should be sent to the stud with the following:

- A well-fitting, comfortable headcollar, with her name or the owner's name on it.

- Her passport, with flu and tetanus certificates.

- A veterinary certificate of cleanliness if she has been swabbed at home.

- A foal slip or headcollar if she is to foal at the stud.

At Stud

She may be out all the time or in at night. She is 'tried' to determine whether she is coming in season. When she is ready, she is served by the stallion. She is 'tried' again two to three weeks later to see whether she has 'held' to the first service. Depending upon the arrangements with her owner, she is returned home.

After Returning Home

- If she has not been tested 'in foal' at the stud, this has to be done (see Pregnancy Testing, page 54).

- She should be kept in good condition, but not allowed to become too fat.

- She should be wormed regularly with a wormer which is safe for pregnant mares.

- She may be ridden gently for a few months if desired. Mares who look well and have shelter from the bad weather may remain out at grass until a short time before foaling. This type of programme is certainly best for mountain and moorland ponies.

- Stabled mares should be turned out as much as possible, but only with other mares or alone, not with colts or geldings. Most mares need to be brought in at night from November onwards, but should still be turned out for exercise during the day. If the fields are too wet, the mare should be allowed to go loose in an indoor or outdoor school.

- After September the grass becomes less nutritious, and extra feed should be given as required.

- Whether in at night or out all the time, as soon as the grass loses its feed value she should be fed good hay ad lib plus a suitable ration. See feeding advice, page 50.

The Last Four Months Before Foaling

- The mare carries the foal for approximately eleven months, and during the last four months the foetus grows very fast, its size and weight increasing three-fold. If she has not already been receiving a special stud mix or cube, this should now be introduced to the diet according to the manufacturer's directions and her condition. Unless she is deficient in some way, which can be ascertained by a blood test, it should not be necessary for her to receive supplements. Good quality forage should continue to be offered ad lib.

- A month before she is due to foal she should have a

tetanus booster. She should also have a flu inoculation, if this has not been done in the last six months. Antibodies are passed to the foal in the colostrum (first milk).

• The mare must continue to be wormed regularly. Worms are lethal to young foals, and can be passed in the mare's milk, or picked up by the foal eating the mare's droppings. It is important that the wormer is safe for pregnant mares, and that the instructions are followed carefully.

FOALING (PARTURITION)

The mare carries the foal for between 320 and 350 days. The average is about 335 days.

If the person in charge of the mare is experienced, and if assistance is available, the mare can be foaled at home. If not, and especially if the mare is valuable and has been to an expensive stallion, it is safer to send her to a recommended stud to foal. If she is to be put in foal again she can go to the stud where the stallion stands.

Foaling Away From Home

It is better to send the mare at least three weeks before the expected foaling date, so that the upsets of the journey do not bring on the foaling, and she can settle down and acquire some immunity to the germs at the stud.

Foaling at Home – Facilities

• A large, safe, disinfected loosebox with as few fittings as possible. A good size is 4.6m x 4.6m (15ft x 15ft).

• No dark corners; new-born foals will nearly always gravitate to them.

• A deep, clean straw bed, well banked up on the walls.

• Good lighting.

• Some means of viewing the mare without disturbing her: CCTV cameras are now widely available.

If she is foaling at home and is the only in-foal mare, it is better for her to sleep in the foaling box a week or two before the expected foaling date.

Signs of Foaling

BAGGING UP During the final few days the udder grows larger, stiffer and rounder. During this time the udder may be handled gently, so that the mare does not resent being suckled. This is particularly beneficial with maiden mares.

WAXING Usually between six and forty-eight hours before foaling starts, the teats exude a wax-like substance. This is not a reliable sign, as it may be closer to the foaling, or the mare may not wax at all.

SLACKENING The muscles on either side of the root of the tail slacken; this occurs usually twelve to eighteen hours before foaling.

When Foaling is Imminent

At this stage, it is wise to put a light, well-fitting headcollar on the mare. The likely signs, which may be spread over a period of about four hours, are:

• Walking the box.

• Pawing the bedding.

• Looking round at flanks.

• Kicking at the belly.

• Swishing the tail.

• Lying down and getting up again.

• Starting to sweat.

At this time the mare should be watched constantly, but without disturbing her. At night, the lights should be left switched on. With modern surveillance cameras it is possible to monitor the in-foal mare without disturbing her and only go in to her if help is needed.

The veterinary surgeon's telephone number and spray as recommended by your vet for the foal's navel should be at hand.

The assistant's hands should be well scrubbed before handling the foal or mare.

Position of foetus immediately prior to foaling.

Normal Foaling

Usually, but not always, the mare lies down.

1. The foetal fluids are discharged as the bag breaks. The foal should then be born within 20–40 minutes.
2. Within about five minutes, the front legs appear, still inside the membrane, with one foot slightly in advance of the other.
3. The head appears, lying along the front legs.
4. The shoulders appear, and then the mare usually has a short rest.
5. The membrane over the nostrils (caul) should break. It is essential that this is done before the navel cord is broken, otherwise the foal suffocates. If the foal has not broken this for himself, the watcher may do so, but not until the foal's ribs are clear of the mare.
6. The hind legs slip out, or are withdrawn by the foal.
7. The foal may struggle to get up, or the mare may get up and the cord will be broken naturally. The stump can then be attended to. After the first discharge (Stage 1 above), the foal has only one to three hours to live inside the mare. If there is any deviation from the sequence just described, veterinary help should be sought immediately. The vet requires hot water, soap and clean towels.

After Foaling

If all has gone well, which in the majority of cases it does, the mare and foal should be allowed to rest, but should be watched unobtrusively. Usually within an hour the foal is on his feet and trying to suckle. It is very important for him to get this early milk (colostrum), as it contains the antibodies which protect him for the first few months of his life. After that time he starts to

manufacture his own. Some foals are slow to find their way to the udder and have to be helped.

Sometimes a maiden mare resents the foal and has to be restrained. The risk of this happening is lessened if the groom has handled the udder on occasions, perhaps giving it a wash with a warm flannel and getting the mare used to being touched in that area. The assistant can hold up a front leg; a tranquilliser may be given; or in very severe cases the mare can be twitched. As the application of the twitch can cause a rise in blood pressure, care must be taken. It is possible to cause a haemorrhage in a newly foaled mare.

Sometimes the foal does not get up. This may be because the cord has broken early, and the foal has not obtained a full blood supply. If he otherwise seems bright and healthy, two people may support him with a clean sack under his belly, so that he can get to the mare's udder. There are cases where it may be necessary to milk the mare and let the foal drink from a sterilised bottle with a calf's teat on the end. If the foal is not bright and alert, or begins to behave strangely, veterinary help should be sought immediately.

The **afterbirth** (foetal membranes) gradually separates from the uterus and is expelled by the mare, often within an hour of foaling. If it is retained for more than three hours, veterinary help should be sought. On no account should any attempt be made to pull it away. If possible, it should be inspected to make sure that nothing has been retained inside the mare. The placenta has a main 'body' which filled the womb and enclosed the foetus, with two 'horns' at the top.

As soon as the mare is on her feet, she should be offered a chilled drink and (if she will take them) electrolytes may be added. Hay may be given, and after an hour or two a small feed. Hay should always be fed loose, so that there is no danger of the foal becoming entangled in the net.

Foaling Outside

ADVANTAGES

- It is nearer to nature.

- There is less risk of infection.

- More natural for native breeds.

DISADVANTAGES

- In an emergency it is difficult to provide human assistance, especially at night.

- The mare may choose a dangerous place to foal, e.g. too near a fence or ditch.

- In bad weather the foal may suffer.

- Once the foal is on his feet the mare may refuse to be caught.

If this practice is to be followed, a safe, level, well-fenced field with no ditches, ponds or other hazards should be chosen. There should be no horses or cattle in the field and it should be adjacent to the stables. There should be shelter, e.g. a thick hedge, or shed.

Usually the system works well with ponies, but for valuable horses it is not advisable.

The mare and foal should be caught and handled each day. In bad weather, driving rain and wind, they should be brought in.

MANAGEMENT AFTER FOALING

The First 24 Hours

Some people like their foals to have an antibiotic injection within the first 24 hours. In any case, it may be a wise precaution for the vet to check the mare, the foal, and the afterbirth. He can also check whether the meconium (foetal dung) has been expelled correctly.

The mare and foal should be looked at frequently.

The foal must be seen to be suckling successfully. He should pass the meconium, which is blackish and may be hard, within thirty-six hours. If this is not passed, veterinary assistance may be sought, or an experienced person can give an enema.

The mare may remain on the same diet as before foaling – i.e. high protein mash-type feeds – but smaller quantities of energy food should be given for the first few days. It is unwise to suddenly introduce bran mashes, as the mare's digestion will not be used to bran. If she has been having flaked barley, mashes may be made from this.

After the First 24 Hours

If the weather is good, the mare can be led out with the foal (see Handling the Foal, page 51) and given an hour's grazing. With an unknown mare it is wise to graze her in-hand the first time she goes out. She should have a headcollar on when she is turned loose with the foal. When the mare is released the foal should be in front of her, where she can see him, so that she will not kick him by mistake as she gallops off. The foal should be led out and not allowed to go loose. He should be released before the mare.

March foals should come in at night with their dams until the weather improves. If the weather is suitable, May foals (after they are one week old) can be left out at night, but they should be caught and handled daily.

When flies become troublesome the mare and foal may be brought in during the daytime. They should also be brought in during bad weather. If a foal is very cold and shivery he should be rubbed down, and if possible put under a heat lamp. It is also wise to bring foals in before a thunderstorm, as horses shelter under trees and are therefore vulnerable to lightning. During storms young horses can panic and may gallop through fences.

Scouring

The foal is likely to scour when the mare first comes into season on the foaling heat. This is quite normal.

However, should he start scouring at any other time, an antibiotic injection may be necessary to deal with any infection. Severe scouring can be serious owing to the danger of dehydration.

The foal's hindquarters should be kept clean by washing and drying them carefully. Baby oil applied either side of the tail can help to prevent the coat being lost.

Worming

Most modern wormers are safe for foals. With foals the danger is usually from roundworms and a wormer suitable for dealing with these worms should be chosen. The instructions should be followed carefully. Worming should be carried out as early as the product allows, usually at four weeks old. Keeping foals as worm-free as possible is a vital safety measure. Much damage, if not death, can result from a worm burden and – even if not evident at the time – can result in serious trouble later in life. Many cases of colic and subsequent death are attributable to worm infestation when young.

The mare should be wormed at the same time as the foal. Thereafter it is sensible to worm them as the vet recommends, but also practice scrupulous pasture care.

FEEDING BREEDING STOCK

The aim when feeding a broodmare or youngster should be the same as when feeding any horse, that is to maintain the animal in a condition score of 2.5–3. The likelihood of fertility problems is greater in horses that are over- or underweight and it is essential to monitor the condition of all breeding and growing animals.

As with any horse, as much of the diet as possible should consist of fibre, such as pasture and forage. This promotes digestive health and lessens the likelihood of colic and other gastro-intestinal conditions. Cereal or hard feeds should be only provided to horses that have a genuine need to receive concentrated energy in order to maintain their body condition at the correct level.

The Pregnant Mare

During early pregnancy, the nutritional demands on the mare are no greater than those on the non-pregnant mare. In the first two-thirds of gestation, the foal will not grow a great deal and the mare should not make any significant weight gain. Most mares will cope well on good pasture and forage during their early pregnancy. If a mare is working, or producing milk for her previous year's foal, some supplementary feed may be required.

The foal increases in size quite considerably during the final three months of gestation and it is at this time that the mare's ration may need to be increased, perhaps with the inclusion of hard feed. By the end of her pregnancy, the mare should have put on between 14% and 15% of her non-pregnant bodyweight and it is useful to monitor her weight to ensure that she remains on track to achieve this. If hard feed is to be introduced to the mare's diet this should be done gradually, starting about four months before her expected foaling date.

The temptation to overfeed a pregnant mare should be avoided. Overweight mares will find the process of foaling more difficult and there is a far greater likelihood of complications than for a mare in correct condition. Obesity will also affect fertility and an overweight mare may have difficulties conceiving if she is to be re-covered following the foal's birth. Conversely, mares who receive inadequate feed during their pregnancy are more likely to give birth to foals with developmental abnormalities or low birth-weights, which may compromise the foal's chance of survival.

Ensuring that the mare remains at a condition score of between 2.5–3 throughout her pregnancy, and adjusting her ration to achieve this, will give the mare and foal the greatest chance of a trouble-free birth.

The Lactating Mare

Lactation is a more energy expensive process than pregnancy and the mare's ration should be adjusted to reflect this. Milk production requires a higher nutritional input than supporting a pregnancy, although the exact amount will vary with the stage of lactation. As the foal grows so does his demand for milk and thus the mare's diet should reflect this. However, as the foal ages and begins to receive his nutrients from sources other than milk his demand will decrease until weaning.

Once again the aim should be to keep the mare at a condition score of 2.5–3 throughout her lactation. Many mares, particularly ponies and native breeds, can support a full lactation on pasture and forage alone, but others will require supplementary hard feed. Particular attention should be paid to ensuring the mare does not gain excessive weight once the foal begins consuming other feeds and is suckling less.

Youngstock

It is imperative that the foal receives colostrum within his first 24 hours of life. Colostrum contains essential antibodies that cannot pass from the gut into the bloodstream after approximately 24 hours has passed. If any circumstance or problem prevents the foal from suckling from his dam within a couple of hours for birth an alternative source of colostrum should be sourced immediately, e.g. from your veterinary practice.

Provided the dam is in good health and receiving the nutrients she requires to lactate sufficiently, the foal will not need any supplementary feed in his early weeks. He will investigate the feed and forage that his dam receives and this is to be encouraged, provided that he does not consume too much of her ration.

Some foals may benefit from the provision of an easily digested creep feed, such as foal pellets. If supplementary feed is to be provided for the foal it is important that the mare is prevented from accessing it. Such feeds will disrupt the balance of a mare's own diet and encourage her to gain weight.

Before weaning, the foal should be eating grass and hay, and any hard feed that he is likely to continue to receive after weaning. His reliance on his mother's milk should also have noticeably decreased. Weaning should not bring about a great difference in a foal's diet; he should simply receive an increase in feeds to which he is already accustomed to compensate for the fact that he is no longer consuming his dam's milk.

It is obviously important that a foal receives sufficient food to allow him to grow. However, a careful balance must be struck. Overfeeding may have serious consequences for the foal's development and implications for his future soundness and career. The over-provision of energy and protein, as well as mineral imbalances, may lead to the foal suffering from a developmental orthopaedic disease, such as epiphysitis or osteochondrosis dessicans. Failing to provide a growing horse with adequate nutrition may result in compromised growth and limb deformities.

As with any horse there are no hard and fast rules for feeding broodmares and youngstock. Each animal is an individual and his or her ration should reflect that. The key is to maintain the animal in the correction condition and a diet may need regular tweaking in order to achieve this. Where there is doubt the advice of a vet or equine nutritionist should always be sought.

HANDLING THE FOAL

Foals should at all times be treated quietly but with firmness. The foal should be handled within twelve hours of his birth. Some foals are very friendly, others very shy.

To catch the foal, two people are required: one to hold and reassure the mare, the other to catch the foal. The foal may try to escape by going in front of or underneath the mare. He should be approached from behind, never from the front. He should be caught with one hand round the front of the chest and the other round the quarters. Once caught, he should be stroked and soothed. Within 24 hours, a foal slip may be fitted. An assistant to hold the foal makes this easier.

The Foal Slip or Headcollar

Opinion is divided as to whether the foal slip should be left on all the time. Many people consider this to be a

The foal may be encouraged to lead for the first few times by cradling him in your arms, one arm behind his hindquarters and the other around his chest.

dangerous practice, as it is easy for the foal to get caught up in it. Whether or not it is worn all the time it should be adjustable over the head and around the nose, and should be made of leather, not nylon, unless fitted with 'panic breaks'.

To put on the headcollar, fasten the headpiece round the neck first, push it forwards to behind the ears, and then fasten the noseband. To begin with it will need adjustment for length and tightness every three or four days. It must be fitted carefully, so that it is not too tight, but must never be loose enough for the foal to trap a hind leg when scratching his face.

Each day the foal should be handled all over, and a hand run down his legs. After a few days his feet may be picked up.

Teaching to Lead

Leading lessons should start in the box. With a very young foal, put a stable rubber round his neck and move him along with a hand around his quarters. As soon as he understands this, a 1.8m (6ft) light rope may be threaded through the foal slip to guide and steady him, but a hand should be kept round his quarters to push him along and to prevent him running back, as he may fall over. The foal should be 'played' like a fish. The rope must be threaded through rather than clipped on, so that should he inadvertently escape, the rope will not be left dangling, which will frighten him. He should never be pulled by the head, but always urged from behind. It is never too early to teach him voice commands such as 'Walk on' and 'Halt', 'Stand' or 'Wait'. (See Methods of Control, page 73, and Leading the Horse in Hand, page 77.)

Foals should not be allowed to go to and from the field loose; they may easily gallop into something and damage themselves. If the leading lessons are started early enough, they learn very quickly. If the training is left too long they become much stronger and, being unused to discipline, will be difficult to control.

When leading them out to the field, the mare should be in front with the foal close to her side. The person leading the mare should watch the foal, and stop immediately if he is left behind.

Feet

When the farrier comes to dress the mare's feet he should handle the foal and pick up his feet, even if they do not need attention. Foals handled only by women can become quite nervous with men. It is important to study the foal's action and to keep his feet correctly trimmed. This will prevent unlevelness of the foot caused by faulty action. If there is abnormality with his legs or feet at birth, the sooner veterinary advice and consultation with the farrier takes place, the more likely is the problem to be remedied. Some foals are born with their fetlocks on the ground and this usually rights itself fairly quickly.

WEANING

There are a number of methods of weaning the foal. If the mare is not again in foal it can be allowed to happen naturally. This usually occurs at seven to eight months but can be later. If the mare is in foal again the foal at foot is usually weaned at between five and seven months; earlier if strong and well grown and later if needing more time with his dam.

Ideally the foal should be quite well handled, be able to lead on his own and be used to hay and foal pellets before he is weaned. If he is used to a little hard feed he is less likely to lose condition on weaning.

Method 1

Ideally two or more foals should be weaned at the same time. Otherwise a sensible pony or quiet horse needs to be introduced to act as 'nanny' at weaning.

The mare and foal are led in from the field and stabled. The mare is removed, preferably out of earshot, otherwise they will call to each other, which is stressful for both. The weanling and his companion need to be shut in a secure stable with a top door that can be kept closed. They should have plenty of hay and water and a good bed. They will need to be kept in for at least 24 hours, perhaps longer. After that they can be let out in a secure paddock. If the mare is within earshot, the foal is likely to throw himself through any hedge or fence in an attempt to reach her. Foals have no sense of danger.

Method 2

This is likely to be less stressful and more successful if it is not possible to remove the mare out of earshot. It works well if she is not in foal and is being brought back into work. It is still preferable to have a 'nanny' if there is only a single foal. Every day the mare and foal are separated for ever-increasing periods, the foal and companion being securely shut in and the mare exercised or otherwise occupied. They are put together again after work. After a few days it is usually possible to leave the foal and companion out whilst the mare is away. After a week or two it should be possible to turn the foal and companion out separately from the mare.

Method 3

The third method is good when there are a number of mares and foals. Gradually, over the course of a few days, the mares are removed, one a day. Start with the dam of one of the more confident youngsters. Again, a steady pony or horse is helpful to teach the youngsters manners and keep them calm. This method means that the foals do not have to be shut in.

After Weaning

The mare must be given a low protein diet and plenty of exercise. If she has a lot of milk, her bag should be examined carefully each day to make sure that she is not developing mastitis. It is not advisable to draw off the milk, as this encourages further production.

Pony foals may winter out as long as there is shelter, but young horses usually lose too much condition. The latter are best turned out in the daytime, and kept in at night. This means that they lie warm and dry without expending food to keep themselves warm, and they are able to take the daily exercise which is necessary to ensure that they grow up strong and active. They should continue to be well fed, but not overfed. They should be wormed and have their feet trimmed regularly. By being handled regularly they will learn manners and be confident youngsters.

STALLIONS

Stallions who are used solely as stud horses have a rather different lifestyle from those who are ridden in equestrian activities, though some do both.

The annual programme for Thoroughbreds, or similar stallions, used solely for stud work begins three to four months before the start of the stud season. At this time, daily exercise must begin, so that the horses are fit before starting their duties. At Thoroughbred studs, mares are covered in February, but at other studs usually not before March.

After the season is over, which may be June, or even later, the stallions should be let down and roughed off. Stallions who are ridden as well as being used at stud should have a particularly strict regime so that they understand what they are required to do in the differing circumstances. It is important to use a different bridle and to choose a special place for serving the mares.

When dealing with stallions, discipline is of paramount importance. Their natural pride and arrogance must not be spoiled, although they must understand that their handler is the boss.

When being attended to, the horse should always be tied up. A chain, rather than a rope, is essential, as stallions by their nature pick up everything with their teeth. People dealing with them should not wear scent or aftershave, as the smell is likely to arouse them.

When holding or leading a stallion it is advisable to carry a stick or whip. If he is being led in a headcollar, a clip chain under the jaw or over the nose, attached to a long lead rope, is a sensible precaution. If he is being led in a bridle, a coupling to the bit and a lead rein 2.4–3.6m (8–12ft long) should be used. The attributes for dealing with all stallions are patience, firmness and common sense. There should be no fear and no loss of temper.

Anyone wanting to work with stallions should apply to work at a well-run stud or establishment where stallions are kept. Working with an experienced stud person and watching experienced handlers go about their duties is the best way to learn.

COVERING MARES

Mares may be covered naturally by the stallion or they can be artificially inseminated either with fresh semen or with semen that has been frozen. The first method is natural but puts some risk on the stallion and also limits the number of mares he can cover. The second method keeps the stallion safe. The collected semen can be diluted allowing it to be used more economically. However, the operatives need training and skill.

The third option allows semen to be sent around the world and is much less risky to both the stallion and the mare than travelling long distances. The fertility might not be quite so high and the operatives need a high level of training and expertise.

Very valuable mares sometimes have embryo transplants. This allows them to produce foals whilst still competing. In this case their fertilised egg is transplanted into a surrogate mare who actually carries and produces the foal.

Thoroughbreds have to be produced from a natural covering in order to be accepted in **The Stud Book**.

PREGNANCY TESTING

MANUAL This is carried out by a veterinary surgeon, from 35 days after service up to the time of foaling.

BLOOD TESTING This is carried out between 45 and 100 days after service. A blood sample is collected from the jugular vein and sent to a laboratory for analysis. The test is a biological one, for gonadotrophic hormones.

URINE TESTING This is carried out at any time after 130 days. A urine sample is collected by the owner and sent to a laboratory to be tested for oestrogenic components.

ULTRASOUND SCANNING This method of testing is now available from most veterinary surgeons who specialise in treating equine breeding stock. It can be used from 17 to 20 days after the last service.

STUD FEES

There are several methods of paying the covering fee for the stallion's services. Some of the most usual are:

• Whole fee paid on completion of covering.

• No foal, free return.

• No foal, no fee.

When the whole fee is paid on completion of covering it can sometimes be a cheaper option, but there is no guarantee of a foal. The other two options are usually calculated on October 1st. If the mare is in foal on that date a slightly higher fee is due. If she is not, there is either the option to return next year or sometimes no fee is due. Sometimes there is the agreement of a live foal being produced before the covering fee is due. In all cases the livery charges, the veterinary fees and the other ancillary charges will all need to be paid, whatever the outcome.

CHAPTER 7

IDENTIFICATION

Brand Marks

Brand marks are used to denote breed or ownership. A hot branding iron carrying the appropriate mark is applied to the horse's skin. Horses imported from Europe often carry a breed mark, which is usually found on the left hindquarter but can be on the shoulder and/or neck.

Many native ponies breeding wild on the hills and in the forests are branded, to denote ownership. A general round-up takes place in the autumn, and ponies in their first year and then still running with their mothers can be easily identified and branded. The brand is usually on the quarters, under the saddle, or on the shoulder.

Freeze-Marking and Micro-chipping

To deter thieves, many owners now have their horses **freeze-marked**. The process has been patented by Farm Key of Banbury, who keep a national register of horses, their owners, and their allocated numbers. The process is quite painless and leaves a permanent white mark. It is applied either under the saddle or under the mane. Freeze-marked animals are less likely to be stolen.

Micro-chipping is still relatively uncommon in Britain but becoming more popular.

EXAMPLE BRANDS

Australian Warmblood	British Trakehner	Irish Sport Horse	Holstein
Dutch Warmblood	Belgian Warmblood	German Riding Horse	Oldenburg
Finnish Warmblood	Danish Warmblood	British Hanoverian Horse Society	Westphalia
Selle Francais	British Warmblood	Hanoverian	Bavaria

Describing a Horse

Consider the following:

• **Colour.**

• **Sex.**

• **Markings.**

• **Height.**

• **Age** – See Chapter 4. Examine teeth: length, tables, shape and condition.

• **Type** – Stand back and check build and bone shape.

Sex and Age

The word 'horse' can be used to describe the whole equine species without reference to sex. The following terms are more precise descriptions:

• STALLION/ENTIRE Uncastrated male horse of any age.

• GELDING Castrated male of any age.

• COLT Uncastrated male under four years of age.

• MARE Female horse of four years or more, if a maiden; any age if she has had a foal.

• FILLY Female under four years of age.

• FOAL Described either as a 'colt' or 'filly' foal and under one year old.

• RIG Male horse who has retained one or both testes in the abdomen due to incorrect castration or failure of the testes to descend. The condition can be rectified, but would probably involve a major operation. Rigs are not suitable mounts. If known at the time of a sale the condition must be declared.

Height

Traditionally horses are measured in hands (4ins/ 10.16cm). All height measurement for competitions and documentation is expressed in centimetres. The measurement is taken from the highest point of the withers in a perpendicular line to the ground.

Height can be measured:
(a) With a measuring stick (see below).
(b) By eye or by touch. Use your own eyes, mouth or chin as a marker, e.g. for a 5ft 3ins (160cm) person the chin is about 14.2hh (147cm). Then stand up to the horse's withers to gauge the approximate height.

For accurate measurement, the following items and conditions are essential:

• A measuring stick with a spirit level on the cross bar.

• The horse should be standing on a smooth and level surface.

• The horse must stand squarely on all four feet. His head should be lowered so that the eyebrows are in line with the withers.

• The horse must be calm and must remain still. If he is tense he should be allowed 15–20 minutes to get used to having the stick placed on the withers.

For the purposes of the Joint Measurement Scheme, the horse must be measured without shoes. For general purposes, the shoes – providing they are of normal weight – may remain on and 12mm (½in) is taken off the measured height.

Correct height measurement is important because:

• It forms part of a correct description of the horse for sale.

• It provides for correct division and sub-division of horses in showing and jumping classes, and in other competitive sports.

• It serves as some indication of size when buying saddlery and clothing, although type and build are of equal importance.

Colours

For the purposes of identification, it is important for a horse's colour and markings to be described correctly. His precise colour can sometimes be difficult to determine, but reference to the colour of his 'points' – muzzle, eyelids, tips of the ears, legs and the mane and tail – should clarify the problem. The legs below the knee can be black or a darker version of the body, but they also may have white markings. A horse with no white markings is said to be **whole-coloured.** When describing horses, any patches of white hair caused by pressure or injury should be noted. These are most likely to occur in the saddle and bridle area or on the legs. Scars should also be noted.

- **A black** horse is black in colour with black points and a black muzzle.

- **A brown** horse is dark brown in colour with similar limbs, mane and tail.

- **A dark bay** horse is mid-brown in colour with black limbs, mane and tail.

- **A bright bay** horse is mahogany in colour with black limbs, mane and tail.

- **A light bay** horse is a paler shade of brown, or pale mahogany, with black limbs, mane and tail.

- **A bay-brown** is a horse where the predominating colour is brown, with bay muzzle and black points.

- **A dark chestnut** is a rich red colour with matching points. He sometimes has small patches of black hair on the body. He may be whole coloured as in a Suffolk Punch, but is most likely to have white markings on his legs.

- A **chestnut** is a paler version of the above and may have a flaxen mane and tail.

- A **liver chestnut** is a rich red brown with similar mane, tail and legs.

- A **grey** horse is one with both black and white hair growing in the coat, with matching points and mane and tail. The skin is black.

- An **iron grey** has predominantly black hairs and can appear nearly black. He may become paler with age.

- A **light grey** has predominantly white hairs.

- A **flea-bitten grey** has dark or brown hair growing in speckles over the body.

- A **dapple grey** has circles of black hair over the body.

NOTE: All grey horses become lighter with age, but are never described as white. On examination, the skin will be seen to be dark coloured. They may be born brown or black.

- A **blue dun** has a very dark, bluey/grey coat which doesn't lighten with age. The mane and tail are black. There may be a dorsal stripe. The skin is black.

- A **yellow dun** horse varies from mouse colour to dark gold with black points. He may show a 'list', a dark line along the back bone and have dark stripes around his legs. The skin is black.

- A **palomino** varies from light cream to bright gold with similar coloured points, and lighter or silver coloured mane and tail.

- A **cream** horse has a light cream coat verging to white in the muzzle area and legs. The muzzle is white. The skin lacks pigment. The eyes may also have a pinkish or bluish appearance. The mane and tail will be a similar colour to the short coat.

- A **roan** has a mixture of white and other colours growing in his coat. There is a tendency to get whiter with age.

- A **strawberry roan** is white and red with similar points.

- A **blue roan** is white and black with black points. The coat has a blue tinge.

- A **red roan** or a bay roan is white and bay or bay-brown with black limbs, mane and tail.

- A **chestnut roan** or **sorrel** is white and light chestnut with matching points. Mane and tail similar or chestnut in colour.

- A **piebald** is a mixture of large irregular patches of black and white. The mane and tail may also be black and white.

- A **skewbald** is a mixture of large irregular patches of white and any other colour or colours.

- A **spotted** horse often has pink or mottled skin. He may have: (a) **leopard spot** markings, when dark spots are distributed over a lighter background; (b) **blanket markings**, when there are dark spots on the rump of a lighter coloured horse; (c) **snowflake markings**, when white spots appear on a darker background.

- An Appaloosa has a pink skin and a silky white or grey coat with darker coloured spots on the coat. These markings can include leopard, blanket or snowflake markings.

- **Odd-coloured** horses are those whose body coat consists of large irregular patches of more than two colours, which may merge at the edges.

A white wall eye.

White upper and lower lips.

White muzzle.

Markings

The Head

- A **star** is a white mark on the forehead. It can be further described as large, small, irregular, etc.

- A **stripe** is a narrow white marking down the face. It may be a continuation of a star, and can be further

Star.

Star and stripe.

Snip.

Blaze, extending to both nostrils.

White face.

described as narrow, irregular, etc.

- A **blaze** is a broad white marking extending from between the eyes and down the face over the nasal bones.

- A **white face** is an exaggerated blaze. It covers the whole of the forehead and front of the face to the mouth.

- A **snip** is a white mark between the nostrils. If extending to a right or left nostril it should be so described.

- A **white upper lip** and **underlip** describes skin at the edges of the lips.

- A **white muzzle** describes where white skin is found on both lips and up to the nostrils.

- A **wall eye** is one which shows a lack of colouring matter. It has a greyish-white or blue appearance. The sight is not affected.

The Body

- **List, dorsal stripe** and **ray** describe the dark lines along the back of dun horses. They are also found on donkeys.

- **Zebra marks** describe any stripes on the body. They occur more frequently on donkeys.

- **Salmon marks** are fine lines of white hair found on the loins and quarters.

- The **prophet's thumb mark** is a pronounced dimple sometimes found on the neck of Thoroughbred or Arab horses. It can also appear in the shoulder or hindquarters. It is said to be a sign of good luck.

- **Flesh marks** are patches of skin devoid of colouring and care should be taken to use this term instead of white wherever appropriate.

The Legs

- White markings on the legs are defined by reference to the anatomy. The traditional terms **'sock' or 'stocking'** are now used only for casual description. Nowadays the terms 'right' and 'left' are used instead of 'off' and 'near'. For example, typical descriptions are: right pastern; left heel; right leg to above knee.

- The term **'ermine'** is used where black spots occur on white markings, usually around the coronet.

Hooves

Any variation in colour of the hooves should be noted, in particular a white stripe or line down the hoof.

Whorls

Whorls are formed by changes in the direction of hair growth. They are an established method of identifying horses, as they vary to some extent in every animal. They occur on the head, neck, body and upper limbs. When describing horses for identification it is the ones on the head and neck which should be noted. Grey and whole-coloured horses, or those with few markings, should have at least five whorls noted, either on the head, neck or body.

Chestnuts

For horses with fewer than five identifying whorls a print can be made of the chestnuts on each front leg. These are like human fingerprints and show a different shape and/or design in every horse.

Certification of Identity/Passport

Official certificates must be completed and signed by a veterinary surgeon. Horses are identified by means of a written description of the horse and a sketch map of his body, together with separate sketches of the front view of the head, muzzle and legs. (See sample description overleaf.) This forms part of the passport.

- **White markings** on the horse should be outlined in red and filled in with diagonal red lines.

Sample description of a horse

NAME SAM

SIRE Scottish Venture.

DAM Breeding unknown.

Chestnut gelding. Foaled 1980. Height 16.1hh with shoes. Mane and tail on. Freeze-marked 6783 under saddle.

HEAD Whorl in centre of forehead above eye level. Small star, narrow stripe and snip to left nostril.

LEFT FRONT Small mark on front of coronet. White stripe on front of hoof. Whorl on posterior-lateral mid-forearm.

RIGHT FRONT Half cannon. White hoof.

LEFT HIND Half pastern to mid-fetlock behind. White hoof.

RIGHT HIND Threequarter cannon. White hoof.

BODY Whorl left anterior crest. Whorl right mid-crest. Whorl left anterior jugular. Whorl mid-trachea.

ACQUIRED Scattered saddle marks on both sides. Girth mark on left side. Scar anterior mid-cannon left hind.

- **Whorls** are shown by an X marked in black.

- **Scars** are shown by a tick marked in black.

- **White marks on a grey** are not noted except for flesh marks.

- The written description of a horse must be in black ink, and should exactly describe the markings, whorls, and scars as shown on the sketch map. The description should start with the forehead.

- The position of head whorls should be exactly described in relation to eye level, centre of forehead, and any white markings. Crest whorls on the neck should be divided into anterior, middle and posterior. Body whorls should be designated by reference to the particular anatomical position.

When describing a stolen horse to the police it is helpful to have a photograph as 'non-horsy' people do not understand such terms as 'dun' or 'chestnut'. Two pictures, one taken in summer and one in winter are useful to keep on file along with photos of freeze or breed brands, to help identification.

All Thoroughbred horses are also blood-typed when registered.

BUYING AND SELLING A HORSE

BUYING

When looking at horses or ponies with a view to buying them, inexperienced persons should always take a more knowledgable person with them. Even experienced people find it helpful to have another opinion.

The owner of the horse should be asked to provide information as to age, any vices and/or bad habits, and suitability for intended use. It can be helpful if this information is written down in the presence of another unbiased person – who can, if necessary, corroborate what has been said.

The National Equine Database (NED), when it is up and running, will be a useful source of information on all registered equines. See Appendix 6.

Breed papers should be available for inspection when the horse is first seen. If he is a show animal he may have a height certificate. If not, and if you intend to show him in height-restricted classes, the vendor can be asked to warrant the height.

It is illegal to buy or sell a horse in the UK without a valid passport. If the vendor is unable to produce this when the horse is first seen, be very careful about agreeing to purchase. If it is not available at the time of purchase do not proceed. Any passport details that are produced should be carefully checked against the prospective purchase and the names and address of previous owners noted in order to verify any information offered. See Appendix 3, Equine Passports.

Before coming to a final decision it is always advisable to have the animal examined by a veterinary surgeon. Unless the vet is personally known to you try to choose one independently from the vendor. Always explain to the vet the purpose of the purchase and any relevant details about the potential rider's ability as this will enable a better judgement to be made as to whether the horse is suitable. Veterinary surgeons will not usually give a warranty as to soundness, and cannot certify height unless able to measure the animal under Joint Measurement Scheme rules. If they consider the animal suitable they will provide a certificate giving a description (including approximate height) and stating that the said animal has no abnormality or injury likely to affect his use for the purpose for which he is being bought. This certificate should be sufficient for insurance purposes.

If possible, the intending purchaser should attend the vetting so that any queries can be answered on the spot. If this is not possible, it is certainly helpful to have a verbal report and to discuss the examination with the veterinary surgeon. Veterinary certificates can sometimes be difficult to interpret, especially for a layman. For an expensive horse required for competition, X-rays or scans of the lower limbs and feet plus blood tests at the time of purchase are a worthwhile investment.

Viewing the Horse

Procedure

First, insist on seeing the horse loose in his stable or, if he is to live out, it might be a good idea to see him caught from the field. Then have him brought out and stood still for inspection, before being walked and trotted up on a hard, level surface. Ask for the horse to be saddled up, and watch whilst this is being carried out. Ask for someone to ride and jump the horse before riding him yourself. If you don't feel able to ride him yourself take someone with you who is able and whose opinion you trust. If buying for a child it is preferable for them to ride the pony after you or your 'expert' have. Note such things as whether the horse stands still to be mounted or to have girth and stirrups altered, if these are relevant. If he is to be ridden out, note whether he will leave the yard on his own. Napping can be difficult to overcome.

Remember, some horses will jump well over coloured fences, some will be bolder over natural fences, and some will perform very much better over known fences at home than they will over an unknown course. It is up to the purchaser to test the horse or to see him perform according to his proposed use.

Information Needed

According to intended use, it is advisable to obtain the following information about the horse in question:

- Is he sound?

- Is he good in traffic? This question should be expanded to cover reactions to heavy traffic, high lorries, main roads, narrow sideroads, etc.

- Is he quiet to handle, groom, shoe, and clip?

- Is he good to box and travel, both in a trailer and horsebox?

- Is he free from any stable vices? These should be itemised. (See page 144.)

- Is he well behaved in company, e.g. with hounds, other horses, dogs, children?

- Is he safe in a field with other horses, and/or happy to be turned out alone?

- Is he free from any known allergy?

- In the case of a child's pony or a horse for a novice

rider, is he easy to catch, both on his own or in company, good to tack up, and well behaved on roads, particularly with regard to shying?

- In the case of a hunter it is preferable to see him ridden out hunting, or to talk to independent people who can vouch for the horse's reliability as a hunter.

- Young event horses should prove their willingness to go through or jump over water. Older horses can often be vouched for by independent testimony or by competition results.

It is preferable to ask these questions over the phone before visiting, as much time can be wasted going to look at animals who are unsuitable. If the questions and answers are written down and the vendor is prepared to sign a copy, this will be an added safeguard.

Procedure After Deciding to Purchase

Confirm your decision in writing and keep a copy of your letter. Agree to complete the sale at the stated price, subject to a satisfactory opinion from your veterinary surgeon. Should the veterinary surgeon give an unfavourable or qualified report, the buyer may still decide to buy, subject to an appropriate reduction in price.

List the information about the horse which has been supplied by the vendor.

State any agreed arrangements which will apply if the horse should prove unsuitable, e.g. return or exchange. (There may be no such arrangements.)

State that no responsibility is accepted for the horse until payment is made.

Confirm arrangements as to payment, and as to when the horse will be collected or accepted.

After payment for the horse, the buyer should take possession of the passport, breed papers and height certificate. In addition to the records of flu and tetanus inoculations (usually found in the passport) it is helpful to know about the worming programme.

The vendor may agree to this letter verbally, or he may write his acceptance, or he may ignore it. In any case, should the horse prove to be unsuitable, the letter may help if the buyer wishes to return the horse and reclaim his money.

There are advantages in buying from reputable dealers, as they are usually willing to exchange a horse or pony should he prove to be unsuitable. With a private owner this is unlikely.

In most cases the buyer should remember the rule of common law – *caveat emptor* – let the buyer beware. In the event of problems, the Trades Description Act and/or the Sale of Goods Act may apply. Legal advice will clarify this and its relevance, as the situation can differ according to whether the vendor is a dealer or private owner.

It is still possible in some instances to have the horse 'on trial' before purchasing. The agreement of what is allowed whilst on trial (i.e. can he be competed during the trial period, who is responsible for worming, shoeing or any veterinary treatment) must be agreed and preferably put in writing before the horse is removed. It is recommended that the horse is insured by the prospective buyer before he leaves the vendor's yard.

SELLING

The vendor can protect his interests in the following ways:

- On meeting the buyer and seeing the horse ridden, he should indicate if he considers that the horse is not suitable.

- He may state that he believes the horse sound, but should not declare him sound. This is a matter for a veterinary surgeon.

- He should state the time limit that he will allow:

> for trial
> to arrange the veterinary examination
> to come to a decision.

If paid by cheque he should ensure that the cheque is cleared or guaranteed before allowing the buyer to take possession.

He should state clearly that possession passes when the cash/cheque is paid, and that the buyer is responsible for the horse from that time.

A Trial Period

From a seller's point of view, this is rarely a sensible procedure. Should any accident or illness befall the animal, the question of responsibility is always a problem. It is wiser to allow the purchaser to make several visits, but not to take the horse home. If necessary, the horse can be taken to an independent yard and tried in new surroundings and over unfamiliar jumps.

If other buyers are interested, the purchaser must be given a definite time limit in which to decide.

AUCTION SALES

When buying or selling a horse or pony at an auction, both the purchaser and vendor are normally bound by the 'Contract of Sale Conditions' as laid down by the auctioneers in their catalogue. All prospective purchasers are advised to study these conditions before bidding in the sale. It is advisable for the seller or his agent to ensure that any statements made about the horse – or information given to the auctioneer to facilitate the sale of the horse – are true and demonstrable. Should the animal concerned fail in respect of some part of the information given by the seller, the purchaser may be entitled to return the animal to the seller, and to have his money refunded. Auctioneers usually retain any monies paid for at least 24 hours, and they should be informed immediately of any breach of sale conditions.

Should the purchaser suspect that pain-killing drugs have been administered to the horse (the analgesic effect usually wears off in 24 hours but may take up to 14 days), he should inform the auctioneer and arrange to have the blood tested.

ALLERGIES AND SEASONAL DISORDERS

Because of prevalence of **'allergic coughing'** it is essential to obtain information about the general management, feed and bedding of any intended purchase.

Head shaking or **'summer asthma'** is another allergy which may escape veterinary detection in the winter months. The animal does not exhibit the tell-tale signs until a spell of warm, humid weather occurs. He will then wave his head up and down and strike at his face with a foreleg. There is no known cure for this ailment. At best, the horse will be uncomfortable to ride, and depressing to compete on, particularly in dressage; at worst he will be dangerous.

Sweet itch is another summer complaint which can go undetected in the winter, particularly if the mane is hogged.

Laminitis, though not an allergy, is a very common cause of unsoundness, particularly in ponies. It is a recurring disease which, if diagnosed in its early stages, can, with careful management, be avoided or controlled. Confirmed sufferers are easily diagnosed by changes in the shape of their feet. However, a mild attack may leave no visible evidence, although the tendency to recur will remain.

Blood testing

As pain-killing drugs can be used to disguise unsoundness, many buyers and their veterinary surgeons now ask for a blood test before a sale is agreed. There can be no valid objection to this from the seller, provided that all expenses are paid by the purchaser, and that the testing is completed without delay and in a proper manner.

X-rays

In recent years it has become common practice for purchasers of valuable horses to ask to have the horse's feet X-rayed. In some cases they will ask for the leg and the knee or hock joint to be included. A foot X-ray can be a wise precaution. Other, more extensive X-rays are justified if an old injury needs investigation.

Many sellers are reluctant to have their horses X-rayed. Should the sale of the horse fall through because of the results of an X-ray, the seller is put in a difficult position with regard to future purchasers. Often an X-ray will reveal old injuries, many of which may never cause unsoundness. Also, a reasonable assessment can only be made by someone who has had considerable practice and experience in the actual reading of radiographs (X-ray plates).

Scans

It is now possible to scan horses but it is an expensive process and is unlikely to be part of a pre-purchase process for the non-specialist.

CARE OF THE HORSE

MANAGEMENT METHODS

Often the management method chosen is governed by the carer's lifestyle. The one-horse owner, who keeps their horse at home and is at work all day, is going to manage their horse differently from the manager of a livery yard or commercial premises with workers available all day. In all cases the well-being of the horses must be the priority. A happy, relaxed and healthy animal is going to perform better.

Areas for consideration

- Owner's lifestyle
- Horse's job
- Finances
- Facilities

Owner's lifestyle

It is not just their lifestyle as discussed above but also their knowledge, inclination and ability that need consideration.

Horse's job

The horse's job, be it racehorse, eventer or child's pony, will be a major factor in deciding how he is kept. The more demanding the job, the more likely it is for there to be full-time care available.

Does the horse live in or out? How much time is spent working/training? How does this affect his feeding regime? These are all questions that need consideration.

Finances

The finances available for keeping horses are sometimes limited. Keeping the horse economically but not skimping on his care is a key part of good management.

Facilities

These are discussed more fully in a later chapter but whether the horse is kept at home or at livery the facilities must be suitable for the lifestyle. Shelter, grazing and opportunities for exercise all need to be considered. Ancillary needs like storage of feed, tack and equipment also need to be catered for.

GOOD PRACTICE

Riding horses is considered a risk sport by insurance companies. As many accidents happen on the yard as when riding, therefore minimising risk in both areas is sensible and good practice.

In the following pages, advice is given on how to handle, groom and move around a stabled horse. The advice is well tried and proven. When young people are being trained it is essential that they get into the habit of working in a safe way. It is in their own interests and those of the horses to do so. During training they usually look after quiet animals, who are easy to handle, but if correct procedure is practised from the beginning, it will become instinctive to do the right thing, even when they are faced with more difficult animals.

Horses are by nature nervous creatures. Most become docile and quiet if they are well handled; others always remain on edge and require quiet, confident handling. The expression in the horse's eye will indicate his state of mind, revealing whether he is calm and relaxed, or worried and frightened. A worried, frightened horse must always be treated with care. He requires firm but kind handling if he is not to become a danger both to himself and to his attendants.

Horses have to be taught good stable manners and behaviour. Well-trained grooms are able to do this. They are also capable of advising and helping other less-experienced staff. Horses are creatures of habit, and they become more relaxed if there is a routine to their life. Every time they have a new handler they will take time to understand that particular person's methods, commands and body language. With a young or nervous horse it is always preferable to keep the same handler, if possible.

Horses, being creatures of habit, like routine. Handling them in a consistent and correct manner, doing tasks in the same order and presenting a calm but authoritative manner around them and always respecting their natural instincts will help to minimise accidents.

Areas for consideration

- Clothing
- Care and use of tools
- Working around the horse
- Hygiene
- Communication
- Record keeping

Clothing

When working around horses the clothing worn should be suitable for the task involved. It should allow movement but not be so loose or flapping that it could catch on something or frighten the horse. Sometimes noisy or brightly coloured clothing will frighten horses. Restrictive clothing that prevents movement such as bending or stepping aside quickly can lead to accidents or work being skimped.

Footwear needs to be comfortable, hard-wearing, protect the feet and not come off when stepping quickly or in poor ground conditions.

Hands need to be protected from damage and infection. Rope burns, machinery and contaminated bedding can all pose a risk. Many people find it difficult to work in gloves but with perseverance it becomes easier.

It is always advisable to wear protective headgear when working around horses, especially youngsters, stallions, highly strung animals or ones who are new to the yard.

Wearing jewellery can lead to accidents. Earrings, neck chains, bracelets and rings can all get caught up in equipment and cause damage. Piercings, in the dusty stable environment, can lead to infection.

Although not clothing, it is unwise to wear scent and perfume on the yard, especially around stallions as they can become excited and/or aggressive.

Tools and Equipment

Anyone working with tools on the yard, even the most basic, needs sufficient training in their correct use. Grooming kits, mucking out equipment and clipping machines all need to be used and cared for correctly.

Developing a good technique will often mean being able to work for longer before becoming tired, prevent physical damage and allow tasks to be completed more quickly. It also means that the equipment will last longer, thereby saving money. Care of grooming kit is dealt with in Chapter 11, Grooming.

Yard equipment should be suitable for the task. A fork suitable for use in a straw bed may not work with shavings, for example. Using the correct equipment for the job makes for efficiency and ease of working. All equipment needed should be assembled before the task is started. It needs to be used in such a way that neither horse nor worker is put at risk. After use, the equipment should be cleaned and stored in its designated area.

Anyone working with electric equipment needs to have specific training in its use and care and initially be supervised when using it.

Working Around the Horse

Correct handling of the horse is vital. Never presume that because a horse has always behaved in a certain way he will continue to do so. Horses are very sensitive to changes in our behaviour. They will pick up on our being tired, nervous, cross, worried or in a hurry. This in turn can make them worried and induce a change in their behaviour. They may also be influenced by outside conditions such as high winds, strange noises or changes in their environment.

The use of the voice is always a good first method of establishing control and reassurance. Horses understand simple words of command such as 'Stand', 'Move over', 'No' and 'Good boy' and can develop quite a large vocabulary with time if the words are used consistently.

Horses respond to the tone of a voice, and in this way they can be rewarded for good behaviour, or corrected for bad behaviour.

When entering the stable, always speak first. Go up to the horse's shoulder and pat him on the neck. Before handling him further, put on a headcollar and tie him up with a quick-release knot (see diagram page 71). He should be tied up sufficiently short to prevent him turning and nipping or biting, but not so short that he feels constrained, is frightened and pulls back.

When dealing with the legs and feet, never kneel or sit, always crouch. If they are frightened or worried, some horses will use their legs as defence and they may:

• Strike out with the front feet – so when holding a horse always stand to the side and never in front.

• Deliver a cow kick with a hind foot.

• Kick out to the back with one or both hind feet.

To minimise the danger of being kicked, never stand behind the horse. When attending to legs or feet, always stand close to the horse. Doing so minimises the impact of any kicks.

Hygiene

Good hygiene should be a routine part of good management in order to maintain the health of both horse and carer.

Dust is one of the most common problems to arise when working with horses. Using a vacuum grooming machine, dust-free bedding, haylage-type forage and mechanical yard sweepers will all help. Workers are often reluctant to wear masks but they should be suggested. Many tasks can be done outside rather than in a confined space.

Workers should be encouraged to wear protective clothing and to cover their hair. The use of gloves is recommended for mucky tasks. Hot water and soap should always be available. The cleaning of tools and equipment after use should be routine. Feed buckets and utensils should be washed after use. If they are to be stacked, remember to wash the bottom as well.

Vermin

Practically all yards will have vermin. A satisfactory programme of control is required. If poison is put down it must be out of the way of dogs, cats and children. A stable cat will help to keep mice down. The feed room needs to be kept clean and all feed properly contained. Birds, especially pigeons, should be discouraged from roosting in the stables as they can carry disease. Bedding and forage can be contaminated by rats, which spread Weil's disease.

Workers should always wash their hands after filling haynets or handling straw. Using bedding and forage in strict rotation will help prevent rats from becoming established.

Communication

Good communication is essential in the efficient running of any organisation and the larger it is the more difficult it can be to maintain. At the very least there should be a daily diary in which all yard staff can write down any occurrence. They should also be taught to answer the telephone in a consistent manner that suits the enterprise. A note pad should be kept beside the phone and all messages written down. Each worker should know the chain of command and who they should refer to with any problem.

Levels of Responsibility

Looking after horses is a very responsible job. However, the level of responsibility asked for and expected of the carer needs to be carefully thought out according to their level of ability and experience.

BHS qualifications are highly regarded throughout the world but often employers' expectations outrun the level of ability of their employee.

At Stage 1 the worker should be able to perform simple tasks with quiet horses, under supervision.

At Stage 2 they should be able to perform routine tasks on quiet horses, without constant supervision.

At Stage 3 they should be capable of all routine care of fit competition horses and be able to perform simple supervisory duties.

At Stage 4 they should have a full understanding of horse care, be able to run a yard, devise new routines and procedures and supervise and organise staff.

CHAPTER 10
HANDLING THE HORSE

SECURING THE HORSE

In a Stable

It is recommended that horses should be tied up whenever a groom is working in the stable or around the horse. Some people always tie up their horses, some never do; again it is consistency of approach that is the key. If the horse is untied, the stable door should be shut. If the horse is tied up it can be acceptable whilst tasks are being done to have the door open.

It is preferable if either the headcollar or the rope has a breaking point. The headcollar can be made of nylon or leather. However, in certain circumstances – particularly while travelling – it is best to use a leather one, with a cotton rope. If home-made baler twine ropes are used, they should be sufficiently well made to untie quickly and not be full of knots and lumps which will prevent a quick-release knot from working. They are extremely strong and should be used with care.

The horse should wear a headcollar; the rope or chain should be attached to the back of the headcollar and thence tied to a string loop on the tie-ring with a quick-release knot (see diagram). The purpose of the string loop is that it will break if the horse pulls back violently. It is important therefore to use string that will break under stress. Modern, strong baler twine usually needs splitting to make it breakable under duress.

In a Stall

Horses kept in stalls are tied up by means of a headcollar, a clip-on rope and a log. This method allows them sufficient room to lie down, but the log takes up the slack of the rope, so that there is no danger of the horse getting his foot caught. The log is a piece of solid wood (preferably circular), with a hole drilled through

string loop

Tying a quick-release knot. This knot will not tighten if the horse pulls back.

Figure of eight knot.

the middle large enough to take the rope. The headcollar rope is passed through a ring or an opening in the fixed manger, and is then fastened to the log by means of a figure of eight knot. This is made to lie across the base of the hole, so that it cannot pull through. A figure of eight knot is ideal because it will keep its shape under pressure but loosens immediately the two ends are pushed together. A tie-ring and string loop above the manger give a shorter tie-up when the horse is being groomed.

PICKING UP THE FEET

To pick up the near fore, stand by the near-side shoulder, facing the tail. Pat the neck, run the hand down the shoulder and leg to the fetlock joint, squeeze above the joint, and at the same time slightly push the horse over with your shoulder so that he puts weight on the off fore. When not picking out the feet, face the horse's shoulder, support the weight of the horse's foot by placing the toe of the foot in the palm of the right hand, and hold it with the fingers. When picking out the feet, face the rear, hold the foot in the left hand, and use the hoof pick in the right hand. The process is reversed for the off fore.

To pick up a hind foot, either of the following methods may be used, but the first is safer if the horse is likely to kick:

(1) Approach the shoulder and pat the neck. When picking up the near hind, run the left hand along

How to pick up a near fore.

How to pick up a near hind.

the body, quarters, and down the back and outside of the hind leg. Squeeze the fetlock, and ease the leg a little forward and up. Keep an arm between your face and the horse's leg. When not picking out the foot, use the right hand to support the foot; slip the left hand round to the front of the leg, and hold the foot in the palm. Do not hold the toe high, as this will unbalance the horse. When picking out the foot, take up the foot as above, then hold it in the left hand. Allow the horse's leg to move to the rear, and pick out with the right hand.

(2) Slide the left hand around the inner side of the hock, and run it down the fetlock. Pick up the foot as before (see diagram).

Never leave the arm supporting the hind leg behind the horse as a sudden kick could result in it being broken.

GROOMING

Sensitive horses, particularly when fit, are often tricky to groom. They require firm but tactful handling. Corrections can be given by the voice or a slap, but only in exceptional circumstances should a horse be hit, and never by junior or inexperienced staff, who are liable to punish the horse at the wrong moment for the wrong reason. Rough handling of horses in the stable is a sign of bad temper or nerves on the part of the groom, and can only have a bad effect on the horse.

When being groomed, horses may bite through irritation, discomfort or over-freshness. Should this occur:

- A muzzle may be put over the headcollar and the horse tied up in the usual way.

- The rope can be put through the stable ring and held with one hand while the other uses the brush. In this way, the horse is kept under control.

- The horse can be tied from both sides (cross-tied).

- If the horse is very touchy, see grooming, page 81.

METHODS OF CONTROL AND RESTRAINT

Control

When controlling or restraining a horse or when leading a horse, especially if he is fit, excited or unknown to the handler, a riding hat, gloves and strong footwear should always be worn.

A headcollar is the most common method of control within the stable environment. They are usually made from leather or nylon and come with a headpiece that buckles on one or both sides.

Yearling headcollars are more adjustable, with buckles on the noseband and also the throatlash.

Foal slips are shaped rather like a figure of eight, held together by a movable ring under the jaw (see drawing page 237). This often has a small strip of leather attached to help in catching up the foal.

All headcollars can be used with either a rope or a lunge line for extra control. For smarter occasions a leather lead rope or a white or coloured webbing lead, sometimes with a length of chain attaching it to the headcollar to stop the horse chewing it, can be used.

When a little more control is needed, the lead rope can be wound round the muzzle underneath the noseband.

If the leader puts their right elbow in the neck

Using a rope around the muzzle for a little more control.

A Chifney bit.

triangle, just in front of the withers, and turns the horse's head slightly to the left, this also helps control.

A bridle is always recommended when leading an unknown horse or one who is fit or excitable. It is often better if the normal reins are replaced by a lunge line. This can be threaded through the left-hand bit ring and secured on the right one for extra purchase. A webbing lead rein with a divided chain is an alternative.

A Chifney bit on its own headpiece with a lead rein can be put on top of the bridle. It is sometimes used on point-to-pointers and racehorses in the paddock. This is taken off once the rider has mounted and is in control.

A halter is made of webbing, often white with an integral lead rope that threads through a loop in the nosepiece. This is adjustable at that point. The rope

must always be secured with a half knot at the nose to prevent the halter becoming too tight. These are still seen on heavy horses and cattle, at shows.

A lunge cavesson is sometimes preferred to a headcollar because it fits more closely to the head. This gives more control when trotting up or when trying to load a reluctant animal. When used in conjunction with the lunge line it gives the handler a better chance of keeping hold if the horse tries to run back.

Control headcollars are available under a variety of names. They are sometimes designed with a bit, and poll pressure is applied by the headpiece being joined to the lead rope and threading though the bit on the near side. They can be extremely effective in preventing a horse from pulling back when being loaded. They should not be left on, nor should the horse be tied up in them. They should be replaced by a regular headcollar once the objective is achieved.

Restraint

There are a number of ways in which to restrain a horse when he is required to stand still. Whichever method is chosen, try to use the mildest that is effective under the circumstances.

- Keep calm and try not to allow the horse to become upset.
- Do not let the horse think that he is being punished.

Control headcollar.

Pressure halter.

Holding up a front leg as a method of restraint.

If you do he is more likely to resist.
- Use for the shortest period of time necessary to achieve the outcome.
- Never abuse the horse.
- The basic rule to follow is that, if possible, the person doing the restraining should stand on the same side as the person giving the treatment. This helps to prevent one or other being jumped on if the horse becomes upset and the restraint is not enough.
- All water buckets and other items should be removed from the stable in order that no one is tripped up by them.

Some methods are:

- Give a feed.

- Hold up a fore or hind leg.

- Pinch a fold of loose skin on the neck.

- Use a twitch.

- Have the vet administer a sedative.

- Use hobbles. Often used when mares are being covered by the stallion.

- Use stocks. More usually seen abroad but becoming more popular in Britain.

Using a twitch

There are two main types; the more usual, a length of broomstick with a short length of cord threaded through one end, and the humane, which is made of lightweight metal. It is hinged in the middle; the two sides are closed together around the horse's lip and fastened together with a length of cord or a clip. They are designed for use when no helper is available. Both types work by inducing the animal to produce endorphins that calm him down. They should be applied for the shortest period of time possible and must never be abused. They should not be applied to the ear as this is extremely painful and will make the horse head-shy, nor should they ever be applied to the lower lip.

Putting on a Cord Twitch

An assistant should hold the horse. The handler takes the end of the twitch in one hand and places the other hand through the loop of cord. He then grips the horse's upper lip with this hand, slips the loop over the horse's lip and twists the end of the handle until the cord is sufficiently tight. The twitch should then be held at the end of the handle. This is the easiest way to hold it securely. When the twitch is released, the horse's upper lip should be rubbed firmly to help restore circulation. A twitch left on too long can cause a permanent scar.

Some horses become adept at getting out of a twitch, particularly if the handler, in an effort to be kind, has failed to put it on sufficiently tightly. They can then often be difficult to re-twitch.

How to put on a cord twitch.

Stallions

Stallions are usually led out in a stallion bridle; this has a bit and the lead rope has a length of chain attaching it to the bit. The primary purpose of the chain is that it won't be damaged by the stallion getting hold of it in his teeth – as a rope might be. The handler often carries a short cane to help maintain respect.

Foals

Some people put a foal slip on the foal soon after birth; others wait a while. Whichever method is used, the very young foal should not be led by the head. A cloth or wide bandage should be wrapped around the foal's neck and held in the left hand; the right arm should be placed around the quarters. With the dam in front, the foal should be urged forward from behind and restrained if needed, by the wrap around his neck. Foals have an alarming habit of leaping forwards when first being taught to lead. As the days progress, a lead rope can be attached to the slip and held in the left hand along with the wrap. Always use voice commands to 'walk on' and 'halt'. As time progresses the foal can be taught to walk beside his dam and then to lead the way. Eventually, as with all horses, he should be taught to lead from both sides. See diagram on page 52.

Attending to the Mouth or Teeth

Some veterinary surgeons use a gag, which is a device placed on the horse's lower face and adjusted to hold his jaws apart so that his teeth can be reached for rasping, scaling or the removal of wolf teeth. When attending to or examining the mouth and teeth it is often necessary to hold the tongue and bring it out to the side of the mouth. Care should be taken that the tongue is not injured by pulling or twisting, or by the use of unnecessary strength. If the horse struggles, let go of the tongue immediately.

Never pass the tongue from one side of the mouth to the other. Let it go and re-take it from the other side. If the tongue is pulled out to the front, there is a danger of the incisor teeth cutting into it. If it is pulled out and backwards, the upper first molar may cut it.

Protective Restraints

Horses often attempt to chew at a wound covering, especially one applied over a knee. Preventive measures include:

CRADLE This is a framework of wood or part metal which is placed on the horse's neck, and prevents him putting his head down. It is secured with leather straps. The crest and withers should be protected with a pad. See drawings below.

BIB Attached to the underside of the headcollar (leather) prevents the horse chewing rugs or reaching his knees.

A KNEE CAP will sometimes solve the problem if protection is only required for the knee.

Two types of cradle.

ADMINISTERING MEDICINES AND POWDERS

By Syringe

Large, used, well-cleaned, wormer syringes are suitable. Most powders can be mixed with water, placed in the syringe and squirted down the horse's throat. This is the most efficient method of dosing the horse, other than by injection or stomach tube. The syringe is placed in the corner of the horse's mouth, pointing down over the tongue, and squirted firmly. The horse's muzzle can be raised to assist swallowing. If any liquid remains in the mouth, food should not be allowed for several minutes. Powders that are difficult to dissolve can be mixed with soft, margarine-type spread. This is then put in the syringe and administered in the usual way.

In Food

Powders can be mixed with a damp feed. Soaked sugar beet or molasses help to disguise the taste. Take care not to spoil the horse's appetite by using this method. It can be difficult to judge if the whole dose has been taken. If the horse is a messy eater it may be wasted.

In Water

Certain soluble medicines can be given in the drinking water. Care should be taken that the horse is not put off drinking, as this could cause other problems. Should the horse choose not to drink, the medication may be wasted.

Administering a worm dose via a syringe.

As an Electuary

Powder is mixed with treacle or honey and placed on the back of the horse's tongue with a smooth wooden spatula or a wooden spoon.

Drenching

Modern veterinary practice is generally not in favour of drenching.

By Stomach Tube

This method should only be used by a veterinary surgeon. A flexible tube is introduced through the nasal tract and passed down the oesophagus and into the stomach. It can be used to introduce liquid paraffin, large amounts of fluid and vitamin supplements, e.g. for colic or dehydration.

By Injection

Intramuscular injections, if authorised by a veterinary surgeon, may be given by an experienced horse owner or trained groom. To give an injection efficiently requires practice and skill. Intravenous injections must only be given by a qualified veterinary surgeon. (It must be the responsibility of the stable manager to ensure that difficult horses are handled only by experienced people. If they are mishandled by nervous or inexperienced staff, they may at best become playful, and at worst frightened and cause an accident. Consult the Health and Safety at Work regulations and see Good Practice, page 67.)

LEADING THE HORSE IN HAND

A horse is normally led from the near side, except when on a road. He should, however, be taught to lead equally well from both sides.

If he is going to be led from another horse, he will be led from his right. If the voice commands 'Walk on' and

'Halt' are regularly used it will be much easier to control him when riding and leading.

In a Headcollar

Put on the headcollar and rope or halter. Tie a knot in the end of the rope. Hold the end of the rope in the left hand, but never wrap the rope around the hand. Put the right hand on the rope, about 30cm (1ft) from the horse's head. With a fresh horse, put the hand over the top of the rope to help restrain him. With a lazy horse, put the hand under the rope to help push him forward. Never attempt to go ahead of the horse and try to pull him along, as his reaction will then be to pull back. The person leading should always be by the horse's shoulder, never in front; the handler should look ahead, not at the horse.

In the case of a fresh or strange horse, it is advisable to lead the horse from a cavesson headcollar with a lunge rein or long rope attached. Horses should never be led from a headcollar without a lead rope. If the horse plays up it will be impossible to hold him and the leader may injure an arm or hand.

It is very poor, sloppy and sometimes dangerous practice to lead the horse with one hand and allow his head to be behind the leader's hips.

- If the horse stops without warning the leader may drop the rein. This could then get either broken or entangled in something if the horse runs off.

- If the horse runs forwards he could tread on the leader or knock him over.

- If rugs or equipment slip the leader is unlikely to notice.

- It does not encourage the horse to walk out correctly and stay alert to the leader's orders.

In a Bridle

Take the reins of the bridle over the head, and hold them in the right hand, with the end of the reins in the left hand, as for a rope, but with the reins separated by the first finger. The stick is carried in the left hand, pointing to the rear. If the horse is lazy, the left hand should be moved back behind the body and the horse tapped on the lower rib cage, just to the rear of where a rider's leg would rest. Use voice commands.

In a Saddle and Bridle

Ensure that the stirrups are run up and secured, as they are for lungeing. The girths should be done up, but not too tightly. A running martingale should be detached from the reins and secured to the neck strap. Then proceed as above. The point of the stirrup bars may be turned up to give extra security to the leathers. These points should never be turned up when the horse is being ridden.

If the martingale is not detached from the reins, they should be left on the horse's neck and the leader should lead by only holding the rein nearer to them. If both reins are held, the bit may pinch in the mouth and the horse will be reluctant to move.

Moving Horses to and from the Field

Moving the horse to and from stable and pasture is often an area where accidents happen. If horses are being led, both horse and leader need to wear the right equipment. A good rope and headcollar for the horse; safe footwear, gloves and a hat for the leader are the minimum required. Do not be tempted to lead too many at one time. Ensure enough help is available. You might be able to lead them together but you will be unable to open or close the gate safely.

If a number of animals are being turned out or brought in at the same time, work out in which order and have your strategy planned beforehand so that one animal is not left alone.

Horses should be trained to stand still whilst having the headcollar removed and never encouraged to gallop away from the gate. Similarly when catching up, train them to come quietly to the gate and wait their turn to be caught up and led out. Horses like to please, remember to praise them when they perform well.

Leading the Horse on a Road

Horses being brought in from the field to the stable may be led back in halters or headcollars. However, if it is known that a horse is difficult to control, or is traffic-shy, he should be led in a cavesson or bridle. If a horse has to be led along a main road, a bridle should always be used for safety and to fulfil insurance requirements in the event of an accident. The person leading the horse should be between the horse and the traffic and on the left-hand side of the road. It is advisable to wear some kind of fluorescent clothing, either a hat cover or a tabard, so as to be more visible to traffic.

Horses Being Led out for Exercise

Whether beside another horse or on foot, horses should wear a snaffle bridle or cavesson. They should be led in the direction of the flow of traffic with the led horse on the inside of the leader, whether the latter is on a horse or on foot. The near-side rein of the bridle can be put through the ring of the bit on the off side, and then both reins should be held with the left hand on top of the rein about 5cm (2ins) from the horse's head. The slack of the rein may be held in the right hand.

The reins of the ridden horse should be held in the right hand. Always put a knot in the end of them. The led horse's head should be kept level with the rider's knee. If the led horse is allowed to move too far forward, or too far behind, he becomes more difficult to control. A cavesson with a short lunge rein attached may be used. The reins of the bridle can be twisted and secured in the throatlash. This keeps them out of the way, and makes the horse more comfortable.

If the two horses tend to argue, a lightweight wire muzzle on the led horse is useful. If the rider needs to carry a stick, a short, showing-type cane is easier to control than a longer one.

Leading a Horse in and out of a Loosebox or Through Doorways

Because the horse is wider across the hips than the shoulders, it is very easy for him, when led by a careless attendant, to knock and bruise his off-side hip on a doorway. After such a mishap he will be nervous and will try to hurry or rush through doorways, thus risking a repeat injury. In bad cases, a fragment of bone can be displaced. It is important when leading a horse in and out of a loosebox to ensure that:

- The horse is securely held and steadied as he reaches the doorway and goes through.

- The horse walks on a straight track through the doorway and into the box and does not approach it at an angle.

- The groom checks that the door will not swing to and hit the horse as he goes through. On windy days, doors should be hooked open.

- The horse is not allowed to go into the box on his own, with the reins thrown over his neck. This will tend to make him hurry.

Trotting out for Soundness

This is best done with the horse wearing a headcollar and no saddle. If the horse is fresh, put on a cavesson headcollar for greater control, and if this is not available, use a snaffle bridle. Check that the yard gate is shut. Trot the horse out slowly, and make allowance for the fact that a cambered yard or corner makes many older horses go unlevel.

To turn the horse, steady him to a walk and turn him away from you. This gives greater control, and the horse stays better balanced and is less likely to step on the leader's foot. If he is allowed to come round towards the leader, his quarters will tend to swing out, and he may well kick.

See also page 31, Assessing Action.

Standing up the Horse for Inspection

For inspection or show, square the horse up and show the near side. The front legs should be level, but the near hind should be a little to the rear of the off hind, not vice versa. The attendant stands at the front, but a little to the side of the horse, with the left hand holding the reins, divided by the fingers, about 30cm (12ins) from the horse's head. The slack of the reins, and the stick, if one is carried, are held in the right hand. To trot the horse up, reverse the hand hold on the reins and stick, and proceed as for leading in a saddle and bridle.

SAFETY PRECAUTIONS

- Never lead the horse out of a stable with the rug undone at the front, and wearing a roller with no breastplate. The rug and roller may slip back and frighten the horse, who may then play up and get away.

- Always tie the horse up when working in the stable or grooming.

- In the case of horses who tend to play with their stable-door bolt and open the door, preferably fit a horse-proof bolt, or at least a spring clip on the bolt.

- When tying up a horse outside the box, make sure that he cannot touch or sniff at another horse, as this will cause squealing and possibly kicking. If two or more horses are tied outside, make sure that they are not within sniffing or kicking distance of each other.

- Never tie horses up to door hinges, window grilles or the rails of fences (use the posts), pieces of machinery, feed bins or anything that might become detached. A frightened horse is immensely strong and can be badly damaged if the thing to which he is tied becomes loose if he pulls back.

- Playful horses, who are likely to chew wood or string, or to pull at stable fixtures, should have their stable checked for likely hazards. If necessary, move the horse to a more suitable box.

- Yard gates leading to public roads should be kept closed.

- Should a horse slip up and not be able to rise easily, lean your knee on his neck, just behind his ears, to keep him still. If possible put a stable rubber or something similar under his head to prevent eye damage. Straw, manure, sacks or old rugs spread on the ground will help him to get to his feet.

- Keep a sharp knife in a predetermined, accessible place in the stable yard. Should a horse become tangled up in a rope, or if he pulls back and is held fast because the safety string fails to break, rapid action will be essential to prevent injury. Parcel string is preferable to baler twine for making loops to tie the horse to.

- When training a young horse to tie up, one method is to put a long lead rope through the ring but hold the loose end in one hand whilst brushing the horse with the other.

GROOMING

To maintain his health, the stabled horse requires regular daily grooming. The fit horse on a high concentrate diet excretes a considerable amount of waste products through the skin, so thorough grooming is essential.

However, there are circumstances when grooming should be reduced. The sick horse, who has to be kept quiet, needs only minimal grooming, while one with an infectious disease, for example ringworm, should not be groomed, since there is a risk of spreading the infection over the horse's body.

When not in work, the grass-kept horse does not require grooming. The natural oils in his coat help to keep him warm.

When in work, he requires only modified grooming: remove surface mud, check his feet and generally tidy him up.

GROOMING

The Objectives of Grooming

Grooming the horse performs a number of essential functions:
- It cleans the horse and improves his appearance.
- It improves blood flow to the skin.
- It may help with muscle tone.
- It allows the groom to develop rapport with the horse.
- It gives the groom opportunity to check the horse over and ensure his well-being.

Areas for consideration

- How the horse is kept
- Temperament/type
- Level of fitness
- Time of year

Whether the horse is kept in or out and whether he is rugged or unrugged will have a bearing on grooming. An animal living out, especially if unrugged, needs to keep the grease in his coat. He should have mud and dust removed and should have his eyes, nostrils and dock washed and his hooves picked out. A horse who is stabled can receive a complete grooming.

How to Groom

Assemble all equipment needed. Tie the horse up. His coat should be dry; if the skin is wet it is almost impossible to get it clean with brushes and, on the thin-skinned animal, mud can be brushed into the skin and cause infection. Remove water buckets.

1. Pick out feet into a skip and wash hooves if muddy.

2. Loosen dry mud or sweat with a rubber curry comb or dandy brush.

3. Use rubber curry comb and/or body brush to loosen and remove deep-seated dust and grease from the main body and neck of the horse. Areas of the body often overlooked are the armpits, loins, belly and between the hind legs. Use the body brush with a

circular motion, clockwise on the left side and anticlockwise on the right. Clean the brush on the curry comb after every 3–4 rotations. Have the body brush in the left hand for the front, left side and right hand for the rear of the horse and vice versa on the right side. This will allow more weight behind the stroke and prevent the arm from getting too tired. This requires practice to get perfect.

4. Don't wear gloves when grooming. This allows the groom to feel any changes in the horse. This is especially important when grooming legs and the head.

5. Untie the horse and use the body brush to clean the head. Support it with the other hand.

6. Sponge eyes, nostrils and mouth. Retie.

7. Brush out and clean the mane and tail using the body brush or fingers. With fine-skinned horses never use a mane comb or dandy brush or the mane and tail will soon become too thin. When brushing the mane take 25cm (1in) sections with one hand and brush down to the roots with the other. When the whole mane has been done, brush it over to one side and lay it with a water brush.

8. To do the tail, brush out the top section in small bits to remove all scurf and then, holding the bulk of the tail in one hand, separate the strands with the other hand or with a body brush.

9. Wash the dock with a second sponge and lay the tail. If required, put on a tail bandage.

10. If wisping, do it now. Wisping, banging and strapping are all terms used for the same thing. Strapping is also the term used for a complete groom plus wisping. A wisp may be made from hay, straw or baler twine. Leather ones may be purchased or a stable rubber can be made into a firm pad and used. Wisping is done on the neck, shoulders and quarters. It should not be used on any sharp or bony areas. Use the same hand as for body brushing; bring the wisp down firmly on the area and then stroke in the direction of the coat. Start with a firm pat until the horse is accustomed to the action and increase pressure gradually. Never hit the horse hard enough to bruise him. If the action is correct the horse will anticipate the stroke and twitch the muscles in the area. This is the desired effect. Travel over the entire area to be wisped, so no two bangs are in exactly the same place. Start with 5–6 strokes and gradually progress to 15–20 in each area. It is advisable to untie the horse for this procedure and to hold the headcollar with the free hand whilst he becomes accustomed. The process should take about 15–20 minutes and is useful for animals with poor muscle development (e.g. a ewe-neck) or horses with uneven muscle development after injury.

11. If required and the hooves are dry, apply hoof oil.

12. Use a stable rubber to polish off the horse and remove any surface dust.

If the horse is clipped, the weather is cold or the animal is sick, keep him warm whilst grooming. Fold the rug back and forth as needed.

The whole grooming process should take about 30 minutes plus wisping time. Ideally it should be done daily, after work when the horse is warm and dry and the pores are open.

Stable stains can be washed off with warm water at the beginning of the grooming process, or powdered charcoal can be rubbed into the area and then brushed off.

Care needs to be taken with a nervous or thin-skinned horse.

Use voice commands such as 'Hoof,' 'Stand,' or 'Over' as appropriate and use one hand to steady the head or leg whilst grooming those areas.

Choose brushes suitable for the type of animal. A nylon or plastic brush may be fine on a hairy pony but irritate a TB, and make him bite or kick. A soft, natural bristled brush would be suitable for the latter but no good on the pony.

Never kneel when grooming. Learn to pick up feet safely. See diagram on page 72. With a young horse, when picking up a hind foot, stand close to the horse's belly, pick up the hoof and bring it towards you. Horses cannot kick forwards, only sideways and backwards! When moving around the horse, untie him if going under his neck and place a hand on his quarters if going around behind him.

Hold the tail if standing behind him; this will give you warning if he is going to move. Always ensure there is enough room between the horse and the wall when picking out the hind feet.

Washing Horses

There are many horse shampoos available and also products that produce an artificial shine to the coat. These should be used according to manufacturers' instructions. They should not be used instead of regular grooming sessions.

Washing a horse off after strenuous or muddy work to remove sweat and mud will prevent 'breaking out' and a lot of hard work later.

If the horse is cold, use warm water; if it is hot use cold water, especially on the large muscle areas.

After washing, use a sweat scraper on the main body areas and dry the legs and fetlocks to prevent water from dripping into the heels.

Walk the horse off until he is dry and/or apply a sweat rug. Do not allow him to become chilled. A drying box with heat lamps can also be used.

Breaking out is the term used when a horse has sweated, dried off and then begins to sweat again. Washing off wet sweat or brushing off dry sweat immediately after work can usually prevent this.

Quartering

This is the term given to a light grooming before work. The main body of the horse is brushed to remove surface dust. The eyes, nose, mouth and dock are sponged. The feet are picked out and the mane and tail laid. The rug, if worn, is folded over the part of the horse not being brushed.

Brushing Off

This is the name for a light groom after work, to remove mud and sweat from the horse and pick out his feet if a complete grooming is not planned. It is often the name given to the grooming of horses living out.

GROOMING TOOLS

Buy the best quality you can afford if they are going to be well looked after. Otherwise buy more cheaply but expect to replace them frequently.

All tools should be cleaned regularly by washing in warm water to which a small amount of disinfectant has been added. They should be rinsed thoroughly in cold water and placed to dry away from direct heat ensuring that water drains away from their backs.

Ideally each horse should have his own set but this is not always possible. Any horse who is ill, especially if he is infectious, must have a specified set.

Dandy Brush

A stiff, long-bristled brush used for removing dried mud, sweat and surface dust. It should not be used on the head, mane or tail. Choose one that has suitable bristle type for the horse. Remember that some animals will become fidgety and bite or kick if irritated by the static electricity generated by some types of artificial bristle.

Body Brush

Short, soft-bristled brush used to remove dust and grease and dried sweat from within the coat. This is the main grooming tool.

Water Brush

This has medium soft texture and length of bristle. It is used to wash off stable stains and to lay the mane and tail.

Curry Comb

There are three types, of which metal is used only to clean the brushes. It should never be used on the coat itself.

The rubber type is good for removing dried mud and sweat from the surface of the skin. It is ideal for removing loose hair when the horse is moulting and it is the best tool for stimulating the circulation and bringing the grease and dust to the surface so that it can be removed with the body brush.

The plastic curry comb is stiff and sharp. It has quite long bristles and can scratch the skin of a sensitive horse and tear the hairs if used on the mane and tail so is best used only on very thick coats.

Hoof Pick

Use to remove mud and debris from within the hoof. It should always be used from heel to toe to avoid damaging the heels.

Sponges

Three are needed. Two small ones, preferably colour-coded, one for the eyes, nose and mouth, the other for the dock. A large one is needed for applying large amounts of water, as when cooling off and also to help remove stable stains.

Stable Rubber

Similar to a linen tea towel, this is very useful for giving a final polish to the horse before he is tacked or rugged up. It can also be used for drying heels, etc.

Sweat Scraper

If the horse is washed regularly this is useful to remove water from the main muscle areas.

mane comb

plaiting comb

Mane Comb

This is not recommended (except for use on very tough manes) as it can tear the hair but a plaiting comb is useful when pulling manes and tails, or plaiting.

EXTRA GROOMING

Mane Washing

- Choose a warm day.

- Collect warm water, horse shampoo, a large sponge, a towel and a sweat scraper.

- Put on a headcollar. To avoid staining his head, it may be necessary to fit a grey horse with a clean nylon headcollar or white rope halter. Do not tie the horse up.

- Wet the mane with the sponge. Starting with the forelock, thoroughly rub in the shampoo, keeping it well clear of the eyes. Continue down the mane.

- Rinse with warm water until all the soap has been removed. Remove surplus water from the neck with a sweat scraper, and rub the ears dry with a towel.

- Brush the mane out with a clean body brush or water brush.

Tail Washing

- Collect the washing equipment.

- Put on a headcollar and tie the horse up. If he is restless, ask an assistant to hold him and to pick up a front leg if necessary.

- Proceed as for the mane, but soak the tail in a bucket of warm water. Take care, because when the water reaches the dock the horse may become disturbed.

- To dry the tail, stand to the side of the horse, hold the tail at the end of the dock and swish the bottom of the tail around in a circle.

- Brush out gently with a clean body brush.

Bathing the Horse

Bathing is a more extensive operation than washing or sponging down after work. It is carried out if there is a non-infectious skin problem, or as a quick measure to ensure a clean horse. Grey horses may have to be washed regularly, as they are difficult to get or keep clean. However, washing should never be a substitute for good grooming. Always use a shampoo designed for horse use and use it sparingly.

It is important for the horse to be thoroughly and quickly dried after bathing, so never wash him on a cold day. Lungeing him with a cavesson and boots on, or walking him out with a clean exercise blanket under the saddle are the best methods of keeping him warm and drying him off.

If possible, enlist the help of an assistant, and proceed as for mane washing. Wash the head first and then dry it with a towel. Tie up the horse and continue the process of washing, making sure that all the shampoo is thoroughly rinsed out as, if any is left in, it can cause an allergic reaction. In warm weather, if the horse accepts it, a hose can be used. The legs should be given a final rinse with cold water. Use towels to dry off the horse, or a brisk rub with straw (though not on greys, as the straw may stain the coat). The legs may be bandaged either with Gamgee and stable bandages, or thatched with straw or hay to help them dry.

Bathing removes oil from the skin, and the horse's coat often looks a little dull afterwards. A good grooming will restore the bloom.

Care should be taken when using products that produce a shine to the coat. They may inhibit sweating if used too liberally and that could be very detrimental to the horse.

Washing White Legs

White legs should not be shampooed in cold weather. Warm water and soap remove the protective oils from the skin, and mud fever or cracked heels may result. However, barrier cream applied to dry, clean legs and heels can assist in preventing this. If there is urgent need, the legs may be washed down individually with cold water, and dried with stable bandages applied over hay or straw.

Sponging Down after Work

Sponging down is used on a sweating horse after exercise. (See also Chapter 36, re cooling off a hot horse after competition.)

Method
- If he is still blowing, lead the horse about until he is calm, and his breathing is normal. The girths should be eased, but the saddle left on. Alternatively, the saddle may be removed and the back gently slapped to restore circulation and then covered with a towel. In cold weather a sweat sheet and light rugs should be put on.

- Pick out the feet. Wash them if necessary.

- Remove the saddle and bridle and put on a headcollar. If an assistant is available, ask them to hold the horse.

- Wash the horse down, using a large sponge and plain water. In hot weather use cold water or, if the horse will accept it, the yard hose. In cold weather, use lukewarm water and sponge only the very sweaty areas. Never use warm or hot water, as it is more likely to give the horse a chill.

- Remove surplus water with a sweat scraper.

- Put on a sweat sheet or cooler. If it is a hot day, walk

dry without rugs.

• Sponge round the base of the ears and face. Dry with a towel.

• Walk the horse about until he is dry. Ensure that the ears are dry and warm. In very cold weather put on stable bandages.

• After 30 minutes, check the rugs. If the horse is dry, groom him and put on his usual rugs.

Introducing the Horse to Being Hosed

In warm weather hosing is a quick and efficient method of cleaning and cooling off a horse. However, at first most horses are nervous of being hosed down. When first introducing hosing to the horse it is helpful to have a second person to hold him. Start gently with little pressure, and apply the resultant trickle around the front feet. Gradually work up the leg. At no time must the horse be frightened. As he begins to accept the sensation, gradually increase the pressure. When horses become used to the water they usually enjoy it, but some never accept it, and where they are concerned it is best to abandon the process.

Washing the Sheath

Some geldings require regular washing of the sheath. The signs that this is needed are a strong smell and nodules of greasy dirt collecting in and around the sheath. An assistant may be required to hold the horse and possibly to hold up a front leg. The equipment needed is a bucket of warm water, mild soap or a proprietary sheath cleaner, a sponge and rubber gloves. Soak the sheath and thoroughly clean out as much as the horse will allow. Then dry it with a towel. Apply baby oil as a lubricant.

GROOMING THE GRASS-KEPT HORSE OR PONY

In Winter

• Tie the horse up.

• Wash and pick out the feet. Check for any nails or stones which might have been picked up, and for cracked heels.

• When the horse is dry, remove the mud from his coat with the dandy brush or rubber curry comb. The latter is more efficient. Pay particular attention to the saddle and girth areas.

• Clean the head carefully, using body brush or hand.

• Sweat marks should have been washed off after work, before the horse was turned out.

• Wet mud on the legs, knees and hocks may be washed off with cold water and the legs left to dry. Do not use warm water and soap, as this will open the pores of the skin, making the legs more vulnerable to cracked heels and mud fever. It is preferable to leave wet mud until it is dry and then brush it off.

• Clean the dandy brush by brushing it against the sharp surface of a wall or door, well away from the horse. The rubber curry comb may be cleaned by knocking it against a similar surface or the floor.

• Sponge the eyes, nose, muzzle and dock area.

• Brush the mane with a body or dandy brush, depending on how thick the mane is.

• If the tail is muddy, wash it then brush it out. If it is dry and clean, brush it out with the body brush. The hairs on a horse's tail, which are easily broken off by rough brushing, take up to two years to grow. Thin-tailed horses and ponies should have their tails brushed out with a body brush, or simply with the fingers.

• The feet, when dry, can be oiled if required.

In Summer

In summer the coat is thinner and, it is hoped, the weather better. Proceed as in the winter, but there should be less mud and less likelihood of mud fever and cracked heels.

When grooming for a special occasion, for instance a show or rally, the procedure is similar to that for grooming a stabled horse, but with less emphasis on cleaning down to the skin with the body brush.

GROOMING MACHINES

There are several different types of grooming machines on the market, such as:

• The **vacuum type**, with a suction head, which can be used for removing dirt/mud or loose coat in the spring.

• The **revolving brush type**, which can be recommended for the large yard, when there is insufficient time for daily strapping. Some are a combination of vacuum and revolving brush and they usually produce the best result. Always bandage the tail before using.

The more modern machines are light and come with a waist belt that fastens round the waist of the operator. This makes them easier to handle than older machines. They have a dust bag attached, which collects all the loose hair and dust.

The stable manager should ensure that staff in the yard do not use the machines as an excuse for inadequate daily care. Some of them are quite dirty to use, especially if the dust bag is not emptied often enough or the animal is very dirty. It is recommended that all personnel wear overalls and cover their hair when using a grooming machine.

A muddy, grass-kept horse or pony required for a special occasion can be effectively cleaned up by the suction-type fixture. This removes mud and dirt, but leaves much of the grease in the coat. Make sure that the coat is quite dry before using the machine.

Because of labour costs, in many racing yards daily strapping has been discontinued. The horses are brushed over and tidied each day. After fast work they are sponged down. They are usually done over with a grooming machine every four to seven days. It has been found that they remain quite healthy and are considerably better tempered in the stable as a result of not being subjected to intense grooming and strapping.

Safety Rules

The operator should wear an overall, with long hair tied back, and rubber boots, and the machine should be plugged into a circuit-breaker. Great care must be taken not to catch the mane or tail in the machine. The tail should be roughly plaited, and then bandaged.

Horses who are difficult to clip often accept a grooming machine and then become easier to manage during clipping. Grooming machines are excellent for cleaning the coat, and the vibratory action of the brush has a stimulating effect on the skin, which is generally much enjoyed by the horse. Care must be taken to use only soft brushes on a thin-coated horse.

The machine should not be used more frequently than once every three days. If it is used too often, the skin may become tender and sore.

CLIPPING, TRIMMING, PULLING AND PLAITING

CLIPPING

Clipping is the removal of the horse's coat by machine. A horse changes his coat twice a year. From mid-September to mid-October he grows a thick winter coat, and between February and April he loses his winter coat and grows a lighter summer one. The old coat may become rough and dull during the period of change, particularly in the autumn. The exact timing varies between different types of horses and ponies, and is also affected by weather and temperature.

The growth of coat also varies for a stabled horse; the temperature of the stable and the number of rugs worn are the major influences. A well-bred horse, stabled and rugged throughout the year, grows a very light winter coat, and if he is not in hard, fast work, he may not require clipping.

Grass-kept horses and ponies are left unclipped to give them protection from the weather. If they are in steady work, they benefit from a semi-trace clip, i.e. the removal of the coat on the shoulder and underneath the neck and belly, in October and early November. This makes work easier and avoids any heavy sweating, which can occur if there is a warm spell of weather in October. Ponies protected by a New Zealand rug can be regularly trace clipped up until January.

The reasons for clipping a stabled horse are:

• To prevent distress when he is in hard, fast work. This is applicable in winter when the coat is thick, and sometimes even in spring and summer if the horse is expected to work at maximum effort, for example in three-day eventing or endurance riding.

• To help keep him in good condition. Sweating leads to weight loss.

• To make drying off after work quicker.

• To save time and labour over cleaning.

• To prevent and/or to control skin disease.

The first clip takes place in late September/early October. The weather is often very warm, and a working horse benefits from the removal of his coat.

Well-bred horses may require clipping only every four weeks; heavy-coated animals may need clipping every two or three weeks, if they are to look tidy and smart.

A horse who is to be shown should not be clipped after the end of January, as late clips spoil the summer coat.

Show Horses

The owner must decide whether or not to clip show horses. It depends on the individual horse, and his type of coat. If the decision is to clip, in all cases the horse is given a full clip. Coarse blades may be used to give a more natural look.

Show Ponies

Ponies who are slow to establish their summer coat, or who have a rough coat, need to be clipped, particularly if they are being shown early in the season.

Competition Horses

Competition horses involved in demanding sports (three-day events, endurance riding, show jumping and polo) may be clipped immediately prior to competition.

TYPES OF CLIP AND THEIR USE

Full Clip

The entire coat is removed, including the legs and saddle patch. A triangle is left at the top of the tail. The clip may be used on coarse-coated hunters. It makes them easier to clean and quicker to dry off, particularly the legs. It is often used only for the first and second clips. Thereafter the horse does not grow such a heavy coat, and a normal hunter clip can be used.

If a coarser blade is used for the saddle patch and legs, some protective hair will be left. Many consider that even with well-bred horses, if the long hair is left on the legs, it makes them slower to dry, more difficult to keep clean and therefore more susceptible to mud fever.

Full Clip with Saddle Patch

The saddle patch is left on to ease saddle pressure. Thin-skinned Thoroughbred horses are often best left with the saddle patch on.

Hunter Clip

The legs (to just below the elbow and stifle joint) and the saddle patch are left unclipped. Hair on the legs

Blanket clip.

Hunter clip.

Chaser clip – sometimes even more hair is removed, leaving only the top of the back and neck covered.

Trace clip.

gives protection from the cold, and from thorns, mud fever and cracked heels. The saddle patch gives some protection from saddle friction.

Chaser Clip

Hair is removed from the head and lower two-thirds of the neck and body. The coat is left on from behind the ear and over the top part of the body to the tail.

Chaser Clip Alternative

Hair is removed below a line starting at the stifle joint, along to the bottom of the saddle flap, up the neck to the base of the ears and down the side of the face.

Blanket Clip

Hair is removed from the head, neck, shoulder and belly and a narrow strip on either side of the dock, thus giving the shape of an exercise sheet.

The above three clips may be used for:

- Horses brought into work during the winter who require walking exercise in cold weather.

- Young horses in their first season's hunting.

- Horses who are cold-backed or who easily catch chills.

- Horses competing in winter in show jumping or dressage who may spend time standing around between classes.

- Riding school horses who may be required to do slow work or spend time standing in line.

Trace Clip

Hair is removed in a strip from the shoulder, belly and thighs, and often from the under-part of the neck and down the side of the face. This clip is used for:

- Horses who resent having their heads clipped. For them, the line of the clip is taken well up the shoulder, belly and thigh.

- Horses in light work.

- Horses and ponies turned out in New Zealand rugs.

- Young horses, as a first clip to familiarise them with clipping.

PREPARATION FOR CLIPPING

- A warm, still day is best. Start as early in the day as possible.

- Good lighting is essential. A utility box with a non-slip rubber floor is ideal. If this is not available, a spare box may be used, with the bed swept back and a minimal amount of bedding left down as this makes it easier to pick up the clipped hair and helps prevent slipping. Horses should not be clipped on a bare floor, because of the risk of slipping and the danger from electricity if the floor becomes wet.

- A haynet can be tied up in the box to keep the horse occupied.

- A strong box or straw bale should be available for standing on when clipping the horse's head.

- The horse should be clean and dry with as much grease as possible removed from his coat. A dirty coat clogs the blades and blunts them, causing overheating, and strains the machine. The blades cannot cut a damp coat. If a horse becomes upset and breaks out in a sweat, it is best to stop clipping until he has settled and dried off. A grooming machine can be a great boon, both to ensure a clean horse and to get the animal used to the noise and vibration of a machine. If a horse is known to be difficult, ensure that experienced help is available, and that sufficient time has been allowed to avoid any hurrying.

- If the horse is likely to get cold during the clipping process, use a blanket or sheet kept for this purpose to keep him warm. This will prevent his own rugs from being contaminated by the clippings, which can cause irritation and discomfort.

- After clipping, the horse can be brushed over with a dampened body brush, which will help to remove any surface scurf. Fit as warm a rug as needed.

- The person handling the clippers should wear rubber boots or rubber-soled shoes as a safeguard against an electric shock. Overalls and a headscarf or cap protect clothes and hair from clipped hair. A circuit-breaker should always be used.

- With a difficult horse, the holder and clipper are at risk. They may have their feet trodden or stamped on, or receive a glancing blow from the horse's head. They should wear strong boots and hard hats. The assistant should also wear gloves, which will make the rope easier to hold. He must never place himself in front of the horse in case the animal should strike out. When required, the assistant should hold up the horse's front foot, standing facing the shoulder and holding the front of the foot in the palm of the hand with the fingers. The rope can then be held in the other hand. (See page 74, methods of restraint.)

ELECTRIC CLIPPING MACHINES

There are two popular types of mains electric clipping machines. There are also smaller battery-driven machines suitable for trimming, clipping heads and for use on thin-skinned, nervous or difficult horses.

Electric Hand Clippers

The motor and clipping head are contained in one machine, with a cable to a mains power plug and circuit-breaker. They are small enough to hold in the hand. They are efficient and excellent for the small yard or private owner clipping clean, stabled horses.

They tend to overheat if worked too hard, especially if the air vents are not kept clean. The larger the motor,

the less strain on it, but it is likely to be bigger and heavier to handle.

Hanging or Heavy-Duty Type Clippers

These are suitable for the large commercial yard where many horses of all types have to be clipped. The machine itself is separate from the clipping head, and is connected by a flexible drive shaft. The machine is heavy and must be suspended from a beam or wall bracket. The actual clipping head is light, but the flexible shaft makes it less easy to manoeuvre, and there is more vibration than with a hand machine. It does give a very clean cut. If possible, such a machine should be kept in a loosebox or utility box reserved for clipping. Grooming machines may also be kept in this box. It will be easier to move the machine about if it is suspended on overhead runners.

Clipping with a heavy-duty machine will be easier if the drive shaft is kept as extended as possible. It requires regular oiling and greasing.

Heavy-duty clipping machine suspended from a beam and fitted with a circuit-breaker. Not generally seen in today's modern yards, which tend to favour electric hand clippers.

Battery Machines

Battery machines are becoming more widely available and efficient. There are two general types – one standard size; the other smaller and suitable for clipping faces, etc.

The standard-size battery clippers usually have a power pack which is attached to the user's back and is independent of any mains cable. This enables much greater freedom of movement and is safer. The clipping head is light and easily handled. As with all clipping machines, it is essential not to overheat the machine by clipping for too long at a time. The blades must be kept clean and oiled.

Electrical Connections

Those machines which are not self-earthed require a three-wire cable correctly connected to a three-pin plug to ensure safe earthing, and they must be connected to a circuit-breaker. The correct cable and working instructions are supplied by the manufacturers. The instruction booklet should be kept with the machine, and the maker's instructions followed.

Self-earthed machines should not be used from a light socket as this is not safe. Should the cable be pulled, either the light socket or the wiring will give way.

Care of the Blades

The clipping blades must be sharp. Blunt blades are uncomfortable for the horse, give an uneven clip and strain and overheat the machine. A spare pair of new or resharpened blades should be available before clipping begins.

Blades quickly become blunt when used on dirty horses and worked hard by those with limited experience of clipping. When used correctly they should last for six to eight clips before resharpening. Blunt blades are one of the most common reasons for horses becoming fidgety or bad tempered when being clipped. Blades can be resharpened as needed.

Blades are packed as a pair. They are ground as a pair and will work best if kept as a pair. They are usually secured together by a flat-topped bolt, a tension spring and a thumb-screw adjustment. Correct tension is essential. If it is too loose, the machine races and does not cut. If it is too tight, the machine is strained and overheats.

When the machine is switched on, light machine oil should be run through the blades and into the oil holes on top of the machine. The machine should be wiped clean before clipping starts. While clipping, the blades must be cleaned regularly. Brush them with a soft brush and then run the machine through a container of blade wash to remove dirt and hair.

Should the machine heat up, stop clipping, clean it and allow it to cool. It may be necessary to fit fresh blades.

When the clipping is finished, remove and clean the blades, then clean and oil the machine, following the maker's instructions. The thumb-screw and tension spring and bolt should be put back on the machine. Wrap the blades in oiled cloth, and store carefully. It is all too easy to drop the blades and chip them. A light knock is sufficient to put them off true, and thus give a strained and uneven clip. When taking clippers apart, do it on a clean stable rubber. This makes it less likely that bits will roll away and get lost.

After clipping, always check the cable for wear. At least once a year have the machine checked professionally for safety and have the motor serviced and overhauled bi-annually.

Electric clippers, and in particular hand machines, are often ill used and prone to strain. They can easily seize up in the middle of a clip. It is sensible to have a replacement machine available in case this occurs.

HOW TO CLIP

- If a mains hand clipper is being used, first assemble the machine. Carry out a safety check, including an inspection for any signs of wear of the cable and the plug. Take the machine to the clipping box. Ensure that there is machine oil, a container of blade wash, a soft brush, spare blades and chalk or saddle soap for marking lines. All this equipment should be placed safely out of the way on a shelf outside the box.

- Plug in the machine, and check that it is working correctly. Switch it off, and put it in a safe place. Ensure that the cable can be suspended over a hook, so that when you are clipping it comes directly to the hand, and does not lie on the floor where the horse can tread on it. Check, too, that the horse cannot reach it with his teeth.

- Bring the horse into a well-lit box and tie him up. If it is warm enough, remove his rugs, placing them well out of the way. If it is cold and draughty, place a blanket over his loins and back. Do not use his own rugs during the clipping process as they will get little bits of hair on them as already explained. Pick up the machine and switch it on. Allow the horse to become used to the noise before starting to clip.

- Switch off the machine and untie the horse, leaving the rope through the safety loop. Hold the end of the rope in the left hand, switch on the machine and then place the left hand on the horse's neck. Start on the near side, and clip the shoulder, running the machine against the direction of the hair. The line taken depends on which clip is required. Keep the machine flat. Do not push it; guide it and allow the machine to do the work. At all times clip against the growth of hair. Make each sweep as long as possible. If there is any likelihood of the horse moving his head, place your free hand between the clipper and his mane.

- When the shoulder, neck and chest on the near side have been finished, the horse may be tied up. The front part of the belly is then done, the blanket moved forward and the quarters, back and belly completed. The off side is then clipped. The machine may be held in either hand and changed if required.

- Ticklish or difficult parts, such as the head, underneath the belly, loins and in between the hind legs can be left to last, when an assistant may be required. When clipping around the elbow and chest,

a front leg should be held up to help stretch the skin and avoid nicking it. Similarly, hold the skin taut when doing the stifle joint and flank area.

- When clipping a front leg of a fidgety horse, the other front leg may be held up by an assistant to prevent the horse snatching up his leg and possibly breaking the clipping blades.

- It is important to check that the machine is not over-heating. This is bad for the machine, and makes the horse fidgety and resentful.

For a Saddle Patch
Draw an outline with chalk or saddle soap around the horse's own saddle. Make sure the outline is even and regular. Clip into the hair and lift the blades to achieve a tidy line. Use the line of the panel, rather than the flaps.

For a Blanket or Trace Clip
Ensure an accurate and matching clip on both sides by measuring over the withers and back, and putting lines on the horse's coat. The top of the front and hind legs should be clipped to the same height and angle. The clip should extend over the elbow to assist cleaning.

To Clip up the Neck
Run the blade as close as possible to the mane hair. It is preferable to leave a narrow edge of coat, rather than risk cutting into the mane. If the clipper places their hand against the mane it will help prevent any unsightly 'nicks' if the horse moves his head at the critical moment.

Trimming the Mane
A small portion of mane may be removed where the bridle headpiece lies over the poll. This should not exceed 2.5cm (1in). A small section may also be removed at the top of the withers. In each case, if too much hair is clipped, it is unsightly. On a fine-maned animal, trimming is often better done with scissors, as it is very easy to remove too much with clippers.

Sometimes hair is removed over the top of the withers although this may encourage rubbing and wear from pressure from the rugs.

DIFFICULT HORSES

Horses who resent having their heads or other ticklish parts clipped often accept a twitch on the nose, and will stand without struggling and allow the clip to be finished quickly and efficiently. The twitch should never be put on a horse's ear. For use of the twitch, see Chapter 9, Restraint.

Some highly-strung horses will not accept a twitch, and become violent if one is used. In such cases it can be dangerous to persevere and attempts to apply a twitch should be abandoned. If it is only a question of tidying up, it may be better simply to leave the horse as he is. If he is treated quietly and calmly, and not upset, he may eventually accept clipping more easily.

Horses may become difficult to clip for a variety of reasons. The most common causes are connected with rough handling and lack of tact, and include:

- Electric shock.

- Over-heated blades.

- Blunt blades.

- Bruising and/or cutting by the machine.

- Rough or impatient handling.

- Clipping for too long a time without rest, especially the first time the horse is clipped.

Remedies

It can be helpful to stand a nervous horse within sight and hearing of another quiet horse who is being clipped.

- Use a grooming machine to accustom him to the noise and vibration. However, some horses will not accept this.

- Before attempting a lengthy clip, trim the horse so that he becomes used to the feel of the machine.

- Music may have a calming effect, or cotton wool in the horse's ears may help.

- The use of a small battery-driven clipper may be less worrying to the horse, as there is less noise and vibration. With such a small machine, it may not be possible to achieve a full clip because of over-heating.

When clipping difficult horses, any rough handling is self-defeating. Personnel involved should be calm, skilled, unhurried and sufficiently strong to hold the horse. It is an advantage if the person clipping is tall, as he can clip the horse's head with greater ease.

Sometimes clipping the horse when he is tired after hard work, provided he is not damp with sweat, can help to keep him quiet.

Sedation

It may be necessary to sedate a very difficult horse. However, in most cases, if patience and kindness are used, this extreme measure may be avoided.

There can be problems connected with the use of sedatives on horses for the purpose of clipping. For the sedative to work satisfactorily the horse must be calm and unworried when it is administered. It is advisable to discuss each individual case with your own veterinary surgeon. Sedatives, orally by syringe or by intra-muscular injection administered by your veterinary surgeon, can be quick and effective but correct timing is essential for the dose to fulfil the clipping time required.

TRIMMING

If trimming is done well, the result should appear natural. Skill is required to trim well but it can considerably enhance the appearance and add to the value. Care should be taken when trimming with machines as it is easy to take off too much.

In winter, horses and ponies at grass should be left

untrimmed, but in summer they may be trimmed in the same way as a stabled horse.

Whiskers

These can be removed to give a smart and tidy appearance. However, it should be remembered that they are the animal's chief means of feel. Many owners will not have them trimmed, as they are of particular use to grass-kept animals.

Ears

The long hair in the ears may be clipped level. To do this the ear is held closed up and the machine is used in a downwards direction from the tip of the ear to the base. The inside hair should not be clipped, because the internal hairs give protection from cold, dirt and infection. Grass-kept animals should not have their ears trimmed.

Cat Hairs

These are long hairs which grow a week or so after clipping, particularly in January and February. They may be removed by clipping lightly in the direction of the hair using a coarse blade.

Heels and Fetlocks

In winter, these may be trimmed if necessary when the horse is clipped. In summer, well-bred horses may be trimmed by hand with a comb and sharp, blunt-ended scissors. The hair is raised by the comb and then trimmed off, so that there are no rough edges, in much the same way that human hair is cut by a good hairdresser. The operation requires practice and skill.

Coarse-coated horses who grow heavy feather are more easily trimmed by machine. A coarse lower blade, called a leg plate, may be fitted. This tidies the hair, but does not clip too closely.

In Mountain and Moorland show classes, native ponies are left untrimmed. Arabs grow very little hair and are left untrimmed.

Jaw, Withers and Poll Piece

These need to be kept tidy throughout the year. Either the normal clipping machine may be used, or alternatively a lighter machine, similar to a dog clipper. This machine is also useful for trimming legs and ticklish, awkward parts of the horse. It is very light, easy to handle, and is quieter and vibrates less than a large clipping machine. Some types are battery powered. Chin hairs may also be trimmed with blunt-ended scissors. When trimming the poll and withers area, great care is needed to avoid the trimmed areas becoming larger and larger. Well-bred animals are often more neatly trimmed with scissors.

Hogging

This is the removal of the mane by clipping. In former years hogging was very fashionable, but nowadays it is not often seen except on polo ponies and for showing cobs. It saves labour, and is a means of keeping tidy a mane which has been rubbed, for instance because of sweet itch, or caught on wire.

To hog, the horse's head should be held low and stretched, so that a clean cut can be achieved. Use the clippers from the withers towards the poll. Once hogged, a mane may take up to two years to grow, and at first will be coarse and upright.

The hogged mane is clipped once every two to three weeks and cleaned daily with a damp brush.

Sometimes the forelock is also removed; sometimes it is left on.

PULLING THE MANE

This is done to:

• Improve the appearance.

• Thin out a thick mane.

• Encourage the mane to lie flat.

• Shorten a long mane.

• Make the mane easier to plait.

Arrange to pull the mane after exercise, or on a warm day, when the pores of the skin are open. This makes the hairs easier to pull out, causing less discomfort to the horse.

To avoid making the skin very sore, it may be advisable to spread the mane-pulling over several days.

Some horses have very thick manes, and these can be the toughest to pull. Well-bred horses usually have thinner manes. Care must be taken in this case that the mane is not made too short.

Do not wash the mane before pulling, as this makes the hair soft and slippery and difficult to pull.

It is customary to encourage the mane to lie on the off side of the horse's neck. The manes of young horses may be trained to lie over by regular brushing, damping down and, when the horse is stabled, by loose plaiting. The manes of older horses are more difficult to retrain. If they lie on the near side and are tidy, they may be left.

The mane should never be shortened by cutting with scissors. This will leave an unsightly and very obvious edge. A very thin mane may be shortened by carefully breaking off the ends of the hair with the fingers. This leaves a natural looking edge. Clippers should not be used to thin a thick mane by cutting the underlying hair.

The manes and tails of all Arabs and Mountain and Moorland ponies, if they are to be shown in breed classes, are never pulled.

Satisfactory mane-thinning combs are now available on the market. These give the mane the appearance of a pulled mane without subjecting the horse to genuine pulling, which some horses strongly resent.

Method

• Thoroughly brush out the mane. A thick, tangled mane requires combing out. Remove the underneath hairs first and then shorten the top hairs. This should allow the mane to lie flat. Start at the poll, with the comb in the right hand. Take a few hairs in the left hand, run the comb up them to the roots, and then with a sharp, firm pull, ease them out. The forelock is done last.

• Alternatively, especially if the mane is long or neglected, take a few hairs from underneath, twist them around the pulling comb once or twice and give a sharp pull. This prevents the fingers getting sore and gets the job done quickly.

• When brushed out and dampened down, the mane should be about 10–12cm (4–5ins) long. If it is still unruly, loose plaiting may help.

PLAITING THE MANE

The mane is plaited to:

• Make the horse look smart, for example for showing, competing and hunting, or when the horse is to be seen by prospective purchasers.

• Train the unruly mane of a stabled horse. Plaiting for this purpose is done very loosely and the plaits are left long and not rolled up. They should be re-done each day. Rubber bands may be used. If the horse starts to rub the plaits, they should be undone and the mane should be washed.

Equipment for Plaiting

• Comb (mane or plaiting/pulling).

• Water brush.

• Needle. Short and blunt, with a large eye. Tapestry needles are ideal.

• Thread of a colour to match the mane.

• Scissors.

• Bucket of water.

• A safe object to stand on, if necessary.

Thread the needle and place it securely in a coat lapel. Double the thread and knot it. Then you're looking for a needle and thread if it is dropped. Much easier to find! Needles are easily mislaid, which can be dangerous. If they are lost the surrounding bed should be removed, the floor swept and fresh bedding put down.

Plaiting a mane.

Method

• Traditionally, plaiting starts at the poll. Many horses settle after the first one or two plaits are in. Comb out the mane and dampen it down. With the comb, divide the mane evenly into as many plaits as are required. Make sure there is a sharp parting between plaits. The number varies according to personal preference, prevailing fashion, the length of the neck and the thickness of the mane. The appearance of a fat neck can be improved with a smaller number of tight, bunched plaits; a poorly developed neck can be improved by thick plaits which are not pulled too tight. In all cases it is customary to have an uneven number of plaits up the neck.

• Take the first section of hair, divide it into three and plait down as far as possible. Take the needle and thread and sew it firmly. Turn the plait under, and roll up tightly. Stitch it backwards and forwards through the plait 3 or 4 times, making sure the thread follows the line of the hair, and cut off on the underside of the plait. There is no need to knot it and it should not be wound round the neck of the plait unless it is then to be taped. No thread should show. Some competitors still plait the top plait around the headpiece of the bridle. The resultant plait should be button-like, preferably with no thread showing. Proceed down the neck. The two plaits in front of the withers require extra stitching, as there may be friction from the martingale, breastplate and reins.

The forelock is done last, and is often laced or plaited down in the same way as the tail.

• To achieve tidy and firm plaits it is essential to stand at an easy height. Short people may need a bale of straw or a strong box on which to stand. Chairs and milk crates are unsafe and should not be used.

• If time is short, rubber bands, of a colour which matches the mane, may be used instead of thread. They should never be used where correct turnout is expected. The rubber band is looped several times round the end of the plait. The plait is then rolled up, and the band looped round the whole plait until it is firm and tight. Two bands can be used, one to secure the plaited hair and one to secure the roll.

• It is not advisable to plait manes the night before an event. Hay and bedding become embedded in the plaits, some hairs break and the result is untidy. Some horses try to rub out the plaits, with even worse results. A mane that is freshly washed is much more difficult to plait.

Style Variations

• For dressage, white tapes are often wrapped around the completed plait for added effect; this practice was developed in Europe.

• Three methods of plaiting a full mane are shown in the diagrams overleaf. In the **Russian trellis**, a rubber

Russian trellis.   Full mane plait.   Iberian plait.

band is put round each bunch and covered with tape. In the **full mane plait**, sometimes a coloured ribbon is plaited into the mane all the way down and then finished with a bow or tassel at the withers. The **Iberian plait** is now very popular. It is similar to the full mane style but the plait lies along the top of the neck.

PULLING THE TAIL

The tail is pulled to:

• Improve its appearance.

• Show off the horse's quarters.

• Save time when turning horses out for showing, competition, hunting, etc., when the tail must be either pulled or plaited. (It is better not to plait the tail the night before, for the same reasons as for mane plaiting.)

The tails of horses and ponies at grass should not be pulled, as the long hair protects the dock area.

Tail pulling should be done when the horse is warm and the pores of the skin are open. Thoroughly brush out the tail, removing all tangles, but do not wash the top of the tail as this makes it slippery and difficult to

pull. The procedure now varies according to the amount of hair to be removed. Well-bred horses should require only a small amount of hair to be removed from each side of the dock for about 15–20cm (6–8ins). The central part should remain untouched so that the natural length of the hair is maintained.

Because the pulling causes discomfort and occasionally bleeding, it is sometimes preferable to take several days to complete it. The hair is removed by using the fingers, or with the help of a mane or tail comb. The hair is pulled out with a short, sharp tug. Resin on the fingers will give a better purchase. After pulling, the tail should be washed and bandaged.

Horses who grow heavy tails need to have a lot of hair removed. Some sensitive horses object, and with these an assistant is needed to hold up a front leg. If the horse is still difficult, it is advisable to place an upended bale of straw in front of the person pulling. Pulling tails is often much more painful for the horse than having his mane pulled. Use of a bladed trimming comb can make the job much less stressful for all concerned and presents a very natural appearance if done well.

Alternatively, it is sometimes possible to hold the tail over a stable door and so complete the task. A twitch may help to control the horse (see page 75). With very resentful animals, it may be more sensible simply to keep the tail well brushed and bandaged, and to plait it for special occasions.

Once a tail has been pulled, it should be kept tidy and well bandaged and the growing hair should be removed regularly. It will require bandaging on a daily basis. Apply for 2–3 hours daily at least when the horse is in the stable. Do not leave on overnight. If the hair of a pulled tail is allowed to grow, it will at first have a bushy and unsightly appearance.

When first learning to pull tails, it is helpful to have an experienced observer on hand. It is easy to pull out too much and to finish with a nearly bald dock. Sometimes tails are shaved in the dock area. This initially gives a neat appearance from a distance, but once shaved it will need constant attention to maintain it. Growing out will involve an untidy, spiky appearance for a long time.

The bottom of the tail can be banged or left in a natural V shape. The length at which it is trimmed depends on the job and time of year and personal preference. Normal practice is to place an arm across the buttocks with the tail draped over it to simulate it being carried. Then cut across, level with the chestnuts. Polo ponies, steeplechasers and hunters often have theirs cut higher so as not to impede the stick or collect so much mud. Some people prefer their horses to have longer tails.

In the UK we prefer the tail hairs to be smooth. On the Continent warmblood horses often have their tails plaited into a loose pigtail when at rest. This results in a bushier, wavy tail when it is brushed out.

PUTTING UP A TAIL

This is done so that in wet, muddy conditions the horse's tail remains comparatively clean and dry. Eventers, polo ponies and occasionally hunters have their tails put up to help keep them out of the way.

The upper part of the tail is usually pulled. The main portion is firmly plaited down to the end, where it may be either stitched or secured with a rubber band. The bottom half of the tail is doubled up underneath and secured by stitching, by tapes or by rubber bands. The latter, if too tight, may restrict circulation. Thread, tape and bands should match the tail in colour.

A neatly pulled and banged tail.

A tail tied up with tape.

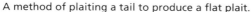

A method of plaiting a tail to produce a flat plait.

A ridge plait.

PLAITING THE TAIL

The tail should be washed and then well brushed out. There are two methods of plaiting: one with a flat plait (this is sometimes called lacing, or a laced tail) and the other with a ridge plait. The latter requires more skill and practice.

Method
• From the top of the dock, take a few hairs from either side and some from the centre. The centre strands can be tied with thread. These are the three locks of hair that make the plait. Plait them together and then work down the tail, each time taking a few more hairs from the side. No more hair is taken from the centre. Continue plaiting approximately two-thirds of the way down the dock. From then on, continue plaiting without taking any more hair from the sides until the end of the plait is reached. The end of the plait is firmly stitched, and then doubled up underneath and again stitched.

• To lace the tail, the locks of hair are brought inwards and passed one over the top of the other. To make a ridge plait, the locks of hair are passed from underneath, so that a ridge line is made on top. For the first method the fingernails face downwards and for the second they face upwards.

THE FOOT AND SHOEING

MODERN SHOEING PRACTICE

Horseshoeing has been an organised craft in Britain since 1356, when the Worshipful Company of Farriers was established in the City of London.

The Farriers Registration Act (1975) states that shoes can only be fitted to horses by persons registered to do so. Registration is confined to persons who have taken and passed the examinations of the Worshipful Company of Farriers (Registered Shoeing Smith until 1977 – now Diploma of the Worshipful Company of Farriers), or persons who at the time of the Act were practising farriery, either on their own or on other persons' horses, with or without reward.

Some farriers operate from a forge to trim and hot-shoe horses brought to them, but many travel around their area and are able to hot-shoe. The majority use factory-made shoes which are available in many sizes, and are finished to a high standard. They save the craftsman many hours of work at the fire and anvil, and are an acceptable substitute for hand-made shoes. The key to successful shoeing is regular and correct trimming of the hooves to maintain the correct balance, length and angle.

The modern farrier is a skilled craftsman. It is the responsibility of the owner to:

- Make regular appointments for attention to his horse's feet.
- Provide a clean, well-lit place with a level floor and protection from the weather.
- Ensure that the horse is trained to stand quietly for trimming and shoeing.

BASIC STRUCTURE OF THE FOOT

Internal Structure

The bones in the foot are:

- The second phalanx (short pastern bone) – half in the foot; half above the coronet band.

- The third phalanx (pedal bone).

- The navicular bone.

Tendons run down the leg and are attached to the bones, the superficial and deep flexor tendons at the back and the extensor tendons at the front. The former flex the joints, the latter raise and extend the limb.

Ligaments hold the tendons and bones in place but at the same time allow necessary movement.

The **lateral cartilages** extend from the wings of the pedal bone towards the heels and form elastic shock-absorbers.

The fleshy structures are tough, elastic pads consisting of:

- The **digital cushion** or sensitive frog, which lies at the back of the foot.

- The **coronary band**, where the hoof meets the skin of the leg and from which the hoof grows.

- The fleshy **sole**, which lies beneath the pedal bone.

The **sensitive laminae** cover the outer surface of the pedal bone, and form a junction between the fleshy and horny parts of the hoof. The fleshy structure and the

PARTS OF THE FOOT

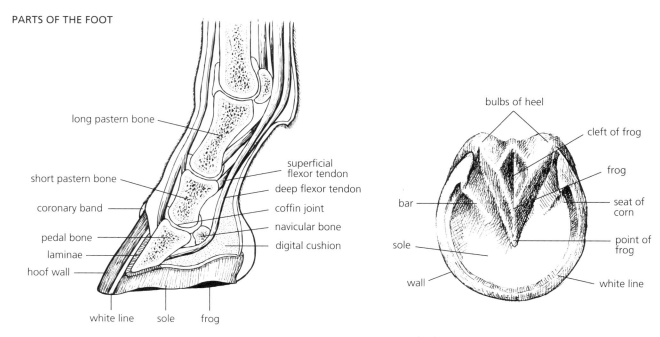

Cross-section through the fetlock, pastern and hoof.

Underside of the foot.

sensitive laminae supply nutrition to their corresponding parts of the foot.

The foot is well supplied with **blood vessels** and **nerves**.

External Structure

The hoof forms a non-vascular and insensitive covering for the internal parts of the foot. It consists of the wall, the sole and the frog.

The **wall** is that part of the hoof which is visible when the foot is on the ground. It is more or less semi-circular, the front feet being rounder in shape than the hind feet. At the extremity of the heels it bends sharply back to form the **bars**. The area between the wall and the bars is called the **'seat of corn'**.

The wall is thicker at the toe than at the heels, and expands slightly at the heel when the foot takes weight. It grows from the coronary band, and takes an average of

nine to twelve months before coming into wear at the toe, and about six months at the heel. When working on hard surfaces, the wall cannot grow fast enough to replace the wear, and shoeing is necessary.

The periople forms a shiny protective layer on the surface of the wall. It prevents undue evaporation; its removal by unnecessary rasping can cause the feet to become brittle owing to excessive loss of moisture. The water content varies from 25% in the wall to 40% in the frog.

The junction between the wall and the sole is marked by a distinct **white line**. This forms an important guide to the farrier as to the thickness of the wall covering the sensitive laminae. It also marks the union between the sole and the wall.

The **horny sole** forms the bottom surface of the hoof. It is softer than the wall, and grows from the fleshy sole. Natural exfoliation maintains a constant thickness to the sole, but its shape and thickness vary between different horses.

The **frog** is of a tough, elastic consistency. It is triangular in shape, and fits into the space between the angle of the heels. The depression in the centre is called the **cleft**. When the foot comes to the ground, the frog expands, acting both as a shock-absorber and a weight-bearing surface. This expansion, followed by contraction, has an important function in maintaining the circulation of the blood in the foot.

CONFORMATION

Good or Normal Feet

The **front foot** should be rounder at the toe than the hind foot, and viewed from the side should usually make an angle with the ground of between 45° and 50°. Although the angle should be the same as the pastern axis, it may vary between horses. The inside wall is normally slightly steeper than the outside wall. The line when the foot is picked up should be symmetrical around an imaginary central mid-line. The heels should be wide apart and the frog large and well developed, with a definite cleft. This should not extend up between the heels. The sole should be slightly concave. Both front feet should match in shape and size.

The **hind foot** is normally narrower and more upright than the front foot, with the toe less rounded. The angle with the ground should be between 50° and 55°. The sole is more concave, and the frog smaller. The hind feet should be a matching pair.

The surface of the wall may have a number of rings. These are normally insignificant in size, and smooth, and merely indicate changes in diet. But they may be larger and ridged, in which case they could indicate a previous illness.

Some horses have unusually high heels. This may be the natural conformation of the feet, or it can be the result of the way in which they are shod. Any excessive lowering of the heel, especially without corresponding cutting back of the toe to maintain the correct foot/pastern axis, can cause problems.

a = angle of shoulder
b = hoof/pastern axis

The well-balanced foot. Weight distribution should be equal in front of and behind c.

When the horse is standing naturally, all feet should point directly to the front. Any deviation affects both the movement of the leg and the wear of the shoe. Sometimes the direction in which a foot points might be a *consequence* of conformation of the limb. Pigeon-toed or 'toed-in' horses show excessive wear of the outer branch of the shoe; those with 'toes out' produce extra wear on the inner branch.

The Hoof/Pastern Axis

It is important to consider the balance of the foot with regard to the relationship between the slope of the pastern and the slope of the hoof wall. To ensure cranio-caudal (forward to backward) balance, the slopes should be similar. It is also important to maintain lateral to medial (side to side) balance, which ensures that the foot lands level on the ground. If the hoof/pastern axis is broken back, for example by excessive length of the toe or by excessive lowering of the heels, undue strain is applied to the flexor tendons and suspensory apparatus of the distal limbs. Any imbalance will furthermore apply undue strain to the bones, joints and ligaments of both limbs.

Foot Balance

The ability to assess and recognise the condition of the horse's feet is an asset to anyone managing horses in whatever state of work or rest they might be.

Understanding the basic structure of the foot is

fundamental to being able to assess the balance of the feet.

To assess foot balance (the principles for assessment apply equally to front and hind feet):

Look at the front feet from in front of the horse. Do they initially look a pair?

Take an imaginary plumb line from the front of the shoulder down through the limb to the floor. Consider the limb alignment when viewing that plumb line. Ideally the line should divide the limb equally, with the line dropping to the centre of the foot on the floor.

Any deviation on either side of the line indicates a lack of alignment through the limb and would indicate more weight taken on one side of the foot at the

from behind (b) from in front

(a) plumb line (b)

imaginary lines can be drawn when the hoof is on the ground to assess whether the balance is correct and the hoof symmetrical

from the side

(c) plumb line (d)

how an imaginary line drawn through the bones of the lower limb would divide them if the hoof/ pastern axis is correct

(e)

hoof picked up and viewed from above

(f)

underside of hoof, viewed from above to assess whether correctly aligned with pastern, and whether the hoof is symmetrical with an even bearing surface, as indicated by the imaginary lines

(a) – (f) How to assess foot balance and alignment.

expense of less weight on the other side.

Looking at the limb from the side, another imaginary line should drop centrally through the forearm, the lower limb and come to the floor immediately behind the heel of the foot. See also diagram on page 103.

Considering the hoof/pastern axis, broken forward it indicates an upright pastern with a tendency for the foot to suffer concussive forces and jarring. A broken back axis indicates a tendency for too much weight to be taken onto the heels and back of the limb, putting undue strain on the tendons.

While considering the hoof/pastern axis it is useful to consider the line or angle of the slope of the shoulder,

broken back   broken forward

Hoof/pastern axis.

which ideally should correspond in angle to the hoof/pastern axis, so that pressure is absorbed evenly through the angles of the joints. See diagram on page 103.

The front angle of the wall of the hoof and the angle of the rear of the foot from coronary band to floor should be the same and parallel to each other if the weight is well distributed over the foot from front to back. See diagram (c) on page 104.

When the foot is picked up and looked at from underneath (diagrams (e) and (f) on page 104), holding the limb by the fetlock or higher so that the foot can hang freely, an imaginary line taken from the ergot through the pastern and the foot from heel region to toe should bisect the foot; any deviation from the line indicates a toe turned in or out.

By making these assessments it should be

straightforward to ascertain whether weight is taken evenly from side to side and from front to back over the weight-bearing surface of the foot (which might include the shoe) and, if the horse's feet are not well balanced, where the deficiency originates.

Poor or Abnormal Feet

FLAT FEET show a decreased angle of the foot with the ground. The heels are low and the sole flat and often thin. The frog compensates for the poor conformation of the rest of the foot, and is usually large and well developed. Such feet are likely to sustain bruising of the sole and if they are not carefully shod, they are susceptible to corns.

BOXY OR UPRIGHT FEET show an increased angle of the foot to the ground. The heels are high, the frog small and the horn texture is often very strong. Many native ponies running unshod on their natural terrain have this type of hard foot, but with a good, well-developed frog.

Boxy foot.

Flat foot with long toe and collapsed heel.

CLUB OR MULE FEET are a more pronounced version of boxy feet, with an even greater angle to the ground.

LONG OR FLESHY FEET can be similar in some aspects to flat feet. The toe is long and cannot be reduced to normal size without risk of injury to the internal fleshy structures.

THIN SOLES are very sensitive soles.

DROPPED SOLES are convex and, in acute cases, below the surface of the wall. Dropped soles are often a sign of chronic laminitis with rotation or sinking of the pedal bone.

PRONOUNCED RIDGES OR RINGS are a sign of an alteration of the growth rate. They can be caused by past or present disease, such as laminitis, or by incorrect hoof trimming. The rings are widely spaced at the heel and converge at the toe. Those associated with a change in diet run parallel to the coronet and are smooth.

BRITTLE FEET can be partly inherited or may be a result of incorrect diet. Careless rasping of the wall – resulting in loss of moisture – or dry weather – resulting in the natural loss of moisture from the hoof without its being replaced – can be contributing factors. Careful balancing of the diet, regular exercise and skilled farriery may improve brittle feet.

CARE OF THE FEET

A horse turned out on good pasture, or a stabled horse on a balanced diet, should be receiving all the vitamins and minerals necessary for the production of strong horn. However, the metabolism of some horses is such that in spite of a suitable diet, they still have weak and brittle feet. Improvement can then be made by adding biotin, a member of the vitamin B complex, to the diet. Methionine, zinc, or glycerine are also useful additions and may help. Stable hygiene and the type of bed used

are also important for the maintenance of strong feet.

Horses need to be exercised on a variety of terrain in order to maintain a large and healthy frog.

Methods of Improving Horn Growth

• Regular attention from the farrier can improve the shape of the foot, and reduce the risk of damage to the wall by a lost shoe. Rasping of the wall must be minimal. The frog and sole should be trimmed, to remove untidy and dead fragments, but not cut back.

• Some people believe that stimulating ointment rubbed daily into the coronary band encourages the growth of horn but it will not improve texture. Care must be taken not to blister the coronet.

• Biotin fed regularly may help.

• Regular oiling of the wall will prevent undue evaporation, but too much oiling of the feet, particularly of the sole and coronary band, restricts the amount of moisture that the foot is able to absorb, and can be counter-productive, causing brittle feet.

Unshod Horses and Ponies in Work

Horses who are ridden on soft surfaces, e.g. in a school, with little road exercise, can work without shoes. Ponies with naturally hard horn often work without shoes, although some may need shoeing in front, particularly if they work on rough or flinty surfaces.

In a dry season most horses' and ponies' feet are hard, and will stand up to wear, although some horses' feet in dry conditions lose moisture and become brittle. In a wet season the feet may absorb too much moisture, and the sole and horn become soft, thus making shoeing necessary.

When the shoes are first removed, the horse/pony may go a little short until the feet harden. If there is no improvement, then the horn texture is not standing up to work without shoes.

Horses/ponies in work without shoes will on

occasions wear the feet down to a degree where they become footsore. It may then be necessary to put on shoes and allow sufficient new horn to grow before removing them again.

An alternative is to rest the animal until the horn has grown, or to work on soft going only.

Care of unshod feet entails:

- Regular inspection of the feet, including removal of small flints and debris which may cause infection and lameness.

- Every four to six weeks the farrier should dress the feet to maintain their balance. Some animals wear the toe, some the heel area, and some wear more on one side than the other. It is important to level up the foot, and to give the animal a level bearing surface.

Horses at Grass and Not in Work

Animals with good, strong horn growth should not require shoes. The feet should be dressed every 4–6 weeks so that the foot does not grow out of shape.

Some horses have poor horn growth and a tendency to flat soles. This type of animal is better kept shod in front. Shoes should be a lightweight pair of normal shoes. The farrier should replace them every 4–5 weeks.

In a dry year when there is little grass, and on a rough or flinty surface, horses can become footsore and may need shoeing.

Young Horses

Young horses with foot and/or gait problems may have them considerably improved if their feet are looked after from an early age by a skilled farrier.

PARTS OF THE SHOE

- The **web** refers to the width of the material from which the shoe is made.

- The **branch** is the part of the shoe from toe to heel.

- The **heel** and **toe** are self-explanatory.

- The **quarter** is the part of the hoof between the toe and the heel.

- The **bearing surface** is the part of the shoe in contact with the foot.

- **Clips** are drawn at the toe of the front shoe, and usually at the quarters of the hind shoe, although some ponies and cobs not used for fast work and jumping may have a toe clip on a hind shoe. The clips should be solid, but not larger than the thickness of the shoe, and rounded rather than diamond shaped. If a shoe becomes loose or dislodged, the horse often treads on the clip, which can cause a serious injury if it is sharp. Clips assist in keeping the shoe in place.

- **Studs** or **nails** can be fitted at both heels but should only be used if extra grip is absolutely necessary.

- Tungsten nails can be very useful for horses doing a lot of road work.

TYPES OF IRON

- **Plain** is heavy, straight-edged, flat iron.

- **Concave iron** has a wider foot-bearing surface than ground-bearing surface. This reduces suction and gives a lighter weight shoe, but it also reduces the ground-bearing surface.

- Fullering refers to the groove made in the ground-bearing surface of the shoe. It provides a secure bedding for the nails and a better foothold.

COMMON TYPES OF SHOE

PLAIN-STAMPED SHOES are made of plain iron with nail holes stamped through the full thickness of the web. Both front and hind shoes usually have one toe clip.

These shoes are only suitable for horses doing slow work, as they give a less secure foothold, and are also more likely to cause interference, such as brushing or over-reaching.

HUNTER SHOES are suitable for most riding horses and ponies. They are made of fullered and concave iron, and have one clip in the front shoes, two in the hind. Dressing the heels of the shoes to the angle of the feet lessens the risk of their being pulled off by a tread. Two clips in the hind shoes allow the shoe to be 'set back', the front edge to be rounded off, and the inner edge bevelled, all of which reduces the risk of an over-reach or of the shoe pulling across the foot when jumping and turning.

Modern farriery favours the balanced foot with minimal interference from introduced studs or heels, and plenty of support for the heels.

Rolled toes on hind shoes are used on horses who drag their toes.The front of the shoe is turned up to make a thick, wide toe. The two clips can still be drawn if required. Reinforced steel or tungsten can be put in the toe to give longer wear.

On front shoes, rolled toes are used for horses with long toes who stumble, but if the foot is short and upright, they can increase the stumbling. The shoe is set back on the foot, and the toe surface is rounded off.

ALUMINIUM SHOES are lightweight shoes used for 'plating' racehorses. They may also be put on show ponies and hacks. Plating is a term for shoeing horses with lightweight shoes for racing. These 'plates' are usually removed the following day and replaced with normal exercise shoes. They are often fitted without clips.

Various REMEDIAL SHOES, for example bar-shoes, egg-bar shoes, heart-bar shoes and raised-heeled shoes, may be recommended in special circumstances; but since these are likely to interfere with the primary requirement of trimming and shoeing – that is, to establish or maintain lateral-to-medial and cranio-caudal balance – specialist advice should always be sought.

SHOEING TOOLS

Forge Tools for Making the Shoe

- The **anvil** should be sufficiently heavy to withstand the blows of a heavy hammer during the making and shaping of a shoe. The beak, or pointed end, provides a surface for shaping the shoe.

- **Fire tongs** are long-handled tongs used to hold hot metal so that it can be turned in the fire.

- **Shoe tongs** have shorter handles and are used to hold a hot shoe on the anvil.

- The **turning hammer** is a heavy hammer used to shape the shoe and to draw the clips.

- The **stamp** is a punch used to make the nail holes. By altering the angle of the stamp, the nail holes are drawn in closer to the inner edge at the toe of the shoe, where the horn is thicker. These are called 'coarse holes'. As the wall becomes thinner towards the heels, the nail holes are made near the outer edge and are called 'fine'.

- The **pritchel** is a long steel punch used to finish the nail holes begun by the stamp. It is also used to hold the hot shoe against the foot.

Tools for Preparing the Foot and Nailing the Shoe

- The **shoeing hammer** is a lightweight hammer for driving in the nails. The curved claw at one end is designed to grip and twist off the point of the nail.

- The **buffer** has a blunt chisel end for cutting clenches, and a pointed end for punching out broken nails.

- The **rasp** is a heavy, flat, steel file about 41cm (16ins) in length. On one side it is coarse cut, and on the other fine cut. It is used to make a level surface for the shoe, and also to smooth off any rough edges of horn after the shoe has been fitted.

- The **drawing knife** has a curved blade with a bent-over, very sharp end. It is used for cutting off ragged bits of horn, and to cut out the small piece of wall for the toe clip. It may also be used to cut away any diseased portions of the frog.

- The **searcher knife** has a lighter blade than the drawing knife, and is used to search and open up a punctured foot or one that may have a suspected abscess.

- The **toeing knife** has a short, flat blade. It is used with the shoeing hammer to prepare and trim the foot surface before finishing with the rasp. It is used for the same purpose as hoof parers, but usually on heavy horses.

- **Pincers** are used to lever off the shoe, to remove nails and to assist in clenching up.

- **Hoof-cutting pincers/ hoof parers** have overlapping blades (one thick, one thin) and are used to trim overgrown feet.

- The **tripod** is a three-legged iron support, which the farrier may use to support the horse's foot when he is cutting the clenches, or when finishing the foot.

SHOEING

The average horse requires a new set of shoes, or must have his old shoes removed and replaced, every four to six weeks. The time interval depends on the growth rate of the feet of the individual horse, and how he wears his shoes. Horses who are heavy on their feet, and who do a lot of roadwork, may need new shoes every two weeks.

Indications that re-shoeing is necessary:

- A lost or loose shoe.

- The shoes are thin, either all over, or in one part.

- The clenches have risen.

- The shoe or shoes have spread.

- The foot is beginning to grow over the shoe, resulting in the heels of the shoes pressing into the seat of corn.

- The wall of the foot has grown and the foot is unbalanced.

The Process of Shoeing

Before shoeing a new horse the farrier should study the horse standing square in his old shoes, and then see him walked and trotted up, so that he can observe any abnormalities of action. When viewed from in front the long axis of the limb should be over the centre of the shoe. He should also check the old shoes for any uneven wear. This may have been caused by faulty conformation or by unsoundness, but it can also result from faults in the dressing of the foot or the fitting of the shoe. When the old shoes are removed, the horse should be observed standing unshod and walking.

To Remove a Shoe

1. The foot is held between the knees, and the clenches are opened, using the shoeing hammer and the sharp edge of the buffer. Risen clenches are easily cut; tight clenches require more skill. The corner of the buffer can be placed against the clench, but on no account should the buffer be driven into the wall to raise the clench. With a heavy horse, it may be easier to place the foot on a tripod when cutting clenches.

2. With the foot between the knees, the pincers are used to ease the shoe at each heel, and then round the toe. The shoe is removed by gripping it with the pincers at the toe, and pulling it backwards towards the frog. On occasions it is necessary to remove the nails individually. In this case the clenches are cut, the shoe is eased at the heels and the shoe is knocked

back with the pincers. This pushes out the heads of the nails, which can then be removed with the pincers.

3. The old shoe should be put out of the way, with the nails hammered flat, or it may be taken to the fire so that the new shoes can be matched up. Any loose nails should immediately be picked up so that the horse cannot tread on them.

Preparation of the Foot

It is necessary to restore the balance of the foot, and to prepare a level bearing for the new shoe. The farrier should look at the shape and angle of the foot when it is on the ground. When viewed from the side, the angle of the foot and pastern should be the same. The foot is then picked up to observe the bearing surface. In most cases it is necessary to remove more horn from the toe than from the heels. In normal circumstances, the foot is reduced with the rasp; first the sides and toes are done and then, if necessary, the heels. If there is excessive growth, it is taken off by using either the hoof cutter or the toeing knife. Any untidy pieces of sole or frog may be cut off, but, apart from this, if they are in healthy condition, neither should be touched. After the final balancing of the foot, the horse should again be observed standing unshod.

Hot Shoeing

The prepared shoe is heated, shaped and then applied to the foot to check for fit and bearing. To avoid excessive burning of the foot, it should be at a dull heat, and should not be left against the foot longer than is necessary to ensure level bearing. It is then taken to the anvil, where any necessary adjustments are made. After a final check on the foot it is cooled in water.

Nailing On

Nails must be of a suitable size (no larger than the wall of the foot can absorb) and must fit into the fullering. The end of the nail is shaped so that when it is driven correctly, it emerges about one-third of the way up the wall. It is usual to have three nails on the inside of the shoe and four on the outside. The shoe is nailed on first at either the toe or the heel, and then on alternate sides. If the foot is broken or weak, it is important that nails should only be driven into sound portions of horn. In this case it may be necessary to drive the nail higher in the wall than is normally desirable, and also to make sure that nail holes in the shoe are stamped so that weak parts of the wall are avoided.

As each nail is hammered home, the point is either immediately twisted off, or bent over and twisted off later. The end of the nail now forms a clench. The closed pincers are held against the clench, and the nail hammered tight. This turns the clench over. The clenches are shaped with the rasp, and then hammered flat against the wall. The rasp is used to smooth off the clenches, and the edge of the wall, thus making it tidy and finishing the shoeing.

Cold Shoeing

Hot shoeing has been preferred to cold, but farriers without a portable forge may have to shoe cold, and as long as it is done correctly it is as good.

Arrange for the farrier to see the horse, measure the feet and see if there are any particular problems. A skilled farrier who makes his own shoes can shoe cold very satisfactorily. However, in the case of factory-made shoes which arrive complete with nail holes, a less satisfactory fit is obtained. Because the nail holes are always in the same position, when the shoe is put on nails may well have to be driven into weak horn. This results in a less secure shoe.

To Measure a Foot

If it is necessary to give the farrier the approximate size of the shoes, measure the foot from toe to heel and then across the widest part. Any broken or weak parts of the wall should also be mentioned. Alternatively, place the foot on paper or cardboard and draw the outline.

THE NEWLY SHOD FOOT

When the Foot is on the Ground

- The foot should be suitably reduced in length at both toe and heel. The line of the pastern should be continued by the foot until the shoe and the ground surface are reached, i.e. straight hoof/pastern axis.

- The frog should be close to the ground.

- The clenches should be in line, well formed and bedded, and the correct distance up the wall. They should not have been driven into old nail holes unless reshoeing after plating.

- The place for the clip should be neatly cut and the clip rounded and well bedded.

- The wall should have been rasped only lightly, and not above the line of the clenches.

- The foot should be level on the ground.

When the Foot is Picked Up

- The shoe should fit the foot. There should be no dumping of the toe (excessive cutting back of the toe). The heels of the shoe should be the correct length, neither too long nor too short, but should support the heels.

- The type of shoe and the weight of iron should be suitable both for the work the horse is doing, and for the size and shape of the foot.

- There should be no unnecessary paring of the sole or cutting of the frog.

- The foot should be evenly rasped down and the heels level, and not opened up by cutting the bars.

- No daylight should show between the shoe and the foot, particularly in the heel area.

- The nails should be of a suitable size and should have been well driven home, so that they do not project above the surface of the shoe.

- The correct number of nails should have been used, usually three on the inside and four on the outside.

- The horse should be sound when he is trotted up.

A well-shod foot.

Foot shod tight to the heel.

Foot shod to support the heel.

FAULTS IN SHOEING

DUMPING The shoe is set back, and is often too small. The toe of the foot is rasped off to make it fit the shoe. The rasping of the wall exposes the soft underlying layers, which then become brittle and will not hold the nails. The foot itself has a neat appearance, but the fault can be easily observed because the angle of the wall changes as it comes towards the shoe. The foot itself has a smaller bearing surface.

NB: Dumping of the toe should not be confused with rasping the toe to obtain a normal hoof/pastern axis.

OVER-LOWERING OF THE TOES raises the heels and reduces the bearing surface. The angle of the wall on the ground is increased, and the balance of the foot, and therefore of the horse, is upset. Frog pressure is reduced and more weight is placed on the front of the foot. The heels should be one-third of the height of the toe from the coronary band.

OVER-LOWERING OF THE HEELS puts weight on the back of the foot, with consequent extra strain on the tendons and ligaments. The angle of the wall to the ground is decreased, and the resultant long toe can cause stumbling, and the possibility of the development of navicular disease.

Opening the heels by CUTTING AWAY THE BARS of the foot causes a weakening of the wall and of the heels, and results in contraction of the heels and in increased concussion.

OVER-LOWERING OF THE BEARING SURFACE can occur through lack of judgement when a farrier first shoes a horse with flat, open feet. The bearing surface is rasped down too much and the horse becomes footsore. An uneven bearing surface occurs when one side of the foot is rasped away too much. When the foot is picked up and the shoe checked, the uneven surface can be seen. It can also result from a lost shoe, when one side of

Dumped toe and short heel.

the foot is worn down or breaks off.

RASPING THE WALLS results in the removal of the periople, and consequent drying out of the foot and brittleness. Ideally, rasping should be minimal, never above the clenches and only sufficient to finish and tidy the foot. However, in the case of long-toed feet, some extra use of the rasp is necessary.

SHOES TOO HEAVY may cause some form of interference, such as brushing, over-reaching, etc. If the horn is not strong, a shoe may come off and often it will take a piece of the wall with it.

NAILS TOO LARGE may split and damage the wall. The resultant loss of holding power may cause problems when the horse is next shod. There is also a greater risk of nail binding. The head of the nail sits above the fullering, and thus receives more wear.

EXCESSIVE BURNING OF THE HORN when applying a hot shoe to the foot. The shoe should be at no more than a dull, red heat, and should be held in contact with the foot only for as long as is necessary. If it is subjected to too much heat, the wall surface is weakened and may well crumble away, leaving a loose shoe. More often, the interior soft tissues of the foot are affected by scalding.

NAIL BIND occurs when a nail is driven too close to the sensitive laminae and causes pressure. When the horse is trotted up after shoeing he goes unlevel or a 'little footy'. The nail must be removed and another nail driven in at a less steep angle. This lameness can occur as long as seven to ten days after shoeing.

NAIL PRICK is when a nail is mistakenly driven into the sensitive laminae. The horse shows pain, and the nail when removed may show traces of blood. Often, the horse trots up sound at the time, and may not go lame for two or three days, by which time pus will have formed in the wound. The shoe will have to be removed, the nail route traced and opened at the base, and the foot poulticed.

STUDS

The use of studs should be considered with extreme caution. They affect the angle at which the shod foot meets the ground, alter the bearing surface and balance of the foot, and increase the wear of the shoe at the toe. These problems can be resolved if the studs are always used in pairs. In this way, the balance and angle of the foot can be maintained.

Studs are made from specially hardened steel, and are used to give a better foothold. Road studs are put in for slippery roads and jump studs for jumping.

Road studs can be hammered in and remain a permanent feature of the shoe. When the horse is re-shod, it is often possible to remove the studs from the old shoes and to use them again. They are usually placed on the outer heel of both hind shoes, but they may be put on the outside quarter of the shoe. For even greater security, they can be put on the front shoes too, although this can cause greater concussion and the risk of tendon strain from steadying too abruptly. There is also a risk of treads (see page 254) if studs are placed on the inside heel.

The **screw-in type road stud** can be used if it is necessary to replace it with a larger stud for jumping.

Jump studs come in several shapes and sizes. Generally, large square studs are used for deep mud, and

road stud – hard ground

small conical stud – added grip on hard ground

maxi dome stud – added grip on soft ground

medium conical stud – soft or slippery ground

mini sharp stud – extra penetration for hard ground

large conical stud – deep going

dressage stud – various ground conditions

large road stud – hard ground

polo stud – good to soft ground

sharp stud - firm or slippery ground

blank stud – travelling

bullet stud – good to soft ground

mini dome stud – added grip for soft ground

Types of stud and their uses. *(Courtesy SupaStuds Ltd)*

smaller pointed studs for hard ground. The actual choice of stud is very much one of individual opinion, and must relate to ground conditions at the time.

On a narrow web shoe, it may be necessary to widen the shoe at the heel to give room for the stud holes, which are made when the shoe is hot. To ensure correct fitting, and because studs can vary, it is important to show the farrier the studs you plan to use.

If the stud holes are not filled by road studs or plugs, they should be greased and packed with cotton wool. This ensures that they are kept clean and facilitates screwing in of studs at a competition.

Studs in a horse's shoe can result in an extra risk of injury to both horse and rider from a strike or kick. For this reason, studs are not permitted in racing. Their use for cross-country competitions must depend on the going and on local conditions. For dressage, again it depends on the conditions of the day. Studs can give more security to the horse on corners and in transitions, but on hard going they may shorten his stride and emphasise any unlevelness. The horse must be allowed to get used to working with studs.

Equipment Required for Fitting Studs

- Nail for removing cotton wool.

- Metal tap for cleaning out and reviving the thread of the screw hole.

- Spanner for removing and screwing in studs.

- Fresh oiled wool for placing in the holes when the studs are taken out.

- Screwdriver to fix or remove plugs, if used.

Drive-in Plugs

These can be more effective than studs on a slippery road surface and in snow and/or ice. They are fitted round the shoe, and therefore give an even bearing and do not upset the balance of the foot.

PADS

Leather or synthetic pads can be used, either temporarily to protect an injured sole, or on a permanent basis to minimise concussion and bruising in the case of horses with thin soles.

Before a pad is fitted, the sole and frog should be treated with Stockholm tar and the sole padded with Gamgee or a similar material.

The synthetic pad is cheaper than leather, but because it is more likely to make the sole and frog sweat, it makes it more difficult to keep these structures healthy. A synthetic pad shaped to the shoe, and continued across the base of the frog, can ease concussion. The bar over the frog can alter the balance of the foot and care should be taken over this. Leather pads are also affected by conditions – when wet, they compress between the shoe and the foot, causing clenches to rise; when dry, they can become rock hard. A more effective protection for bruised or thin soles, and one which minimises concussion, is a rubber or plastic cushion, which fits under the shoe but leaves the frog area clear.

Wedge-shaped pads can be used to ease the pressure on the tendons and to reduce concussion. In snow or freezing conditions, pads fitted under the shoes help to prevent snow balling in the feet.

NEW TYPES OF SHOES

Alternative shoeing methods and types of shoe

A number of new styles of trimming feet and shoeing horses are now available. Very careful consideration should be given before any new style of foot trimming is instigated.

Ensure that the practitioner is experienced and qualified and preferably look at examples of their work and talk to owners who have had it done to their horses before having it done to your horse.

Cytek shoe.

Glue-on 'plastic' shoe.

The Cytek shoe has a lot of devotees amongst horse owners and some farriers only practice this type of shoeing. The foot is trimmed slightly differently from normal and the shoe has a very pronounced 'roll' at the front. Many horses who have suffered for years with foot problems work extremely well in Cytek shoes. They are more expensive than ordinary shoes.

There are various 'plastic' shoes available. Those designed to be nailed on are not always satisfactory as the plastic 'plays' between the nails.

There are some now on the market designed to be glued on. If the instructions are followed with extreme care the shoes stay on as long as normal shoes. One make is Easy-Glu by Mustad. These are aluminium shoes encased in high grade polyurethane. The aluminium core prevents the 'play' in the shoe. They are kept in place by polyurethane tabs that extend up the wall of the foot and are glued in place.

They are designed to absorb high frequency shock. They can have studs fitted and are excellent for use when the hoof wall is of poor quality. Some styles are especially designed to be used when the horse is being treated for laminitis or navicular. They are excellent when some of the hoof has had to be replaced with filler because of an accident or surgery.

There are also designs for racehorses and for foals who need remedial foot care. As with any 'alternative' management method, research carefully before deciding to use it and ensure that the practitioner is qualified and experienced.

CHAPTER

BEDDING

REASONS FOR BEDDING

Bedding is material that is put on the floor of a loosebox or stall to:

- Encourage the horse to lie down and rest.
- Enable him to do so in comfort, without risk of injury.
- Keep him warm and minimise draughts.
- Encourage him to stale.
- Reduce jar to his legs from standing and moving around on a hard surface.
- Prevent him slipping up when moving about the stable.
- Minimise ammonia fumes.

Bedding is also sometimes used in a trailer or horsebox when a horse is travelling, to cover the floor and give a softer and less slippery surface.

CHOICE OF BEDDING

When choosing bedding consider the following:

- Cost
- Availability
- The type of stable floor
- Ease of use

- Suitability for horse
- Suitability for type of stable
- Ease of disposal
- Palatability
- Storage
- Need for machinery

Cost and Availability

As the cost of bedding material is unlikely to be recouped, consider not only the cost of buying but also of delivery and disposal. A better deal can usually be made when purchasing by buying in bulk but there needs to be sufficient storage space available.

Bedding bought locally should not be so expensive to transport and some suppliers may be prepared to store it for you and deliver it piecemeal as required if storage is a problem.

Whatever bedding is chosen, ensure that it is readily available, and preferably locally. Some, such as locally produced sawdust or straw, may only be available at certain times of the year.

Floor Type

A stable with drains needs bedding which allows moisture to run away and which will not block them up. A stable without drains needs absorbent bedding that will also minimise odour.

Basically, straw bedding allows drainage and most paper and wood derived beddings are more absorbent. Many stables use rubber matting very effectively. Some also have the walls lined to help prevent injury. Rubber matting is expensive to fit but some types can be used without any other form of bedding or need only a small amount on top, to encourage staling or to absorb ammonia fumes given off by stale urine. Many horses do not like to splash their legs when staling.

Rubber matting is very cost-effective in many cases as spending on other forms of bedding is reduced and the time spent mucking out is also cut, therefore allowing staff to use their time more productively. However, if large amounts of water are used to wash off the flooring this could lead to extra expense and/or problems in times of drought or water shortages.

Some designs of matting allow urine to drain through them and quickly become very smelly if the surface underneath is rough or uneven and difficult to clean.

The matting needs to be either easy to lift and wash or completely sealed so that moisture cannot penetrate.

Matting should only be laid on a smooth, correctly prepared base. Manufacturers will usually provide guidelines for their products.

Ease of Use

The type of bedding chosen needs to be easy for the user to move when dry, from store to stable, preferably pale in colour so that droppings are more easily seen and not too heavy to move when wet. It is also better for both horses and grooms if it is dust free. Some bedding, paper is an example, can blow about when dry and add considerably to time spent sweeping up, if not managed carefully.

Suitability for the Horse

It is preferable for all horses to live in an environment as dust free as possible and bedding obviously can add to the dust problem. Any horse with a dust allergy or wind problems should have bedding as free from dust as possible. However, there is little point in providing him with dust-free bedding if other animals in the same building are not on dust-free materials.

Bedding for horses should be non-slip and encourage them to stale and to lie down.

Horses with leg and joint problems need bedding that is comfortable and easy to walk on.

When animals are ill and need specialist care, the type of bedding used needs to be considered in consultation with the veterinary surgeon.

Suitability for Type of Stable

In barn-type stabling it is often easier to deliver fresh bedding and remove muck by using machinery. Some barns are highly automated and the muck is moved by machinery from the aisle to the muck heap or skips. However, this involves a greater risk of dust and allergic reaction to some types of bedding, and if the ventilation is inadequate the stables may be smelly.

With the stables opening onto an open yard there is more likelihood of the bedding blowing around and it may not be so easy to remove the waste to the muck heap. On the other hand, the environment is likely to be less dusty.

Disposal

Disposal of bedding needs to be safe, legal and cost-effective. In some districts the building of muck heaps is not allowed, nor is burning of waste. If muck is stored, care needs to be taken that effluent and run-off cannot contaminate any rivers or water sources. EU laws mean that waste from commercial yards may incur charges if it is stored, processed and then sold as garden manure. At the time of writing, private yards are exempt.

TYPES OF BEDDING

Bedding can be divided into two types: drainage and absorbent. There are many types on the market, almost all of them the byproduct of another process. Traditional beddings, such as straw and wood shavings, are still popular and can be cost-effective if sourced locally and of good quality.

Wheat straw is considered the best type of straw for bedding, being more hard wearing and less palatable than barley or oat straw.

Barley straw is now combined in such a way that there are few 'awns' left to irritate the horse.

Oat straw is the softest of all and can sometimes get tangled around the horse's legs and be more trying to muck out.

Both barley and oats are sometimes fed as part of the forage ration and are often eaten by horses when used as bedding.

Sawdust and wood shavings produced locally are fine as long as they are checked for foreign bodies before being used. They may be dustier than the same product which has been produced commercially.

Various commercially produced beddings made from **paper, hemp, wood and flax** are also available and, being dust free, are worth considering.

They vary considerably in cost and not all are available nationwide but most of them are highly absorbent, easy to use and, once the initial bed has been put down, do not require much topping up if the bed is well managed and regularly skipped out.

Palatability

As well as having the qualities already mentioned, the bedding chosen should not be palatable, but if eaten should not be injurious to the horse.

Storage

The storage of the bedding needs consideration. It needs to be kept dry so, if there is insufficient storage under cover, consider a product which comes pre-wrapped.

Needs for Machinery
Some bales are so large and/or heavy that they need

machinery to move them safely. If this is not available they should not be chosen; the workforce might be injured if asked to move them by hand.

MANAGING THE MUCK HEAP

If muck is to be stored on the premises the area chosen needs careful planning. Ideally it should have a concrete base and three solid walls.

It is easier for a worker if the barrows can be tipped from above, i.e. the site is cut into a bank, or, if tipped on a level site, that the waste can be pushed up together by machine. The old way of building the heap without supporting walls is very time-consuming and may not meet present Health and Safety guidelines. It is also not satisfactory for certain types of bedding, such as paper, which might blow about. An untidy muck heap gives a very poor impression to visitors.

If a free-standing muck heap is managed properly it may take at least one hour each day to build.

Horse manure should not be put on horse pasture as it will add to the worm burden and will tend to make the soil more acidic.

Rather than storing the muck it may be preferable to load it straight into a trailer or skip and have it removed on a regular basis. In some areas mushroom growers will take fresh, straw muck, and some farmers are diversifying into composting waste and selling it to gardeners. Bagging muck and selling it at the gate is only possible for the smallest enterprises.

It is important that only waste bedding is put on the heap. Plastic bags and baler twine will not rot down and will damage any machinery used on the heap.

EQUIPMENT

Choose carefully when buying equipment. Make sure it is suitable for the type of bedding chosen and for the workforce who have to use it. In yards with student workers make sure that there is enough to go round.

Tools which might be required are:

FOUR-PRONGED FORK with either a short or a long handle. The tines should not be sharp. This fork is used for mucking out straw beds, digging out riding surface tracks and spreading other types of bedding.

MULTI-PRONGED FORK sometimes found with the tines joined together across the points. This is used for removing droppings from bedding made from fine particles, such as shavings or sawdust. Some designs can be heavy and unwieldy for workers to use.

SHOVEL used for collecting up piles of detritus. Can have either a short or a long handle. Should be sufficiently sturdy to cope with prolonged damp and scraping on hard ground.

BROOMS come in two forms. Stiff-bristled ones, for sweeping up muck and wet areas, often have smaller heads and nylon bristles to withstand the wet and to get into corners and over rough surfaces. Soft-bristled ones may have a head up to 1m (3ft 3in) wide. They are extremely useful for sweeping up aisles and passages but will not last long if used in wet areas. Soft brooms with small heads are handy for sweeping down walls and removing cobwebs.

BRUSHES with very short handles are good for cleaning out feed bins and brushing off rugs. Scrubbing brushes are useful for cleaning out feed and water buckets.

SKIPS are used for the daytime collection of droppings from the stable and collecting up the sweepings from aisles and passages. Some people improvise with plastic laundry baskets but these soon break and need two hands to lift them. Purpose-built skips, made from heavy duty rubber-type material, can be carried with both handles in one hand and last longer. They should be emptied immediately after use and washed out as necessary.

WIRE RAKES can be used for tidying up shavings and sawdust type beddings and keeping the surface level.

RUBBER GLOVES are extremely useful for collecting droppings when skipping out. Heavy duty ones should be chosen, and ones with extra-long wrists can be handy when carrying out wet tasks. Disposable ones will also be useful for certain tasks.

WHEELBARROWS need to be chosen with care. The types sold for garden use are seldom a good choice in the stable yard. Single-wheel barrows need to be of sturdy construction and large enough to carry the waste from at least one stable. The wheel should be large enough to travel easily over the ground and be easy to maintain. They are less stable and prone to tip over if used on rough ground. Two-wheeled barrows are much more stable to push. They usually carry more and if properly cared for will last for many years. They are considerably more expensive to buy.

All wheelbarrows should be swept clean after use and stored so that they do not fill up with water. The wheels should be checked on a weekly basis for tyre pressure and to see that no baler twine is caught up in them. If the main body is painted annually with a good quality protective paint, they will last for years.

MUCK SACKS are not recommended for carrying stable waste to the muck heap. They are, however, very useful for carrying dry, loose bedding or forage from the storage area to the stable, especially if two people help each other. They are also useful for covering barrows and trailers to prevent their loads from dropping onto the ground. They can be bought ready-made, from tough, easily washed material and with a loop handle at each corner, or they can be made from the large bags in which fertiliser is delivered to farms.

MUCKING OUT

The method used needs to be quick, efficient and create as little dust and smell as possible. Some horses are really messy and others quite tidy. Knowing their individual habits helps to make the process easier. The more regularly skipping out is done during the day, the less bedding will be contaminated and the easier mucking out will be.

General Rules

It is easiest and better for the horse if he can be removed from the stable while mucking out is done. If he remains, he should be tied up.

All relevant tools should be collected and the barrow so placed that the handles are not in the way of horse or worker. There are two main methods: complete, usually used for straw and drainage bedding, and partial deep litter, often used with dense, absorbent bedding.

Complete Muck Out

1. Remove all obvious droppings, as if skipping out.

2. Sort wet and dry bedding in one half of the bed.

3. Put wet bedding in barrow and dry under the horse if he is in the stable.

4. Sweep floor and return dry, used bedding to clean area.

5. If possible move horse across.

6. Repeat steps 2 to 4 on second half of the box.

If fresh bedding is being introduced at the same time, build it into the sides of the bed during the day and put it down when the bed is set fair for the night. Most people like to keep some bedding on the floor during the day. Horses left to stand all day on hard floors are more likely to slip, less likely to stale and often the box

becomes very smelly. Older horses often like to lie down and rest their legs, as do animals which have been out all night. If the bedding is pushed well back from the door during the day it will not be trodden out when the horse is moved.

Semi-deep Litter

This is often used for absorbent bedding such as paper, shavings, Aubiose, etc. Use a shavings fork or sturdy rubber gloves.

• Remove the droppings and the wettest patches and pack any holes with drier bedding from the walls.

• Make sure the bed is level and of equal firmness throughout.

• Build fresh bedding into the walls.

• Sweep the entrance on a daily basis but properly dig through the whole bed once a week and rebuild it.

Whichever method is used, keep the barrow handles well out of the way of horses and passers by. Do not overload the barrow, and stack it correctly so that the weight falls on the wheel not the handles. Pack it down

Cross-section through stable.

raised bedding wall

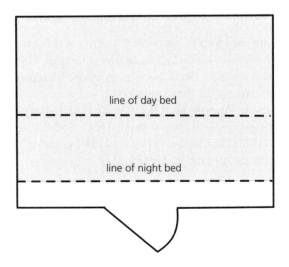

Stable seen from above.

line of day bed

line of night bed

so that the bedding is not blown over the yard, thus making more work. If windy, cover with a sack.

Tools should never be left in the stable with a horse. Use the muck fork away from the animal's legs, not towards them. Remove water buckets before work begins and clean and refresh them when work is complete. Remove bird droppings and dust from the stables on a regular basis.

When setting fair for the night, bring bedding nearer the door to prevent draughts and maintain walls to a minimum height to help prevent the horse from getting cast.

To test if the bedding is of a sufficient depth, turn the fork over so that the tines face downwards and pat the bed. The tines should not hit the floor. Less bedding is needed if rubber matting is underneath.

It should be possible to muck out a 4m x 4m (13ft x 13ft) box inside ten minutes once the worker is practised.

In many yards it is still the practice to wash out the boxes on a weekly basis. The floors should be allowed to dry completely before the bed is put back. In many areas water is in short supply or expensive. Relying on large amounts to clean stables may not be possible. However, where hygiene is paramount, such as in foaling boxes and isolation boxes, the use of a pressure hose is recommended.

Drains

It is vital that the drainage system is able to cope and will not be blocked with detritus. The type of sump shown, outside a stable complex, offers three ways in which debris can be prevented from blocking drains.

They will still need to be checked regularly and cleaned out as necessary. It is preferable not to sweep up outside stables on to the top of deep drains.

When mucking out is finished, clean the tools. Brush off shovels, barrows and skips. Pick straw out of brooms. Hose off anything that is very mucky and wash off gloves. If barrows are stood on end and tools stacked in a designated area they will last much longer and always be ready for use. Always empty skips immediately after use. In some large barn complexes the muck from all the boxes is forked out into the central aisle and then pushed straight out to the muckheap by machine. After the initial expense of buying the equipment, this can save considerably on time and effort.

Avoiding Dust Allergies

During the process of mucking out and shaking up a straw bed, there is considerable increase in the number of fungal spores in the atmosphere. This is not good for any horse and can be especially bad for one that suffers from COPD or similar wind problems. If possible, whenever straw is shaken up, the horse should be

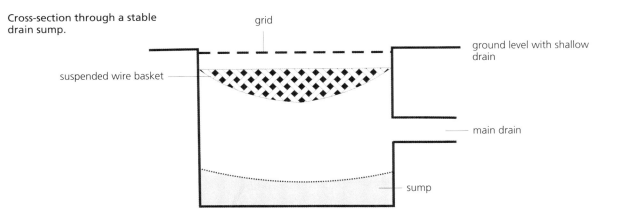

Cross-section through a stable drain sump.

grid

ground level with shallow drain

suspended wire basket

main drain

sump

removed from his stable. Consideration should also be given to animals in adjacent boxes.

Workers who suffer from asthma or who are allergic to dust should consider wearing dust masks.

Setting Fair

This is the term used when the bed is made ready for the night. It is most usually done at evening stables but can be done just as well in the morning if the horse is out all day.

- The bed is thoroughly skipped out.

- If a full bed is being used, the existing bedding is levelled and drawn further towards the door to minimise draughts. The side walls are well packed and if extra bedding has been stored on them during the day, it is spread evenly over the top of the bed to provide a dry, clean surface. If more bedding has to be carried in it will be used in the same way.

- If rubber matting is being used, ensure the horse has a clean and dry area to lie on. If the horse lies on a wet, soiled floor his rugs quickly become very smelly and unpleasant to handle.

- The water buckets should be emptied and refilled.

- The horse's hay or forage may also be carried in at this time, depending on the feeding regime.

Deep Litter

It is not recommended practice to deep litter horses. It is almost impossible to keep the fungal spores in the atmosphere down to acceptable levels. If it must be done, such as when yarding ponies or young stock, or when a horse is too ill to be disturbed, consider the following:

- The available fresh air: always choose the airiest available stable.

- It is better to rug the horse in an open-fronted stable than compromise on the volume of air.

- The type of bedding.

- The management.

- How to get rid of the waste.

- Make sure the access is good for when the time comes to remove the bed.

- Choose a light, non-dusty, absorbent bedding that compacts readily.

- One of the wood-derived beddings is likely to be ideal.

- The bed must be kept clean.

- All droppings should be removed each day.

- The bed should be kept level and any wet or soggy patches removed and the resulting hole filled with old bedding from around the edge.

- It must be well packed down.

- A regular, light sprinkling of fresh bedding over the whole surface will help to keep the stable free from ammonia fumes.

The whole bed should be removed when appropriate. This might be:

- When it gets so deep that it is difficult to get in and out.

- When the horse has recovered.

- If the bed gets too difficult to manage or becomes wet or smelly.

- At the end of the season.

It is easiest if it is removed by machine. A tractor with a fore-end loader or something similar is ideal. There will be a considerable amount of waste so ensure there is some way of getting rid of it. It will be quite well rotted at the base so may be saleable for garden use.

Deep litter is not an easy option. It may well suit some owners' lifestyles but still requires daily management if it is to succeed. It is essential that the horse's feet are kept clean and free from muck and bedding.

SIGNS OF GOOD AND ILL-HEALTH, AND SICK NURSING

Condition is the bodily state of the horse. An experienced manager with a trained eye will be able to recognise the condition of all the horses in his care, and will be quick to observe any change. He should look at each horse at least once a day, preferably twice, once in the morning and once in the evening, and each leg should be inspected manually.

See also page 27, for condition scoring.

SIGNS OF GOOD HEALTH

- A bright, alert expression.

- Clear eyes. The membrane under the lids should be pale salmon-pink in colour.

- No discharge from the eyes or nose. Discharge from eyes in summer could indicate irritation by flies.

- Mobile ears.

- A glossy coat which lies flat.

- Loose skin, which moves easily over the underlying bones.

- The horse stands with all four feet evenly on the ground or, if relaxed, resting only one hind leg.

- No visible sign of sweating when at rest, except in very hot weather or in humid conditions.

- Cool limbs, with no unusual swellings.

- Fairly opaque and colourless or pale yellow urine, which should be passed several times a day.

- Droppings that are free from any offensive smell and are passed several times a day. They may be of various colour and consistency, according to the diet.

- Normal appetite and water consumption.

- A temperature of 38°C (100.5°F). This can vary by up to half a degree night and morning (usually lower in the morning).

- A pulse rate at rest of 36 to 42 beats a minute.

- A respiration rate at rest of 8 to 12 inhalations a minute.

SIGNS OF ILL-HEALTH

It is important to recognise signs of ill-health as quickly as possible in order to minimise distress and damage to the horse. It is another reason why keeping the same carer with each horse is good practice. The carer should notice any change more quickly than someone less familiar with that horse's normal behaviour.

Signs which may signal a problem are:
- Feed/forage not eaten.
- Dust on water, indicating it has not been drunk recently.
- Bed disturbed.
- Scuff marks on the walls.
- Droppings of a different consistency from usual and/or

evil smelling.

- Horse distressed.
- Sweating.
- Kicking belly or just looking around at it.
- Rolling.
- Flatulence.
- Grinding teeth.
- Raised pulse, temperature or respiratory rates.
- Unusual behaviour – e.g. not coming to the door.
- Laid-back ears.
- Standing or lying down alone when in the field.
- Mucous membranes not salmon-pink. They may be pale, bright red or dark bluish in colour.
- Coughing.
- Runny nose – thin clear liquid or thicker yellow mucus.
- Bleeding from the nose.
- Standing awkwardly or unable to move easily when asked.
- Unable to get up.

The first task of the groom each morning is to look over each horse in their charge and to notice any of the changes already mentioned.

If any are noticed, look more carefully. As a rule of thumb, if there are three or more adverse signs or if any of the signs are severe or acute the stable manager should be informed and the decision made as to what further action to take.

WHEN TO CALL THE VETERINARY SURGEON

The decision as to when to call the veterinary surgeon is dependent on a number of factors, the two most obvious being:

- The severity of the symptoms.
- The knowledge/experience of the groom.

A veterinary surgeon should be consulted when:

- There is profuse bleeding.

- There is profuse, unexplained sweating.
- The horse is unable to stand or move.
- He shows any of the classic symptoms of colic.
- He has an unexplained raised pulse or temperature.
- He has very pale mucous membranes.
- He is grinding his teeth or showing other signs of acute pain.
- There are signs of choke.

Less acute symptoms which have persisted over one or two days or less and have not responded to treatment also need to be referred. With the new Welfare Bill now law, it is illegal to subject horses or other animals to abuse or neglect either on purpose or through ignorance.

Always consult a veterinary surgeon if in doubt as to the horse's well-being. It may be that a telephone call alone will solve the problem.

As carers/grooms become more expert they will notice signs and symptoms more quickly and should be able either to rectify the problem before it becomes serious, or to give the veterinary surgeon much useful information about the health of the animals in their charge.

SICK NURSING AND THE CONTROL OF INFECTION

At all times the attendant must be observant and use common sense to ensure the horse's welfare. Close attention must be paid to comfort, cleanliness and diet. The veterinary surgeon's instructions should be written down and followed carefully.

Stable

A very sick horse may well settle and be more peaceful if he is put in a loosebox in a quiet or separate part of the yard. Ideally it should be easily accessible at night and have well lit paths, etc. However, some horses become upset if they are required to change boxes, and are better left in their own environment where they have company.

Horses with eye trouble should have light restricted and smaller windows, and the top-door openings should be covered. Essential ventilation must be maintained.

Warmth

In cold weather, or in some forms of illness, warmth is essential and should be achieved by using extra lightweight clothing, rather than by restricting ventilation. There must be an ample supply of fresh air; the atmosphere in the box must never feel stuffy. Outside looseboxes may have the top door closed, provided that there is another adequate form of draught-proof ventilation. Stable bandages, warm, lightweight rugs and, on occasions, a hood, all help to combat the cold. An infra-red lamp fixed in the ceiling adds to the horse's comfort. This can usually be run from a suitable light fixture if no permanent socket is available.

In warm weather there must be an ample supply of fresh air but no draughts. Light rugs may be put on, but care must be taken that the horse does not become overheated, as excessive warmth can be damaging. A sweat rug or wicking rug is often ideal for both day and night-time use. The sweat rug may may need a light cover at night.

Bedding

An ample bed, with banked-up walls, should be provided. It should be kept clean and regularly skipped out. A weak or injured horse's leg may become entangled in deep straw, so this type of bedding should be well flattened and not shaken up unnecessarily. If an absorbent bedding is used, the problem is avoided and there is also less disturbance and dust when the bed is mucked out. If the horse is very sick a full mucking out may not be possible. In this case, semi deep litter with scrupulous skipping out is the answer. Using rubber matting, as long as it can be thoroughly disinfected once the box is vacant, is excellent. Shavings or sawdust are not suitable when a wound has to be left uncovered, or during foaling.

Grooming

In the case of very sick horses, grooming should be restricted. The eyes, nose, sheath and dock area should be sponged clean, and the horse may perhaps appreciate a light body brush or hand rubbing over his head and body. Stable bandages should be removed twice a day, and the legs hand-rubbed towards the heart. The feet should always be picked out carefully. A clean cotton sheet worn under the rugs can make a horse more comfortable.

In the case of infectious or contagious diseases, grooming should be discontinued, as brushing can only assist the spread of the infection.

In cases of lameness, or in convalescence, a thorough grooming can be beneficial and is usually enjoyed by the horse.

Hygiene

In cases of infectious or contagious disease, stable tools, grooming equipment and food utensils should all be kept separate. The attendant should wear a special overall, headgear and rubber gloves when looking after the horse. A bucket of strong disinfectant should be kept outside the door for washing boots. Jeyes Fluid is suitable. All articles, tools, buckets, etc. should be kept by the isolation box.

All hay, forage and bedding should be taken to the box, rather than the haynet being taken to the hay barn.

All used bedding and uneaten food should be burnt. All feeds should be prepared in a separate container and then emptied into the horse's manger, rather than the manger being taken to the feed room.

Ask your vet's advice on antiseptic for cleaning feed bins etc., but Milton is good and doesn't leave an unpleasant taste and smell.

Water

A constant supply of clean, fresh water must be available. In all cases where the horse's water intake has to be monitored, automatic watering bowls should be disconnected and water supplied by bucket. All water containers must be cleaned out and filled with water several times a day. This is particularly important where there are nasal discharges.

Diet

In all cases a low concentrate diet will be necessary. If possible it should be based on the one which the horse is used to, with the forage level being increased and the concentrate level decreased. It should include nutritious and easily digestible ingredients. Soaked sugar beet with chaff or molassed chaff, plus hay or vacuum-packed forage would provide an open yet balanced diet. Forage should be offered ad lib but only in small helpings – as soon as one haynet is finished it is replaced with another to avoid contamination. A horse with a nasal discharge will quickly contaminate the forage and then it is wasted. Meadow hay is easier to chew and to digest than seed hay, and horses with respiratory diseases are best fed from the ground, with the feed damped and the hay soaked. Fresh-cut grass makes a suitable and appetising ration. Apples, carrots or other roots may also tempt the appetite.

It is essential to appreciate the preferences and needs of the particular animal. All food should be freshly prepared and offered in small quantities. In some cases, hand feeding may be necessary. Uneaten food should be removed after half an hour and discarded.

Feed bowls and mangers should be washed out after every feed.

For special cases the veterinary surgeon may suggest a suitable diet.

Administration of Medicines

If medicines are mixed in feeds or added to the water, they may put the horse off his food or discourage him from drinking. It is better to mix them with water and administer them by syringe into the mouth, or mix them with treacle or soft margarine-type spread and put this on the tongue (see Chapter 10, Handling the Horse).

All administration of medicines or treatments needs to be recorded and the record kept by the stable. Then there is less likelihood of mistakes being made.

ROUTINE CARE

The horse's **temperature, pulse and respiration** should be taken morning and night and noted on a chart. This chart should also contain information as to the state of the dung and urine, how often they are passed, and also details of water consumption, food eaten and the horse's appetite.

In epidemic situations it is sensible to chart the temperatures of all horses in the yard morning and night.

As stated earlier, the **normal temperature of a horse is 38°C (100.5°F)**, although there can be slight variations from horse to horse.

To take the temperature
The horse should be held by an assistant. Sharp horses should have a front leg held up. The thermometer should be the type with a short, stubby end. Shake it until it registers below 37°C (99.5°F). Grease it with Vaseline or wet the thermometer and, standing to the side of the horse's quarters, insert two-thirds of it into the rectum. Leave it for half a minute, or as directed. The thermometer should be held firmly, as it can be drawn into the rectum and be difficult to recover. After taking it out and noting the reading, shake the thermometer down, wash it in cool disinfectant, dry it and replace it in its case. Modern digital thermometers obviate the need for shaking down before or after use and are quicker and easier to read.

To take the pulse
The **normal pulse of a horse at rest is 36 to 42 beats to the minute**. The pulse can be taken by a light feel of the artery as it crosses the horse's jaw bone. It is a skill which needs practice. It is helpful to have a watch with a second hand and a large, easily seen face.

Respiratory rate

The **normal respiration of a horse at rest is 8 to 12 inhalations per minute**. This can be observed by watching the movement of the horse's flank.

CONTROL OF INFECTION AND CONTAGION

It must be accepted that in many cases it is not possible to prevent the spread of airborne germs, or to stop other horses from becoming infected. The offending animal may be infectious for several days before showing any signs of illness. In any case, an isolation box is unlikely to be of use unless it is at least 400m (¼ mile) downwind from the yard. Birds and flies also carry germs.

Contagious conditions, for example ringworm, are passed by contact (direct – touch, or indirect – e.g. via a brush), and can be successfully isolated with strict care.

Isolation boxes should be used for housing animals new to the yard, particularly those bought from sales or any who have travelled long distances.

Precautions

- The person attending the horse should not be in contact with any other horses. They should wear overalls especially kept for the sick horse, rubber or disposable gloves and cover their hair. They should take care not to touch their face whilst ministering to the horse or wearing the contaminated clothing. All protective clothing should be stored by the isolation box and not worn on the general yard. It should be washed regularly.

- The veterinary surgeon should see other patients in the yard before seeing the infectious horse.

- Overall washing facilities and paper towels should be provided.

- A door grille prevents any passer-by from handling the horse and helps to prevent infection by contact.

- A warning notice should be pinned to the door.

- A supply of paper towels and cotton wool should be available for dealing with nasal discharge.

- Used material should be burned. Rubber gloves should be disinfected after use, or plastic disposable gloves used.

- In the case of contagious skin diseases, for example ringworm, the most likely points of infection and contact should be carefully watched on all other horses, for example the girth, saddle and bridle areas and where the rider's leg rests. Early signs of the disease can thus be noted and treatment given before it spreads. All riders should disinfect their boots before riding another horse.

- Horses with ringworm may be rideable. They should have their tack kept separate, and this should be disinfected each day. If numnahs and nylon tack are used, disinfection is easier and leather saddlery will not be harmed. Attendants and riders should bath each day, and if possible wash their hair. Special soap can be obtained. Particular attention should be paid to any place where there is friction from clothing, for instance the wrists, neck, etc.

CONVALESCENCE

A horse who has had a serious illness may need several months' convalescence before being brought back into work. If he has been on box rest for any length of time he will probably start by being walked in hand once or twice a day for increasing periods. He will then benefit from a period out to grass which may be for a number of weeks or months as recommended by his veterinary surgeon. After that he can be gradually brought back into work. Exercise may start with five minutes walking out and progress gradually as the horse gains strength. When work is resumed, it should progress in very slow stages, so that at no time is the horse put under strain.

The vet will recommend a suitable programme.

The horse must be kept warm without being overheated. Hill work of any sort should be avoided. Walking on long reins can give more control and less strain than lungeing. Work on a circle can put undue pressure on slack muscles.

CLEANING AND DISINFECTING STABLES AND EQUIPMENT

• Competition and racing yards usually employ professional cleaning services, and the buildings concerned can be steam cleaned. This is an expensive process, and the private owner or the small yard is more likely to do the work personally.

• To remove grease and dirt, use washing soda and bleach. Used together these are also an effective disinfectant, and kill fungus. A strong disinfectant, such as Jeyes Fluid or Lysol, also kills fungus.

• The Jockey Club recommends Halamid. DEFRA recommends creoline derivatives (synthetic Phonolee disinfectant, e.g. Hycolin).

• Always check before use as old products are superseded by new ones.

• All bedding should be removed and burned.

• The roof or ceiling should be washed down with a jet hose to remove all dust. The walls, doors (inside and out), windows and mangers should be scrubbed clean with washing soda and bleach.

• Brick or block walls may be Snowcemmed or emulsion painted.

• Clothing and grooming kit should be soaked in disinfectant (not bleach or soda) for six hours, then washed in detergent and carefully rinsed.

• Stable tools, buckets and portable mangers should be washed with strong washing soda and bleach.

• Leather saddlery which has been in contact with a fungal infection (for example, ringworm) should first

be cleaned with washing soda and water, then with a strong disinfectant. It can then be oiled. Soda is bad for leather, but a daily application of glycerine soap should restore it. Non-leather girths, numnahs and nylon tack should be soaked in strong disinfectant (Jeyes Fluid or Lysol) for six hours and then washed.

SOME BASIC TREATMENTS

POULTICES

Poultices may be used warm or cold, and can be applied anywhere on the horse where they can be kept in place successfully.

Warm Poultices
• Soften the tissues, so that pus can escape.

• Increase the blood supply to the injured area, and thus assist healing.

• Soothe bruising.

• Should be put on at a heat just bearable to sustained contact with the back of the hand.

Cold Poultices
• Reduce inflammation.

• Constrict blood vessels and arrest internal haemorrhage.

NOTE: Both warm and cold kaolin poultices eventually return to blood heat.

As a basic principle, cold poultices are for immediate use to ease inflammation; warm poultices are for infections, deep puncture wounds and to help the healing process once the original inflammation has subsided. Poultices are usually left on for twelve hours and then renewed. The poulticing of wounds on a joint, particularly the knee, should be done only on veterinary advice. Poultices are usually only applied for a maximum of 3–4 days. Any longer and there is a risk of proud flesh forming.

Types of Poultice

- **Kaolin** is a natural clay with medicinal properties. It may be applied warm or cold. It can be used on open wounds, but is better encased in muslin. It is used for bruising, strains and all foot injuries. It is economic to use when several days' poulticing are required.

- **Animalintex** is a prepared medicinal lint. It is applied warm or cold. It is used where there is an open wound, or for a punctured foot. It has less of a clogging effect than kaolin. It is more expensive than kaolin.

- **Glycerine and Epsom Salts** mixed to a paste may be applied cold, and are of particular value for coronet abscesses and swollen cannons.

- **Bran and Epsom Salts** 227g (½ lb) bran and 57–85g (2–3oz) of Epsom salts are mixed with hot water to form a stiff dough which is used for foot problems. The horse may be tempted to pull off and eat the bran poultice. A poultice boot usually prevents this. This type of poultice is less often used today. Few yards have bran readily available.

Leg Poultices

KAOLIN If applied warm, kaolin has to be heated in its tin or in a small container in a saucepan of boiling water. The lid should be eased so that steam can escape. The water must not be so deep that it can overflow into the tin. To test for temperature, stir well and then test a small portion on the back of the hand to ensure that it is not too hot. An over-hot poultice will blister the horse's skin. Kaolin may also be heated by spreading it approximately 6mm (¼ in) thick on a suitably sized piece of cotton or linen, or brown paper. This is then put on a flat container and placed either in an oven or under a grill on a low heat. It heats very quickly, and care should be taken that it does not dry out.

If kaolin is heated in a tin, the poultice is then spooned out on to a suitably sized piece of plastic, tin foil or brown paper. Test it again for heat and then place it on the injury; cover with thick Gamgee and secure with a stable or crepe bandage. This must be firm, but not tight. If the kaolin has previously been spread on cloth, this is placed on the injury, covered with plastic and Gamgee and bandaged as above. The purpose of the plastic is to keep in the heat, exclude air and retain moisture, thus allowing the poultice to work.

ANIMALINTEX A suitably sized piece of Animalintex is cut off and placed on a plate or other clean surface. The Animalintex is then saturated with boiling water. The surplus is removed either by placing another plate of equal size over it and squeezing, or by placing it between plastic sheets and squeezing. Test the Animalintex for heat on the back of the hand and apply directly to the injury, dressing side down. The Animalintex is covered and kept in place in a similar way to kaolin (the plastic covering is essential). It can also be used as a dry poultice, or dampened with water if applied cold (see instructions on packet).

GLYCERINE AND EPSOM SALTS Place the paste over the wound, cover with plastic, and bandage, as for kaolin.

Foot Poultices

All surfaces of the foot should be scrubbed clean.

USING AN EQUI BOOT The selected poultice is placed over the area of the foot to be treated. Plastic is put on top and the Equi Boot then put on and secured to the foot. If the boot fits well, it is sometimes possible to allow the animal to be turned out.

USING A POULTICE BOOT The poultice is put on as above. Bran or Epsom salts or yeast may be used instead. Place the poultice over the sole of the foot, cover with plastic, place the foot in the poultice boot and fasten securely. The leg should be protected with Gamgee and a stable bandage. The heel of the foot, if not the seat of injury, should be protected by a layer of thick grease.

USING A THICK PLASTIC BAG AND/OR SACK The selected poultice is either placed on the sole of the foot or, if it is bran based, is placed in the bottom of a strong plastic bag. The foot is then placed in the bag, which may be covered with sacking. This is then wrapped round the fetlock and leg. The leg should be protected with Gamgee. The sack and/or bag can be tied round the pastern with an old crepe bandage or string. A stockinette bandage is then put on to secure the Gamgee and the top of the sack or plastic bag. This is made more secure by putting on a stable bandage. With heavyweight horses it may be necessary to reinforce the bag or sack. The pressure of weight quickly wears through a thin layer of sacking or plastic. It is advisable to apply the poultice as near to the stable as possible to prevent undue wear. A cradle may be needed to prevent the horse from removing the dressing.

Cold Kaolin Poultices

These should be chilled in a refrigerator before use. They can be applied with advantage to all four legs of a horse after any type of severe work. The kaolin is put on the leg by hand, then covered with brown paper and thick Gamgee. A secure, but not tight, stable bandage is then put on. Various forms of prepared bandage for use as a cold poultice are now available.

Inflamed Backs

Inflammation under the saddle can be reduced by putting cold kaolin on the area and covering it with plastic. This can be held in place by Elastoplast.

Cut Animalintex to shape, pour on boiling water, leave until cool enough to handle, then squeeze out water.

Place on sole, push into frog, and cover with plastic, e.g.clingfilm.

Secure with Vetrap bandage, using heel as anchor; cross Vetrap over foot towards toe.

Keep bandage low on heel, to avoid pressure on tendons; secure with Elastoplast.

Place foot in Equi-Boot or poultice boot, or encase in thick plastic bag and/or sack.

Apply stable bandage for support and to prevent possible filling of the leg; a similar bandage should also be applied to the 'good' leg.

Poulticing a foot using Animalintex.

KNEE, HOCK AND HEEL BANDAGES

Knee or Hock Bandage

Apply the dressing or poultice as directed, and cover all surfaces of the joint with thick Gamgee. With the knee, it is the bony projection (pisiform bone) at the back of the knee joint which may become susceptible to friction, particularly when the joint is moved. This area must be kept free from bandage pressure.

The bandage, preferably crepe or 'Vetwrap' type, is started above or below the joint with two secure rounds.

It is then put into a figure-of-eight around the joint, leaving the back of the knee or point of the hock free. If the front of the knee is the area injured it must always be kept free from pressure, with the crosses being at the sides. The bandage can finish above or below the joint but should end with one more round to complete and assure security. A stable bandage should be placed on the leg below the joint to prevent the upper bandage slipping down.

Putting on knee and hock bandages requires considerable skill and experience. It is advisable to practise beforehand, so that should the necessity arise the bandaging itself will cause no problem.

Horses often attempt to chew at a knee covering, especially over a wound (see Chapters 8 and 10).

Various patented forms of leg support and protection are now available, some of which can be used to retain poultices and dressings, particularly on awkward areas such as the knee or hock (e.g. Tubigrip or Vetrap bandages).

NB: In all cases of leg or foot injury, thick Gamgee and a support bandage should be placed on the opposite leg to prevent filling and to ease strain.

Heel Bandage

This is very useful to apply a dressing to an over-reach or to prevent over-reach boots rubbing the bulb of the heel. A small dressing is placed over the wound if necessary and then Vetwrap is applied starting at the front of the coronary band, over one heel bulb, twisted, applied over the other heel and back to the front. Two rounds should be enough. As it does not cover the shoe it should stay in place during exercise.

PRESSURE BANDAGES

This type of bandage is used after a suspected tendon injury. The bandage helps to limit any swelling caused by the injury. Such swelling interferes with the healing process. The bandage, preferably crepe, should be put on over a thick layer of evenly applied Gamgee. It should be removed each morning and night, and the leg should be given a brisk massage by hand, the hands working in an upward direction towards the heart. Veterinary advice should be sought before long-term treatment with pressure bandages.

TUBBING

This is useful for puncture wounds in the foot. It draws out pus without softening the horn and can help relieve pain from a bruised sole.

METHOD

• Scrub the foot clean. Grease the heel with Vaseline.

• Use a clean container of heavy duty plastic or rubber. The handle should be removed.

• Dissolve 227g (8oz) of Epsom salts in hot water.

• Place the Epsom salts and water in the container and reduce to blood heat.

• Place the horse's foot in the container and soak for ten minutes. Top up with water if required.

• Repeat three or four times a day.

• It is not advisable to tie the horse up whilst tubbing.

• always dry the heels after treatment.

FOMENTING

This is a method of applying heat and/or cold to areas which cannot be poulticed.

METHOD

• Dissolve 227g (8oz) of Epsom salts in hot water.

• Place the Epsom salts and water in a bucket and reduce to blood temperature.

- Soak an old towel in the water, wring it out and apply to the affected area.

- Repeat every minute and continue for fifteen to twenty minutes. Top up with hot water as required.

This is useful for drawing out infection. If used too much proud flesh may form.

Hot and Cold Fomenting

Hot and cold fomenting is useful to reduce pain and swelling in cases where the skin is unbroken, such as lymphangitis.

METHOD
- Have two buckets of water, one a little more than hand hot, the other with cold water and ice in it.

- Have two cloths, one for each bucket. Wring them out alternately and apply to the area, as one returns to neutral temperature, replace with the other. Repeat for ten minutes three or four times a day.

COLD HOSING

This treatment is appropriate for the immediate relief of bruising, for instance following a kick, or a bang when jumping. It is also appropriate for cleansing a wound and assisting in restricting blood flow to arrest bleeding.

METHOD
- Ask an assistant to hold the horse, who may need to be bridled for extra control.

- Run the water gently over the foot at minimum pressure.

- Gradually work up the leg to the bruised area or wound, and allow a slight increase of water pressure.

- For bruising continue the treatment for ten minutes, and repeat four or five times during the day. There is little point in hosing for longer than ten minutes in

Fomenting a forearm.

any one session, as the capillaries will have reduced in that time.

- An alternative, if available, is to stand the horse in a running stream or in the sea.

- Always dry the heels when the treatment is over.

Pressure bandages, if practicable, may be applied between hosing sessions.

COLD BANDAGES

Patented forms of cold pack are now available. Makers' instructions should be followed. These packs can be held in place on the leg with a light bandage. Gamgee, or similar, should be placed underneath the bandage.

An ice-pack can be made by crushing ice cubes in a cloth and placing them in a plastic bag. Cover the leg with Gamgee, or similar, and put the ice bag on the leg and secure with Gamgee or a light bandage. Purpose-made 'ice' preparations are widely available. Vetrap bandages are light, versatile and effective, though expensive.

Great care should be taken with any type of frozen/iced application that 'burning' does not create greater problems than the curing effect.

CHAPTER 16

BASIC SYSTEMS OF THE HORSE & HOW TO GET A HORSE FIT

In order to maintain basic good health the horse needs regular exercise. He is not designed to be cooped up in a stable for twenty-three hours a day. His basic functions and systems such as digestion, his respiratory, circulatory and lymphatic systems, all benefit from regular exercise and fresh air and his muscles will only maintain or improve their function if they are used. See simple facts about muscles, page 17.

If the horse lives out he will be less bored than if he is in but he will not maintain much fitness – although a sloping field will help a little.

It is important to have a basic understanding of the systems mentioned above.

• The Respiratory system, page 135

• The Circulatory system, page 136

• The Lymphatic system, page 137

• The Digestive system, page 161

Definition of fit

The horse is fit when he is able, without undue strain, to perform his normal work. Obviously a horse required for gentle hacking will not require the same level of fitness as a competition horse.

See Chapter 36 for specialist fittening.

Basic fittening programme

To create and maintain a satisfactory level of fitness a regular and sustained exercise regime needs to be in place.

Alongside the exercise, thought has to be given to the feeding and general welfare.

Even the horse who is only used for gentle hacking should have his own annual programme of care and management.

An easy way to organise this is to use a wall chart. On it, fill in all unalterable dates such as vaccination dates. Next, fill in holidays or times when he won't be worked. Then fill in shoeing check dates, approximately every six weeks, and worming dates possibly every six to eight weeks.

By now you will be able to see a pattern emerging.

Although the horse is not working hard it is preferable for him to have a regular day off – possibly a weekday if his owner works.

When designing a fittening programme the following need to be considered:

• Age.

• Present level of fitness.

• Desired level of fitness.

• Soundness.

• Temperament.

• Whether he has been fit before.

• Opportunities for exercise.

When fittening from scratch, start by checking the horse over to ensure that he is in good health. Check the following:

- Teeth – have them checked by a veterinary surgeon or horse dentist.

- Feet – have him shod by a good farrier.

- Skin – ensure it is clean and healthy and harden the saddle and girth areas with saline solution.

- Worming programme, see Chapter 17.

- Vaccinations – start the vaccination programme if needed. See Appendix 4.

The fitness programme can now be worked out under the following headings: exercise, feeding and care.

EXERCISE: In the first week start with walking, about 20 minutes the first day, increasing by about 10 minutes a day until walking for about 45 minutes a day on level ground.

FEED: Only a maintenance ration is needed at this time. See Chapter 20.

CARE: If possible keep the horse living out. Prevent coughs, colds and sore skin. Do not let the horse sweat. In the second week continue to increase work time by about 10 minutes a day. Stay in walk but include slight slopes uphill, if possible. Feed and care stay the same. In the third week increase exercise until he is doing between 1 and 1½ hours. Once he has been working for 40–50 minutes a day for a week, introduce trot on level ground. Start with 5 minutes and increase by 5 minutes daily until he is trotting for 15 minutes and walking for the rest of the time.

FEED: By now he will feel in need of more energy and can start on hard feed. Begin with ½-1 kilo (1–2lb) of coarse mix or horse and pony cubes and ad lib forage or grazing.

CARE: If he has to be stabled he can start now, but keep as much ventilation as possible and ensure all bedding and feed is dust free. If he is stabled begin to groom thoroughly and get the coat and skin clean.

FOURTH WEEK: By now he is working for his maximum time of 1–1½ hours a day. By now his skin is more accustomed to the tack and he can start to sweat. Walk and trot on more undulating ground. Do most trotting up hills but some downhill on good going will help teach self-balance. Introduce canter. Start with 1 minute and increase by 1 minute until 5 minutes is reached. Canter two or three times a week.

FEED: Increase his concentrates in line with his energy requirements.

FIFTH WEEK: Continue to improve on the work of the previous week. He is now fit enough to begin schooling if required. Start with two or three times a week for 10–15 minutes.

SIXTH WEEK: The horse is now at a level of fitness which can be maintained or increased if he is needed to go on to compete. He should be able to work in each gait for a third of the time he is out. He can be schooled two or three times a week, if required.

FEED: He should be on a diet of approximately 30% concentrates and 70% forage and/or grazing.

CARE: He will need shoeing. Check fit of tack, as he becomes fitter he will change shape.

A varied programme of work with changes of environment and ground, and a balance of hacking and schooling and plenty of turnout time will keep most horses happy and at a reasonable level of fitness. A horse with this level of fitness could occasionally work for 2 or 3 hours a day if the work was mainly walking and trotting. If he was required to canter and gallop as in a hunter trials he might need another two weeks with a bit more canter work.

Training and schooling does not always have to take

place in an arena. The horse can be ridden forwards from leg to hand and work on the bit out hacking. By changing diagonals regularly to follow the bends in the road the horse can be encouraged to improve his lateral suppleness, and by working over uneven ground he will learn to work in self-balance.

Walk is an important gait and should form at least one third of the horse's exercise time. Walking at the beginning of exercise allows the muscles to warm up gradually. Walking breaks during work are a reward and prevent muscle strain. Walking at the end of work allows the horse to warm down and arrive back in the stable in a cool, dry and relaxed state. The walk should be active, on the aids and have a regular 4:4 rhythm.

Trot is the gait to improve musculature as it is possible to work specific groups of muscles. Muscles only develop with work and then need continued work to maintain or increase their development.

Canter is an excellent gait for improving the cardio-vascular system. The horse's breathing works alongside its action. Every time the leading leg hits the ground the horse will exhale (breathe out), therefore the rider can control the respiratory rate by the speed and quality of the canter. Canter work is very important if the horse is going to small competitions, long, fast hacks, hunter trials or fun rides. If any of these form part of the horse's programme, put them on the chart and use the two weeks before to bring him up to the required fitness level.

The fitter a horse is for the level of work he normally does, the less likelihood there is of him breaking down.

The timings given are suggestions only as each horse is different. Always monitor progress, make a note of anything worthwhile and if in doubt take the programme back a bit, allowing an extra day or two before progressing to the next stage. Consider whether the feeding regime needs changing if the horse is too idle, lazy, excitable, thin or fat.

Feel the horse's legs every day and note any changes. Keep an eye on his skin. Keep to the care routine that you planned in the beginning.

Note also when things are going well as you may want to repeat the same programme next season.

RESPIRATORY SYSTEM

The primary function of the respiratory system is to provide oxygen for the body and to eliminate carbon dioxide.

It also eliminates water all the time; this can be easily seen on a cold day.

It assists in temperature control by breathing out warm air and taking in cool air.

There is some sensory application through smell and touch and it is involved in voice production.

Oxygen is taken into the **nostrils** only (not the mouth) through the **nasal passages**. The air is warmed and is filtered by very fine hairs. The mucous membrane lining the nasal passages also assists in making sure that the air reaching the lungs is clean. The nerve endings which detect smell (**olfactory nerve endings**) are in the higher part of the nasal passage.

The **pharynx** or throat is the common area at the back of the mouth where the food coming from the mouth and the air from the nostrils share the passage before passing down the oesophagus and windpipe respectively. The **epiglottis** closes automatically over the **windpipe** when the horse swallows to prevent food passing into the wrong tube.

From the pharynx, air passes through the **larynx (voice box)** which is the organ producing voice. The larynx also further filters foreign bodies from the air entering the lungs.

The **windpipe or trachea** runs from the larynx to the lungs, it branches in the chest into two **bronchi**, one **bronchus** passing into each lung.

The **bronchi** then continuously subdivide again and again into **bronchioles**, ultimately ending in **alveoli (air sacs)**. The multitude of **alveoli** provide a huge surface area of cells which allows for exchange of gases through the cell walls. The **lungs** are large, elastic organs; they fill the thoracic cavity and are enclosed by the protection of the ribs, and lie above the diaphragm. The lungs are enclosed by their own protective membrane (**pleura**). The lungs are flexible and able to expand and contract with the intake and expulsion of air. The fine system of blood vessels allows oxygen in air to diffuse through the alveolar walls into the blood, and carbon dioxide and water to diffuse from the blood to the air. The carbon dioxide laden air is then exhaled along the same route as inhalation.

The thorax expands through muscular action, which draws air into the nostrils and down to the lungs. In exhalation the air is expelled through elastic recoil of the rib cage. At rest the horse's respiratory rate is in the region of 8 to 12 breaths per minute. In extreme sustained exertion this rate may increase to 120 breaths per minute. The horse takes in more air as exertion makes greater demands on the system.

THE CIRCULATORY SYSTEM

The circulatory system functions as follows:

• Carries oxygen from the lungs to all parts of the body.

• Carries carbon dioxide from all parts of the body back to the lungs.

• Carries water and nutrients from the gut to the body cells.

• Carries waste products from the body cells to the kidneys.

• Transports hormones from the endocrine glands to other organs in the body.

• Provides a defence system for the body.

• Maintains body temperature.

Blood is made up of:

PLASMA, which itself is serum carrying fibrinogen which assists in the clotting of blood.

PLATELETS also assist in the clotting process.

CELLS which are further divided into red cells or white cells. Red cells originate in the bone marrow. They contain haemoglobin and this substance has the ability to combine with and carry oxygen to the organs in all parts of the body; the oxygen is then released and carbon dioxide is picked up to return to the lungs. White cells defend against infection by attacking and destroying harmful germs.

The heart is a cone-shaped muscle contained in a protective cover called the pericardium. It is in the thoracic cavity slightly to the left of centre. The heart has four chambers. The upper chambers are atria (or auricles) and the lower chambers are ventricles. The heart maintains the circulation of the blood.

Oxygenated blood leaves the heart through the **aorta** from the **left ventricle** and is transported to all parts of the body through **arteries.** The arteries subdivide into arterioles and ultimately into capillaries to supply all parts of the body, where the oxygen is given up to the body tissue. Deoxygenated blood then returns through capillaries, venules and into veins to carry the carbon dioxide back to the right side of the heart, arriving through the **vena cava** into the **right atrium.** Blood then passes into the **right ventricle** through the **mitral valve** and from there is pushed via the **pulmonary artery** to the lungs, where the carbon dioxide is deposited and replaced by a new uptake of oxygen (see Respiratory System). Oxygenated blood passes through the **pulmonary vein** to the **left atrium** and from there it passes through a one-way valve (the **tricuspid valve)** into the right ventricle and the whole cycle starts again. Both sides of the heart work in parallel so both atria fill and then contract and blood passes into the ventricles, both ventricles contract and send blood under pressure into the aorta and the pulmonary artery.

Arteries are thicker blood vessels than veins as they take blood under pressure from the heart away to other parts of the body. Veins are returning blood to the heart and therefore the blood is under less pressure.

Structure of the heart.

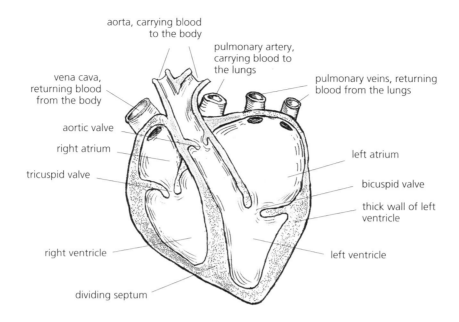

aorta, carrying blood
to the body

pulmonary artery,
carrying blood to
the lungs

vena cava,
returning blood
from the body

pulmonary veins, returning
blood from the lungs

aortic valve

right atrium

left atrium

tricuspid valve

bicuspid valve

thick wall of left
ventricle

right ventricle

left ventricle

dividing septum

THE LYMPHATIC SYSTEM

The lymphatic system works closely with the circulatory system. Its function is to retrieve the fluid which diffuses from the capillaries into tissues when bringing white blood cells, nutrients and oxygen to the cells. The lymphatic vessel walls are extremely thin and the lymphatic fluid should pass between the blood vessels and the lymphatic vessels with ease. The blood supply is pumped around the body by the heart. The lymphatic system has no pump as such and has to rely on movement from other body functions, especially movement from the limbs, to keep the fluid moving back towards the heart. It has a system of one-way valves to ensure the correct direction of flow. The vessels also have bean-shaped lymph nodes or filters to check the lymph for infection and to trigger the production of lymphocytes and antibodies if required. These nodes increase in size when there is an infection and are particularly prominent under the jaw and inside the thigh.

When there is inflammation the lymphatic system cannot remove the lymphatic fluid and the inflammation increases. The horse is then often in discomfort and reluctant to move, thus perpetuating the problem.

INTERNAL PARASITES

'Worms' are the common name given to an important group of internal parasites of the horse. All horses and ponies, except newborn foals, may suffer from a worm burden.

Worms cause anaemia, debility, unthriftiness and colic. This means that horses are not able to work up to their true potential, food is wasted and young horses do not grow properly. Almost 90% of all colic cases can be traceable to worm infestation. In some cases they lead to death.

A proper routine to control worms is, therefore, an essential part of any horse-care programme. Money spent on wormers (anthelmintics) is excellent insurance for cheerful, healthy horses and ponies, who can enjoy their work and give of their best.

Symptoms of Worms

The following symptoms should be cause for concern, although some may occur for other reasons:

- The horse eats well but doesn't put on condition.

- He has a large belly but very little condition along his top line.

- His skin feels dry and inelastic. His coat is harsh and 'staring'.

- He is anaemic. This can be confirmed by veterinary investigation.

- He has little energy and tires quickly.

- His droppings are loose and smelly; sometimes there may be diarrhoea.

- He has recurring attacks of colic.

- He has a short, dry cough.

Any, or a combination of these symptoms, warrants veterinary investigation.

NB: It is possible for horses and ponies to have a serious worm burden without visible outward signs.

Worm Egg Count

Worm infestation can be assessed by counting the number of eggs per gram of faeces. If any eggs are counted this indicates that there are adult worms of some species 'passing'/laying eggs. These eggs can be hatched out in a laboratory and the larvae allowed to develop to be identified by a specialist.

The number of eggs per gram can vary from as few as fifty to tens of thousands. A high count would indicate a large number of adult females. A low count simply tells the story on that day and the number could rise rapidly within a few weeks.

The number of eggs per gram is usually required by the veterinarian either to investigate a current problem and/or to help plan a control system.

Horse owners should accept the fact that all horses at grass have some worms. There is no 100% effective way of eradicating worms, only reducing numbers to a manageable level.

If a horse is not thriving, the veterinary surgeon may well recommend a blood test. This can also help to confirm the level of the worm burden.

Life Cycle

Under conditions of moisture and warmth in the sward, eggs can hatch in a few days or lie dormant for many months or years. The optimum time for hatching and development is spring and early autumn. Hatching larvae are called first stage larvae and, subject to moisture and temperature, these moult to become second and third stage. The interval between stages varies with the time of year.

There is a large loss of eggs and larvae under normal conditions, particularly in excessively hot and dry weather. The weather in the UK is unlikely ever to be cold enough for long enough to do the eggs any damage in cold weather. Eggs and larvae in stages one and two cannot develop further if eaten; they are digested. Stage three cannot feed, and unless consumed within a few days, they will die. They take up position in droplets of moisture on grass and these droplets travel up the blade to be more readily eaten. Once consumed, irrespective of species, the third-stage larvae penetrate the mucosal lining of the gut, where they moult again to become fourth stage. After a variable period within the gut lining they leave to live on the surface of the bowel, and there become adult males and egg-laying females.

There are variations once larval penetration into the gut has taken place.

Strongylus vulgaris (Large Redworms)

As a result of the development of the drug Ivermectin, which kills migrating larvae, the incidence of worm infestation has greatly reduced. The worm larvae pass through the bowel wall into the blood vessels and travel along them until they reach the junction of the gut artery and the aorta. Here they may sit for up to three months before returning to the bowel to become adult egg-laying worms. The waiting larvae can cause a thrombus (blood clot), which may partially or completely block the blood supply to the large intestine, impairing the gut's ability to digest food, and in the worst scenario causing death.

SYMPTOMS
Loss of condition may be visible if the horse has a heavy infestation of redworm. Intermittent colic for no apparent reason is the most common symptom.

CONTROL
Ivermectin, dosed every 8–10 weeks.

The other species of large redworm (*Strongylus edentatus*) migrates through the peritoneal cavity, setting up streaks of peritonitis with adhesions which could entrap parts of the small intestine. The migration of edentatus is not so long as that of vulgaris. Symptoms and control are as for *Strongylus vulgaris*.

Cyathostomes (Small Redworms)

There are forty species of small redworm, not all appearing in any one horse. Although they do not leave the gut they can become encysted within the mucosa and remain in that dormant situation for weeks or months. In this state they are much less easy to kill and their numbers increase. It is the sudden release en masse of these encysted worms into the lumen that causes acute enteritis, often with diarrhoea, but more frequently the pathological effect is one of abdominal shock.

SYMPTOMS
Poor condition and sometimes very acute weight loss accompanied by the onset of diarrhoea. This may indicate a life-threatening situation.

CONTROL
Treatment as for large strongyles.

Parascaris equorum (Roundworms)

These are most common in foals and yearlings. The predilection site is the small intestine. The eggs are deposited in stables and pasture. They can live for many years and are resistant to most chemical disinfectants. The eggs are taken in by the mouth during suckling from a contaminated teat, from udder skin or when grazing. The eggs hatch in the intestines; the larvae penetrate the gut wall and enter the lymph stream, travelling through the liver and then via the blood to the heart and the lungs, then into the airways to the throat and so back to the small intestine.

SYMPTOMS
Unthriftiness, emaciation, dry staring coat, pot belly. Sometimes there is an unexplained respiratory illness and coughing.

CONTROL
All common anthelmintic drugs are effective. Foals should be treated from six weeks of age every four weeks with a wormer safe for foals.

Gasterophilus Species (Bots)

The predilection site of these larvae of horse bot flies is the stomach. The female fly lays eggs on the hairs of the horse's legs. They cause irritation and, when licked by the horse, hatch and migrate to the stomach. They are passed out in the dung as mature larvae which pupate and develop into flies during the summer.

SYMPTOMS
Very unlikely to show specific symptoms unless present in huge numbers, when colic could result.

The eggs can be seen on the legs in summer and autumn. They appear as small yellow dots on the leg hairs and should be removed by scraping off with a blunt knife or clipping off the hairs and then burning them.

CONTROL
Ivermectin should be given in one annual dose. If eggs are seen on the legs during the summer, they can be inactivated by washing vigorously with warm water containing an insecticide; alternatively they may be shaved off.

Strongyloides westeri (Threadworms)

The predilection site is the small intestine. These parasites can be free-living, especially in warm, humid conditions such as deep-litter beds. They are of importance in foals. Infection can occur by two different routes. First, and most common, is via the dam's milk. The second is via penetration of the skin.

SYMPTOMS
There is persistent scouring in the foal after the foal heat. The mare is simply a carrier of infection and shows no clinical signs.

CONTROL
The stables should be kept clean and dry. With very young infected foals, veterinary help should be sought. Thiabendazole or Ivermectin are the usual drugs used. It is difficult, if not impossible, to control the larvae in the mare and therefore the resultant infection in the foal.

Oxyuris equi (Pinworms)

The predilection site is the large intestine. The eggs containing larvae are taken in by mouth. These hatch and the worms develop in the wall of the large intestine before returning to the lumen of the gut. When mature, the female moves to the anus to lay her eggs.

SYMPTOMS
Because of the irritation caused by the egg-laying females, the horse rubs the top of the tail and sometimes breaks the skin. Similar signs are seen in sweet itch and louse infestation.

CONTROL
The treatment for other worms also deals with

pinworms. The eggs should be washed off from under the tail with a disposable cloth.

Dictyocaulus arnfeldi (Lungworms)

The predilection site is the major airways of the lungs. Lungworms are particularly common in donkeys, who are the main carriers of infection, although they may show no symptoms. The larvae are taken in from pasture and migrate through the lymphatic and blood system to the lungs. Mature worms produce larvae which then pass up the throat, are swallowed and hence excreted in the dung to develop to the infective stage on pasture. In horses over a year old the worms remain small and immature, and do not produce larvae, which makes diagnosis from the dung impossible. This is not so in foals and donkeys, where infection can frequently be diagnosed by finding larvae in the dung.

SYMPTOMS

These only show in horses over one year old. A horse develops a persistent, chronic cough. Often, diagnosis is retrospective, after a favourable response to treatment with an anthelmintic effective against lungworms.

CONTROL

Donkeys should be routinely treated in the spring. A single dose of Ivermectin, or twice the normal dose of Mebendazole for five days running, has been found effective. Treatment of horses may prove difficult, and veterinary advice should be sought.

Tapeworms

There is evidence that horses can suffer problems from tapeworms, although clinical symptoms are relatively uncommon. A double dose of Pyrantel should be given in September.

WORM CONTROL

The worming of all horses, ponies and donkeys, especially those living at grass, should be carried out on a regular basis, in accordance with veterinary advice. It is a false economy to cut back on worming, especially with young animals.

Some parasites can build up a resistance to the group of Benzimidazole drugs. If a Benzimidazole compound is used then worming should be carried out every 4 weeks; if Pyrantel is used then every 6–8 weeks is advisable; with Ivermectin, every 8–10 weeks should suffice. If the wormer being used does not control bots (see Methods of Dosing, below), Ivermectin should be given once during the winter. Ivermectin is lethal to large and small strongyles and will kill bots. There is evidence that it will control blood-sucking lice. Two doses, eight weeks apart, between November and January are worthwhile.

Foals are particularly susceptible to worm damage, as they have little immunity. This damage, apart from stunting their growth or even killing them, may affect them throughout their working lives. They should be dosed every month from six weeks onwards with an anthelmintic safe for foals and effective against *Parascaris equorum*.

As grass is the commonest method of access for worms, the importance of clean grazing cannot be over-emphasised. Rotation of pasture, cross-grazing, preferably with cattle but also with sheep, especially during the spring and summer, helps reduce the population of infective larvae on the grass.

The daily picking up of droppings in small paddocks greatly reduces the chances of infestation and increases the amount of palatable grass.

Taking a crop of hay from fields also reduces infestation.

All new horses should be routinely dosed and kept in for 72 hours before being turned out and preferably turned out onto 'clean', rested pasture.

Even one untreated horse can contaminate the pasture and cause reinfestation of his companions. With grass-kept horses, all in any one field should be wormed on the same day, preferably kept in for 24 hours and then turned out on fresh, clean pasture. The old pasture should be cleaned of droppings, top-harrowed, grazed by sheep or cattle and then rested until the grass has regrown to a suitable height.

It is not sufficient to spread the droppings out onto the pasture unless the weather is very hot and dry for some weeks and the grass is very short.

At present, nothing is known which can be put on grassland to kill the eggs or larvae.

Studs and any enterprise that has a reasonable acreage should consider investing in a vacuum cleaner to keep the fields clean.

It is important with stabled horses to prevent their feed and hay from being contaminated by eggs or larvae from the faeces. If they are fed on the ground the stable hygiene must be impeccable.

Methods of Dosing

Powder (as such or in suspension) – added to feed
Granules – added to feed
Pellets – added to feed
Paste – in a dosing syringe

Active Principles of Anthelmintics

It is very important to read the name of the active principle as well as the trade name, so that the correct anthelmintic is used.

Benzimidazole Group
The advantages of this group of drugs are that they are of a broad spectrum, that is, they deal with many species of worms, and they are very safe. However, resistance to the whole group may be caused by using one of these drugs exclusively over a long period. Their use must be monitored with faecal egg counts, measured before and after worming. If the egg count does not noticeably drop then this compound should be abandoned and an alternative type of drug should be used.

The present range includes:

- Thiabendazole
- Mebendazole
- Fenbendazole
- Oxfendazole
- Oxibendazole
- Febantel

NB This group of drugs is not effective against bots.

Ivermectin
This is a broad-spectrum drug, which also kills bots. It is unrelated to the Benzimidazole group. It is sold under a number of different brand names.

Pyrantel
This is a broad-spectrum drug which, like Ivermectin, has the advantage that it is not related to the Benzimidazole group. It has no activity against bots.

Frequency of Dosing

The interval between treatments recommended for routine parasite control programmes is four to eight weeks. For this period the dung will be free of eggs so that further pasture contamination is prevented. There are so many variations in the effects worms have on horses, in conjunction with environment, age, grazing, numbers, etc. Not only should suspected parasite infestation be under the guidance of a veterinary surgeon but a programme of control should be planned between veterinarian and yard owner.

Some modern veterinary thinking has raised concerns about using chemicals on such a frequent basis. It has been found that in some yards which have a stable horse population, satisfactory worm control is maintained with mature horses only being wormed twice a year.

By using a mixture of scrupulous pasture cleaning and not feeding on the ground, combined with careful monitoring of the worm burden by egg counts of the faeces and blood tests if recommended by the veterinary surgeon, it is possible to keep the worm burden down to an acceptable level.

Sample about 10%–20% of animals, or as advised by your vet. They should be a variety of ages, sizes, weights, etc. and should include any who show signs of worm infestation. This will give a good indication of whether the worm programme is satisfactory.

Any animals fresh to the yard should be wormed before being introduced to the rest of the herd unless you are satisfied that they have been wormed regularly.

Adult horses who are well managed and fed particularly on pasture where there is a faecal clearing programme rarely suffer from what should be a comparatively small adult worm burden. The aim of routine treatment is to reduce the number of eggs passed out throughout the year and thus reduce the number of larvae which mature on the pasture. Especially nowadays with the small redworms, it is the level of consumption of their larvae which can prove dangerous to stock, in particular young horses.

18 STABLE VICES AND PROBLEM BEHAVIOUR

Most stable vices may be classed as nervous habits. They are acquired by the horse as a result of stress or boredom, or by imitation. The tendency may be inherited, that is it may be a question of temperament, but it can often be avoided through good stable management and firm but considerate handling of the horse. The following measures help to relieve stress and to avoid boredom:

- For feeding, grooming, exercise and stable routines a regular timetable should be adhered to.

- Sufficient bulk food should be provided to occupy the horse when he is in his loosebox. Many nervous habits start when horses in training have their hay reduced.

- Extra care must be taken with a horse who is on complete nuts and reduced bulk. A lump of rock salt should be put in his manger. To prevent chewing of wooden stabling, place a length of tree branch in the stable and allow the horse to bark it.

- Since most horses like music, transistor radios played quietly are acceptable.

- Because travelling can cause stress, whenever possible long journeys should be avoided. Never drive too fast, or travel a horse in a noisy trailer.

- Avoid subjecting the horse to undue pressure during training, by either the trainer or the rider asking too much.

- Try to get the horse out of his stable as much as possible. Either turn him out, put him on a horse walker or walk him in hand between periods of riding/training.

Many horse 'toys' are now available to help prevent the onset of boredom.

Things to consider:

- Dividing feeds into smaller, more frequent portions.

- Feeding hay in a double haynet to slow down eating.

- Working the horse twice a day.

VICES

Weaving

This is a nervous habit most common among well-bred horses. The animal rocks himself to and fro, the head swinging with the movement. Confirmed cases lift each foot in turn as the forehand is swayed from side to side. As a result, extra strain is placed on the tendons of the front legs, and lameness can occur. Established weavers give themselves little rest, and often lose condition. The habit can be catching, being quickly imitated by some other horses.

Animals sometimes continue the habit even when they are tied up in a loosebox or stabled in a stall. In the latter case, if they are turned round and put on pillar chains (chains or ropes attached to the rear side pillars of the stalls and then hooked to the headcollar), they may become less bored if there is more to look at and so lose the habit.

Anti-weaving bars fitted on a stable door.

Some horses weave when they are first brought up from the field; others only when they become fit and are competing or racing. Some start weaving when they are stabled on their own, others when they are in a line of boxes. There are no fixed rules or indications; each animal reacts in his own particular way. Some only weave at feeding time.

Remedies

- Try to find out the cause, and rectify it. A confirmed weaver is incurable, but if a young horse is caught in time, the habit may be checked.

- Fix an anti-weaving grid to the top of the lower door of the loosebox. This allows the horse to put out his head, but prevents him moving from side to side. Some yards have these grids fitted on all doors to discourage horses from starting the habit.

- Alternatively, fix a grille to the top of the lower door to prevent him putting his head out. But bear in mind that although this prevents a horse weaving over the door, boredom may still lead him to continue the habit while standing back in his box.

- Take a length of wood, slip the top half through the handle of a rubber dustbin lid and bolt the bottom half firmly to the door. This cheap, easy-to-make

device allows the horse to put his head out over the door, but prevents him weaving.

Crib Biting and Windsucking

The original cause is usually boredom, though both habits can also be developed by one horse watching another. In crib biting, the horse seizes hold of any projecting edge or object with his teeth, arches his neck and gulps down air. In doing so, he makes a distinctive grunt. When windsucking, the horse does not seize anything with his teeth, but gulps air in a similar manner. A crib biter placed in a loosebox with no suitable surfaces to seize often turns to windsucking.

Crib biters often continue the habit when turned out to grass. The top of fence posts and gates make convenient surfaces. Other mature horses turned out in the same field rarely develop the habit, but young animals may easily do so.

There appears to be no infallible remedy for these two habits. Numerous preventive measures can be tried. In some cases they may work, but in others they are only successful until the horse learns to outwit the prevention. If caught in the early stages and if no suitable surface is made available, a crib biter sometimes loses the desire and hence the habit.

To prevent crib biting, the loosebox should have no projecting surfaces. A metal grille fitted to the door allows the horse to look out but protects the top of the

Windsucking.   Crib biting.

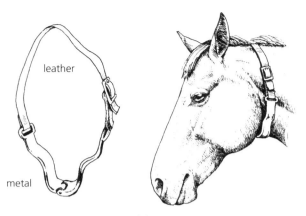

Anti-crib biting strap.

door from his teeth. It must be sufficiently fine that he cannot seize hold of it.

Should a suitable box not be available, a muzzle is an effective deterrent. The horse should wear it at all times in the stable, except of course when he is being watered or fed or having his hay.

There are various patterns of anti-crib biting straps, of which the Meyers pattern is probably the best. It is made of vulcanite and has a leather strap which runs over the poll and fastens to the headcollar. The vulcanite or metal section has a V-shaped part, which fits tightly up into the gullet, and prevents the horse arching his neck (see diagram). The Matthew Harvey Grinder's Bit is also reputed to stop horses crib biting. When it is removed they do not resume the habit.

A flute bit may be used, fixed to the headcollar. This has a perforated, hollow mouthpiece that disperses the gulp of air and prevents it being sucked in.

In recent years, a surgical operation on the neck was at first thought to be effective, but this has since proved less successful.

Weaving, crib biting and windsucking are all stable vices. They must be declared at the time of sale, and should be noted on the veterinary certificate. If this information is knowingly withheld, the sale can be declared null and void.

PROBLEM BEHAVIOUR

Kicking the Stable Walls

This sometimes starts when mares become irritated by the presence of a neighbouring horse. It can also be a sign of ovary trouble in a mare. Moving the horse to a different box may help. Some horses do it only when they are stabled on their own, others only when they are stabled in company.

Rats or mice in the stable can also start the habit, or it may be a sign of frustration. The noise seems to be addictive.

It may be caused by parasite infestation of the heels. This is more likely in horses with feathers. More usually they stamp rather than kick. A veterinary surgeon will provide an appropriate shampoo. Once cleared, scrupulous grooming of the feathers, or trimming them off if not required for show, is recommended.

Remedies

• Line the box with rubber matting.

• Hang a sack of straw from the roof, so that it rests just behind the horse's hindquarters.

• Hang a bunch of gorse or a broom head in the same position as a sack of straw – although the horse may eat it.

• Fit kicking hobbles – though these may cause other problems and need to be used only by an experienced person as a last resort.

Try to arrange for the horse to spend several hours in the field each day.

Rug Tearing

Remedies

The skin and mane should be checked for skin infection and/or parasites. If present, these should be dealt with. It may begin with a rug that is too small, too tight around the shoulders or that has been pulled too far back. Rugs

Bib fitted to headcollar to prevent rug tearing.

that have a build-up of static electricity, especially with clipped horses, can cause discomfort, as can rugs that have hair clippings in them. This happens when the horse's own rug is used to keep him warm whilst being clipped, before the little hair shards are brushed off the coat.

This habit is often caused by boredom, and the provision of toys, such as a ball in a haynet or plastic bottles hanging on pieces of string, often helps. A bib of strong leather fastened to the back and side squares of the headcollar, so that it lies behind and below the chin, checks most offenders. Those who persist can be muzzled. A bar muzzle, which allows the horse to pick at hay, is the best type.

Banging the Stable Door

This is an irritating habit, which can quickly spread round a yard if it is not checked. It is usually started by horses impatient for feed, particularly if some are fed and others are kept waiting. However, it can become addictive, and horses will bang doors with a front foot or knee as a nervous habit. It can cause bruising and concussion.

Remedies

• Fix a grille over the door, so that the horse is kept back and is unable to reach the door with his foot or knee.

• Fix an iron bar or a chain across the doorway, so that the door can be left open in working hours. This is usually successful, as long as the arrangements are secure.

• If it is essential for the door to be kept closed, set a bar at an angle across the doorway. This will also keep the horse back from the door.

• Because many horses appear to enjoy the noise, fix thick matting or lining on the door. This will muffle the noise and may discourage the horse from persisting with the habit.

Gnawing Wood

Remedies

• Apply Jeyes Fluid, or some other strong-flavoured mixture, to wooden stabling.

• Cap all accessible surfaces in the stable with metal.

• Check the fibre and mineral content of the horse's food because in some cases it can be a diet problem.

• A strand of electric fencing inside post and rails will prevent the horse reaching the fence to chew.

Eating Droppings

This is usually considered to start as a diet problem, but it can become an addiction.

Remedies

• Check the mineral and vitamin content of the horse's diet and correct any deficiencies.

• Put a forkful of turf, with its roots and earth, in the box.

• Worm the horse regularly. Seek veterinary advice on a programme of worming and diet supplementation.

Eating Straw Bedding

Most horses bedded on straw eat a certain amount of it, but a greedy horse eats so much that it affects his condition and wind.

Remedies

• Bed the horse on shavings, sawdust, paper or a wood derivative bedding.

• If straw bedding has to be used, spray it with non-toxic disinfectant.

• Muzzle the horse.

Pawing the Ground and Stamping

The attraction of this habit appears to be the noise which it creates, but it can also be a sign of internal discomfort and/or pain. Heavy, solid rubber matting put down at the front of the loosebox by the door can help to check it. The concrete flooring underneath will sweat, so it should be swept daily and, when possible, exposed to the air.

Biting

Horses who bite when being handled and groomed can be controlled by a muzzle, or by being tied up to two rings across the corner of the box. The cause may be rough grooming – some horses are very sensitive – poor handling when young, or the feeding of tit-bits.

Tail Rubbing

A horse may rub his tail, either because of the presence of whipworms in the area of the anus and rectum or, in summer, because of sweet itch caused by midges.

Remedies

• If the tail rubbing is caused by worms, the horse should be dosed with an appropriate wormer. Keep the area around and under the tail clean, and the tail itself regularly shampooed.

• If the cause is sweet itch, a special lotion should be applied. Seek veterinary assistance.

• Do not turn out at dusk or dawn.

• Use anti-sweet itch clothing.

Refusal to Lie Down

This puts extra and unnecessary strain on the legs. It is usually caused by one of the following:

• Insufficient bedding.

• Getting cast.

• Slipping when getting up.

• Worry in a new stable, especially if there are no other horses.

• Old age or stiffness.

Remedies

• Put the horse on a deep shavings bed or, if straw is used, adopt the deep litter system.

• Provide a pony or donkey in a neighbouring field or loosebox for company. This often helps.

• Use rubber matting with a good bed on top.

Once the horse has overcome his nervousness and has lain down, providing the above precautions are taken, the problem should not recur.

Tearing Bandages

A muzzle, cradle or crossed side-reins are the most effective remedies for this. In the latter the horse will not have freedom to lie down at will. The muzzle must be removed for feed, water and hay.

Pulling Back When Tied Up

This habit arises from fright. It usually starts because the horse, when first tied up in a stable, possibly with too short a rope, pulled back and frightened himself. Therefore, always attach a safety loop of string to the ring and tie the rope to the string, never to the ring itself. Unfortunately, once learned, this habit is difficult to cure, and many remedies have attendant risks.

Careful handling in the stable may eventually effect a cure. When grooming, try threading the rope through the ring, but not actually tying it. The problem often arises when a horse is being tied up in a trailer if he is allowed to pull back before the back strap is done up, or before the back of the trailer is closed.

Halter and Headcollar Slipping

This habit is often acquired as a result of pulling back, tilting the head and learning that the halter or headcollar slips off. Ponies and cobs can be checked by being tied up with thick neck straps instead of a headcollar. This is not wise with young or highly strung horses, as they may pull back, lose their footing, and give themselves a fright and, often, an injury. Such horses should never be left on their own when they are tied up. If they are not allowed to persist in the habit, they may in time forget it.

PROBLEMS IN THE STABLE

Choking

Choking results when there is a blockage of the tube down which food passes from the mouth to the stomach. The obstruction can usually be felt by examining the left and lower side of the neck.

Possible Causes

- An apple or a large piece of root fed whole and not chopped.

- A greedy horse bolting his food.

- A tired horse who is suffering from mild dehydration and whose mouth is not salivating.

- Feeding certain foodstuffs dry, when they should have been soaked.

The symptoms are salivation and frequent attempts at swallowing, causing a gurgling sound. The head is either drawn in tight to the chest, or stretched out towards the ground. The neck muscles are tense. There may be a discharge from the nose. The symptoms are alarming.

Treatment

- Do not give water.

- Do not try to drench the horse.

- Smear a lump of butter on the tongue. It may help to ease the obstruction.

- Lightly massage the left side of the jugular groove.

Stay with the horse. If he can relax the spasm, the obstruction may move itself. Should the condition not be relieved within half an hour, seek veterinary help.

Horses who are known to bolt their food, particularly cubes, should have their feed mixed with bran or chaff. An alternative is to soak the cubes before feeding, and then feed them mixed with soaked sugar beet.

A Cast Horse

If a horse rolls over too close to the wall of his loosebox and has insufficient room in which to right himself, he may become cast. Many horses become very frightened and/or violent, and by kicking and struggling do themselves injury. Other more placid horses lie quietly until help arrives.

Horses often become cast at night. The tell-tale signs in the morning are a disturbed bed and scratch marks on the wall. This shows that horses, given time, often right themselves without help. If a horse has been cast, he must be closely examined for injury, and then walked

Dealing with a cast horse.

out and trotted up in hand.

Horses may roll in their box at any time, but are more likely to do so:

• When clean bedding has been added.

• When first put back in after work.

• When they feel the onset of an attack of colic.

The sight of a cast horse is alarming. As he tries to right himself, his thrashing hooves put a helper at risk. The task of righting a cast horse should not be attempted by inexperienced persons.

Anti-cast ridges or grooves, which help a cast horse to right himself, can be placed on loosebox walls. His hind feet will catch on the ledge, and he can then push himself over.

He can be fitted with an anti-cast roller. This has a metal hoop across the withers and prevents the horse from rolling right over. Make sure there is sufficient bedding, with banks built up around the edge.

Methods of Getting a Horse Up

One person on his own may well be able to right a pony or lightweight animal under 15hh. Considerable strength is required to right a large animal, and two or three people are required, particularly if the horse is very violent.

One person on his own restrains the horse by sitting or kneeling on the horse's neck, just behind his head. Make sure the animal's nostril is free. A cloth placed beneath the head will help prevent damage to the eye on the underside. Reassure the horse with voice and hand, and consider the situation. Sometimes the horse will remain quiet and in a few minutes is able to right himself. If he does not, stand up and release his head. Remove any ridges of bedding immediately behind his back and shoulders. Then take hold of his tail and pull his quarters round. The horse will pivot slightly on his middle and shoulders, which should give him room to extend his legs and get up without trouble.

Two or three people: Collect one or two strong ropes or webbing lunge lines. One assistant sits on the horse's neck as before, and the second removes the bedding from behind the horse. Most experienced people fasten the ropes round the front and hind legs nearest the wall using a slip knot. The first assistant releases the horse's head and is then ready to help pull. By pulling on the ropes the horse can be rolled over. He is then able to stand up. Release the ropes as soon as possible.

WATERING AND FEEDING

19 WATERING

THE NECESSITY FOR WATER

Water is essential for life and health. Horses can stay alive without food for a few weeks but without water they would probably die after five to six days.

Water makes up approximately 65% of an adult horse's body weight and almost 80% of a foal's body weight. Every cellular activity requires water. It is present in all body fluids, which are in three compartments: blood, intercellular fluid (between cells) and intracellular fluid (inside the cells).

Water is essential for:

DIGESTION – as saliva, which helps swallowing; water also provides a fluid medium for the food to pass along the digestive tract and provides the basis for digestive juices.

BLOOD – the fluid containing blood cells and nutrients etc., which circulates round the body and also carries waste from the tissues.

LYMPH – to drain tissue and help maintain the right balance of body fluid. It is important for defence against disease.

URINE – to excrete the waste products, and as a vehicle to regulate levels of sodium, potassium and other electrolytes as determined by kidney function.

FAECES – to supply fluid to aid excretion.

BODY – to regulate the body temperature by transferring excess heat to the surface.

SKIN – to get rid of surplus heat as sweat.

EYES AND NOSTRILS – in the form of tears and mucus as a lubricant.

JOINTS – in the form of oil as a lubricant.

MILK – to make 91% of the milk of lactating mares.

Stabled horses eat conserved food, with a water content averaging about 14%. It is therefore necessary to have water always available so that they can make up this deficiency. Some horses will drink between eating mouthfuls of their concentrate food. Most will drink after eating concentrates and roughage, especially the latter.

A stabled horse on dry food requires 20–40 litres (approximately 5–10 gallons) of water a day depending on the work he is doing and the weather. A lactating mare with a foal at foot requires considerably more.

An 8% deficiency of water, however lost from the horse's body, causes sub-acute illness. A loss of 15% causes dehydration and possibly death, especially if associated with heat exhaustion.

The Principles of Watering

Horses should have clean, fresh water available at all times. If this is not possible, for example after exercise or when travelling, they should be offered some water as soon as possible and before they are fed. Horses who have free and constant access to water rarely drink very much at one time.

Care should be taken that horses do not drink excessively before fast work. For racing, when maximum effort is required for only a short time, water may be removed before a race but never for longer than 2 hours (see also watering competition horses, page 155).

Purity of Water

Horses are extremely fussy about water. If it is tainted in any way they will go thirsty rather than drink it. Even a change of water may cause rejection.

Any suspicion of dung in the water will prevent a horse drinking.Water may be contaminated by ammonia (NH_3) absorbed overnight from a soiled stable. Fresh water should therefore always be available in the morning. It is sometimes recommended that medicines are put in the drinking water. This can be unwise as the horse will usually refuse to drink it. Water that has stood for any length of time in plastic containers may be rejected. Sometimes the addition of a little glucose or molasses will persuade horses to drink.

'Hard' water is probably preferable to 'soft' but the important point is that it is clean and fresh. The main storage tank for the stable yard should be regularly checked, and a dust-and vermin-proof cover used.

If horses are seen to play and fuss with their water this is likely to be because of contamination, but could be a sign of a sub-acute colic attack.

SYSTEMS OF WATERING FOR STABLED HORSES

Automatic Water Bowls

ADVANTAGES

- Water always available.

- Labour-saving. May be essential in a large yard.

DISADVANTAGES

- Can cause physical injury unless boxed in.

- Liable to destruction from horse activity.

- Liable to freeze in cold weather, or malfunction. (It is possible to fit devices to the water pipes to prevent freezing.)

- Unable to monitor amount of water being drunk unless each individual bowl is metered.

- Not suitable for mares and foals.

- Difficult to clean.

- On a communal gravity-fill system supplying a number of stables, the risk of infection passing from horse to horse would be greater.

Water bowls must be large enough for the horse to get his muzzle in with ease. They should be of the self-filling kind with a small ball-cock, and preferably with a plug to facilitate emptying and cleaning. The inlet pipe must be well insulated to prevent freezing and should have a stopcock. They should be so fitted that the horse cannot sit on them.

Gravity-filling bowls are sometimes installed but can prove troublesome. Also, bowls that have a plate for the animal to press with the nose are not suitable for horses.

Water bowls must be emptied and cleaned daily. In big yards they must be inspected daily by a single competent person as well as by the groom.

It is easier to fit them along the back wall of barn stables but preferable to fit them along the front. They are less likely to freeze. Horses are less likely to sit on them and, if well designed, they can be cleaned from the gangway or centre aisle.

Buckets

ADVANTAGE

• Water consumption can be monitored.

DISADVANTAGES

• Labour-intensive.

• Can be knocked over.

• Horse may be without water at times.

Buckets should be large (14 litre/3 gallon for preference) and of heavy-duty material. They are usually made of PVC.

Buckets should be emptied and refilled twice daily. They should be topped up at midday, or more often. Cleaning should be daily with plain water and a brush kept specially for the purpose. If light colours are chosen for the buckets it will be easier to see if they have been properly cleaned. They should not feel slimy to the touch.

Buckets should be put in a corner of the box with the handle turned away from the horse. They should be well banked up with bedding to prevent them from being knocked over. They should not be put by the door but preferably near the drainage outlet.

Buckets with handles are not suitable for foals.

WATERING COMPETITION HORSES

See also Section 5, Specialist Care of the Competition Horse.

Event Horses

Provided that horses have had free access to water they will not need a long drink before the competition starts. This will particularly apply at a three-day event where the horses are stabled nearby, but at a one-day event, if the horses have travelled some distance, they should be offered water immediately on arrival. Half a bucket of water drunk 20 minutes before starting work will do no harm because the dressage phase requires no fast, strenuous exertion. Event horses should be allowed a small amount of water between each phase to maintain their body fluids. More may be given if the gaps between phases are very long.

At a three-day event most veterinary surgeons now consider that horses should be offered a few mouthfuls of water – 1 litre (2 pints) – in the box before the cross-country. This is especially important in warm, humid conditions.

After the cross-country is completed, and as soon as the horse's breathing is recovering steadily and he shows no signs of distress, he may be given 2¼ litres (½ gallon) of water every 15 minutes until he is satisfied. Electrolytes may be given, but plain water should also be offered. It is important that the horse drinks and if he appears distressed, veterinary advice should be sought immediately. (See Signs of Dehydration, next section.)

Endurance Horses

Much veterinary research has been done on endurance horses. It has been found that the best method of avoiding dehydration is to allow the horse ad lib water whenever possible during the ride. If this has been done the horse should be allowed 2¼ litres (½ gallon) every 5 minutes after finishing the ride. If water has not been available on the ride 2¼ litres (½ gallon) every 15 minutes may be allowed. Electrolytes may be added but the horse must drink, so plain water should also be available.

Hunters

Hunters should be allowed unrestricted access to water before hunting.

If the journey home in the box or trailer is longer than 30 minutes, the horses should be offered water before they start travelling. On arrival home, if they are cool and dry and do not appear distressed they should be allowed water ad lib.

If they are hot they should be allowed 2¼ litres (½ gallon) of water every 15 minutes. If they are distressed, veterinary help should be sought. (See Dehydration, below.)

DEHYDRATION

Dehydration results when more water and salts are lost from the body than are taken in and the horse has not enough fluid in his body to maintain normal physiological conditions. It is usually associated with fast, energetic work but there are many other situations in which dehydration can occur.

Possible Causes of Dehydration

- Lack of available water or failure to drink.
- Sweating – prolonged and marked.
- Diarrhoea – especially in foals.
- Excessive urination when not accompanied by a compensatory thirst.
- Haemorrhage.
- Heat exhaustion.
- Overlong or delayed journeys.
- Excessive heat and humidity.

Dehydration may result in:

- Reduced performance.
- Muscle damage.
- Colic.
- Reduced kidney function.
- Laminitis.
- Azoturia (rhabdomyolysis).
- Coma.
- Death.

Signs of Dehydration

- Skin loses its pliability (see Pinch Test, below).
- Lack of inclination to graze or eat.
- Listlessness.
- Loss of normal colour from the membranes of gums and eyes and reduced membrane refill time.
- Muscles quiver.
- Pulse becomes small.
- 'Thumps' (see below).
- Thick, patchy sweat.
- Panting (only if in association with heat exhaustion).

Any horse showing the above symptoms after severe exertion should have veterinary attention immediately. Dehydration can be confirmed by blood-testing.

Pinch Test

A fold of skin on the neck is picked up between finger and thumb. If, when released, it does not return to normal in 5 seconds, the horse is dehydrated to some extent.

'Thumps' (synchronous diaphragmatic flutter)

The diaphragm contracts in the same rhythm as the heart beat so the horse's flanks synchronise with the pulse. The contractions may even be heard. Veterinary advice should be sought immediately.

Causes of Dehydration

Lack of Water

This may be a chronic, ongoing, low-grade dehydration

where animals are not provided with a sufficient supply of fresh, clean water over a long period of time. Poor performance will follow and is one cause of the horse's fitness being 'over the top'. It is likely to occur in the following situations:

- Ponies at grass, particularly those on tethers, who are watered from a bucket or other inadequate supply.

- Stabled horses who are only offered water at set times.

- Stabled horses whose water bowls are not cleaned regularly.

- Stabled horses whose buckets are not cleaned, emptied and refilled regularly and thereafter kept full. The available water may be tainted.

- Water being withheld deliberately.

It is not unknown for dealers, and riders, especially in dressage, show jumping and showing, to withhold water so that the horse becomes partially dehydrated and therefore quieter. This is inhumane and can result in permanent damage. If this happens at a three-day event, even if the horse is given water ad lib after the dressage, he will start the cross-country below par.

Sweating

Humans and horses are the only animals that regulate their temperature by sweating. When the horse sweats, he will lose valuable electrolytes, the most important being sodium, chloride and potassium.

Excess sweating is usually caused by long-term strenuous work such as long-distance riding. It is the duration of sweating which is important but temperature and humidity are important factors.

Other causes of sweating include:

- Travelling.

- Illness, especially obstructive colics.

- Stress.

- Fear.

- Pain.

- Excitement.

- Airless hot stable with high humidity prevents evaporation and may lead to heat stress.

If these cause dehydration, water and electrolytes (essential salts) are necessary for recovery. In severe cases veterinary assistance is indicated.

Travelling

Travelling, even short distances, can be a stressful experience for the horse. Some horses, however accustomed they are to travelling, will refuse to eat while in the vehicle and will not drink even when stationary. These horses must be treated with great care as there is a danger of dehydration and colic is more likely when they start eating at the end of the journey. During any breaks in travelling, watering is a top priority and, if possible, some grazing.

Horses can also suffer dehydration through excessive sweating on the journey. This is particularly likely with young horses unaccustomed to travelling. It is not always appreciated how much they have sweated as the air blowing through the vehicle may dry them off and hide the extent of the sweating. Many horses will not drink strange water. Always take some from home if this is a problem.

Diarrhoea

Diarrhoea will cause dehydration. It is especially serious in the case of foals. Acute diarrhoea will require replacement therapy urgently. Horses who are ill or are suffering from the effects of worm infestation causing chronic diarrhoea should have electrolyte salts added to their diets in addition to the anthelmintic treatment given under veterinary supervision.

Excessive Urination

This may be the result of over-prolonged dosing with a diuretic. Veterinary advice should be sought. However, the horse with polyuria (excessive urination) will usually develop a compensatory polydypsia (increased thirst).

Electrolytes

These are a mixture of body salts which are added to the water or feed after strenuous exercise. It is pointless giving them a long time before a competition, but to get horses used to the taste in water they may be offered daily after work for a week or so.

With a commercial preparation it is important to check that the proportions are correct. If glucose is incorporated, it is there to increase absorption and not as a source of energy.

Electrolytes as powders added to the feed or in an oral paste in a syringe (similar to a worm dose) are an easier way of guaranteeing that the horse takes in the dose. Veterinary advice regarding electrolyte supplementation is worthwhile.

If electrolytes are given after a competition, plain water should also be offered. It is extremely important to get the horse to drink. In cases of extreme exhaustion the veterinary surgeon may give the horse fluid intravenously as in this case oral rehydration can be dangerous.

FOOD AND DIGESTION

THE NECESSITY OF FOOD

Food is needed by the horse for:

• Maintenance of life.

• Growth and/or work.

• Repair of tissues.

It is the source of energy. Energy is needed to sustain life, and for the production of all body tissues (e.g. muscle and blood). Energy is needed for the maintenance of muscle activity, digestion, excretion, reproduction and all body processes.

DIGESTION

In this chapter the emphasis is on those particular features of the horse's system which are practically related to a better understanding of the rules which govern the art and the science of feeding. Knowledge of these features can be considered to be a basic requirement of responsible horsemanship at any level. Such responsibility is directed towards the skills concerned with feeding, which is one aspect of the welfare of the horse.

The aims of feeding are to:

• Maintain health.

• Maximise performance.

• Minimise nutritional mistakes.

• Reduce the risks of malnutrition in all its aspects.

The more advanced the athletic performance of the horse, the greater the attention needed to detailed application of the skills. Although background knowledge, as distinct from this essential knowledge, is not necessarily required, it is assumed that stable managers so involved will wish to increase their theory. The 'what', 'when', and 'how' are more efficiently put into practice if the 'why' is also understood.

Any theoretical knowledge gained should be primarily directed towards the practical ability to:

• Appreciate when all is well, and that the horse is at ease.

• To recognise quickly when all is not well, and the horse is at 'dis-ease', as judged by the clues produced by the structures and functionings of the system(s) involved. See Chapter 15 for signs of good and ill-health.

The 'feeding of the horse is in the eye of the master'!

The art of feeding horses has been practised and taught for over 3,000 years. The scientific understanding is much younger, since most research into the subject has been carried out during the last fifty years. It must not be forgotten, however, that the horse has not basically changed in many thousands of years. His instincts and behaviour as a nomadic, gregarious herbivore, his appetite and his digestive system, have not altered since he became *Equus caballus*, an established plains dweller living by grazing and browsing.

The horse is still constructed and 'programmed' to survive by eating vegetation, and although the vegetation to which he has access has changed, it has done so only to a degree. These changes first occurred as the various 'types' of horse spread out into Europe and Asia to settle in different climatically controlled areas:

- Mountain and moorland.

- Lush lowland pastures.

- Steppes and prairies.

- Deserts.

Early domestication within these broad locations still depended upon 'natural' eating.

Farming practices in those countries where seasonal changes in grass growth occurred (temperate zones) eventually produced methods of conserving herbage for over-winter feeding, followed by the development of harvested indigenous grains.

More recent centuries recognised the need for energy intakes on a daily basis in excess of that which hay and unimproved grain could supply, and horsemen learnt how to concentrate the ration by using progressively more improved cereal crops of denser, therefore richer, starch content so that they met the energy requirements within the limitations of the horse's daily capacity. Thus began 'unnatural' feeding practices.

Modern feeding may seem to be a complicated business of permutations of many indigenous and foreign materials but, with few exceptions, these are all vegetations and their by-products and they are basically similar to the horse's 'natural' foods but with marked differences in starch content and mineral ratios. It is these which make such rations 'unnatural'.

MAIN INTERNAL ORGANS

The major internal organs of the horse are found in the thoracic cavity and the abdominal cavity, which is divided by the diaphragm. The **heart** and the two **lungs** are found in the thoracic cavity or chest cavity and these fill much of the area between the forelegs, protected by the scapula (shoulder blade) and the fore part of the rib cage. The abdominal cavity behind the diaphragm holds the **stomach, intestines, liver, spleen, kidneys (two)** and **bladder**. These vulnerable 'soft' vital organs are protected by the skeletal frame, which encloses and protects them.

The **liver** is the largest gland in the horse's body and has several functions in metabolism.

- It assists in the formation and storage of glycogen or animal starch, which the horse can use in future for breakdown into glucose.

- It produces bile, which is alkaline and assists in digestion in the small intestine and neutralising the intestinal contents.

- It assists in protein metabolism.

- It assists in the digestion of fats and oils.

The **pancreas** secretes important digestive juices into the small intestine, but vitally its endocrine function is to produce insulin, which regulates glucose metabolism

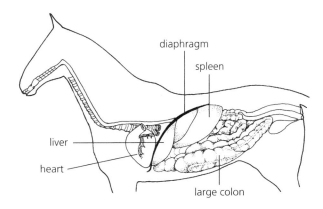

Abdominal contents, simplified. Note the greater volume occupied by the abdominal contents relative to heart and lungs (see also illustrations above right).

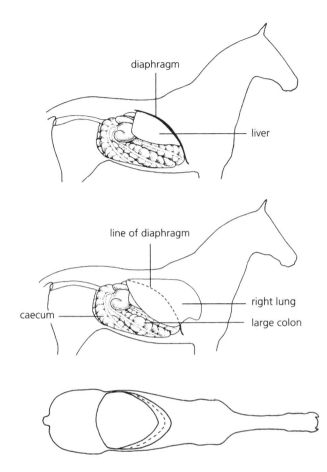

ABOVE: Relative positions of digestive organs and lungs. Lungs project backwards over either side of the 'dome' of the diaphragm, whose contraction and relaxation causes inspiration and expiration.

and its use. Its second endocrine function is to produce glucagon, which is involved in the breakdown of glycogen.

Digestion involves the breakdown of the food which the horse eats into its main component parts. These are: **carbohydrates, fats, proteins** and **vitamins.**

Vitamins, which are either fat soluble or water soluble, can be absorbed through the gut wall once in solution. Carbohydrates, fats and proteins must first be broken down through the digestive process: carbohydrates to glucose, fats to fatty acids and glycerol

and proteins to amino acids. They can then pass through the gut wall at appropriate sites. Once absorbed they can then be anabolised or built up into compound substances for specific use.

DIGESTIVE SYSTEM

The horse's digestive system is adapted to function effectively for this herbivorous mammal. The 'wild' horse would have access to food over a 24-hour period of browsing and constant but usually quiet mobility. The manager of the modern day horse, who may live in circumstances quite far removed from this natural state, must understand the way the digestive system is designed and functions most effectively. They will then be able to manage the modern horse in a way which maximises the horse's welfare.

Parts of the Digestive System

The digestive system starts with:

- The **lips** (select food).

- The **incisor teeth**: tear food (e.g. grass).

- The **tongue**: pushes food to the back of the mouth.

- The **molar teeth**: grind the food into a 'bolus' (chewed food mixed with **saliva** which renders the mass able to be swallowed).

- The saliva secreted in the mouth is alkaline in pH and helps to neutralise the acidity of the gastric (stomach) secretions. It helps to moisten the food, which lubricates the mass to ease swallowing.

The food is passed over the **pharynx** at the back of the mouth and passes down the **oesophagus** with the help of **peristalsis** (involuntary muscular actions which aid the 'swallowing' process to take food to the stomach).

The digestive parts:

- The **stomach**. Has a capacity of about 9–12 litres (2–3

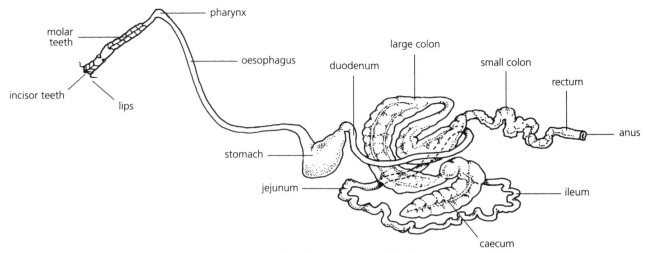

The digestive system, simplified.

gallons). It is roughly the shape of a rugby ball (oval) and is situated behind the diaphragm and the liver, slightly to the left of the midline through the horse. The gastric secretions contain mucus, hydrochloric acid and digestive enzymes. The stomach produces powerful muscular contractions, which help propel the food mass towards the intestine through the **pyloric sphincter**.

- The **pyloric sphincter** is a one-way valve, which allows semi-digested food through into the small intestine. It is activated by chemical messengers and by local reflex stimulation of the nerve structure lining the stomach.

- The **small intestine** is made up of three parts. The **duodenum** is the smallest portion at 90cm (3ft), quite short and closely attached to the stomach, it is S-shaped and has the pancreas in close proximity in one of the bends. The pancreatic and bile juices are secreted through ducts into the duodenum. The **jejunum** is the main part of the small intestine, 18m (60ft) long, and the **ileum** is the smaller portion, 2m (7ft) towards the end of the small intestine. In addition to the pancreatic and bile juices, there are important secretory cells in the small intestine which

are active in the breakdown of sugars and starches into glucose, proteins into amino acids and triglycerides into fatty acids and glycerol. Absorption of nutrients begins to take place in the small intestine as they become available. The mixture of digested material from the stomach and small intestine is known as **chyme**.

- The large intestine is also made up of three parts. The **caecum** is a 'blind' sac about 1m (3¼ft) long and has a capacity of about 35 litres (8 gallons) The **large colon**, 4m (13ft) long, has a 108 litre (24 gallons) capacity. The **small colon**, 3m (10ft) long, is only about 7.5cm (3in) in diameter.

- Within the **large colon** and the **caecum** particularly is a large habitat for microbial flora, which act upon the cellulose in the food to break it down into volatile fatty acids. Large amounts of water are reabsorbed in the large colon, leaving just enough to smoothly facilitate the passing of faeces.

- Within the **small colon** the undigested residue is formed into faecal balls and pushed towards the rectum by peristalsis.

- **The rectum** holds the faeces and the **anus** expels

them; they have no digestive function.

The Micro-organisms

There are several species always present in the digestive tract. The relative proportions vary with the predominant pasture strains. Some are adapted for fermenting lush grass cellulose, others for the stemmier types and yet others for the husks of seeds. Yet again other strains are concerned with those undigested solubles and starch that reach the large intestine.

This is partly why the horse's ration should be changed gradually, to allow the micro-organisms to adapt to the new foodstuffs.

The Horse and His Herbivorous Diet

Grass, even when fresh, succulent and high in water content, is still a fibre-rich plant containing comparatively small amounts of solubles. The horse must ingest large quantities: on average, approximately 2½% of his own body weight as dry matter intake. He eats for the greater part of a 24-hour day and for long periods at a time. Such is called **'trickle feeding'**.

An inherited instinct is the desire not only to eat but to eat foodstuffs which have the stimulus to instigate **mastication.** The horse 'feels the need to chew' and the fibrous nature of even wet grass guarantees this satisfaction.

Mastication takes time and requires powerful jaw muscles to move the lower jaw across the upper, and long jaws to accommodate large molar teeth.

Characteristically the grazing (eating) horse eats and chews continually.

The stomach is relatively small and so is liable to overfill, especially when feeds are lush and suddenly available after periods of scarcity. Its construction is such that burping (eructation) and vomiting cannot occur.

Mastication serves other important functions besides stimulating saliva:

• It breaks up the stem, leaf, flower and seed.

• It liberates the sap with its solubles.

incidentally, a horse does not salivate at the sight, smell, taste or 'sound' of foodstuffs.

Under 'natural' grazing the horse may show herbage variety preferences but all the nutrients in each and every grass, legume or plant are ingested and utilised. There is, of course, a residual indigestible component.

Changes in nutrient ratios related to growth rates of the herbage are minor or slow in onset, associated more with the seasons than with weather variables. The micro-organism colonies, once established, therefore remain fairly steady and they suffer no 'dis-ease', as can happen with sudden and dramatic feed intake changes. Consequently gut function, subsequent metabolism, and ultimate life and work remain in a 'steady state'.

Stabling, winter feeding and feeding for high performance require quite marked changes for the horse's digestive system. Grass is replaced by hay and allied products with their higher dry matter, stemmier consistency, i.e. more cellulose and fewer solubles, now collectively called **roughage.**

The energy input is obtained from increasing use of grains – cereal seeds – which are rich in starch, densely packed, hence the name **concentrates.**

It is any change to the dietary regime which demands good stable management.

Hay, haylage, oat or barley straw can all be fed as roughage and might accurately be termed forage which as a general rule should not be less than 50% and never less than 30% by weight of the total ration. It is eaten slowly.

Corn is eaten quickly. It should be mixed, 'opened', with chopped roughage, bran or soaked sugar beet to slow up ingestion and encourage better chewing.

The effect of mistakes in these changes are dealt with elsewhere but always:

• Offer hay after grain whenever possible but include chaff or chop in the bucket feed. Alternatively offer hay half an hour before the concentrate feed to stimulate the digestive system, e.g. in early morning.

- Offer the largest amount of forage after the evening feed.

- Change from grass to hay slowly over 7–10 days.

- Establish on forage before introducing concentrates.

- Offer no more than 500g of concentrate (roughly 1lb) for a 500kg (1100lbs) horse on day one and increase daily by no more than 200g (½lb) daily till the maximum is reached. Remember that the work which requires concentrates progresses slowly anyway.

- Never put more than 2kg (4½lbs) of feed in the manger at one time.

- Feeds should be divided into at least two per day and more as feed is increased.

- Make sure that there is always plenty of water.

ROUTINE HORSEMANSHIP

Once settled on to a pasture, a horse will graze for up to 16 out of 24 hours. This will be broken up into variable sessions, more at night in warm weather but usually the longest periods in daylight. It is not known what regulates the horse's appetite. Ideally grass should be 7–10cm (3–4ins) high. With a laminitic animal it may be shorter to prevent him eating too much, or too quickly.

There are various designs of muzzle on the market which allow the laminitic pony/horse to graze but limit the amount taken up at any one time.

Horses tend to walk forward as they graze. Occasionally they will lift their head and neck to check out the environment, but continue to chew. Most will stop grazing and come to, or at least heed, a call from the owner/handler.

At the end of a grazing session various activities will follow:

- Close contact with a 'friend' for mutual grooming.

- Exercise with other horses.

- Movement to excretory areas, but horses rarely void urine and faeces at the same time.

- Rest: standing, lying down.

Deviations from known behaviour should attract attention. Interpretation and assessment is described in other manuals but beware the horse who stands 'away from herd', refuses to stand up on stimulation, or shows no interest in his preferred tit-bit or plucked grass. It is fortuitous if defaecation is observed during any visit to inspect the horse. The sudden appearance of a soiled tail and bottom in the grazing animal should be investigated.

In the stable, evidence of a horse 'off food' is seen in the manger and haynet, if feed and hay are untouched or thrown on to the floor.

A badly disturbed bed and marked alteration in the number of droppings, especially if down to nil, and changes in their colour, consistency and smell are all important clues.

Partially chewed, dropped out wads of hay, grass, etc. may indicate an acute mouth problem.

Copious salivation, especially down the nostrils, with intermittent marked swallowing attempts, indicate oesophageal choke which requires urgent veterinary attention.

See also page123, Signs of Ill-health.

IN THE STABLE

It takes a horse about 40 minutes to consume 1kg (roughly 2lbs) hay; straight hard feeds take about 10 minutes for 1kg (2lbs). When openers, especially chaff, are added, this time will be doubled or trebled.

A horse will defaecate eight to twelve times in 24 hours. (During working hours there is no excuse for more than one 'pat' in the bedding at any one time, assuming that the stable is regularly skipped out.)

The horse can be seen to eat, seen and heard to masticate, and seen to swallow (the bolus passes down the left jugular groove at intervals during eating and chewing). He can be heard to produce intestinal rumbles (borborygmi), heard and smelt to have passed wind (flatus), and seen and heard to pass faeces.

FAECES

Faeces is the undigested residue of the feedstuffs consumed. Even the dry-looking droppings of the horse contain a percentage of water, at least 15% by weight.

The small colon and rectal wall secrete a water-based mucus to lubricate the faeces' passage but the bulk of the water content is that left after reabsorption of the water in the large colon.

The water found in the digestive system consists of:

- that drunk;
- that extracted from the foodstuffs; and
- that secreted by the many glands:

  salivary

  biliary

  pancreatic

  gastro-intestinal wall mucus and digestive enzymes

During the passage along the digestive tract there is also a two-way (secretion/absorption) movement of water across the gut wall to transport:

- the digested constituents **inwards**; and
- the exchange of electrolytes involved primarily in determining the pH level of the different regions of the tract, from stomach to small colon.

This considerable quantity of water, greater than that in the blood and in the extracellular fluids, has to be reclaimed.

The residue of water is a reflection of:

- The water content of the original food eaten, e.g. spring grass gives wetter (softer) faeces.
- The 'health' of the digestive system.

It is recognition of **unusual** consistencies of faeces which is important in horsemanship. Beyond this is the appreciation that the rations fed (and eaten) according to the rules have maintained the desired condition in the light of work, temperament and weather.

To maximise this end result, regular attention should be given to dental care: the 3,500 jaw movements per 1kg (2lbs) food masticated soon wears the molars to produce sharp points in both upper and lower jaws in stable-fed animals.

21 THE RULES OF FEEDING

The rules of feeding are based on scientific fact and it is important for the horsemaster to know and understand them:

1. Feed according to the horse's condition, work, size, temperament and age.
2. Feed only good quality foodstuffs.
3. Feed sufficient roughage (fibre).
4. Feed little and often.
5. Make no sudden changes in the type of food fed.
6. Keep to the same times of feeding every day.
7. Feed something succulent every day.
8. Do not work immediately after a full feed.
9. Water should be freely available at all times. Where this is not possible, water should be given before feeding.
10. Keep all watering and feeding utensils clean.
11. Know the weight of the volume of food in the stable scoop or bucket so that weight is the basic measurement.

The reasons for these rules are as follows:

1. Feed According to the Horse's Condition, Work, Size, Temperament and Age

It is important that the rations are suitable for the horse in question bearing in mind:

• Present condition.

• The individual's metabolism, i.e. difficult to keep in condition, or puts on weight too easily.

• The workload.

• The ability of the rider.

• Whether extra food is needed for growth.

• His general behaviour.

2. Feed Only Good Quality Foodstuffs

It is a false economy to feed poor quality food. Poorly harvested forage or cheap or badly stored concentrates can cause many problems and these include colic and COPD (chronic obstructive pulmonary disease). Performance will be affected and fussy feeders will reject food.

For competition horses, the higher the level at which they compete, the greater the care required in assessing the quality and overall composition of the ration. In terms of performance the ratios of the major nutrients and that of minerals, trace elements and vitamins become critical.

3. Feed Sufficient Roughage

The horse requires plenty of roughage in his diet in order to digest his food properly. Even fit competition horses should never have less than 30% by weight of the ration made up of bulk food and this only for a limited period; 50% or 60% is preferable. This is mostly hay or its equivalents, but also includes chaff.

4. Feed Little and Often

As already stated, the horse is a trickle feeder. If the stomach is overloaded with food, some will be pushed into the small intestine without being properly prepared for digestion. Not only will this be a waste of food but it may also cause colic through fermentation.

The small size of the stomach (see previous chapter) means that not more than 2kg (4½lbs) of concentrated food should be given at any one time and part of this should be chaff or soaked sugar beet.

It follows that the total daily concentrate ration must be divided into separate feeds to adhere to this 'not more than 2kg (4½lbs) at a time' rule and the feeds spread as evenly as possible over a working day – a long day may be necessary.

5. Make no Sudden Changes in the Type of Food Fed

Because the bacteria (micro-organisms) in the horse's gut are 'food specific' it is important that any new foodstuff is introduced gradually. A new supply of hay should be mixed gradually with the old supply so the change is not sudden.

When a new horse enters the yard enquiries should be made as to his previous diet. If possible, it should be adhered to and only changed slowly. However, if a horse is suddenly unable to work through lameness or illness, his concentrates must be cut immediately to a maintenance ration, and be replaced by forage.

When horses travel and compete it is important that all the rations they require are taken with them. A new supply of hay or a different brand of cubes must not be introduced suddenly.

6. Keep to the Same Times of Feeding Every Day

The horse is a creature of habit and will do much better on a regular routine.

Make the timetable suit the yard routine. It is no good arranging for a late night feed unless it can be given regularly every night.

For the one-horse owner who is at work all day the feeds should be given early and late, with the horse having plenty of hay to keep his digestion working.

Regular feeding times should also apply to horses living out otherwise they are apt to spend much time waiting at the gate.

7. Feed Something Succulent Every Day

Ideally all horses should have some grazing each day. To the horse, green grass is the acme of enjoyment. Grazing old pasture will give him the chance to find different grasses and valuable herbs. Carrots, turnips, swedes, etc. are appreciated by the horse, as are apples.

Carrots are very high in carotene and a good source of vitamin A for horses who are stabled all the time.

Succulents will help to tempt the appetite of the poor feeder and will provide a natural source of minerals and vitamins. Many vitamins are present in fresh, green food. In the spring, dandelions, both leaves and roots, are much relished by stabled horses.

Some yards now feed barley grass. This is hydroponically grown in a purpose-built cultivator.

8. Do not Work Immediately After a Full Feed

It takes approximately 20 minutes for a horse to eat a full feed and at least 1½ hours to process it through the stomach and small intestine.

Blood is involved in the digestion of food. If there is a simultaneous work effort with muscle activity, the digestion will be impaired. A full stomach will also restrict room for lung expansion, which could cause strain if hard work was expected.

It follows that if it is necessary to exercise early in the day, either the first feed should be after work or it should be very small. Feed should be given early enough to allow time for digestion. This is especially important for competition horses or hunters whose workload is extra demanding.

This rule also applies to the bulk food. Whilst bulk food takes a short time to pass through the stomach and small intestine, it can dwell in the caecum and large intestine for up to 72 hours.

9. Water Should be Freely Available at All Times

This subject is covered in detail in Chapter 19.

10. Keep all Watering and Feeding Utensils Clean

Horses are very fussy feeders with an acute sense of smell. All water buckets and feeding utensils should be kept scrupulously clean; all stale food should be thrown away. Food must be kept free of contamination from mice, rats and other vermin. Some horses will starve themselves rather than eat tainted food.

Warmth and humidity enable micro-organisms to flourish and manufacture toxins. Regular emptying and cleaning of all food containers is essential.

11. Know the Weight of the Food in a Scoop or Bucket

Weigh the empty scoop/bucket, then fill it with each food and re-weigh it. Subtract the weight of the empty scoop/bucket to find out the weight of the food. Feeds can then be measured out in terms of scoops/buckets rather in kilos or pounds, which is quicker.

However, when talking about the ration always do it in kilos or pounds, especially in exam conditions.

FOOD – COMPOSITION AND TYPES

COMPOSITION OF FOOD

Broadly speaking, there are five categories into which the horse's food can be divided. They are:

• Carbohydrate – which includes starch, sugar and cellulose (fibre).

• Protein.

• Fat/oil.

• Minerals, including trace elements.

• Vitamins.

Carbohydrate

Carbohydrate is a food substance found in vegetable tissue comprising starch, sugar and cellulose (fibre). In the feeding of horses carbohydrates are important and should be the main source of energy for the horse (two-thirds of the weight of the concentrate feed ration should be carbohydrate).

• STARCH is the major energy store in plants.

• SUGARS are the simplest form of carbohydrate.

• CELLULOSE (fibre) is insoluble carbohydrate.

Crude fibre contains cellulose, and lignin. The horse can digest cellulose fibre but not lignin.

Fibre is an essential part of the horse's diet: without it he cannot digest his food properly. It stimulates the contractions of the gut. At least 40% of his rations must be fibre – but more is preferable.

The main sources of fibre for the horse are grass, hay, haylage and straw, which are known as bulk food, or forage.

Protein

Protein is a complex organic compound containing nitrogen. Different proteins are formed from varying combinations of twenty-two amino acids and their derivatives.

Protein is necessary for growth and replacing tissue wastage. It is made up of chains of amino acids linked together. Some of these amino acids can be synthesised (made) by the horse. Others are made by the micro-organisms in the gut. However, others known as essential amino acids must be included in the diet. An ordinary hay/cereal ration is low in these essential amino acids, so for growing or working horses, additions should be made to the ration.

Lysine, methionine and tryptophan are three of the essential amino acids, which are not available in 'straight' grain feeds.

Foods that are high in lysine are:

• Peas and beans, including soya-bean meal.

• Fish meal.

• Lucerne/alfalfa.

Not all high protein foods have easily digestible protein.

Reputable compounders making up a mix usually ensure that the protein is digestible.

Some nutritionists maintain that the total percentage of digestible protein in the ration should not be over 10% except for lactating mares, foals and young stock.

The protein levels will naturally alter with the changes in the quality of cereal fed. There is no evidence that athletic horses require high protein supplements, although individual National Hunt and three-day event horses might. In fact it is thought that the overfeeding of protein to competition horses can be detrimental to their performance.

Fats and Oil

All foods will contain some fat/oil as an integral fraction of their composition (i.e. their analysis).

Fat and oil are important for the growth and maintenance of cell membranes, the metabolism of cholesterol and the formation of prostaglandins. They are also used by the horse as a source of energy but, as far as is known, only after metabolism from body fat deposits. Such fat deposits play a role in control of body temperature.

Traditional rations are low in oil and many feeders now add corn oil to the diet.

Dietary fat, in the form of corn oil, is digestible and can reduce the requirements for cereal carbohydrate (starch). Recent studies show that it also lessens the decline in blood glucose during endurance rides and seems to accelerate the recovery of heart and respiration rates during the first 10 minutes of rest.

Since corn oil, along with other oils and fats of plant and animal origin, provides twice as much energy as does starch per g/oz fed, it is a useful part-substitute for cereals in endurance and three-day event horses on high rations.

Minerals (including trace elements)

These are essential elements of the diet but are required in very small quantities. They are inorganic substances.

Macro-minerals

The major minerals are as follows (their abbreviations are in brackets):

- Calcium (Ca)
- Phosphorus (P)
- Potassium (K)
- Sodium (Na)
- Chlorine (Cl)
- Magnesium (Mg)

Micro-minerals

These are the trace elements of importance to horses:

- Zinc (Zn)
- Manganese (Mn)
- Iron (Fe)
- Fluorine (F)
- Iodine (I)
- Selenium (Se)
- Cobalt (Co)
- Copper (Cu)
- Sulphur (S)

Wild horses roaming over large, open areas were able to choose variable herbage and were 'naturally' certain of a reasonably correct intake of minerals in terms of range and quantity. Properly balanced feeding and good pasture management are therefore essential for the domesticated horse's well-being.

Both minerals and vitamins interact with one another, so an imbalance can affect the correct functioning of many body processes.

Adding minerals to the horse's diet should always be

carried out with great care. Many of them can be very harmful if given in excess and 'guestimates' of what should be fed may well produce serious imbalances. A horse being fed compound feed is unlikely to need extra supplementation unless he has a specific problem. Veterinary advice is recommended.

Calcium and common salt may have to be added to the diet, especially for performance horses and young stock who are fed on straights i.e. oats or barley, rather than a balanced compound feed, but magnesium, manganese, copper, fluorine, iodine and cobalt are usually present in sufficient quantities. Sometimes potassium, zinc, iron, sulphur and selenium may be deficient.

Some experts consider that extra iron may be needed in high performance horses.

Calcium (Ca) and Phosphorus (P)

These are the commonest minerals in the horse's body and it is particularly important that they are correctly balanced and are supplied in the correct proportions.

Calcium and phosphorus should be present in the diet in a ratio of 2:1, i.e. 2 parts calcium to 1 part phosphorus. Most cereals have a very poor calcium to phosphorus ratio, so seek advice from a reputable feed merchant or from your veterinary surgeon.

Bran inhibits calcium uptake. A calcium supplement, possibly in the form of ground limestone, will be needed if much grain or bran is fed. Calcium-rich foods such as lucerne/alfalfa and sugar beet are the best way to introduce calcium into the diet. The body can more efficiently utilise calcium within a food substance rather than as a supplement.

Potassium (K)

Potassium is needed for body fluid regulation. It is likely to be deficient in water-extracted foods but is high in lush pastures. Well-saved forages are higher in potassium than cereals. Supplementation may be necessary when horses are working hard on a high cereal diet but care is required. Molassed sugar beet is a good source of potassium.

Sodium (Na) and Chlorine (Cl)

Sodium and chlorine are also needed for body fluid regulation and are likely to be lost in sweat. The best supplementation is probably common salt.

Iron (Fe)

Essential in the formation of haemoglobin, the means by which oxygen is carried by the blood. Lack of iron causes anaemia.

Magnesium (Mg)

Magnesium is an important element in the blood and in most cellular activities. Its major interaction is with calcium, phosphorus and vitamin D.

Soya-bean meal, good permanent grazing, well made hay and other forages are all good sources of magnesium but most cereals, especially maize, are poor.

Problems such as poor performance syndrome and obscure muscle stiffness have been shown to be associated with imbalances of these major minerals but not necessarily in the rations. Individual animals seem to be unable to make full or correct use of what is present.

Veterinary advice based on laboratory findings is necessary before attempting to supplement the diet.

Selenium (Se)

When horses graze pasture which is low in selenium there may be problems and diets should be supplemented with selenium and vitamin E. A deficiency of either selenium or vitamin E can cause muscle disease in young horses. As with most trace elements an excess can be toxic.

Cobalt (Co)

Cobalt may be used in cases of anaemia. It is a component of vitamin B12. A deficiency may cause liver dysfunction or poor appetite.

Copper (Cu)

There are parts of the British Isles where copper deficiency occurs. Copper is necessary for the formation of the blood pigment haemoglobin. A deficiency may cause anaemia or reduced growth.

Macro-minerals play important parts not only in tissue structure but also in metabolic processes and some in the electrolyte balances of intracellular and intercellular fluids.

Micro-minerals (trace elements) play important parts in enzyme action.

Vitamins

Like all mammals, horses need vitamins, although in very small amounts. Most of these will already be present in the diet of the correctly fed horse, although supplementation may be necessary under some circumstances. Little research has actually been done into the amounts required by the horse although the signs of deficiency are known.

The main vitamins are: A, C, D, E, K and the B complex. They can be divided into two groups: fat soluble and water soluble.

- A, D, E and K are all fat soluble and can be stored in the body.

- B complex and C are water soluble and cannot be stored.

FAT-SOLUBLE VITAMINS

Vitamin A (Retinol)
May be referred to as beta-carotene.

The horse obtains vitamin A naturally from green herbage which contains carotene. This is converted into vitamin A. There is some carotene present in newly made hay and other preserved grass but this deteriorates considerably with age.

A summer out on good grass will provide enough vitamin A, which can be stored in the horse's liver, to last through the winter.

Horses living in throughout the year and not receiving any green food may benefit from the addition of cod liver oil to their rations, although the amount must be carefully controlled.

Succulents such as carrots, apples, etc. also supply some vitamin A.

Broodmares and young stock, particularly newly weaned foals, may also require supplementation.

Lack of vitamin A can cause anorexia, poor growth, night blindness, inflammation of the cornea, infertility and respiratory disorders. Excess vitamin A is toxic.

Vitamin D (Calciferol)
The horse can obtain vitamin D naturally from sunlight on the skin. However, this is limited by: (a) the strength and amount of sunlight; and (b) the amount of time the horse is outside unrugged.

The amount of sunlight in the British Isles in winter is probably of little value but the vitamin can be stored by the horse.

A horse living out during the summer will probably accumulate enough to last him well into the winter but thereafter he may need supplementation. A horse who lives in all the time, or is turned out only occasionally, or who is out in a New Zealand rug, will require vitamin D added to his diet. Cod liver oil is a natural source. Synthetic vitamin D can be very potent and needs adding with great care as too much is toxic.

Vitamin D is necessary for the metabolism of calcium and phosphorus. Lack of vitamin D can cause bone and joint problems, as can excess vitamin D.

Vitamin E (Tocopherol)
Fresh food such as grains, seeds and herbage are all natural sources of vitamin E. Its level in stored foodstuffs falls daily as it is 'used' by the foliage and grains as a protection antioxidant.

More vitamin E will be needed when selenium is deficient and in an oil-rich diet. Late winter supplementation with vitamin E and selenium may be necessary. Synthetic vitamin E deteriorates and all compound food and supplements should be date-checked when buying new supplies. Wheatgerm oil is a good but expensive natural supplement.

Vitamin K

Vitamin K is synthesised by gut micro-organisms. It is also present in leafy matter.

Vitamin K is involved in the blood-clotting mechanism and supplementation is normally unnecessary.

WATER-SOLUBLE VITAMINS

The water-soluble vitamins include:

- B1 – thiamine
- B2 – riboflavin
- B6 – pyridoxine
- B12 – cobalamin
- niacin (nicotinic acid)
- pantothenic acid
- folic acid
- biotin
- choline
- C – ascorbic acid

Most of these vitamins are either present in high-quality food, especially green food, or are synthesised by the gut bacteria. Horses on good quality rations should not need supplementation but horses suffering from disruption of the gut bacteria because of sudden changes of food or antibiotic treatment will need additional supplementation. The important vitamins in this group are thiamine, folic acid and biotin.

THIAMINE is important for horses in hard work as it assists with the breakdown of lactic acid.

FOLIC ACID is high in good grazing, especially that with a high legume content. Stabled horses may be deficient, in which case a form of anaemia may develop. This

shows after approximately three months of stabled feeding.

BIOTIN is thought to be of value for horses with poor hoof formation.

TYPES OF FOOD

The modern horse's food can be divided into four groups:

- Roughage (bulk food).
- Concentrates.
- Succulents.
- Additives and supplements.

ROUGHAGE (BULK FOOD)

Grass

Grass is the most natural food for horses. If the quality and quantity are adequate grass is a complete maintenance food from April to September. This is why, if not otherwise organised by man, mares have their foals in late spring.

As the season progresses the energy value falls. In May it may be as high as 12MJ per kg of dry matter, falling in July to 9MJ (MJ = megajoule – a measure of digestible energy). Sometimes the value may rise again in the autumn. If saved at the optimum time it will supply suitable amounts of fibre, protein and minerals for the resting horse.

Grass is conserved by various means so that it is available as a basic ration throughout the year. The earlier in the spring it is cut, the higher the protein value. It can be saved in the following forms:

- Hay.
- Silage.

• Vacuum packed (as haylage).

• Dried and cubed.

Hay

The most common way of saving grass as hay is to cut it, allow it to part dry in the field, bale it and bring it under cover.

Hay that is grown for sale is usually setting seed and therefore depreciating in food value. It is cut at this stage because the bulk will be larger, the grass more stemmy, and easier to 'save'.

The way the hay is made is of almost more importance than anything else. If it is rained on, this washes out valuable nutrients. It should be dry when it is baled otherwise mould spores will generate inside the bales. Hay baled too wet may also cause the bales to overheat and some stacks can even catch fire.

Judging the value of hay by looking at it is almost impossible. Knowing its 'history' does help. In a large establishment, particularly one with competition horses, where a large quantity of hay is bought as one lot, it is worth the expense of having the hay analysed. For small establishments or the single horse owner, the cost of a full analysis would be uneconomic, so in this case it must be judged by the following criteria:

• It should be a good colour. Hay varies from greeny/grey to pale fawn but the greener it is, the better.

• It should smell pleasant, not musty, nor of vermin.

• It should shake out well and not stick together.

• It should be free from dust and disintegrating leaf, especially clover.

• It should not have any trace of damp or mould. To test this, it is essential to check the centre of the bale.

• It should have a good proportion of flowering heads.

• It should be free from weeds such as docks, thistles, nettles, bracken and, most particularly, ragwort.

Ragwort, when dried, becomes palatable to horses but it is very poisonous, causing liver damage which will eventually result in death.

New Hay

New hay can be harmful to horses. This is because grass made into hay continues to mature chemically in the bale. Although the maturing process uses up some of the sugars, it converts the unwelcome nitrates into amino acids.

The basic sward from which hay is made is rich in sugars and nitrates. New hay is still maturing and horses fed on it are likely to develop digestive problems. These can result in colic, laminitis and other metabolic disturbances. Filled legs are a typical result.

Hay should not be fed until two to three months after it has been made. It should then be introduced gradually by mixing it with the 'old' ration in increasing amounts proportionally over three to four days.

Types of Hay

Hay can be made from grass or lucerne. It may be specially grown or taken from permanent pasture. Grass hay is usually divided into two types:

• Seed or hard hay.

• Meadow or soft hay.

Seed Hay

Seed hay is made from grass that has been sown specifically as a crop. The grass is usually left down for only one to five years before being ploughed in. It consists of only a few varieties of grass or, in some cases, one variety only. The grasses commonly used are rye grass, timothy or cocksfoot. Some red clover may be added.

Seed hay feels hard to the touch and looks quite 'stalky', hence the alternative name 'hard' hay.

ADVANTAGES

- The grass used for the hay will be of a variety that is nutritionally valuable.

- Because it has been grown for re-sale, it is likely to have been made with more care.

- It is unlikely to have weeds in it.

DISADVANTAGES

- Because only one or two types of grass are included, the horse may be limited in mineral intake.

- It is expensive.

- It is less palatable.

- It is often mistakenly considered to be of greater nutritional value than meadow hay. In fact it contains more fibre.

Meadow Hay

Meadow hay is made from fields that are down to permanent grass and as a result contain many more types of grass and in addition herbs and possibly weeds as well.

The grasses are usually much finer and shorter in the stalk; thus it is sometimes known as 'soft' hay.

ADVANTAGES

- It is made up of many different types of plant, so the horse has access to a wide range of minerals.

- It is less expensive.

- It is more palatable.

- It is usually less fibrous than seed hay and of greater nutritional value.

DISADVANTAGES

- The optimum time for cutting is difficult to determine as the grasses flower at different times.

- Weeds, such as docks and thistles, may be

incorporated. Worse still, there may have been ragwort in the field.

Clover Hay

Clover hay is seldom seen in Britain as it is hard to make and inclined to break up and become dusty. If used, it should be fed with care as it is high in protein.

Lucerne/Alfalfa

Lucerne, or alfalfa, is very high in protein and is ideal for young, growing horses, especially if they are working. Many racehorse trainers use it for the two-and three-year-olds in training. It is usually very expensive but less concentrate food will be needed when lucerne is fed. It can, however, be low in phosphates so may need supplementing.

OTHER ROUGHAGE FOODS

Silage

Silage is made from young cut, but not dried, grass and either put into a clamp with the air excluded, or sealed in large, airtight bags (known as big bales). It is often made with additives of different kinds. It is important to check that any additives used are suitable for horses. Deaths from botulism after eating big-bale silage have been recorded in horses. Bacterial contamination is more of a risk if the silage has been cut very close to the soil. Unless it has been specifically made with horses in mind it is not recommended.

Vacuum-Packed Grass (Haylage)

This comes in sealed plastic bags, and to differentiate between hay and silage, the vacuum-packed contents are known as haylage, although there are many trade names. If it is used sensibly, horses seem to do well on it.

Haylage is of particular value for horses with respiratory problems. It should not be used for two months after cutting. It is made on the same principle as silage, although it is wilted for one or more days before being baled and sealed in plastic. It is important, therefore, to make sure that the bags are not punctured. Mice and rats chewing the plastic can be a problem.

Haylage is usually higher in protein than hay so a horse's concentrate ration should be reduced. The manufacturer should state the protein level. Haylage may have molasses added; this is not necessary.

Because of the higher water content in both silage and haylage it is important that pound for pound the weight of forage compared to hay is not reduced or the fibre intake for the horse would be affected and this must be maintained. If the horse thrives on haylage then the concentrates could be reduced accordingly.

Silage or haylage, whether in big or small sealed polythene bales, must be stored carefully and once opened the contents should be used in two to three days. Particularly in hotter weather, once opened the haylage/silage will begin to deteriorate in quality as the presence of air allows breakdown and chemical changes to start again. Whether in small or large sealed plastic bales, it is always wise to purchase it from a supplier who has made it specifically for horses. Some, especially when in big bales, may be of inferior quality and should not be bought. Any bale that shows earth when opened should not be fed to horses as the bacteria that cause botulism may be present and could prove fatal.

Dried Grass or Lucerne Cubes

These are made from grass or lucerne which has been cut at intervals during the growing season, usually when it reaches about 20cm (8ins) high. It is taken straight to a drier and then made into cubes.

It cannot really be classed as a bulk food as it is high in concentrates, both carbohydrate and protein. It is, however, a valuable food and can be mixed with soaked sugar beet to make a mash. The cubes are best soaked before being fed.

Oat or Barley Straw

This can be a useful bulk food in certain circumstances. Its value is often equal to poor hay and, in a bad hay-making year, it is better to feed clean, dry straw than musty, mouldy hay. In this case, however, the horse will need more concentrates as straw's energy value is low. Straw can be very useful for ponies, and for horses turned out on rich, succulent grazing. Made into chaff, it can be added to the feed to prevent bolting and to give bulk. It is also useful to mix with haylage or alfalfa hay to slow down the eating process and thus help prevent boredom and maintain the fibre ration.

Barley straw used not to be acceptable, as the awns, which are very irritating, were left on the straw. Now combine-harvesting removes the whole top of the stem, leaving only the straw behind.

Chaff

Chaff, or chop, usually comes ready cut. Few yards are large enough to warrant the expense of a modern chaff cutter. Hand-operated ones do not comply with Health and Safety recommendations. Chaff is an essential part of any ration as it provides the vehicle through which much digestion takes place. It can be made from hay, oat or barley straw, alfalfa or any other forage cut into approximately 2cm (1in) lengths. It does not need to be molassed or flavoured in any way if the material from which it is made is of good quality. Between ½ and 2 kg (1–4½lbs) can be fed at each meal. There are many ready-made products on the market, mostly of excellent quality but sometimes quite costly.

CONCENTRATES

This is the term given to the feedstuffs fed in a bucket. Most of them have a relatively high nutritional value and form a major proportion of the carbohydrate and protein intake of the horse.

They can be fed in two ways either as straights or as a

compound feed.

Seeds contain a high energy store of carbohydrate as starch. Farmers select those plants which carry a high proportion of seed to stem. The harvested crop of seeds is grain and is the additional energy part of the horse's ration.

The amount given should be balanced with the roughage to enable the horse to carry out the work required of him.

FEEDING STRAIGHTS

Feeding straights is the term used when the feed ration is made up from the various cereals: oats, barley, maize, and perhaps peas, and beans, mixed with sugar beet and or chaff and mineral, and vitamins by the owner or yard manager, to their own specifications.

It is the traditional method of feeding and was practised by all yard managers until the introduction of cubes and factory-made mixes. There was a great skill in getting it right and a good 'feeder' was a much-valued member of staff. Reasons for feeding straights are:

- May be cheaper as you are not paying for the processing.

- It is possible to see and assess the quality of the ingredients.

- You know exactly what is in the ration.

- You are able to design a ration specific to each horse.

- The ration is not adulterated with too much molasses.

- May be useful in a large yard with a number of horses all needing a similar ration.

- Useful for preparing a specific ration for old, sick animals or horses after surgery, or ones with a poor digestive system.

Arguments against:

- All cereals have a poor calcium/phosphorus ratio, which needs to be balanced by feeding something

high in calcium such as sugar beet pulp or adding ground limestone flour to the ration.

- Although it is possible to assess the quality of the various ingredients by sight, smell, weight and sometimes taste, it is difficult to get a proper analysis of the feed value of the ingredients used.

- It is difficult to ensure that vitamins and minerals are present in the right quantities.

- A variety of different feedstuffs need to be stored to make up the ration.

- Depending on how they have been treated, they will need to be used up in a specific time. Whole grains can be stored for months in the right conditions but any that have been rolled, bruised, crushed or micronised should be fed within three weeks of being treated, as the feed value is quickly depleted.

- If all the ration components are locally grown, any deficiency in the soil will be reflected in the ration.

- It is difficult to ensure the components are free from contaminating substances considered illegal in competition.

However, there are instances where the ability to make a bran mash, cook cereals or linseed or add particular ingredients to the diet can be useful. See page 181, Methods of Preparing Feedstuffs.

Oats have always been the traditional cereal fed to horses in the UK. They can be fed whole, boiled, bruised, rolled or crushed and oatmeal can be used to make gruel.

Ideally they should be assessed for quality whilst whole.

- They should be pale in colour unless they are black oats, which some claim to be superior.

- They should be smooth, shiny and hard to the touch.

- They should not smell.

They are seldom fed whole in Britain unless they are

cooked. Up to 1kg (2.2lbs) can be fed per meal. Bruised is the term given when the grain has been lightly passed between rollers. On looking at a sample, some grains will still be whole, some slightly cracked and some so squashed you can see the flour. This is the ideal way to feed them.

Rolled is when they have been squashed a bit more. There are no whole grains, some are cracked and some are well squashed.

Crushed is when nearly all the grains are well flattened.

The more the flour is exposed to the air, the quicker the sample will deteriorate and the feed value is lost.

Oats supply energy for work without putting on too much weight. They should only be fed according to work otherwise the horse can become quite excitable and strong. They are an excellent feed for fit horses required to work hard or fast and ridden by experienced riders. Up to 6kg (13lbs) can be fed per day but it is more usual to feed up to 4kg (9lbs). Most ponies are unable to cope with oats and can become quite unmanageable.

Barley is a shorter, plumper grain than oats and because it is usually kiln dried it is not always shiny. It is much harder than oats and needs to be crushed, micronised or boiled before being fed. It is more fattening than oats and is less likely to make the horse excitable. It is a good feed for excitable horses or ones who need to put on or carry a bit more weight and are not required to do too much fast work. Barley is usually more expensive than oats. Up to 3kg (6½lbs) are usually fed per day. It is possible to feed more but it might be better and cheaper to feed fewer oats to get the same energy levels.

Maize is usually fed flaked. It is good for maintaining body temperature and therefore makes a useful addition to the feed of horses living out in winter or animals such as hunters who may have to stand around in the cold. Up to 3kg (6½lbs) per day can be fed to young stock living out or ½kg (1lb) to animals living in.

Wheat is not usually fed to horses except as **bran**. This is the outer husk of the inner kernel of wheat. The milling process is now so efficient that there is little, if any, feed value in bran and it is expensive. However it is a useful source of fibre and can make a very palatable feed if mixed with boiled grains or linseed. It is often recommended by veterinary surgeons for horses after colic or gut surgery.

All the above need to have the calcium/phosphorus ratio made up to 2:1.

Sugar beet comes in various forms but all are essentially the shredded remains of the sugar beet after the sugar has been extracted. It needs to be soaked for anything from one hour to 24, depending on how it has been processed. When ready to feed, each shred should be separate and soft and there should be little excess water in the container. In hot weather care needs to be taken that it does not begin to ferment. You can tell because bubbles occur on the surface. Normally two measures of water to one of beet, by volume, will provide an adequate mix. Anything from ½–4kg (1–9lbs) of the soaked beet can be fed per day. The beet does not need added molasses. Some research suggests that too much sugar may predispose towards azoturia in horses doing medium or fast work. Beet provides slow release energy for work, is palatable, helps maintain weight and balances the calcium/phosphorus ratio as it is high in calcium.

Peas and/or beans are high in calcium and very high in energy. They need to be crushed before being fed and are seldom fed to horses as part of a straight ration unless they are in very hard work, such as racing. A quarter to half a kilo (½–1lb) would be the maximum fed per day.

Oil can be readily digested and utilised by horses and soya oil is a popular source. Research has shown that there are many benefits including improved stamina and endurance, reduced fatigue and less heat production during digestion. It is said to make excitable horses calmer and reduce the risk of diet-related ailments. It is very popular with the owners of endurance horses.

ADDITIONAL FEEDSTUFFS

Carrots, apples or **whole beet** are all good sources of something succulent. They are excellent to add to the feed of horses, especially if they are unable to be turned out.

Carrots can be fed whole, cut into long strips or minced if the horse is sick. Up to 1kg (2.2lbs) per day can be fed.

Apples are much enjoyed by horses. They should be ripe, not too green and hard. Slightly bruised or soft ones are fine as they are less acidic. They can be fed in the same quantities as carrots. They are best if cut into quarters.

Whole beet need to be sliced lengthwise in to quarters or eighths depending on their size. They provide a good distraction to a horse on box rest and are especially liked. Not more than ½kg (1lb) should be fed per day as they are inclined to give the horse the runs!

Salt should always be available. A tablespoon can be added to each feed, or a salt lick can be hung on the wall. They do not need to be flavoured. The horse will take it if he needs it and should not be encouraged to take too much.

A general **mineral/vitamin supplement** is sometimes recommended, fed according to instructions on the packet. Consult your veterinary surgeon. Sometimes a balancer can be fed instead – see page 181.

Sometimes owners like to feed **extra supplements**. Unless the horse is suffering for some deficiency diagnosed by a veterinary surgeon they are not usually necessary. Consult your veterinary surgeon.

Beer or stout is occasionally fed, also **eggs** fed raw. Both are said to add a shine to the coat. They should not be fed to excess.

Linseed is the seed of the flax plant. It is a traditional feed for horses. It is high in protein and oil but the quality of the protein is poor, being low in lysine. It must always be cooked before being fed, this deactivates the hydrocyanic acid, also known as prussic acid, which is present in the raw seed. Linseed is used to improve the coat condition but as a source of energy there are better oils.

Milk pellets are seldom recommended now. After the foal has been weaned his digestive system is not well suited to digesting milk.

Herbs

Herbs will be selected by horses from whatever grazing is available. Usually these herbs are high in valuable minerals and especially trace elements. When land is re-seeded for grazing horses, it is recommended that a strip be sown with herbs.

Dried herbs can be mixed into the horse's food. If minerals have been added to dried herbs, it is necessary to check the balance of the ration.

GARLIC is usually fed as a powder and is more readily accepted by horses when mixed with molasses. It is useful for horses with respiratory problems and is said to be helpful in the control of sweet itch. Its regular use is effective as a fly repellent. It can be used to disguise the taste of medicines.

COMFREY is known as the 'healing herb' and has been used for many years. It is the only plant known to metabolise vitamin B12 from the soil. It has a high content of easily absorbed calcium.

DANDELIONS, both leaves and roots, are much relished by horses. They are high in minerals and vitamins.

NETTLES, if cut and allowed to dry, are often appreciated. They are a good source of minerals, especially iron.

COMPOUND FEEDS

Compound feeds, in the form of cubes, pellets or mixes, are manufactured by a number of reputable firms. Between them they manufacture an enormous variety formulated especially to suit widely differing types and temperaments of horses and ponies working in all disciplines, at all levels.

Each compound is specially formulated with the correct levels of energy, protein, fibre, vitamins and minerals to suit the average equine of any given type.

Any one firm may manufacture between ten and forty differing compounds and if the range of one maker doesn't suit, another's might. Most firms publish a catalogue giving the specifications of their various products and the type of animal they are designed for.

They are scientifically formulated to produce a balanced diet and usually only need the addition of succulents and chaff in the bucket, along with the forage ration and water, to supply the horse with all his nutritional needs. There should not be any need to add extra cereals or minerals and vitamins. If the horse requires more energy look for a different compound that has a higher energy ratio. Similarly, unless the horse is deficient, extra additives should not be needed and should not be added without veterinary advice.

Reasons for feeding:

• Consistent quality in each bag.

• Scientifically formulated.

• Competition mixes are usually guaranteed free from forbidden substances.

• Ingredients specially formulated and treated to be easily digested, palatable and particularly suitable if the right formula is chosen.

• Specified shelf life.

• Suggestions on how much to feed are usually printed on the bag. (These are sometimes over-generous and may need to be modified.)

• Convenient for horses who travel a lot.

• Convenient for the less experienced owner.

• Particularly suitable for the one-horse owner as only one bag of feed is needed.

Reason against feeding:

• Often expensive.

• In yards with a wide range of horses, many different mixes may be needed.

• May take time to find the right formula.

• Not all formulas readily available.

Compound feeds were originally produced in cube form but strong owner pressure resulted in most manufacturers producing 'mixes' as horse owners wanted to see what made up the ration. Most mixes are more expensive than the cube of similar feed value. Originally many mixes were heavily molassed but the trend is now away from this. It is sometimes difficult to incorporate much oil into the ration, so it is important to read the analysis if this is a requirement.

There are compound feeds available for the whole range of equines from foals, broodmares, young stock, horses at rest, horses with awkward temperaments, animals working very hard such as race horses and competition horses, through to the great majority of animals who do not aspire to great things, perhaps only working a few hours a week or who have digestive problems and need an easily digestible ration.

Although compound feeds make the feeding of equines much easier, all horse owners should have a basic knowledge of the horse's digestive system and the feed components and the part they play in the horse's nutrition. The horse's digestive system is not designed for a rich diet and nowadays it is as likely to be overfed as underfed and this can lead to many digestive problems, which can lead to serious illness. The first rule of feeding, '**feed according to work**', must always be adhered to.

Some cubes are designed to be a complete feed with only water being additional to the diet. However, this can lead to horses becoming bored if they are stabled for long periods. Ideally, if these are fed, a small amount should be fed every one or two hours, which is often impractical.

Some cubes are designed to be fed with the addition of forage and water. Often called 'Horse and Pony Cubes' or 'Cool Cubes' or 'High Fibre Cubes' they may contain as little as 8% protein and are ideal for ponies, animals on a maintenence diet or ones doing very little work.

Other cubes or pellets (little cubes) are available for specific groups of animals such as brood mares and foals or competition horses. They will have a much higher protein specification, up to 14% for competition horses, 15% for brood mares and 17% for foals. It is vital, whatever form of feeding is chosen, that the protein level is correct; too little is better than too much.

Balancer cubes are also made to be added to a 'straights' feed ration or a high forage diet with little or no concentrates. This ensures that horses are receiving all the nutrients they require.

Compound 'mixes' usually known as 'coarse mixes' are exactly that. A loose mix of various ingredients many of which, like cereals, peas and beans, can be recognised by eye. Usually mixes and cubes can be found that have exactly the same feed values. It is a personal choice and many horse owners prefer to buy mixes even though they are sometimes more costly; they feel that their horse prefers them to a dry cube. Cubes occasionally have a longer shelf life than the equivalent coarse mix.

- When selecting a compound feed, always check the details on the bag.

- It is a legal requirement to state the name and purpose of the feed.

- There should be guidance on how much should be fed each day and to what sort of horse. Sometimes the amounts recommended are on the generous side and the feeder needs to modify them.

- The weight should be stated.

- The required storage conditions should be stated.

- It should have a detailed analysis of the protein, oil, fibre, and ash. It may show DE MJ/kg which is megajoules of digestible energy. All are shown as percentages.

- It is also mandatory to declare any added vitamins A, D and E as well as the total content of the trace elements selenium and copper.

- It may also list the ingredients such as oats, barley, grass meal, etc., usually with the greater percentages first. These are not required by law but market research has shown that most owners like to know. It is extremely unlikely that any animal derivatives are used in horse feed.

- Any synthetic antioxidants used to prevent the oils and vitamins from deteriorating during the shelf life must be declared.

- The 'best before' date will refer to the vitamin content. However the manufacturer must also ensure that the whole product does not go off within that time.

- There will also be a manufacturer's number that shows that the factory is licensed to produce animal feed.

METHODS OF PREPARING FEEDSTUFFS

- Steam pelleting

- Steam flaking

- Extruding

- Micronising

These are all commercial methods of processing concentrates with the purpose of making them more easy to digest, therefore having improved palatability, better feed value, longer shelf life and destroying any natural toxins that may be present. They are often included in coarse mixes although some, micronised barley is an example, can also be bought as a 'straight'.

Extruded grains have been super-heated with steam at 120°C for one minute. Extruded foods are broken down much more quickly as the feeds are instantly water soluble. This allows the stomach and small intestine to have a greater chance of utilising the important carbohydrate part of the ration. It has been found that horses fed on extruded food have much more water in their digestive system and therefore run less risk of impaction. However there is no increase in the water content of the faeces.

Micronised grain has been subjected to infra-red radiation which causes the grain to swell and gelatinate, thereby avoiding a high starch concentration in the large intestine.

METHODS OF PREPARING FEEDSTUFFS AT HOME

The following are methods of preparing feedstuffs at home to make them either more palatable or more easily digested, sometimes both.

• Gruel

• Bran mash

• Boiled barley

• Boiled oats

• Boiled linseed

Gruel

This is an excellent way of getting nutrients into a tired horse. Widely used before electrolytes, it is still helpful after hunting or long, tiring work, to prevent the horse from tucking up and preparing him for a more substantial feed later.

Put a double handful of porridge oats or pin meal in a bucket with a dessertspoon of salt. Mix to a paste with **cold** water. Add sufficient hand-hot water to half fill the bucket, stir around until it looks like milk and offer to the horse instead of his normal first drinks, until his thirst is quenched, in the normal way. Once the initial half bucket has been drunk, more tepid water can be added as needed until there is little or no oatmeal left and the horse is back on normal water.

Bran Mash

Bran mashes are seldom given as a regular feed nowadays but they are often recommended by veterinary surgeons after bowel surgery and if mixed with palatable additives can encourage a sick horse or poor feeder to eat.

Put between ½ and 1kg (1– 2lbs) of broad bran in a bucket. Add up to a tablespoon of common salt and enough boiled water to moisten the whole when mixed. It is easy to add too much so add gradually and mix well before testing. When it is correct, a portion squeezed in the hand will stick together and no moisture will drip out. Cover the steaming mash with a cloth and leave until hand-hot throughout. Always test with a bare hand: horses are not used to hot feeds and will be put off if it is hot to the tongue. Always mix it again before feeding to ensure it is an even temperature throughout. If it is left to get cold it will quickly become sour and unpalatable.

A mash can be made much more nutritious and interesting if it is made with something other than plain water. If feeding on veterinary instructions always ask before doing so. Some things to consider are:

• Warm molasses

• Very sloppy sugar beet.

• Boiled oats

- Boiled barley

- Boiled linseed

- Grated carrot or apple could be added but would not be damp enough to make the mash on their own.

Boiled Barley or Oats

Boiling whole oats or barley is a method of adding a palatable, easily digested alternative to a faddy or thin horse's diet. It is possible to cook bruised or crushed grain but it makes a claggy porridge that most horses do not seem to enjoy. Whole barley and whole oats can both be prepared in the same way. If cooking a large amount, a metal bucket and an electric boiler or substantial cooker will be needed. Smaller amounts can be cooked on the domestic cooker in a large saucepan. Allow between ¼ and ½kg (½–1lb) of dry grain for each horse. Cover with the same amount of water, by volume, and bring to the boil. This can take a long time if a big bucketful is being cooked. Once boiling, simmer gently until each grain can be cut in half by your thumbnail being pressed across it. This is similar to cooking rice and should not take longer than half an hour. Once all the water has been absorbed, the grain should be soft; if not, add a little more boiling water and after a few minutes test again. Care must be taken when using an electric boiler that it does not boil dry before the bucketful of grain is cooked. About ½ litre (just under a pint) of the cooked grain can be added to each feed. It can be fed warm but not hot.

Boiled Linseed

Whole linseed is tricky to cook and there are easier methods of feeding linseed oil – and there are other oils that are better feed value. However, horses usually love a cooked linseed mash, it can be used to disguise medications and many owners of show horses use it to improve the coat and put weight on their horses without them becoming 'hot' to handle. Too much will have a laxative effect. Traditionally it was fed as a first

feed after hunting or other very hard work. Whole linseed must never be fed raw to horses as the hydrocyanic or prussic acid that is present in raw linseed is toxic. It is safe to feed once prepared.

Allow about two tablespoons of the raw linseed and half a litre (1 pint) of cold water for each horse.

There are three methods of preparation to choose from:

1. Soak the linseed for twenty-four hours. This is the least satisfactory method.

2. Bring to the boil and simmer for three hours.

3. Soak overnight, bring to the boil and simmer for an hour.

The last is the easiest method and is to be recommended. The result should be a thick, grey jelly with the seeds suspended in it. Up to half a litre (1 pint) of this mixture can be fed per meal but only once a day and usually not more than three times a week unless the horse needs a laxative diet. It can be fed mixed with bran or chaff or added to the normal ration.

Linseed is notorious for boiling over and needs to be watched carefully as it comes to the boil and then simmered very gently to prevent it burning.

Linseed can also be fed as a gruel, in which case the jelly is diluted with warm water or as a tea, then the seeds are strained out and the jelly diluted even more. Neither method is any more beneficial.

SUPPLEMENTS

The horse owner is at present deluged by manufacturers advertising all sorts of mixtures to add to horses' and ponies' feeds.

If horses in medium work are being fed their concentrate ration as a compound food, plus good quality roughage, they should require nothing extra except possibly salt (NaCl).

Horses on home-mixed diets should have their rations checked. Many such diets are low in salt and calcium so competition horses should certainly have salt added to their rations and may need calcium, lysine and methionine. Vitamins A, D, E and folic acid may be necessary in the winter or where horses are permanently stabled.

However, vitamins and minerals cannot be considered in isolation. There are complicated interactions between them and between other nutrients, especially between vitamin D, calcium and phosphorus, and vitamin E and selenium, and the B vitamins and carbohydrates. The specific manipulation of vitamin levels in the diet should only be undertaken with professional guidance. Many of these interactions are not yet clearly understood or identified.

Supplements include:

• Minerals, including trace elements.

• Vitamins.

• Herbs.

• Bacterial cultures (probiotics).

• Feed balancers.

Reputable manufacturers of compound food will incorporate the necessary minerals and vitamins in their products and provide details of their analysis. Horses living out on land known to be deficient in some minerals will need supplements unless bought-in feeds contain the specific minerals.

Common Salt

Salt may be given by any of the following methods:

• Rock salt in the manger.

• Salt-lick on the wall.

• Added to the feed.

• Salt block in the field.

• It does not need to be flavoured.

There are advantages and disadvantages to all methods.

Rock Salt in Manger

ADVANTAGES

• It is cheap to buy.

• It stops horses from bolting their feed.

DISADVANTAGES

• Horses may not gnaw at it every time they have a feed and so will not ingest sufficient salt.

• Metal feed pans become corroded.

Salt Lick on Wall

ADVANTAGES

• Salt is always available.

DISADVANTAGES

• Some horses do not use it.

• It is very messy on walls and tails.

• Empty holders can be physically dangerous.

• There is a danger of infection if horses with coughs and colds are moved from box to box.

Salt Added to Feed

ADVANTAGES

• The amount given can be monitored.

Salt Block in Field

ADVANTAGES

• It is readily available.

DISADVANTAGES

• Some horses may not use it.

• If placed on the ground it will eventually dissolve and kill the grass on which it lies.

• It needs a special non-metal holder, with drainage holes; or it can be hung on a fence, thereby limiting the grass damage.

Probiotics, Antibiotics and Feed Balancers

PROBIOTICS are supplements designed to promote the performance of the existing digestive micro-organisms and also to add to their number. They are now used, under guidance, to assist in the better use of the food given to some horses.

Their usefulness and perhaps their risks are not yet fully evaluated. It is wiser not to consider them as a supplement but as a therapeutic or prophylactic medicine (e.g. to counteract the stressful effects of worming or travelling).

Similarly with ANTIBIOTICS, including those used against ringworm which are 'in feed' medications. Horses on antibiotics may have to be given extra vitamins. This is because oral antibiotics can kill the good 'bugs' in the gut. The horse will take some time to build up the flora. During this time some degree of indigestion may occur.

FEED BALANCERS (such as Blue Chip or Equilibra) are designed to be added to the chosen ration. They come as small cubes which contain a balance of vitamins and minerals, some probiotics, and perhaps some good-quality protein.

CHAPTER

23 DECIDING ON A RATION

Art Versus Science

Although the science of horse feeding has increased with new-found knowledge, it is important not to forget the practical aspects.

Weighing or measuring horses can be very useful, but nothing quite takes the place of the person who, just by looking at the horse, can alter his feeding a little to keep him in top condition. This takes much practice. The changes in amount should still be done by weight.

It is useless saying that the horse must have X amounts of this and Y amounts of that if (a) the horse does not look or do well on it; or (b) he does not like the food. Two horses of the same type and size both eating identical rations may look completely different because one is a good converter of food and the other a bad one. This is where the practical horsemaster comes into his own.

It is almost impossible to give exact amounts of food for different horses doing different jobs. For example, it is possible that one three-day event horse may be fit to run for his life on 5kg (11lbs) of concentrates while another of the same size and type may need 9kg (20lbs). However, **as long as the horse is not losing condition it is better to under-feed than over-feed**.

Deciding what to feed can seem very complicated to the less experienced person. The simplest way of doing this is to decide on a maintenance ration by considering the horse's size, age and type. Then it is necessary to work out what energy ration the horse will need to carry out his task, either for work or growth or both. The tables on pages 189 and 191-3 give a guide, and the approximate amount of the concentrates the horse will need can be calculated from them. It is then necessary to decide on the type of concentrates, bearing in mind their energy and protein value.

THE RATION

The ration can be divided into two parts, maintenance and ration for work.

The **maintenance ration** is what is required by each horse to maintain bodily functions and replace body tissue, i.e. to keep the mature horse at optimum weight and condition. This may well be provided just by grass in the spring and summer and include hay/forage, with perhaps some added sugar beet and hard feed in the winter, when more feed is needed to maintain body temperature and the grass has less nutritional value.

The **ration for work** will vary according to the amount and type of work.

Working horses include brood mares in the last stages of pregnancy and when lactating, young stock who are growing and developing and breeding stallions, as well as animals being ridden or driven.

Animals breeding and developing will require a higher protein diet to help with their development.

Horses being ridden and driven will require energy for exercise which will come mainly from carbohydrates.

CALCULATING RATIONS

The following considerations should be taken into account when deciding on a ration:

• Amount and type of work.

• Present state of condition and health.

• Size and type.

• Age.

• Conditions under which the horse is kept – inside or out.

• Weight.

• Temperament.

• Ability of rider.

• Economy (cost-effectiveness).

• Availability of foodstuffs.

• Feed storage and handling facilities.

Condition

The condition of the horse is assessed by using a scoring system (see pages 26–27). This measures the weight distribution over the neck, back, ribs and quarters.

Fat should not be confused with muscle bulk, or vice versa. Often, apparent muscle bulk is, in fact, excessive fat which has 'hardened', such as on the crest of ponies or overweight stallions. (Note: when standing relaxed, the horse's muscle, when palpated, feels soft and pliable.) Contrary to popular belief, fat will not turn into muscle with work.

Horses vary in their bulk of muscle, and the type of work they do can also influence their shape. For example, the muscle fibres in the horse trained for stamina and endurance, such as a three-day eventer or long-distance horse, are less 'bulky' than those of a sprinter, dressage horse or show jumper. The fit eventer will look lean and streamlined, whilst the show jumper

will have a more rounded appearance.

The muscle groups in a fit horse are clearly delineated.

Excessive weight puts unnecessary strain on the heart, lungs and limbs, and can shorten the useful working life of the horse or pony.

CALCULATING WEIGHT

Size and Type

Size and type should be considered together, as the more 'common' type of animal, although heavier, will usually have a better food conversion rate than the more Thoroughbred type of horse.

Size (height and weight)

The height and weight of the horse can provide a guide to feeding. Determining the height is not a problem. To discover the weight, the following methods can be used:

• Weighing the horse on a horse weighbridge.

• Driving the horsebox or trailer on to a public weighbridge with and without the horse.

• Using a specially calculated equine weigh tape (available from tack shops and feed merchants).

• Calculation using the following equation:

$$\text{Weight (kg)} = \frac{\text{girth}^2 \text{ (cm) x length (cm)}}{11900}$$

Girth is measured around the barrel immediately behind the elbow, after the horse has breathed out. Length is measured from the point of the shoulder to the point of the buttock.

Once the body weight of the horse has been determined, it is important to decide whether the animal is overweight, underweight or showing a lack or loss of muscle tissue, i.e. wasting.

As a rule, weight loss or gain relates to too much or

too little body and subcutaneous fat. If wasting is obvious, or if an animal is plainly obese, weight as such is of little consequence. Over-feeding or under-feeding of the average-conditioned horse has no (immediate) effect on muscle mass.

It has been suggested that for the resting horse, i.e. one on a maintenance ration, 1½% of body weight is required in food; for light work, the horse requires 2% of his body weight in food, and for medium to strenuous work from 2½% to 3%. Young horses and pregnant mares in the last three months of pregnancy need between 2½% and 3% as dry matter weight. However, these rough guide percentages depend on the type of food supplied. Horses do vary in the use they make of their food according to their type and individual metabolism. There is also a minimum requirement of 1.5% of the body weight as long fibre for correct gut function.

Establishing the Diet

• Amount and type of work will establish whether the horse is on a maintenance or a work diet. As soon as he is out of work his 'work' ration must be reduced.

• His present state of condition and health need to be considered. If the animal is underweight, unless the feeder is very experienced it is best to have a full health check and consult a veterinary surgeon. If the amount and type of food is increased and changed too suddenly complications can occur.

• If the horse is overweight, his total ration will need to be reduced until the optimum weight is reached. He will still need sufficient energy for his work but too many horses are overweight and this puts strain on their limbs, heart and lungs.

• Feed according to work is arguably the **most** important rule of feeding. The horse will always require the minimum weight of feed according to his body weight etc., but as soon as the work load is reduced the amount of energy food for work must be cut, also the

ration returned to a maintenance one. Even on a day off, the hard feed should be reduced and if the horse becomes ill or lame the hard feed should be cut immediately and be replaced by a more suitable ration and increased forage. Many of the common digestive problems are caused or exacerbated by horses being on too much hard feed.

• When building up the work ration always build up the work slightly in advance of the ration and when decreasing work – say before a holiday – decrease the ration beforehand.

• Calculate the total ration using the following method:

$$\frac{\text{Body weight (kg)} \times 2 \text{ or } 2.5}{100} = \text{amount per day}$$

Age

The age of the horse will have a bearing on the rations chosen. Young horses who are working as well as growing will need more food to cover the extra requirements for carbohydrate and protein.

Older horses may also require extra rations, but this can be decided by assessing their condition. Very old horses whose teeth may be poor or who are living out and taking very little exercise, will require an easily masticated and digestible ration of high-quality food. Old horses who are unable to graze properly or to keep themselves warm should never be left out in the winter. Keepers of these horses should appreciate that it is far kinder to have them painlessly destroyed than to allow them to linger on when they are not happy and cheerful.

Temperament

Placid, easy-going horses who 'take little out of themselves' will be easy to feed but must not be over-fed and allowed to get fat. They are likely to turn extra food into fat. However, it is important to differentiate between naturally 'laid-back' horses and those with an illness or suffering from a deficiency. Any alteration of

Percentages of body weight as total dry food requirement

Height in hands	Girth in cm	Girth in inches	Body weight in kg	Body weight in lbs	2%/3% in kg	2%/3% in lbs
12hh	145cm	57ins	260kg	573 lbs	5.2–7.8	11–17
13hh	155cm	61ins	320kg	705 lbs	6.4–9.6	14–21
14hh	165cm	64ins	390kg	860 lbs	7.8–11.7	17–26
15hh	180cm	71ins	490kg	1080 lbs	9.8–14.7	22–32
16hh	195cm	76ins	580kg	1279 lbs	11.6–17.4	27–38
17hh	205cm	81ins	640kg	1411 lbs	12.8–19.2	28–42
18hh	215cm	85ins	710kg	1565 lbs	14.2–21.3	31–47

temperament requires investigation.

Horses with a difficult, excitable temperament can be a problem to feed as they lose condition through excessive energy expenditure. Giving them more food to replace lost condition can often make them more excitable. They require plenty of roughage and are usually better on energy foods that do not contain too much cereal, e.g. sugar beet and lucerne.

Conditions Under Which the Horse is Kept

The weather must be considered when deciding on the amount of food that horses require. Food is used to maintain body temperature. In very cold weather horses will use more food to keep themselves warm. This is particularly so for clipped horses. If no extra food is given they will use stored fat and thus start to lose condition.

Under-fed horses, because of loss of insulating fat, will more readily lose body heat by radiation and convection and will, of course, feel cold. This results in shivering and further energy expenditure.

Food as such does not produce heat, but the act of eating does produce muscle activity heat. The cellular work necessary for digestion, absorption and metabolism and other vital activities are all heat-producing. It is the risk of loss of body fat in cold weather which necessitates extra winter feeding.

Economy (Cost-effectiveness)

Quality should never be compromised by cost, but one of the skills of a good manager is to be cost-effective in the purchase of forage and hard feed. See Chapter 53.

Simplifying the feed regime, ensuring there is no waste and monitoring stocks are all methods that are cost-effective and maintain quality.

Owners often prefer 'coarse mixes' because they can 'see what is in them' but usually it is possible to find a cube of the same feed value and possibly with a longer shelf life. Cubes are often cheaper. The majority of horses will eat either.

The more complicated the feed regime, the more time is taken in implementing it and the more opportunity exists for mistakes to be made.

Availability of Constant Supplies of the Same Quality

This applies particularly to hay, and, to a lesser extent, cereals such as oats or barley. If storage is available, enough forage should be bought to last for several months. If not, arrangements for storage may be made with the supplier, but this will make the food more expensive. Having a reliable supplier is essential for the welfare of horses and smooth running of the operation.

If compound foods are bought it should be ensured that further supplies will be available when required.

Supplementing the Ration with Grazing

Some daily grazing will benefit the horse's health but will make the balancing of rations more difficult. The quality and quantity of grass will fluctuate with the seasons and this must be taken into consideration. The richness of spring grass can easily lead to feeding too much protein and carbohydrate, with too little long fibre. Conversely, winter grass has lots of long fibre but little in the way of carbohydrate and protein. The possibility of infestation by the various forms of parasites must also be considered.

Ease of Handling

The considerations here are:

• The staff.

• The layout of the feed and hay shed.

• Access.

Other points might include:

• Size of bales.

• Size and weight of bagged concentrates.

• Movement of loose food (such as oats).

• Time taken to bring food to feed shed.

• Time taken to make up feeds.

HOW TO CHOOSE WHAT TO FEED

The main points to consider when choosing what to feed are:

• Energy.

• Protein.

• Fibre.

• Calcium/phosphorus ratio.

Measuring the Value of Foodstuffs

Food should always be fed by weight. The weight of a 'scoop' of oats or cubes should be known. As an example, a scoop of oats will weigh less than a scoop of cubes. Hay or vacuum-packed grass should be weighed before being fed unless it is being fed ad lib, i.e. to appetite.

The nutritional value of the food should also be known: straight foodstuffs such as oats, barley or hay can vary enormously in quality and for competition horses it is worth having these analysed – although this is seldom possible or practical except in a large yard, buying in bulk.

The value of the food is expressed as:

• The digestible energy (DE) of the food.

• The crude protein.

• The Ca/P ratio.

• The vitamin and mineral content.

Concentrates made up by food manufacturers have their values listed on the label and these should not alter, although the actual constituents may vary in amount owing to the economics of the market.

Digestible Energy

Digestible energy (DE) is computed in megajoules (MJ). (A joule is a measurement of energy. Energy is expressed as the number of joules in a kilogram of food.

Because there are so many joules in a kilogram they are measured in megajoules.)

For example, if oats are measured they are likely to have digestible energy levels of around 14 megajoules per kilogram; this is written as DE = 14MJ/kg. (See the table opposite.)

As a rough guide, for maintenance, a horse or pony needs 18MJ of digestible energy plus an extra 1MJ for each 10kg of body weight. For work, add 1–8MJ for each 50kg of body weight, according to how hard the horse is

Nutritive value of some common foods

	Crude Protein %	Digestible Energy MJ/kg
Cubes		
Horse and pony	10	10
Racehorse	13	13
Cereals		
Oats	12	14
Barley	11	15
Maize	9	17
Protein foods		
Soya meal	49	16
Linseed	26	24
Field beans	26	16
Grass meal	12–18	13
Intermediate foods		
Wheat bran	16	12
Sugar beet pulp	9	14
Forage		
Good grass hay	9	11
Average grass hay	8	9
Poor grass hay	4	8
Grass silage	3–17	12
Haylage	16	11–12
Hydroponic barley 'grass'	16	17

NB: This table is a guide – in practice a lot of variation will be found.

working. Add extra MJ for lactation, pregnancy and growth, as shown later. Thus a 500kg horse doing 1 hour of work per day (including cantering and jumping) requires:

$$18MJ + \frac{500MJ}{10} + \frac{4 \times 500MJ}{50} = 108MJ \text{ DE/day}$$

i.e. maintenance + work = energy required

Protein

Suggested percentage of protein in the total ration:

• Light work: 7.5–8.5%.

• Medium work: 7.5–8.5%.

• Hard work: 8.5–10%.

• Strenuous work: 8.5–12%.

• Adult horses: not above 10% in total ration including roughage – but see exceptions mentioned below.

Suggested protein percentages required for brood mares and young stock:

• Pregnant mares: 8–10%.

• Mares in last three months of pregnancy: 11–13%.

• Lactating mares: 14% gradually decreasing to 12%.

• Foals not receiving enough milk or spring grass: 16–18% in a compound ration. On good grass with sufficient milk from their dams no extra food is necessary. (Thoroughbreds will require special consideration, especially if bred for flat racing.)

• Weaned foals 6 months old: 14.5–16%.

• Yearlings 12–18 months old: 12–14%.

• Two-year-olds: 10–12%.

• Three-year-olds: 8.5–10%.

NB: There is evidence that overfeeding foals and yearlings may cause epiphysitis and/or contracted tendons. The significance of excess protein, excess energy and/or imbalanced minerals is not yet resolved but must be important as distinct from just one nutrient being blamed.

Work

The work the horse is required to do, the rider he has to carry, and his own temperament all have to be considered under this heading.

Work per day

Work can be defined, on a scale of 1 to 8, as follows:

Scale points for levels of work

Category	Scale Point	Activity
Light work	1	1 hour walking
	2	Walking and trotting
Medium work	3	Some cantering
	4	Jumping, schooling, dressage, driving
Hard work	5	Eventing, cross-country driving, hunting, endurance riding
	6	Hunting 2 days a week, three-day eventing
Fast or	7	Racing
strenuous work	8	Racing

Feed requirements for work

The following table is an approximate guide and must be altered to suit the horse. However, the 'bulk food' ration should never be less than 40% of the total ration. This ratio should only be sustained for short periods around a specific time of competition or strenuous work. If other types of roughage are used in the place of hay, the concentrates may well have to be decreased.

A horse at rest will require only a maintenance ration but if the horse is working, not only is it necessary to feed him so that he has enough energy for the job, but also so that he remains sensible enough to carry it out without harming himself or his rider.

A guide to feed requirement for work

Work category	% Hay	% Concentrates
Maintenance	100	0
Slow light work	85	15
Light work	80	20
Medium work	70	30
Hard work	50-60	50-40

FINALISING THE RATION

When the horse is on 100% forage, unless he is out at grass on good pasture he will require forage throughout the 24 hours, this is termed 'ad lib'. When living in it is preferable if this is given in 2–4kg (4½–9lbs) portions. When one helping is finished the next can be offered. If the ration is served in larger helpings, many horses will contaminate it by dropping it on the ground and treading on it. If it is fed on the ground initially it is even more likely to be rendered unfit to eat by coming into contact with faecal remains and being trodden on.

If it has to be fed in larger amounts, a rack at the correct height for the animal is often the best method.

Horses who are coughing will often contaminate the forage with their own mucus and then be unwilling to eat it.

If haylage is being fed, many horses tend to eat it very quickly. To slow them down, putting it in a double haynet or one with very small holes, or mixing it with good-quality oat or barley straw will often solve the problem.

Once the horse receives hard feed, i.e. from a bucket, this ration should be calculated for the whole day but then be divided up into portions. The forage might be divided into 2–4 portions, i.e. small portion – 2kg (4½lbs) before work, 2kg (4½lbs) after work, 2kg (4½lbs) in the afternoon and the rest in the evening haynet or overnight.

The hard feed will work itself out. For every 1–2kg (2–4½lbs) fed in a bucket, the horse will need another feeding time. If chaff or chop is fed with the horse feed, this is calculated as part of the roughage ration but is also counted as part of the hard feed when deciding on how many feed times are needed.

Research has shown that more smaller feeds are preferable to fewer larger feeds in preventing digestive disorders and allowing the feed stuffs to be digested more efficiently. It is also preferable if the forage is fed 10–30 minutes before the concentrates and this is even more important if chaff is not mixed with hard feed.

It is difficult to calculate the amount of grass a horse

eats when he is turned out. In the winter it may provide some roughage but have little nutritional value. In the spring and autumn it can have a high nutritional value and therefore the concentrates in the 'bucket' can be reduced or even cut completely.

If in doubt always reduce the hard feed and increase the forage.

Suggested ratio of hay to concentrates during fittening work

Week 0	The horse is on maintenance alone	100% hay or grass
Week 1	Walking exercise 1 hour	Hay to concentrate 90%:10%
Week 2	Walking exercise about 1½ hours	Hay to concentrate 85%:15% to 80%:20%
Week 4	1½ hours walking and trotting	Hay to concentrate 80%:20% to 70%:30%
Week 6	1½ hours walking, trotting and cantering	Hay to concentrate 75%:25% to 60%:40%
Week 8	2 hours walking, trotting and cantering	Hay to concentrate 70%:30% to 50%:50%
Week 10	As before but including some fast work	Hay to concentrate 60%:40% to 40%:60%
Week 12	Starting competitions	Hay to concentrate approx 50%:50%

Hay has been used in these tables as the 'roughage' ration. If other forages, such as vacuum-packed grass or lucerne, are used the protein level will need to be checked and the ratio altered to balance the ration.

Having considered all the above points the ration is worked out as follows, using a 500kg (1100lbs) horse as the example:

- Because he weighs 500kg (1100lbs) it is estimated that he needs about 13kg (29lbs) of food daily (2½% of his body weight).

- Because of the work he is doing he probably requires a concentrate: roughage ratio of about 25%: 75%, or roughly a quarter of his ration in energy food made up with three-quarters of hay.

- His suggested ration might be:

> 2.6kg (6lbs) horse and pony cubes at 10% protein
>
> 0.5kg (1lb) sugar beet weighed before soaking at 9% protein
>
> 9.5kg (22lbs) quality hay at about 8% protein

- As a compound food has been used no extra supplementation should be necessary.

- According to condition, behaviour and the work being done the ratio of concentrates to roughage may be altered.

(For the sake of simplifying calculations in this chapter, figures have been 'rounded up'.)

RATIONS FOR DIFFERENT TYPES OF HORSE

Horses Living Out and Not Working

A horse who lives out and is not working requires maintenance rations, i.e. he must be given enough food to maintain him in good condition.

Spring and Summer Maintenance

From May to October grass is an adequate ration for all horses and ponies if in sufficient quantity and quality. Native ponies may need their grazing restricted if the grass is very good, owing to the danger of laminitis. Always ask veterinary advice. Laminitic animals must not be starved – they need fibre going through their gut. There are a number of muzzles on the market designed for use on laminitic animals. All stock benefit from additional long fibre when on lush grass.

If the grazing is limited, or of poor quality,

supplementary feeding will be necessary.

Winter Maintenance

Horses and Thoroughbred-type ponies will require supplementary feeding. The grass will have little feed value and they will need food to keep themselves warm. Oats and sugar beet with a mineral/vitamin supplement and hay ad lib is a suitable ration. A ratio of between 10% and 20% concentrate to 90% or 80% hay should be adequate, but a careful watch should be kept on the animal's condition. Winter coats can easily disguise any loss. If an 'oat balancer' (a concentrate mix specially made to feed with oats) is fed with the oats no mineral supplementation should be required as this will contain the necessary minerals. One of the many 'cool mixes' on the market will serve equally well.

Native ponies grazing on a sufficiently large area may not need any extra food but those on restricted or possibly poor grazing will need hay. In years when hay is difficult to obtain, clean oat straw and sugar beet is an acceptable alternative.

Animals being fed haylage may eat their ration quite quickly. They can have the ration mixed with good quality straw to make it last longer and also to make up the fibre that is lacking in haylage.

Competition Horses

The horse in hard competition work will require more energy food than the same horse in medium work. However, it should be appreciated that each horse will have a level of required energy. Food and feeding above that level will not produce extra fitness. Food does not create fitness.

The fittening chart on page 193 should be studied, but note that fitness can go on increasing after the level of food remains the same.

It used to be thought that horses doing strenuous work required considerably more protein than other horses. This has been found not to be so. The level of protein in the whole diet should not add up to more than 10%. (National Hunt and three-day event horses may, as individuals, benefit from a determined amount of extra protein.)

The rations for competition horses doing fast or energetic work are all very similar although the type of work is often very different.

Blood-testing at the beginning of the fittening programme, and then again when the horse is fit, is a sensible investment. Some successful racehorse trainers test as often as once weekly.

Competition horses become less bored and digest their food better if more of their bulk food is chaffed.

They also benefit from having a larger number of small feeds – sometimes as many as five or six if working conditions allow. Their overall roughage intake should generally be 50% of their ration. There are now enough good-quality compound feeds on the market for it not to be necessary to restrict their roughage intake as they can obtain enough nutrition from a smaller concentrate ration than in earlier times.

Prohibited Substances

Racehorses in Britain and horses running under FEI rules anywhere in the world may be tested for prohibited substances. This also applies to some national competitions. It is therefore very important that these substances do not get into horses' food by mistake. Contamination usually occurs during transit or at the milling plant. Cocoa is the most likely contaminant. Many of the top feed suppliers produce their competition equine mixes on production lines used solely for that purpose. They guarantee their products but it is important that they are not contaminated once reaching the yard. Tools, feed bowls, buckets and storage bins must all be specific and scrupulous hygiene practised.

Event Horses

Event horses should be fed so as to maintain trained muscle bulk without becoming fat, yet so that they have enough energy to do their work in a sensible, economical way. Feeding them so that they are jumping out of their skins is not only a waste of food but may cause them to injure themselves or their riders.

Keeping them on a very low hay ration can cause them to run up too light and lead to digestive problems.

Event horses are subject to doping rules, so if they are fed cubes or a coarse mix it is important that the supplier is prepared to state that these products are free from prohibited substances.

Event horses need very little extra protein. The normal rules for feeding should apply and the total protein ration should not go above 10%.

Advanced, energetic competition horses should have their hay/roughage analysed and properly balanced rations made up in conjunction with quoted or determined analyses for concentrates and supplements.

Novice event horses are often given too much concentrate food. They are not being asked to do a great deal and should be fed according to the rules based on the recommendations given earlier. Most novices do not need more than 2.5–4kg (6–9lbs) of event cubes of, say, 11% protein, plus hay. For some horses this may have to be stepped up, or for others decreased.

Advanced three-day event horses probably do not need more than 4.5–6.5kg (10–14½lbs) of concentrates. Several Badminton winners have had less than this. Too much concentrate food can result in toxicity problems and the horse refusing his food. Feeding per se will not produce fitness: this must be built up through work. The energy spent must be replaced by appropriate feeding.

Horses must be watched to see they are not losing condition and the ration adjusted accordingly.

Roughage/concentrate ratio – event horses

	Roughage	Concentrate
Novice eventer	75% to 50%	25% to 50%
Advanced 3-day eventer	50% to 40%	50% to 60%

The roughage part of the ration should not be less than 40% and then perhaps only for a few days before an event.

Endurance Horses

Endurance horses need more energy than any other type of competition horse. Although they are not working at high speeds they have very long distances to cover at a consistent speed.

These horses must not be allowed to become fat. They should be very well muscled, but without the round outline of the dressage horse or show jumper, and should carry no excess weight.

They require easily digestible high-energy food with not too much bulk food. The addition of oil (such as corn oil) to their daily ration may be of benefit. Usually 100 ml (2–3 fl oz) is fed but much more has been given successfully.

Roughage/concentrate ratio – endurance horses

60% to 40% Roughage: 40% to 60% Concentrates

If a grain diet is fed a broad-based mineral supplement should be given. This should not be given with compound foods as they already have added vitamins and minerals. Salt (100mg) given daily is important. Endurance horses lose water and electrolytes since they sweat for much longer (distance/time). Na and Cl (salt) are two of the electrolytes lost. More advanced horses will benefit from a more comprehensive mixture of minerals (precursors of electrolytes) but specialist advice should be taken.

Dressage Horses

The dressage horse needs to produce slow power and does not need speed (it must be fit for this job but must not carry too much fat). He must be sensible and obedient, yet have enough energy for the job. The more advanced the training the more energy the horse will require. Dressage horses, unlike hunters, have to remain fit throughout the whole season, so a careful check must be kept on their condition and behaviour.

Point-to-Point Horses

Getting the point-to-point horse fit for racing is rather different from getting other horses fit because the point-to-pointer will have been hunted and will be fairly fit but may well be rather lean. After hunting he may benefit from being let down slightly for one to two weeks with slow exercise. During this time he should be on reduced rations but not if it is judged that he requires to put on some fat before serious fittening starts. (See also Chapter 42.)

Because he is now partly fit his feeding can start as at the sixth week with a ratio of 50% roughage:50% concentrate.

The traditional method of feeding point-to-point horses was good quality oats and hay. This is still practised with much success. However, it is suggested that if this diet is chosen an oat balancer and some sugar beet should be added. Salt and a general-purpose supplement will help to make up for any deficiencies in the diet.

If compound foods are preferred it is important that they are free of banned substances.

By the time he starts racing the horse should be on a ratio of 40% roughage:60% concentrates, or even 35%:65% briefly around the race date.

Show Jumpers

Show jumpers are required to make a considerable muscular effort for a short time. They need to stay fit for a good length of time as the season is now very long. When horses are travelling for so much time it is sensible to feed compound foods. This will mean that it is necessary to carry only one kind of concentrate food and hay.

It is important that feeding times are carefully adjusted to fit in with jumping times.

Polo Ponies

Polo ponies have to work very hard and fast for short intervals. They need to be muscularly very fit and need high energy food to enable them to achieve this.

Because of the usual time of play, the afternoon, the feeds on playing days need adjusting. Polo ponies should be fed four times daily if possible – morning, early lunch, tea and late night.

On a non-playing day the larger feeds should be lunchtime and late night. On a playing day only a very small feed should be given at lunchtime. Hay should be given first thing in the morning and taken away at least three hours before playing.

Any pony who stops eating should have his mouth carefully examined. Owing to the severe bitting used on some ponies there may be damage to the mouth which will make the animal reluctant to eat.

Usually cubes or coarse mix are more suitable than a straight cereal ration as, although polo ponies need to be very fit, they must be sensible.

Hunters

Hunters should be fed the same sort of rations as event horses but with more bulk food. They require between 3.5 and 5.5kg (8–12lbs) of concentrates plus good hay. Thoroughbred horses need hay or bulk food ad lib but the usual rules still apply.

They must be fed so that they are well behaved, can gallop for short distances, and remain out of their stables all day, probably for three days in every fortnight from November until March. Once fit it is not easy to keep them looking and feeling well throughout the season. Their rations will need careful adjustment so that they do not lose condition. A late night feed, if it can be given regularly, can be of great benefit. On hunting days they will almost certainly miss their midday feed and perhaps the afternoon one, as well. These should be made up later in the day.

On rest days after hunting, their concentrate ration should be reduced and their roughage ration increased. They should be walked out and, if possible, grazed in hand.

Traditionally a bran mash was given after hunting; this is seldom done nowadays but giving an oatmeal gruel (see page 182) or electrolytes immediately on return from a hard day can prevent the horse from running up light. Always offer forage before hard feed – it encourages the horse to relax and therefore the digestive system to work more efficiently.

The first hard feed after return should be small and easily digestible. The second can be of normal size and contain the remainder of the ration.

Riding School Horses

Economy has to be a prime consideration. It is essential to shop around and compare the prices and contracts that are available from feed merchants and farmers. Large discounts are often offered for yearly contracts. However, low cost must not be the only criterion. The horses and ponies must look well, their manners must be impeccable and they must stay healthy and content.

Good, clean, affordable hay is the basis for feeding riding school horses; good hay will lower the necessity for large quantities of expensive concentrates. Meadow hay is usually cheaper than seed hay and if well saved is just as nutritious. In years when good hay is scarce and very expensive, alfalfa pellets fed with clean oat straw make an acceptable alternative.

Big bale haylage makes an excellent alternative to hay when there are enough animals to finish the bale in between 3 and 4 days and where it has been well made.

Most commercial riding schools have found that horse and pony cubes provide the best type of energy food. These cubes are low in protein and high in fibre and are ideal for animals doing 2–3 hours of slow work daily. They will already contain the necessary supplements. Soaked sugar beet, although sometimes difficult to manage in large quantities and rather messy, is a good non-heating addition.

It is impossible to give amounts of food without knowing the weight, size, type and the work the horses are going to do. If students are being trained it will be necessary for them to experience the use of some other kinds of foodstuffs – possibly these could be used for special liveries or any competition horses at the school.

The 'One-horse Owner', Non-competitive Horse

For the one-horse owner whose animal is not going to do anything very strenuous it is sensible to choose a reputable manufacturer and feed their compound food, either as cubes or mix. In this way all the necessary nutrients will be automatically included in the diet. Usually manufacturers are apt to be too generous in the quantities of food that they suggest for the various sizes and types of animals, so, as always, it is necessary to consider the condition of the horse and his behaviour.

Between 70% and 80% roughage should be fed, as little energetic work is being done.

Children's Ponies

It is of prime importance that children's ponies are fed so that they are quiet and sensible. They should look well, but their manners are paramount.

They can be divided into groups and then divided again as to the work they are doing:

GROUP 1 – The small woolly native pony, such as the Welsh or Dartmoor types.

GROUP 2 – The larger native pony, such as Highland, Dales, Fells and Welsh Cobs.

GROUP 3 – The more finely bred pony, such as Connemara, Arab or Welsh riding ponies.

GROUP 4 – The Thoroughbred or nearly Thoroughbred pony.

All these groups blend into one another but it should be remembered that Groups 1 and 2, the native ponies, are much better converters of food than their aristocratic cousins. If being fed with the pony's weight as a guide, Groups 1 and 2 will probably only require 2% of body weight. The ever-present danger of laminitis in over-fat ponies in Group 1 must be kept constantly in mind.

Groups 3 and 4 will need about 2½% of body weight. The roughage:concentrate ratio will depend on the other factors already discussed but particularly on the work they are doing. This can be divided into:

• **Beginners' ponies** – Whatever their size, as long as they have sufficient roughage, they usually require little or no concentrate. If it is necessary to give them a tit-bit to catch them or some food in the stable so that they are keen to come in, this should be a small handful of the lowest-possible energy food. If they start to lose condition, the roughage should be increased or some sugar beet and dried grass or alfalfa added. The last should not make them excitable and will help to put condition on again.

• **Family ponies** – The energy food required will depend on the amount and kind of work being done. Their concentrates will probably be between 5% and 20% of the total ration. A compound mix of about 10% protein is most useful.

• **Riding-school ponies** – Those working 2–3 hours daily may need between 10% and 20% of the total ration fed as concentrates. Their concentrates are likely to be whatever is fed to the other school horses.

• **Hunting ponies** – Those living in at night and hunting every Saturday may need between 15% and 30% of their total ration as concentrates. A compound mix is better for them than a ration based on oats.

• **Competition ponies** – These may vary from top-class JA jumping ponies to show ponies in lead-rein classes and their rations must depend on the type of competition for which they are used.

It must be remembered that cereals such as oats have a hotting-up effect. A horse and pony type of mixture is a safe food. It will contain a reasonable amount of fibre and have all the necessary vitamins and minerals added. Soaked sugar beet pulp is a good source of digestible energy and does not have the same hotting-up effect as the cereals.

Mares, Foals and Young Stock

Mares

Although pregnant and nursing mares should be well fed with good quality, easily digestible food they should not be over-fed. The size of the foal is determined by the genes from the sire and dam and not by the amount of food the mare is given. A higher protein ration should be given in the last three months before foaling (especially if foaling early) and while the foal is on the mare. If the grass is very good this extra protein may not be necessary. During the last three months, feed a specialist mix or compound developed specifically for 'in foal' mares. There are many good products now available.

Foals

The feeding of the foal should depend on the response of the foal to the dam's milk. Some mares give a large quantity and others very little. In the latter case the foal should start eating concentrates as soon as possible. Early weaning may cause a loss of condition so foals who are to be weaned early should be eating well and will have to have their energy and protein ration increased when they are taken away from the mare. Foals who are weaned at five to six months should need little extra if they are eating concentrates and grazing. Mares who are not in foal again may be allowed to run on with their foals. As the mares dry off they will wean the foal themselves, when they may be separated with little trauma.

A balanced diet must be fed to growing animals if their full growth potential is to be reached whilst achieving healthy bones and teeth. Incorrect or over-feeding of foals may cause epiphysitis or contracted tendons. A good appropriate pre-mixed feed, specially prepared for young stock from a major horse feed manufacturer and fed at recommended levels, is really the most efficient way to feed foals and young stock. Foals cannot digest whole oats and need quality foods suitable for their limited digestive ability. Because of the immature nature of the foal's hind gut, proteins produced by the gut flora in the adult are not available to the youngster.

Young Stock

Young stock will require supplementary feeding from August right through to the end of April, and possibly longer if there is little grass. They need extra protein for growth and carbohydrates for maintenance. They should be fed so that they always look well covered but not too fat. Too much protein may cause lameness problems. Their diet must be well balanced with sufficient minerals, especially calcium, to ensure steady healthy growth.

Young stock, particularly weaned foals and yearlings who are living out in the winter, will require extra feeding to make up for the loss of condition through adverse weather conditions. Given sheltered conditions and good grazing they can be left out until the end of December and then brought in at night until the weather starts to improve in the spring. However, even Thoroughbreds, provided they have enough proper food and available shelter, will do perfectly well kept out all the time. The disadvantage is that they do not have daily handling and may object strongly when they are eventually brought in. Whether they are in at night or out all the time, good hay, sugar beet, stud cubes of about 14% protein, plus a good supplement will provide a good ration.

Growing horses require a higher level of protein than mature horses and the younger they are the more they will need.

Stallions

Stallions may be divided into two groups:

- Those used only as stud animals.

- Those who are ridden or competition animals as well as used at stud.

Stallions Doing Stud Work Only

Stallions should be on a rising plane of nutrition as the stud season (spring) approaches. During the season and depending on the number of mares they are to cover, they should have high-energy food but must not be allowed to become fat. When the season is over they should be let down gradually and returned to a maintenance ration.

Stallions Being Ridden and Used at Stud

Sometimes the competition stallion is retired to stud for the season and afterwards continues with his ridden work. In this case, depending on the work that he has been doing there is usually no necessity to change the rations. For the stallion who continues to do his ridden work as well as his stud work, his concentrate ration will have to be increased. In all cases, the condition and behaviour of the stallion will determine the changes that should be made.

FEEDING PROBLEMS AND NON-ROUTINE FEEDING

Sudden Refusal of Food

If a horse who usually eats normally refuses to eat, it may be a sign that something is seriously wrong with the horse. Should refusal persist for more than two feeds, especially if hay is also refused, the veterinary surgeon must be called. If other signs of illness appear, this professional help should not be delayed. However, there are other reasons such as:

- Stress – horse usually shows little desire for food and won't eat.

- Over-feeding – horse usually shows little desire for food and won't eat.

- Lack of clean, fresh water over several days – horse usually shows little desire for food and won't eat.

- Contaminated food – horse will usually show a desire to eat but appear fussy.

- Dirty feeding utensils – horse will usually show a desire to eat but appear fussy.

- Acute tooth problem, sore mouth, tongue, etc. – horse will usually show a desire to eat but appear fussy.

- Bullying from other horses

- Being disturbed whilst eating – too much coming and going of people and/or horses.

In the absence of clinical illness check on the above.

'Bad Doer' (Thin Horse)

A bad doer is the horse who eats all he is given but does not look well. The more common reasons are:

- Worms.

- Sharp teeth.

- Lack of adequate food.

- Poor quality food, especially hay.

- Unbalanced diet.

- Poor metabolism, often caused by being incorrectly fed or starved in the past.

- Over-stress.

- Bullying – he may not be getting his share, if out in the field with others.

The bad doer should be checked by the veterinary surgeon.

There are serious reasons for horses being thin or losing weight. They include:

- Heart abnormalities.

- Chronic pain.

- Anaemia.

- Ragwort poisoning and other liver pathologies.

- Cancers.

• Kidney disease.

• Worms (internal parasites). See also Chapter 17 and consult your veterinary surgeon.

The Sick Horse

It is essential that veterinary advice is taken when there is doubt about diagnosis and especially treatment.

Illness can be acute or chronic. The acute form could be colic, sudden viral infection or something resulting in a high temperature. The chronic form could be liver damage, anaemia, or cancer of some part of the digestive system. Some of these can be diagnosed by blood testing.

The veterinary surgeon will advise on a ration in cases of acute illness.

Recent work suggests that feeding certain types of fats may stimulate healing mechanisms.

For ill and convalescent horses, feeding little and often is of prime importance. Any food not eaten within 10 minutes must be removed. Containers must be washed with plain water between each feed. Many sick horses prefer to eat from the ground.

They require nourishing, easily digestible food and should not have large quantities of cereal-type food. Anything that they are prepared to eat is generally the answer, and molasses is often of assistance to tempt them. Some freshly cut grass, if it is available, is usually acceptable and many horses enjoy dandelions, which are full of minerals. Chopped dried lucerne is often appreciated and is a valuable food. A mash may be made of soaked, dried grass cubes and sugar beet. Carrots are also good.

See sick nursing, page 123.

Enforced Rest

For fit horses who are going to be off work for perhaps only a few days, reduce the concentrates the first day by 75–80%. Give more roughage and cut out any oats after three days, and adjust down to maintenance rations.

Horses who have to be kept stabled with no exercise for some time, perhaps from lameness, should be given a maintenance ration with no additional energy food. They must have all the necessary minerals and vitamins to aid recovery, and the diet must be sufficiently laxative. Hay or its equivalent plus sugar beet and some additives should be sufficient. A slight loss of condition is of less importance at this time than the maintenance of a calm attitude and prevention of conditions such as azoturia.

Stress

Excessive stress may result in loss of condition. The causes of stress can be:

• Strange stable.

• Disturbance in yard.

• Poor handling.

• Travelling.

• Pain.

• After hard work or competition.

Discover and minimise the cause as far as possible. Give most of the food at night. If this is only a short-term problem, do not worry; although the horse may run up a bit light he will not be harmed by not eating very much for two or three days.

The horse suffering from long-term stress may show this by weaving, box walking or other stable vices. He needs to be kept in a quiet box and have a strict work and feed routine. A slightly larger, late-night feed, that he can digest quietly, may be of help. The more he can be turned out, even if the grass is poor, the better.

Travelling

Water and food should always be carried and enough time should be allowed for stopping to water and feed the horses en route. Horses who travel regularly will usually learn to drink and eat when it is offered. On long journeys offer water at least every three hours, more often if it is hot or if the horse did not drink last time. Many horses will drink water from home but not strange water. Always carry a few canisters but ensure they are not contaminated, e.g. smell sour because they previously contained milk. Horses should be given time to finish their feeds before proceeding. Some horses will not eat when on the move and there is a risk of choking should they do so.

When travelling very long distances, such as across Europe, care must be taken during the journey that the food is easily digestible and is not likely to cause metabolic upsets. The quantity of concentrates should be halved and the roughage increased. Extra electrolytes may be necessary. It is essential when travelling abroad to find out what feed is and is not allowed into the countries that the horse is travelling through. (See also Dehydration, in Chapter 19.)

PROBLEMS AND AILMENTS CONNECTED WITH DIET

There are several ailments that may be directly caused by incorrect feeding and others on which incorrect feeding may have a bearing. They include:

- Under-feeding.
- Over-feeding.
- Colic.
- Diarrhoea.
- Azoturia.
- COPD.
- Electrolyte losses.
- Anaemia.
- Choking.
- Lameness, including laminitis.
- Lymphangitis.

- Poor teeth.

Under-feeding can cause:

- Starvation – resulting in death.
- Chronic malnutrition.
- Weakness and inability to work.
- Deformity of bones in young horses. Stunted growth in young horses.
- Dehydration.

Over-feeding can cause:

- Bone disorders in young horses – mainly epiphysitis. (See feeding young horses, page 198.) Contracted tendons in young horses.
- Reduction of fertility; problems in foaling mares.
- Problems in strenuous exercise owing to carrying excess weight.
- Lameness from added strain on the legs and feet.
- Inability to carry out proper work.

The over-feeding of concentrates is particularly common with event horses, who may suddenly go off their food. The answer is to cut the concentrates by half for one day and by another half the next day and then gradually alter the diet so that the quantity and balance are correct.

Colic

The word 'colic' simply means abdominal pain of some sort. It may be severe, sudden or gradual in onset, or of a low level of pain. There are many different kinds of colic and many causes, including those listed below:

- Incorrect feeding, e.g. wrong times, variations in type, wrong amounts.
- Windsucking, which may cause indigestion.

- Mouldy food.

- Poor teeth.

- Too large feeds.

It is now accepted that feeding mistakes are less commonly the cause of colic but the risk should not be ignored. A sudden change to cereals will readily produce large gut acidosis, producing electrolyte imbalance, bacterial proliferation and colic as well as laminitis.

A sudden change to long fibre is more likely to induce colonic impaction.

Diarrhoea

Can be caused by:

- Worms.

- Stress.

- Oral antibiotics.

- 'Upset' micro-organisms in the gut, caused by sudden change to cereal or lush grass feeding.

In all cases of diarrhoea there will be dehydration, particularly in acute cases. Fluids containing electrolytes may be required. Veterinary advice should be sought; this is particularly important in the case of foals, and in adults if it persists for more than 24 hours, or less if general signs of illness are present.

Azoturia, Set Fast, Tying Up

These are all names for more or less severe symptoms of the same process. Equine rhabdomyolysis is the name used to encompass the whole syndrome. This may range from muscular cramp to actual degenerative changes in the muscles.

It is usually associated with exercise after a short period of rest on full rations, or if the horse is asked to work much harder or longer than usual. Symptoms range from stiffness and sore muscles to a refusal to move, severe sweating, high pulse and respiration rates and obvious pain.

Often the horse appears lazy and reluctant in his work. Care needs to be taken to rule out azoturia before urging him to greater effort.

The horse should not be moved and veterinary assistance should be sought immediately. Permanent damage to muscles can occur if the horse is moved.

Mares are said to be more prone to azoturia than are stallions or geldings.

Horses should always have their concentrate ration reduced on their rest days and should be warmed up slowly before work and allowed to unwind gradually after fast work.

The following have all been suggested as possible predisposing factors:

- Faulty metabolism.

- Vitamin and/or mineral deficiencies.

- Hormone abnormalities.

Some success has been achieved in the treatment of constantly recurring rhabdomyolysis by feeding extra calcium and/or salt.

Lymphangitis

Lymphangitis is inflammation of the lymphatic system. It is also known as 'Monday Morning Disease', a name often given incorrectly to azoturia. Lymphangitis usually occurs after a rest day, so often on a Monday, when the horse's hard feed has not been cut back on the rest day and he has been left in his stable.

The lymphatic system relies considerably on movement to work efficiently. When the horse is kept in his stable the system is unable to remove the waste products and inflammation is the result.

This results in filled legs. Usually the insides of the hind legs above the hocks appear the worst affected but all the legs can be filled and warm to the touch. The horse is often in considerable discomfort and reluctant to move. Cold hosing or hot and cold fomentations will help reduce the swelling, and then walking in hand until the swelling is reduced.

Reducing hard feed and turning out, walking in hand or time on a horse walker on the day off should prevent a recurrence.

If the horse is in discomfort a veterinary surgeon should be called. (See page 137, the Lymphatic System.)

Feeding a Horse with Wind Problems (COPD)

This horse will almost certainly be allergic to the fungal spores in hay and straw and also to dust. As far as possible he should live in a dust-free environment, and be bedded on shavings, sawdust or paper. His food should be chosen or treated so that he does not inhale any mould spores or dust. The bulk food should be either hay that has been immersed in water for 10–20 minutes, or vacuum-packed grass. He should be fed on cubes and sugar beet and if other food is given it should be damped. Good ventilation is of prime importance .

He should be taken outside to be groomed and for mucking out. The more he can be outside, the better he will be. The addition of garlic to the ration has proved beneficial in some cases.

When travelling, straw should not be used on the floor of the vehicle and the haynets of any travelling companions should also have been soaked.

Lameness

Lameness which can be caused by incorrect feeding includes:

- Laminitis.

- Epiphysitis.

- Contracted tendons.

- Poor hoof formation.

- Lymphangitis.

25 MANAGING FORAGE

How horses are fed is important. Forage is expensive and it should be carefully stored and prepared so that none is wasted.

HAY/FORAGE

Hay can be fed:

- Loose on the ground.
- In haynets.
- In hay mangers.
- In hay racks.

Loose

ADVANTAGES

- Natural for the horse to eat off ground.
- Labour-saving.
- Safe.

DISADVANTAGES

- Difficult to soak but can be tipped out of soaking net.
- Difficult to weigh but slices of a bale of known weight can be measured off reasonably accurately.
- Wasteful.
- Untidy in yard.
- Liable to contamination.

Haynets

ADVANTAGES

- Economical.
- Can be prepared in advance.
- Easy to weigh.
- Tidy to handle.
- Easy to soak.
- Horse takes longer to eat, therefore improves digestion and helps prevent boredom.

DISADVANTAGES

- Time-consuming in labour, and if soaked, difficult to lift unless a pulley is fitted.
- Can be dangerous, especially in young stock boxes.
- Expensive to buy – poor 'life'.
- Unnatural eating position.

Hay Mangers

If correctly designed, they can be the ideal method of feeding forage. They should be set at about chest height and off the floor.

ADVANTAGES

The same as for feeding loose and less wasteful **and prevents contamination from the bedding/floor.**

DISADVANTAGES

Horses must not be able to get feet stuck under them nor should they be able to stand in them.

Hay Racks

Because of the possible danger of hay seeds entering the horse's eye there are reservations about the use of hay racks, particularly those which are high.

Soaking Hay

Mould Spores

Certain horses are allergic to the mould spores found in hay, straw and chaff. These spores are a danger to these horses, not because they are eaten and swallowed, but because they are inhaled. All hay and straw contains some spores, but visibly mouldy products contain considerably more. Horses fed and/or bedded on mouldy material run a greater risk of inhaling more spores than the natural mechanism of their respiratory system can cope with. Sooner or later some spores reach the bottom of the airways (alveoli). Although the healthy horse may be able to cope with this, in the allergy-prone horse a disease state is stimulated.

It is advised that such horses should be fed soaked hay. Soaking hay keeps the spores' surface tension high and so prevents them from escaping from the eaten fibre into the airway. They are masticated and swallowed and do not enter the lungs. Another school of thought suggests that soaked spores swell to become too big to gain access to the sensitive alveolar area. When exhaled they are wiped off on to the throat and swallowed. Of course, the welfare of a known COPD horse should be discussed with a veterinary surgeon.

Soaked Hay

The prevalence of allergic coughing has encouraged the feeding of soaked hay. This is hay soaked in water for about 10–20 minutes before being fed to the horse. The easiest method is to put the hay into a net, which is then immersed in a tank of water until no more air bubbles escape. The haynet is then hung up and allowed to drip before it is given to the horse. It should not be allowed to dry right out. Another advantage of soaking is that it washes out much of the dust, which in many horses causes 'hay cough'. It must not be soaked for longer than 30 minutes maximum or valuable soluble nutrients will be lost to the water in which the hay is immersed.

In a large establishment where all the hay is soaked (a sensible precaution) a long tank not more than 1–1.2m (3–4ft) high is essential. The nets are lifted from the water and allowed to drain before being hung up. They are very heavy and a pulley system saves the staff considerable strain. In a one-owner yard a dustbin makes a suitable receptacle for soaking.

When travelling, boiling water poured on to hay in a plastic sack will be a suitable alternative to soaking. This is not practical for large numbers of horses.

All hay should be weighed before being soaked.

The water in which hay has been soaked needs to be disposed of safely into the drainage system. If tipped on the ground it can pollute water courses.

Feeding Hay Loose on the Ground or in a Manger

Hay to be fed loose should be shaken up and placed on a sack that has handles at each corner. The sack can then be picked up by the handles, weighed on a weight hook and carried directly to the horse's box. Hay should not be carried loose in the yard; it is both wasteful and untidy.

Managing hay/forage

Having decided on the type of forage to be fed it is important to devise a practical, labour-saving method of feeding.

On large yards where haynets are being used, they can be colour coded according to weight and type of forage with the same colour being marked on the stable door.

If mangers are being used it may be possible to load nets or bales onto a motorised vehicle and drive through the building off-loading as you go.

When a number of animals are fed in paddocks it is preferable to use cattle forage racks or something similar. Ensure they have a safe, hard standing. They are especially good if big-bale forage is being used.

Forage, especially hay, should always be shaken up before being fed. This ensure no dried weeds such as ragwort are introduced into the diet.

There is a growing tendency to feed by 'slice'. This is an inaccurate and unsafe way of feeding and should be avoided except in fields where it might prevent the hay from being blown away.

A 'slice' can vary in weight by 100% which can be wasteful and it is not possible to check for 'foreign bodies' within the slice.

Nets, either full or empty, should never be left on the ground. Bad accidents have been caused by horses getting caught up in nets. In the box they should be hung as high up as possible and tied with a quick-release knot.

Haynets are unsafe for foals and young horses, who should be fed from mangers or loose on the ground.

Horses who have a dust allergy are probably best fed haylage to prevent the problem of dust.

Haylage

Haylage can be managed in the same way as hay except that as it is dust free it will not need soaking/steaming. It is excellent for horses with a dust allergy or who are in hard or fast work.

26 THE FEED SHED AND STORING FOOD

FEED SHED LAYOUT

In the layout of the feed shed the following points should be considered:

• Saving time.

• Cleanliness.

• Storage.

• Security.

• Ease of management.

Time

Feeding, especially in a large establishment, can take up a lot of time. It therefore makes sense to design a layout that is as labour-saving as possible. Everything should be easily to hand.

Cleanliness

The feed shed should be easy to keep clean, in the interests of hygiene and appearances. It should be possible to sweep the floor easily without having to move any of the contents. The walls should be smooth and easily dusted. Shelves should be of painted wood or melamine or metal.

The storage bins should be brushed out or vacuumed between refills. Stale feedstuffs will contaminate new. It is difficult to dry bins throughly after washing and this should be avoided if possible.

Storage of Concentrates

All types of concentrates can deteriorate if kept in poor conditions. Ideal conditions are:

• Low temperature.

• Little or no variation in temperature.

• Low humidity.

• Good ventilation.

• No direct sunlight.

• Protection from infestation by rats, mice, birds, insects and mites.

Suitable containers are:

• Metal bins, which should be raised off the floor on small wooden blocks or pallets.

• Plastic dustbins – these hold about one 25kg (55lbs) bag of feed but sometimes are vulnerable to rats. Metal dustbins are better if available.

In ideal conditions whole grains can be stored for many months without deteriorating. Once they have been crushed, bruised, rolled or treated they deteriorate very quickly and should be ideally used up within ten days.

Prepared concentrates and mixers will have their shelf life stated on the packaging. Again, once the bag is open the contents should be used within ten days.

When choosing a feed merchant it is wise to discuss your requirements with them. Usually a better deal can be made for larger amounts bought at regular intervals.

In a small yard try to buy concentrates at the beginning of their shelf life in order to have longer to use them. On a big yard it may be possible to buy in bulk and have the feed transferred into a hopper.

Make sure that all feedstuffs are used in rotation.

Storage of Vacuum-packed Forage

Because these bags are airtight, the storage considerations are rather different from those of other foodstuffs. Under no circumstances must the bags be punctured. It is important to protect the bags from:

• Rats and mice, who chew the plastic.

• Sharp edges, which may puncture the bags.

• Sunlight.

Storage of Salt

Salt absorbs moisture from the atmosphere; it is therefore important that it is kept airtight.

It is usually bought in plastic bags and, even when opened, it is sensible to keep it in its bag inside a container such as a dustbin.

A week's supply should be taken out at a time and kept in a large plastic jar. Do not leave it in contact with metal as it is corrosive.

A plastic spoon should be used for measuring.

Security

It should be possible to secure the feed room in order to prevent:

• Theft – this may happen in a livery yard with many owners feeding their own horses and 'borrowing' from the main yard or career thieves coming in with a van.

• Loose horses/ponies helping themselves; this can lead to colic or laminitis.

• Vandalism – this is an ever-increasing problem especially in urban areas.

Ease of Management

The siting of the feedroom should be considered carefully. If feeding is mechanised and all feeds are carried on a vehicle it is probably better to have it at one end of the yard. If feeds are carried by workers it may be better to have it sited centrally or, in very big yards, to have more than one.

If the feed store is separate from the feedroom, consider how easy it is for deliveries to be made and transferred from one to the other.

See page 404, Design of Stables.

Storage of Hay, etc.

Even well-saved hay deteriorates with age but good storage conditions will keep it palatable for a longer time. The important points to consider are:

• Protection from weather.

• Protection from damp, especially from the ground.

• Good ventilation.

• Protection from vermin such as rats and mice.

• Safe stacking.

Further information on hay storage can be found in Chapter 53.

EQUIPMENT IN THE FEED SHED

Feed Containers

These may be buckets, which are then emptied into mangers, or feed pans, which are given directly to the horse.

Buckets should be fairly heavy-duty 10 litre (2 gallon) size with names or numbers on them. These can be painted on or put on with Dymo tape. The contents should be emptied into a more suitable manger in each loose box.

ADVANTAGES

• Easy to keep clean.

• Easy and light to handle.

• Easy to store by stacking.

DISADVANTAGES

• Some food is liable to be left and wasted in the bucket.

• The feed is difficult to mix.

• Buckets may be piled inside one another without checking that the bottoms are clean.

Feed pans should be difficult to knock over yet not too heavy.

ADVANTAGES

• All the mixed food goes straight to the horse.

• Owing to their large size the food is easy to mix.

• They can be fitted into a rubber tyre which prevents bruising and tipping over.

DISADVANTAGES

• They can be difficult to keep clean.

• They are bulky to store.

• They must be removed from the boxes after the feed is finished. This can be a problem with late night feeds. Rubber bowls as distinct from metal ones are not so dangerous but even these can be stood in and kicked up, bruising cannon bones.

• They can be difficult to label.

• Difficult to carry.

Mangers

Many modern yards have mangers set into the stable wall or partition, or that hang over the stable door.

These can ease management and speed up feeding. They must be kept clean.

If mangers are set permanently into the partition it may be possible to feed by taking a bulk carrier around the yard and dishing straight from that into the mangers. This minimises labour but may mean some horses have to wait a while, in a large yard.

Whatever form of container is used to take the feed to the horses, when they come back and are washed out, the feedroom floor should remain clean and dry with no spilt food to encourage vermin. It may be possible to devise a rack to keep the clean containers on if the yard is not too large.

Do not prepare feeds more than an hour before feeding especially if damp feedstuffs such as sugar beet are being used. The feed will quickly become sour. If only dry feedstuffs are being used, ensure that birds, rats and mice cannot reach them between dishing up and serving. Stable dogs are also often partial to horse food.

Water

It can be useful to have a tap and a drain either inside or just outside the feed shed. This can be used for washing utensils, for providing water for soaking sugar beet or for damping feeds. A sink is always useful. Hot and cold running water is ideal.

Power point

This should be well away from the water supply and should be used with a circuit breaker. A power point can be useful for boiling a kettle or for a linseed or barley boiler if used.

Kettle

An electric kettle can provide hot water for washing. If used it must comply with up-to-date requirements for safety at work.

BOX NO	HORSE NAME	COARSE MIX			OATS			COMPETITION MIX			HAY/HAYLAGE		
		7AM	1PM	5PM	7AM	1PM	5PM	7AM	1PM	5PM	7AM	1PM	5PM
1													
2													
3													
4													
5													
6													
7													
8													
9													
10													
11													
12													
13													
14													
15													

Example feed chart.

Feed Chart

In any but the smallest yard a feed chart is recommended. It should show the box number and name of each horse along with his daily concentrate and forage ration. These need to be divided into the requisite number of feeds.

Cupboard

This is essential for storing small items, supplements and oral medicines that are currently in use. It should be fitted with a lock and be out of children's reach.

Scales

It is essential that scales are large enough to hold the contents of a scoop. Fold-up, hanging wall scales are tidy and unobtrusive. Spring-loaded balances are required to weigh hay; these may be more appropriately sited in the hay barn.

A Shelf

A separate shelf for supplements, additives, oil, etc. is advisable.

Other Useful Additions

- A damp-proof container for salt.
- Scissors or snips.
- Knife.
- A big mixing spoon for molasses, etc.
- A ml measure for medicine.
- A dustpan and brush for cleaning out bins.
- A short, soft broom for sweeping the floor.

A Feed Trolley

In a large yard this can be a valuable piece of equipment. The buckets or feed pans can be placed on the trolley and the food then put directly into them.

The trolley can be wheeled along the yard to the boxes. If a trolley is used, ensure all surfaces are smooth and not too steep.

SECTION

4

SADDLERY AND TACK

THE SADDLE

LEATHER

Most leather used for saddlery comes from the skin or hide of cows. To meet the demands of the saddlery and leather trade, much of it is imported. Because cattle come to maturity more quickly nowadays much of the leather is softer and does not last as long as previously.

Tanning

The hide requires considerable preparation before it is ready for use. The process is called tanning and currying. The hide should have plenty of substance – i.e. thickness – thus ensuring that it will last and will also stay flexible, because of the added fat content of the leather.

Texture

Leather has a grain or outer side, and a flesh or inner side. The grain side is shiny, and is sealed to make it more waterproof; it is therefore less absorbent to any soap or dressing. The flesh side is unsealed, and has a rougher, slightly dull surface. It is more absorbent and is the side of the leather (except for the underneath lining of the saddle) which is usually nearer to the horse's skin. In use it loses fat and oil, and this is the side which, being more absorbent, should receive greater care during cleaning.

Colour

The colour of leather can be varied during the tanning process, but is confirmed by the use of dyes during curing. The most widely used colours are **London tan**, which is yellow, **Havana**, which is the colour of a good cigar, **Warwick**, which is much darker, and **Black**.

Some saddle manufacturers can offer many more colours including red and blue. Synthetic saddles, especially those used in racing, come in many bright colours.

Types of Leather

RAWHIDE is cowhide which has undergone a special vegetable tanning process. This makes the leather very strong and leaves a light, untanned central strip. Rawhide is used for stirrup leathers, girth straps, etc.

BUFFALO stirrup leathers are red in colour, greasy and soft to the touch. They are exceptionally strong and last many years, but they usually stretch.

CHROME-TANNED LEATHER is pale blue-grey, and is produced by using salts of chromium. It is very strong, withstands wet, and remains supple. It is often used for New Zealand rug straps.

HELVETIA LEATHER is yellow in colour, and very greasy and tough. It is often used for reinforcing martingales, nosebands, etc.

Quality

When buying saddlery, it is important to be able to judge the quality of leather. Good leather should have plenty of substance, unless a special request has been made for a lighter weight – e.g. show bridles and racing saddles. This light type of leather wears much more quickly than a heavier sample.

Good leather should feel smooth and firm. When bent in the hand, neither side should form bubbles on the skin. The grain or sealed side should not crack.

When examining a bridle, note that the flesh or unsealed side of the leather should be smooth in texture, with no rough fibres visible. Poor leather, seen in a cheap bridle, has rough edges and may feel spongy. Such bridles often have poor-quality fittings.

STRUCTURE OF THE SADDLE

The Saddle Tree

The tree is the framework around which the saddle is built. Trees were traditionally made from beech wood, but this has now been superseded by laminated wood, which is bonded under pressure, and then moulded to the required shape. The resulting tree is both lighter and stronger. Other materials, such as fibreglass and plastic, are also used, though these are not as easy to work with as laminated wood. Fibreglass is exceptionally strong and light, and is used in some racing saddles. Plastic appears to lack strength, and another disadvantage is that nails or tacks cannot be driven into it.

Trees are made in different shapes and sizes according to the intended use, the shape of the horse, and the preference of the rider. The shape of the tree dictates the main outline of the saddle.

Trees can be either rigid or sprung. The rigid tree has a larger, more solid framework than the spring tree.

The **spring tree** has two flat panels of steel, which run from the underneath of the pommel to the cantle, and are set to lie about 5cm (2ins) on the inside of the

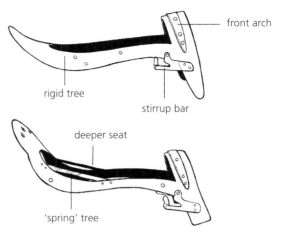

Saddle trees.

broadest part of the seat. These steel panels are thin enough to give greater resilience to the seat of the saddle, and a more direct communication between the seat of the rider and the horse's back. On occasions, there can be a risk of damage to the back, and it is advisable always to use a numnah. However, no numnah should be used to make the saddle fit. Always fit a new saddle without anything underneath it. The pommels of both types of saddle are reinforced on top and underneath with steel plates. For very heavy work, they can be reinforced further.

Some manufacturers now produce saddles with adjustable trees. Some can be adapted by the horse owner, others need suitably trained staff to do the alterations. It enables the width of the tree and the shape of the panels to be altered at will. These can be useful in a yard where the horse population changes frequently or where the horse is difficult to fit.

Treeless saddles are also available and popular with some riders. They can be a useful solution for horses difficult to fit with a treed saddle.

The Stirrup Bars

The bars are riveted to the points of the tree.

'Cast' stirrup bars are found on cheap saddles, and

their strength is suspect. The words 'forged' or 'cast' can be found stamped on the bar. The bar itself should be of the regulation type, and straight.

There has been discussion as to whether the safety-catch hinged on the bar is of any value. It is suggested that the length of the bar should be slightly extended, and with a slight upward curve.

Recessed bars are used on most spring tree saddles, and on some rigid trees. They are placed under, rather than on top of, the tree, so there is less bulk to the stirrup leather under the rider's leg.

The bars on jumping saddles are placed well forward, and on dressage saddles they are positioned further back.

The Seat

Pre-strained webbing is fixed from the pommel to the cantle, and over this is placed stretched canvas or linen. Bellies – short pieces of felt or leather – are placed round the broadest part of the seat to support the edge. Serge is stretched down to form the seat shape. Wool or plastic foam or synthetic padding are added to give resilience and extra cover to the tree, so that the rider cannot feel it through the seat. Of these three materials

wool is most popular, and lasts indefinitely.

Pigskin suede or hide is then stretched on as the final seat cover, with attached skirts. The **saddle flaps** are attached, followed by the **girth straps**. Two of the girth straps should be fixed to the web strap. The third strap is fixed independently. Girth straps should be of best quality leather, as their strength and attachment are vital to the safety of the rider.

The Underneath Panels

These panels vary in design. The **full panel** gives a greater weight-bearing surface, and is probably the most comfortable for the horse as it makes the waist wider; however, this can be uncomfortable for the rider. The **side panel** must be kept thin to allow the rider a close contact with the horse's sides. **Continental-type panels** are narrow at the waist and allow the rider a much closer contact. They go by various names and are used on all modern deep-seated saddles, together with knee and thigh rolls.

The **short**, or **half**, panel is now mainly used in the cheaper pony and cob saddles. It has no knee or thigh rolls and does not help the rider as much as the other types to establish a balanced position. As there is less

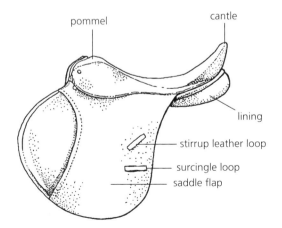

General-purpose saddle.

bulk under the leg, allowing a closer contact than a full panel, it is also used for show and polo saddles.

Girth Straps

Many modern saddles, in particular those for dressage, have long girth straps to avoid bulk under the knee and thigh. These saddles require a shorter girth. The design is not as suitable for cross-country riding and hunting, as the straps are difficult to adjust from the saddle and are more likely to cause sores from mud around the buckle and guard area. They must be adjusted so that the buckles are clear of the elbow.

Linings

LEATHER is the usual lining for leather saddles. It is easy to clean and wears well, as long as it is well looked after. It is usual to use a numnah or saddle cloth underneath. This helps preserve the lining and feels warmer to the horse when the saddle is first put on. It also absorbs sweat.

SERGE AND LINEN LININGS are rarely seen in modern saddle manufacture; they may still be seen on side-saddles. Serge is warm, absorbs sweat well but does not wear well. Linen is easier to clean and longer-wearing than serge.

SYNTHETIC LININGS are used with synthetic saddles. They are easy to clean but are still usually used with a numnah or saddle cloth.

MAIN TYPES OF SADDLE

Traditional Jumping

This saddle is shaped to help the rider stay in balance when riding in a forward position over a jump. It has forward-cut flaps to accommodate the knees of the rider with his relatively short leg position, and it has

Forward-cut jumping saddle.

Dressage saddle.

Racing saddle.

appropriately placed knee and thigh rolls to assist in maintaining the leg position. The depth of seat varies: the choice depending on the individual's style of riding – some riders favouring a much deeper seat position.

Close-Contact

Many show jumping and event riders now favour the close-contact saddle. These have a flat seat and are designed with the minimum of padding between rider and horse. The aim is to allow the rider maximum contact with the horse and versatility in his position in any situation.

Dressage

This saddle helps the rider to sit close to the horse with a long leg. The saddle flap is cut much straighter, with only a slight curve in front. The stirrup bar is placed further back than on a jumping saddle. The saddle flap may need to be correspondingly longer, so that it does not catch the top of a tall rider's boot. It is no longer popular to have saddles with very deep seats, which keep the rider in too fixed a position and concentrate their weight too much on the horse's back. The amount of knee and thigh roll can vary considerably.

General Purpose

This saddle is a combination of the jumping and dressage types, with a less forward-cut flap. It is the saddle used by the majority of riders who do not wish to specialise. It is important that the panel and flap are wide enough to accommodate the varying leg position of the rider and that the seat is long enough to allow the rider's seat to slide back when the stirrup leathers are shorter.

Endurance

Special saddles are now available for endurance riders, and are designed to spread the rider's weight over as

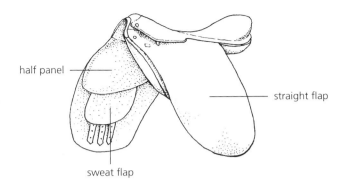

half panel

straight flap

sweat flap

Show saddle with half panel.

wide an area as possible so that pressure points are minimised. The various designs incorporate features of cavalry and Western saddles, and they are placed over very thick, specially designed numnahs.

Showing

This saddle has a very straight-cut flap to show off the horse's front and the seat is relatively flat. It is always used without a numnah, so the fitting is of even more importance than usual.

Racing

This is a lightweight saddle with a sloping head and very forward-cut flaps. Exercise racing saddles are built more substantially, although the design is similar.

Polo

This saddle may have a reinforced pommel. It is built with a short panel, extra long sweat flaps, and no knee or thigh rolls.

Competition Saddles

Many top competition riders now design saddles to their own personal specifications. These are then marketed by saddlers under the rider's name.

Synthetic Saddles

There are a number of saddles on the market made from synthetic materials. They usually follow traditional designs but are considerably cheaper to buy and easier to maintain.

They are particularly useful in riding schools, trekking centres and for child riders. Racing saddles are also synthetic.

Synthetic saddles can sometimes encourage the horse to sweat if worn for long periods and can also be uncomfortable for the rider if the seat does not allow him to move in the saddle. Care must be taken to ensure that the stirrup leathers and girth straps do not stretch or tear.

Modern Saddle Design

There are some alternative saddle designs on the market. Some have carbon fibre trees. The material is very strong and flexible and is designed to allow the horse greater freedom through his back and shoulders.

Some have air flocking; this can be adjusted to ensure that the rider sits squarely and in balance. The amount of air can be altered as the horse develops.

With some saddles the headplate is interchangeable so can be chosen to specifically fit any horse or design of panel or flap.

ACCESSORIES

Girth

The following types can be used:

LEATHER GIRTHS, if well cared for, last much longer than any other type. The main types are: three-fold, Balding and Atherstone. The latter two are shaped so that there is less risk of causing girth galls.

SHORT GIRTHS OF LEATHER OR MAN-MADE FABRIC suit dressage and jumping saddles with long girth straps.

NYLON is a good general-purpose material, which is easy to wash. Care should be taken that the girth does not get twisted.

STRING is similar to nylon but of softer texture.

LAMPWICK girths are soft and comfortable but not commonly seen these days. They are not suitable for demanding work.

WEBBING is generally preferred for racing, and by some riders for eventing. It is less restricting than leather. Two girths should always be used, as one can break without warning under strain.

WHITE TUBULAR SHOW GIRTHS can be used on hacks and ponies.

LEATHER OR WEBBING GIRTHS WITH ELASTIC INSERTS at the buckle ends are popular. They are less restrictive to a horse when he is galloping than the conventional girth. The elastic needs regular checking for stretch and wear. They must not be adjusted too tight.

ELASTIC INSERTS which are sometimes used for racing, require careful adjustment. Sweat rots them in time.

SYNTHETIC GIRTHS ('COTTAGE CRAFT' type) are soft and comfortable yet hard-wearing and durable. They are versatile and widely used.

Stirrup Leathers

These should be made of the best-quality leather. They should be chosen to suit the size and weight of the rider. It is dangerous to put a heavy leather on a lighter stirrup iron because if the rider falls, the iron will not easily be freed from the foot. Lightweight leathers are often more comfortable for the rider and easier to handle. For racing, hunting, eventing and jumping, buffalo or rawhide leathers are the most suitable as they are less likely to break.

Synthetic leathers usually come with synthetic saddles. They must be checked regularly for stretch and wear.

All stirrup leathers should be changed regularly from side to side on the saddle to prevent uneven stretch.

Stirrup Irons

Materials used are:

- Stainless steel, which is the best.

- Composite, which is satisfactory.

- Nickel, which is dangerous, as it bends and breaks. It can be recognised by its yellow colour. It requires regular polishing to stay bright.

The normal basic pattern stirrup iron is suitable for all purposes. The important factor is that the stirrup should be of suitable weight and size.

With the foot in the stirrup, there should be 12mm (½in) clearance on either side. In the event of a fall, too light and/or small a stirrup may jam on the foot. Conversely, too large a stirrup can permit the rider's foot to slip right through. The correct size and weight of iron is therefore important, and should always be checked by the rider and/or attendant.

Alternative Designs of Stirrup

There are a number of alternative designs on the market. They are mainly designed with either comfort or safety in mind.

THE BENT TOP IRON OR POLO IRON This is designed for the rider who keeps his foot well forward in the stirrup. Fitted so that it slopes forward, it removes pressure from the front of the ankle. Fitted sloping backwards the reverse action occurs. The stirrup leather is placed through the iron with the curve away from the leather.

KOURNAKOFF The eye of the iron is offset to the inside, and the sides slope forward with the tread sloped upwards. This helps to keep the heel lower than the toe, and the knee to be tight, with the lower leg off the horse. As it does not encourage an effective position of the rider's lower leg, it cannot be recommended. If it is used, however, it is essential to put the irons on correctly, and it is advisable to mark the left and the right.

PEACOCK IRON These have a thick rubber band replacing the metal on one side of the iron. The band should always be to the outside. A leather loop fitted to the bottom of the iron helps to hold the rubber band and to prevent its being lost if it comes off the top hook. As the weight is uneven, these stirrups do not hang straight, but they are much safer than standard irons, and as such are advisable for young children. They are not safe if the rider is over 54kg (8½ st).

THE AUSTRALIAN BENT LEG or SIMPLEX IRON has an S bend shape on the outside. The bulge of the S should be forwards. They are excellent safety irons for all ages and sizes.

THE STIRRUP CONTROL SYSTEM S(SCS3) is a system more suited to adults. It consists of boots, quick release stirrups and treads that can be used separately or together for added security.

Peacock

Simplex

Safety stirrup irons.

MDC, called the intelligent stirrup, has a Fillis iron with a rotating top which can be fixed in any of three positions.

SPRENGER IRONS are designed to absorb concussion and therefore are easy on the ankle joint.

RACING IRONS are usually made of lightweight stainless steel or aluminium. Because of their lightness they are not easily dislodged during a fall and are not suitable for general use.

CAGED STIRRUPS These stirrups, used by endurance riders, are fully enclosed to prevent the foot from sliding through the stirrup. This allows the rider to wear soft footwear without a heel, e.g. trainers, which are more comfortable for long hours in the saddle and give the rider the option of being able to run more easily beside the horse if required.

Treads

Rubber or plastic treads are used to help the rider maintain his foot position. They are also warmer to the foot than metal. It is preferable that they are flat and not wedge-shaped. Anything that forces the ankle or foot into a certain position is likely to be detrimental to the rider in the long run.

BUYING AND FITTING SADDLES

Buying

Always buy the best you can afford, and one made by a reputable saddler. Good saddles, well looked after, last for years and retain their second-hand value. A cheap saddle may look suitable, but it has a limited life and trouble can be expected from the tree. The leather of the girth straps, saddle flaps, and seat may rapidly show signs of wear. A good second-hand saddle is usually a better buy than a cheaper new one, as long as the tree is undamaged.

Nowadays there is a much more holistic approach to the choice and fitting of saddles. Far more is known about the effect and distribution of weight over the horse's back, and this can be taken into account when choosing a saddle for a specific discipline.

If you are buying for a riding school, remember that rigid-tree saddles are stronger and stand up to hard wear and heavy weights better than spring-tree saddles. They are also likely to be less expensive. A wide-seated saddle, cut generously to spread the rider's weight, is kinder to the horse's back. The general-purpose type is preferable.

When buying for private use, many people prefer a spring-tree saddle as it is more comfortable for the rider and gives a better feel of the horse's movement; also the seat aids are felt more directly by the horse.

Before deciding on a saddle, it is essential to ensure that it fits both the horse and the rider, and suits the latter. For the average rider, a general-purpose saddle is the most practical.

Fitting

A good saddler, who is a member of the Master Saddlers Association, should always be happy to come out and fit a new saddle. He can then advise as to whether the tree is the correct shape and width, and can often adjust the panel-stuffing on the spot.

When you are having a saddle fitted, remember that the outline of a horse's back can change according to his management and work, and that the padding of a new saddle flattens during use. It may therefore have to be set up (padded) by the saddler.

A good fitting and comfortable saddle is essential if a horse is to perform well and avoid such problems as pressure and girth galls. A badly fitting saddle can easily be a cause of poor performance.

Always fit a new saddle without a numnah underneath.

Procedure for Examining a Saddle

- Test the tree for signs of breakage or distortion both across the waist and the front arch. Many saddles, even some new ones, are twisted along the gullet (see below).

- Up-end the saddle and examine the underneath for any unevenness of padding or outline.

- Place the saddle on a saddle horse and check that the padding is level and even, both from behind and in front.

- Make sure that the gullet is wide enough – 63–75mm (2½ to 3ins) – so that there can be no pressure close to or on the spinal vertebrae. This must be checked again when the saddle is on the horse's back.

- To avoid marking the leather, a stable rubber should be placed on the horse's back under the saddle. To avoid marking the saddle flap, buckle guards should be fitted on the girth straps. The saddle should sit level and even, with no tilt either towards the cantle or the pommel when girthed up. Either would affect the rider's position and make it difficult for him to stay in balance with his horse.

- The saddle should fit the horse with the weight evenly spread over the lumbar muscles, not the loins.

- It must not hamper the movement of the horse's shoulder. This can occur with a forward-cut jumping saddle. The tree points should follow the line of the withers/top of the shoulder and also align with the panel.

- A rider, preferably the future owner or one of similar height and weight, should be legged up on to the horse. With traditional saddles, in both upright and jumping positions it should be possible to place two fingers under the pommel without feeling any pressure.

- There should be ample clearance under the cantle and along the gullet.

- When looked at from behind, it should be possible to see a clear channel of daylight.

To Test for a Damaged or Broken Tree

The Front Arch

The first indications of trouble are usually when the arch of the saddle widens and comes down on the withers. There may or may not be a squeaking or grating noise when the saddle is used; such symptoms are more likely to be heard with a heavy rider.

Place your hands on either side of the pommel and try to widen and move the arch. Or hold the cantle and grip the pommel firmly between your knees.

Any movement or clicking sound usually indicates damage.

Damage to the front arch is often caused by the saddle being habitually placed on the top of the stable door or somewhere similar, when saddling and unsaddling. The weight of the saddle needs to be supported on the padded part of the saddle, not the gullet.

The Waist

Rigid Tree Place the pommel against the stomach and, holding the cantle with both hands, try to press it upwards and towards the pommel. A movement in the waist indicates a break or crack. If the tree is seriously damaged, the rough edge can usually be felt when the gullet is examined. Damage can occur either on both sides of the tree or on one side only.

Spring Tree There should be some give in the seat of a spring-tree saddle, but when it is tested, as for a rigid tree, it should spring firmly back into place. A weak or broken tree feels slack and without spring.

It can be difficult for an inexperienced person to detect damage in a saddle with a spring tree. If you are in doubt, ask a saddler for advice.

Damage to a saddle caused by careless mounting by the rider can be observed by putting the saddle on a saddle horse and checking if there is a twist and/or if the saddle does not sit evenly.

With either type of saddle, if the damage has been present for some time there may be a crease across the seat.

Cantle This should feel rigid. Any movement indicates damage.

Points As these are the continuations of the front arch, they can be tested in a similar manner to that of the arch. Some saddles have flexible points, which should not be confused with damaged points. If the damage is below the stirrup bar, it is possible to see it.

To Measure a Horse's Back for a New Saddle

- Obtain a piece of soft lead or flexible plastic or wire, e.g. a coat hanger about 46cm (18ins) long.

- Place this just behind, and at right angles to, the horse's withers – in the position where the saddle would rest.

- Shape it into the required outline, then trace round it on a large sheet of paper.

- The next measurement should be taken about 23cm (9ins) further back and similarly traced.

- A third outline should be taken from the top of the

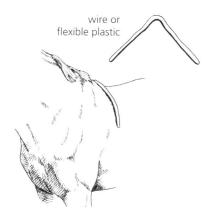

Measuring the shape and size of the back for saddle fitting.

withers along the spine.

- When ordering a saddle, it is helpful to give the rider's height, weight and length from crotch to knee.

Horses with Problem Conformation

The following are problems which need special attention in the fitting of saddles:

HIGH WITHERS A narrow tree is necessary, well padded at the withers, and preferably 'cut back'. The saddle may have to be set up at the rear to give a level seat.

STRAIGHT SHOULDER The saddle is likely to work forward, with a possible risk of girth galls. This is more likely if the horse is at grass and has a big belly. The rider feels insecure. The saddle needs careful padding to encourage it to stay back. A point strap can be fixed (see below).

FLAT SIDES These encourage the saddle to slip back, which can be a problem when horses become fit. Careful padding of the saddle and the use of a breastplate should resolve the problem.

FAT PONIES WITH LOW WITHERS The only satisfactory solution is to use a crupper. A point strap can also be fixed to the points of the tree, and the girth attached to this and to the first of the girth straps. This may help prevent the saddle sliding forward over the withers and on to the neck.

One of the modern treeless or air-flocked saddles may well solve the problem more easily than a more traditionally built saddle.

Typical Examples of Ill-fitting Saddles

- **Too much padding.** This causes the saddle to rock, with a risk of saddle sores, particularly on either side of the backbone to the rear of the saddle.

- **Too wide in the pommel.** This causes sores on the top

of the withers and possible damage to the spine.

- **Points of the saddle too long.** This causes undue pressure on either side of the withers.

- **Uneven padding or a twisted tree.** This results in a crooked rider, uneven weight distribution, and the development of pressure and friction sores. It may also

damage the muscles of the back. The tree often becomes twisted if the rider habitually holds the cantle when mounting.

- **A crooked rider** can also cause uneven muscle development of the horse's back, thus aggravating the crookedness.

CHAPTER

28 BRIDLES

Leatherwork must be of a suitable size and weight. Show and dressage bridles can be of lightweight leather. Bridles for hunting, eventing, show jumping and riding school work should be of a heavier type.

Bridles can be made of synthetic material, which is cheaper, hard-wearing and does not require the care needed by leather. These bridles are very popular with endurance riders and are a practical solution for children's ponies, riding schools and trekking centres where regular tack cleaning is a low priority. Good-quality leather, well cared for, remains the first preference for most other disciplines. All buckles should be of good quality metal.

Parts of a Snaffle Bridle

- Headpiece and throatlash.

- Browband.

- Cheek pieces.

- Noseband – plain cavesson or specialist type depending on requirements of the horse.

- Reins.

- Snaffle bit.

Parts of a Double Bridle

- Headpiece and throatlash.

- Browband.

- Cheek pieces.

- Plain cavesson noseband.

- Bridoon headpiece (or 'sliphead' – has no throatlash).

- Bridoon cheek piece.

- Bridoon rein, often thinner than a snaffle rein. It may be laced, plaited or covered with rubber.

- Curb rein (thinner than the bridoon rein).

- Bridoon.

- Bit (curb bit).

- Curb chain (metal or leather).

- Lip strap (optional). Some bits do not have the necessary Ds.

Snaffle bridle with loose-ring bit and plain cavesson noseband.

Parts of a Pelham

- Headpiece.

- Browband.

- Cheek pieces.

- Plain cavesson noseband.

- Bridoon rein and curb rein as for double bridle above. or Pelham rounding and one rein.

- Pelham bit.

- Curb chain.

- Lip strap.

REINS

Reins should be chosen according to intended use. A full size rein should be 1.5m (5ft) in length: i.e. the longest strip which can be cut from a hide. Reins for show jumping or flat racing – when a shorter hold is taken – can be 1.4m (4½ft). Pony reins can be 1.3m (4ft 3ins) or shorter. Long reins on a pony can result in the child getting his feet through the reins.

Simple double bridle.

Types of Rein

LEATHER REINS can be plain, plaited, laced or rubber-covered. The last-named when used for steeplechasing or eventing should have enough plain leather at the buckle end to enable them to be knotted. If the rider should slip the reins to the buckle end, the strain can be taken on the knot, not the buckle.

OTHER MATERIALS are webbing, linen, plaited cotton and nylon. These are all popular for jumping. Some have leather slots stitched every 13–15cm (5–6ins) to provide a more secure hold. All the reins should have a fastening in the middle. If they do not they can cause an accident if the horse runs free, especially if they are nylon which does not break easily.

FITTING A SNAFFLE BRIDLE

When the bridle is on the horse, check the following points:

- The fit of the **browband**. This must be comfortable. If it is too tight it will pinch the ears; if too loose, the headpiece may slip back causing the browband to look untidy.

- The **headpiece** should be broad across the poll and when the browband is fitted it should not interfere with the point where the throatlash divides.

- The **cheek pieces** should be a pair, fit the headpiece and be long enough to allow for adjustment up and down, depending on the bit being used. Each one should have one keeper (a fixed loop just below the buckle) and a runner (a movable loop) to keep the end of the headpiece from flapping.

- The **bit** can be attached in a variety of ways. Whichever is chosen it should not interfere with the actions of the bit or the noseband or rub the corners of the horse's lip or the muzzle.

- The **snaffle bit** should be adjusted so as to slightly

wrinkle the corners of the horse's mouth and not to protrude more than 6mm (¼in) on each side. The horse's mouth should be opened to make sure that the bit is high enough in his mouth to clear the tushes. The bit should be pulled straight in the mouth to measure its width. A bit that is too wide can cause great discomfort to the horse.

- The **throatlash** should be buckled so that it is possible to place a hand between the leather and the horse's jaw when the head is flexed. Some thick-jowled horses may need it looser than this. The purpose of the throatlash is to keep the bridle on. Therefore consider the likelihood of the rider falling off when fitting it. If the horse is doing dressage he will be flexed at the poll therefore needing a longer throatlash, but his rider is unlikely to fall off. Conversely, if the horse is going cross-country he is unlikely to be so flexed but more likely to lose his rider, therefore the throatlash should be tighter. It should not be able to slide over the horse's jaw.

- The **cavesson noseband** should be fitted two finger breadths or 2.5cm (1in) below the cheek bone. When it is fastened at the back, allow two fingers' width between the jaw and the leather. It should never be so tight as to cause discomfort to the horse.

- The **reins** should have about 38–51cm (15–20ins) spare when the rider is holding them. They must never be so long that the slack part can be looped over the rider's foot. They should always be buckled together at the ends.

FITTING A DOUBLE BRIDLE

- The fit of the **browband, headpiece, throatlash** and noseband should be similar to that of a snaffle bridle.

- The **bridoon bit** should be fitted on a separate headpiece, known as the **sliphead**, which should buckle on the off side a little below the buckle of the main headpiece, at a height which will slightly

wrinkle the horse's lips. It should be fitted between the headpiece and the noseband.

- The **bit** should lie below the bridoon so that both can act independently. The word curb should not be used on its own when referring to the double bridle bit, either bit or curb bit is correct terminology.

- The **curb chain** should be hooked on the off side of the bit, so that when twisted clockwise to the right the fly link, through which the lip strap passes, will hang down. The first link of the curb chain should be put on the near-side hook with the index finger underneath and the thumb on top. The selected link should be taken up and attached with thumb nail underneath and maintaining the twist to the right. If it is shortened more than three links, take up an equal number on both sides. When correctly fitted it should lie with the front edge of the chain in the curb groove, and when the rein is applied it should lie flat in the groove. (See diagram on page 251.)

- The end links of a **leather-covered chain** should be put on in a similar manner.

- There must be no risk of rubbing the horse on this very sensitive part of the jaw. Double link or leather curb chains are preferable. The curb chain must never be fitted through the rings of the bridoon. Its action must be quite independent of the bridoon. The curb chain should begin to act, exerting pressure in the chin groove, when the cheek of the bit forms a **45° angle** with the horse's mouth.

- The **lip strap** should be put through the fly link of the curb chain and buckled on the near side. It is primarily decorative, rather than functional. With some types of bit, e.g. the Banbury, it will prevent the bit cheeks from rotating too far forwards. If used, there is less danger of losing a curb chain when the bridle is being carried.

The Reins

- A **bridoon rein** may be slightly shorter than those of a snaffle bridle. If so, the bit rein should be 20–30cm

(8–12ins) longer than the bridoon rein. The reins should be bought and used as a pair. The bridoon rein is likely to be slightly thicker than the bit rein. It is much more difficult to maintain a correct balance in the rein if they do not work as a pair.

FITTING A PELHAM BRIDLE

This is fitted so that the bit lies close up against the corners of the lips without wrinkling them. The curb chain, when fitted, should lie in the curb groove. The curb chain should be hooked on as for a double bridle and should have a lip strap. Most Pelhams are so designed that the curb hook should be outside the snaffle ring of the bit with the chain threaded through. This prevents the hook from pinching the side of the lip when the rein is used.

If this is not done, assess carefully if it is going to cause discomfort or damage to the horse.

Care must be taken that the length of the Pelham cheek is correct for the horse and that the chain is not lifted out of the curb groove when in use.

Ideally only a cavesson noseband should be used with a Pelham although Grakles and flashes are frequently seen.

Pelham with roundings. *Above left:* curb chain fitted behind the snaffle bit ring. *Above right:* curb chain passed through the snaffle bit ring.

FITTING A KIMBLEWICK

This is fitted in a similar manner to a Pelham. The correct fitting of the curb chain depends on the length of the horse's jaw. The action of the Kimblewick can be quite severe and vice-like because the 'square eye' attachments for the cheek pieces exert stronger poll action.

NB: Curb chain hooks must open outwards, away from the horse's face. See diagram on page 253.

NOSEBANDS

Drop Noseband

This is used to prevent a horse opening his mouth so wide that he can evade the action of the bit.

Correct fitting is essential. If it is fitted too low, it interferes with the horse's breathing and can cause distress. The front of the noseband should lie on the bony part of the nose. The strap at the back should drop down to be fastened below the snaffle bit. The noseband should allow the horse to flex and move his jaw, but should prevent him from opening his mouth too wide. The buckle should not be by the bit but behind the jaw.

Rings which connect the front nosepiece to the back strap have small hooks which, when the leather is firmly stitched, hold up the front nosepiece and prevent it dropping down. Alternatively, short leather straps can be attached from the nosepiece to the headpiece.

Some nosebands have adjustable fronts to ensure a better fit over the nose.

Common Faults in Manufacture

- The front strap is too long, which makes fitting difficult, and the horse's face and lips can get pinched.

- The buckle end of the back strap is too long, making adjustment difficult. The buckle end should be short and the strap end long.

Flash noseband.   Grakle noseband.

- The front strap is not on fixed rings, and therefore drops down.

- The headpiece is too long, resulting in an untidy and unnecessary length of strap.

Flash Noseband

This is a cavesson noseband on to which a light strap is sewn, or is passed through a small loop on the front of the cavesson. The strap fastens below the bit, and acts in a similar way to a drop noseband. It is easier to fit than a drop, and is generally more comfortable for the horse. The flash should not ride up over the bit rings. The buckle should not be on the lip and the nostrils should not be interfered with.

Grakle, Figure-of-Eight or Cross-over Noseband

This is made of lighter-weight leather than a drop noseband. Its action is similar, but it is also effective in preventing a horse from crossing his jaw, as it acts over a wider area of the head. It is also less likely to affect the

horse's breathing. It acts from a headpiece, which ends immediately above the horse's cheekbone or just below. Two straps cross over the bridge of the nose, where they are stitched together and are usually padded underneath. They then pass round the horse's nose, and are buckled above and below the bit. They can be adjusted as required, but must allow some freedom to the mouth, although not being so loose that the lower strap drops down under the horse's chin. A small adjustable strap can also prevent this.

Kineton Noseband

This may help in the control of a strong horse. It acts by transferring some of the rein pressure from the mouth to the bridge of the nose. Note that it can also restrict breathing. It consists of two metal loops, one end of which is attached to a short, adjustable, centre strap, the other to a long headpiece. It is worn with a snaffle bit. The metal hoops fit round the mouthpiece between the bit ring and the horse's face. The centre strap should rest on the bony part of the horse's nose.

Other Nosebands

The **Australian noseband** is made of rubber. It attaches to the headpiece at the top and runs down the front of the face. It divides into two in the centre of the nose and ends in two rubber rings. These attach one either side of the bit. It is often seen on hard-pulling point-to-pointers and racehorses.

Sheepskin nosebands are formed by covering the front of a cavesson or drop noseband with a sheepskin sleeve. They are said to encourage the horse to concentrate on the job in hand and can be helpful with a one-eyed horse to help him to carry his head straight.

OTHER SADDLERY

MARTINGALES

In theory, the educated rider on a well-schooled horse should not need auxiliary aids such as martingales. There are occasions, however, when they can be used with benefit, to prevent the horse or pony putting his head above the angle of control, and so to help the rider to manage his horse as well as to improve the safety factor. Ideally as the horse's schooling progresses the martingale can be removed.

Running Martingale

The running martingale consists of a thin neck strap buckled on the near side and with a loop at the base of the neck. A wide strap called 'the martingale' is put through the loop. At one end it has an adjustable loop through which the girth is threaded. At the other end it is divided into two, each end having a ring through which the reins are threaded.

This acts via the reins and should be adjusted so that it only comes into action when the horse puts his head up too high; above the point of control. It also can be used by a novice or unbalanced rider who carries his hands too high, as this ensures that the action of the rein is kept lower, which is less likely to upset the horse.

A rough guide to fitting is to hold both the ring ends of the martingale together and to draw them towards the withers when the loop end is through the girth. If they reach the withers, the fit is loose. It should never be adjusted so tightly that it pulls the rein downwards when the horse carries his head correctly. When adjusted too tightly martingales can cause insensitive hands to damage a horse's jaw – as they have a very

Correctly fitted running martingale. It will have no action when the horse's head is in the correct position.

This running martingale is far too short and is continually putting pressure on the horse's mouth through the reins.

severe action with strong downward pressure on the bars of the mouth. As a running martingale affects the rein contact with the horse's mouth, two reins may be used, with the martingale attached to the bottom rein, thus leaving the other rein free to maintain direct contact (although this is a practice rarely seen). When attaching the reins, to ensure that they can slide smoothly through the rings, stand on the near side, hold the rings up with the right hand, and thread each rein through separately. Then buckle the reins together.

Reins not sewn on to the bit should have rubber or leather stops to prevent the martingale rings catching on the fastenings. The stops will also be necessary if a martingale is used on the curb rein of a double bridle or Pelham on which the bit rings are smaller than the martingale rings. This practice is not recommended. A running martingale on a bridoon rein is more effective and less severe.

A strong rubber ring or stop should also be used to secure the neck strap to the martingale.

The girth strap loop should have two keepers which should be adjusted to hold the loop flat.

The loose end of the neck strap should hang down on the left hand side of the neck.

The running martingale detracts from the correct use of the open rein.

Standing Martingale

A standing martingale prevents the horse from putting, or throwing, his head up above the angle of control: a bad habit which can result in the rider receiving a bang on his nose.

The martingale is secured to the neck strap and girth in a similar manner to the running martingale, but it is then attached directly to the back of a cavesson noseband. It should never be attached to a drop noseband. It is adjustable either:

• At the girth.

• By a buckle under the neck.

• At the noseband.

When the horse's head is in a normal position, it should be possible to push the end of the martingale up into the horse's gullet. It should not be fitted so tight that it exerts continual pressure, as this will encourage the horse to lean up against it. It can also restrict a horse's action, particularly over a jump.

Combined Martingale

This is a combination of a standing and running martingale and has the action of both. It is more often used for show jumping.

Bib Martingale

This is similar to a running martingale, but with a centre piece of leather between the two rings. It can be used on an excitable or overbent horse who is likely to catch his teeth in the strap or ring of an ordinary running martingale. It is more restrictive, as an opening rein cannot be used. It is often used on racehorses at exercise.

Irish Martingale

This consists of a short leather strap about 10–12cm (4–5ins) long, with a ring at either end. The reins are

Bib martingale.

Irish martingale with rein stops.

threaded through the rings, and if the reins are not sewn on, stops must be used. It is positioned under the horse's neck. In the event of a fall, it helps to prevent the reins going over the horse's head. It is more generally used on racehorses. It can also help a horse who shakes his head and gets the reins over his head when being ridden. It can adjust the angle of the rein contact down if the hands are too high. It can be very useful to steady the rein contact of a novice rider on a horse with a sensitive mouth.

BREASTPLATE

This is used to prevent the saddle slipping back – usually on horses who are very fit or on those whose conformation fails to prevent the saddle from slipping back (i.e. flat-sided or herring-gutted horses). It is also used when hunting or in very hilly country.

There are various types of breastplate:

1. A hunting breastplate consists of a leather neck strap attached first to the girth by a leather strap and then to the 'Ds' of the saddle by two narrow leather straps on either side of the withers. The neck strap has buckles on both sides so that it can be adjusted evenly. It should fit comfortably and not be tight around the neck.
   If a martingale is used, a short attachment can be added, either in the design of a running or standing martingale. This can be buckled to the centre ring of the neck strap and then put on to the reins or the noseband as required. This centre ring should have a leather 'safe' or protecting pad to avoid any rubbing of the horse.

2. 'Aintree breastgirth' – more often used on racehorses or eventers. It consists of a band of webbing or wide elastic which is passed round the horse's chest and attached to the girth on either side by adjustable leather loops. Another strap is passed over the horse's withers, which prevents the breastgirth from dropping down. The breastgirth must be carefully fitted so that neck movement and the windpipe are not affected.

3. There are a number of new designs which combine some of the features of the two mentioned. They are used mainly by event riders in the cross-country phase.

SPECIAL GIRTHS

Surcingle or Overgirth

This is essential equipment for racing and eventing, but is also used in show jumping. It is a high-quality webbing strap, long enough to fit over the top of a saddle and weight cloth. It helps to hold everything in place, and acts as an extra girth in an emergency. Some may have a small but very strong elastic inset, which makes for easier fitting. It should go over the saddle at its deepest point and over the top of the girth (some girths have a special loop through which to thread it) and be fastened under the belly. On no account should it lie or slip behind the girth as it will pinch the horse.

Foregirth

This has a metal arch positioned in front of the saddle to stop it slipping forward. It is attached to a surcingle, which must be buckled up tightly before the saddle is put on. It is used particularly in dressage to ensure that the saddle does not come too far forward, thus putting the rider's weight on to the shoulders.

WEIGHT CLOTH

This is necessary when a rider has to carry weight to conform to competition rules, e.g. in racing. It consists of a strong linen or synthetic fibre saddle cloth secured to the saddle by straps, and with stitched pockets for holding lead. The pockets can be placed in front of the saddle on the shoulders, or behind the saddle flaps and against the horse's ribs. When fitting a leaded weight cloth, care must be taken that it does not press down on the withers, or interfere with the rider's position.

NUMNAHS

These are protective pads worn under a saddle to add to the horse's comfort and to protect his back from friction and pressure. They follow the line of the saddle. Saddle cloths may serve the same purpose but may be purely decorative. They do not follow the line of the saddle and may extend below and behind it.

They are especially valuable:

• When first riding the horse after a long rest.

Quilted numnah.

• When riding for a long period of time with the rider's weight continually on the horse's back.

• With learners, who find it difficult to sit quietly and in balance, particularly if they are of heavy build.

• With inexperienced or novice riders who do not sit straight and square in the saddle. The uneven distribution of weight can encourage the saddle to rock, and creates additional friction.

• With a modern saddle which has a spring tree, narrow waist and deep seat, and which concentrates pressure over a smaller area.

• When the shape of a horse's back changes. A numnah will then make the saddle fit more comfortably. This should only be a temporary measure, as the stuffing of the saddle has to be altered.

• When jumping. A numnah under the saddle may add to the horse's comfort and encourage him to jump with a rounded back.

• To make the saddle more acceptable to a cold-backed horse.

NB: The saddle should fit the horse's back before the numnah is put on. Except in emergencies, a numnah should not be put on to make a badly fitting saddle usable.

Types of Numnah

There is a considerable range of numnahs on the market, some of which are made from natural materials such as cotton or wool. Others are a mix of synthetic and natural and some are wholly artificial.

NATURAL SHEEPSKINS are seldom seen nowadays as they are difficult to clean and maintain.

Pure wool numnahs with the appearance of sheepskin are available. They are not cheap and can become very heavy when wet. They are very good looking but need care with their cleaning.

ARTIFICIAL 'SHEEPSKIN' NUMNAHS come in a variety of thicknesses and colours. They are not as expensive as natural wool. They are easy to wash and dry.

QUILTED NUMNAHS, often with artificial padding and a cotton cover, are utilitarian and practical. Thicker padded numnahs may be difficult to keep in place. The artificial padding is always trying to flatten out.

All numnahs and saddle cloths should be fitted so that there is still a passage of air through the gullet of the saddle. They must not press down or cut into the withers.

A WOOLLEN BLANKET folded in four makes an effective back protector if a saddle has insufficient padding.

NATURAL FIBRES – wool, linen, cotton – are the best choice as some horses are allergic to man-made fibres.

Numnahs are secured in place by:

• Light leather straps and buckles.

• Nylon loops, which fit round the girth straps.

• Velcro straps.

• Strong elastic.

• Leather loops, which are the most satisfactory type for hard or competition work.

Quilted saddle cloth.

Saddle Pads

Saddle pads come in a wide variety of synthetic materials and range from gel pads, through Polypads to riser pads. They are used under the saddle and are purchased according to individual preferences or needs. Most are designed to increase the horse's comfort and provide protection; however, riser pads can affect the balance of the saddle by raising the area under the cantle. They are often used in conjunction with a saddle cloth.

Caring for Numnahs and Saddle Cloths

Ceremonial numnahs and saddle cloths made from natural sheepskin or pure wool cloth need specialist care.

Everyday numnahs and saddle cloths must be kept very clean, even if it means daily washing, in order to prevent sore backs and skin disorders.

On clean, well groomed horses a daily brush and weekly wash will suffice.

On horses living out or who have thick coats it is best to use thin cotton numnahs or saddle cloths and wash them daily.

The articles are best washed in a machine on a cool wash using a washing powder or liquid suitable for people with allergies as horses are very susceptible to chemicals.

At the end of the day all numnahs should be removed from their saddles, brushed and placed upside down either over the top of the saddle or on a rack where they can dry and air.

Dirty, greasy numnahs are a major cause of sore backs.

WITHER PADS

These are used under the front arch of a saddle, which would otherwise press on the horse's withers. They should be considered an emergency remedy, as their use often upsets the balance of the saddle and encourages the rider's seat to slip back. The saddle should be restuffed to make the use of such pads unnecessary.

They can be used successfully under stable rollers and breaking rollers.

CRUPPER

This is usually worn by small, fat ponies or donkeys to prevent the saddle or roller from slipping forward.

The crupper consists of an adjustable leather strap put through a metal ring or 'D' on the cantle of the saddle. The other end of the strap is a padded and rounded leather loop, through which the tail is placed. This may or may not have a separate fastening.

When fitting the crupper, place it over the tail first, well up under the dock. Then connect it to the saddle and adjust it to a comfortable length. Care should be taken when first fitting, as ponies not used to a crupper may buck or kick. If they are worn frequently, the skin under the tail may become sore, and this area should be examined regularly. The crupper loop must be kept soft and supple.

GRASS REINS

These are adjustable narrow leather, nylon or cord reins which are attached round the girth straps or clipped to the saddle 'Ds'. They are then crossed over the withers and attached to the bit rings, or they may be fitted through the browband loops and down to the bit. They are used to prevent a pony from putting his head down to eat, thus pulling off a small rider. They also help to control a pony who bucks.

NECK STRAP

This is a strap which is fastened round the horse's neck and buckled on the near side. It can be a stirrup leather. It is used (a) to give unbalanced, novice riders something to hold on to rather than the reins, and (b) to help more experienced riders on young or fresh horses who might buck. If required, it can be attached to the front 'Ds' of the saddle and/or to the girth between the front legs.

It is often preferable to get a leather strap made up with a buckle at either end that fits onto the saddle 'D's. It is more secure and keeps the rider's hands in a more normal position.

Many stirrup leather neck straps are too short and too thick for small riders to reach comfortably and hold onto.

HEADCOLLAR

A good-quality headcollar is an expensive item because of the amount of leather and stitching involved. Various designs are available, brass-mounted with buckles on both sides being the smartest (as well as the most expensive). A cheaper headcollar with galvanised or tin fittings and less stitching is perfectly adequate; in many cases the stitching is now replaced by rivets. On some designs the front may unbuckle, which makes it easier when brushing the face and when putting on a bridle.

Yearling headcollars have buckles on the headpiece, noseband and behind the jaw. They are excellent on young horses as they can be adjusted to fit.

Nylon headcollars are a cheap and suitable substitute for leather but they can be dangerous, particularly if left on in the field, as the nylon is virtually unbreakable.

A headcollar should be fitted so that the noseband lies 5cm (2ins) below the cheek bones and allows a hand to be held between the leather and the jaw bones. Tight headcollars cause discomfort and result in sore patches.

Foal slips should be made of leather, with adjustable buckles on the headpiece and noseband to allow for growing. Nylon foal slips are unsafe. A 16cm (6ins) strip of leather, which a hand can hold, should be attached to the back of the noseband.

ROPES

These are made of:

HEAVY JUTE, which is strong and stands most wear.

COLOURED COTTON, which is attractive but can snap. Best for use with nylon headcollars and easier on the hands. They are cheap to replace when they get worn.

NYLON, which is strong but which should be discarded when frayed; a frayed rope, when knotted, can be impossible to untie. If used, they are better with leather headcollars. A nylon headcollar with nylon rope is virtually unbreakable and can lead to accidents.

PLAITED BALER TWINE. This, if carefully plaited, with no loose ends or knots, is effective and is also easily and cheaply replaced.

Ropes are made with an eye, or are fitted with a spring hook which, when attached to the headcollar, should face away from the horse's chin and towards the neck. On occasions, spring hooks have been known to catch in a horse's face.

HALTERS

These are made of webbing or rope, and usually have the rope as an integral part of the halter. The 'Yorkshire' type of webbing halter is very strong and has a string throatlash which prevents the halter from being pulled over the head. Rope halters are adjustable and can be altered to fit any size of head.

It is important to ensure that the nose section of the halter cannot pull tight and panic the horse. After fitting, a knot should be tied by putting the lead rope round the noseband and pulling it back through the loop. This prevents the halter from tightening and also from working loose.

Control Halters

There are a number of devices on the market designed to exert pressure and/or control over the horse. Usually to prevent him from rearing or from running back, especially when being loaded. They can be extremely effective but as they exert extra pressure on the nose or the poll they must be used with care and the horse should not be tied up in one.

See also page 74.

Foal slip.

Halter with knot to ensure security.

LUNGEING EQUIPMENT

Cavesson

Modern lungeing cavessons are lightweight and made of either leather or synthetic fibre. They must be well padded in the nose area, so that pressure will not cause a sore. There are two patterns:

1. The nose piece is made like a drop noseband with the back straps attached to rings, so that they can be fitted either above or below the bit. This is also known as a Wels cavesson.

2. The nose piece is made like a cavesson noseband, and fits round the nose above the bit.

Both patterns have a jointed metal plate on the front of the noseband with a central swivel-mounted ring. They may also have small rings on either side. They should be

Modern lungeing cavesson with nose piece fitted above the bit.

The Wels cavesson has a nose piece made like a drop noseband.

fastened firmly or they will cause rubbing on the front of the nose.

A securing strap is set about halfway down the headpiece. This passes over the cheek bones and fastens on the near side. It holds the cavesson in place and must be fastened firmly. If it is set too high, its firm hold causes discomfort and affects the horse's ability to flex at the poll.

With both types, take care to ensure that the cheek strap does not pull round into the eye on the outside when lungeing.

Lungeing Roller or Pad

This is made of leather, man-made fibre or strong reinforced webbing approximately 10cm (4ins) wide, and should be well padded over the back. It can be shaped in the elbow area to avoid rubbing the horse's sides. It should have two buckles on either side to ensure that when the roller is fitted the rings on either side are at the same height. It is also safer to have two buckles when dealing with a young horse who may play up as the buckles are tightened.

Rings should be fixed on to the roller:

• On the front and back of the top.

• Approximately 5cm (2ins) below the top on either side.

• On the girth section near the buckles.

• Underneath the girth.

• 'Ds' should be fixed as for a rug roller, to hold the breastplate.

• It may have 'terrets': raised, fixed metal rings set high on the pad either side of the withers.

If required, a pad may be put under the roller. For a young horse, who may buck, the pad should be attached to the roller.

Breastplate

This is a leather or webbing strap placed round the chest and fastened to the lower rings or 'Ds' of the roller to prevent it from slipping back. For lungeing young horses it should always be used, even with side reins. It should always be fastened before the girth.

Side Reins

These are adjustable straps about 1.8m (6ft) long, which run from the roller or saddle to the bit. They are used:

- To teach the young horse to accept the bit.

- To help to keep the horse straight, and if lungeing in a paddock to prevent him from snatching at a mouthful of grass.

- To increase control over a fresh or strong horse.

- To improve the trained horse's way of going.

- To work the horse in hand from the ground.

- To lunge a rider and so help to keep the horse in better balance and give the rider a better feel of the gaits.

There are a number of types:

1. At one end the leather strap fits through the rings on the roller (or round the girth of a saddle), and returns to buckle on itself. To allow for adjustment, there should be at least twelve numbered holes. At the other end, strong spring clips facing outwards and away from the horse are clipped to the bit rings, or on occasion to the side rings of the cavesson.

2. Similar to (1), but with a loop to go round the roller or girth and an adjustable fastening in the middle.

They can also be made from nylon or other synthetic webbing. Ensure that there are enough holes and that they are not too far apart.

Some side reins are made with rubber rings or strong elastic inserts. If the elastic becomes stretched, it must be replaced.

Some trainers prefer not to lunge in side reins, because they feel that the horse should be free to adjust his head and neck position according to his natural balance. This applies particularly in the early stages.

When leading the horse in and out of the stable or when the horse is not being worked, side reins should be unfastened and put over the withers or clipped to the side 'Ds'. Whether training the horse, or when lungeing the rider, the side reins must never be fitted so tight that free forward movement is hampered. Side reins should not be attached until the rider has mounted the horse, and they should be fitted with care. It is advisable to lunge an unfamiliar horse without side reins for a few minutes before fitting the side reins.

Lunge Reins

A lunge rein, unless for ponies, should not be less than 10m (33ft) in length. It should have a loop at one end and an attachment to the cavesson at the other.

Materials for lunge reins

- Tubular or flat linen webbing.

- Nylon.

- Rope.

- It is possible to get expanding lunge lines rather like dog leads. These are not recommended as serious damage to horse and lunger can occur if they go wrong.

Webbing is strong but may be a little heavy. Nylon is strong but very light – this can make it difficult to handle, and even with gloves on it can cut into or burn the hand. Rope is strong, and lighter than webbing, but can be more difficult to handle and may burn the hand.

Cavesson attachments for lunge reins

- Swivel joint with buckle or strong clip.

- Strong clip.

• Leather strap and buckle.

If the cavesson has a swivel it is not necessary to have a swivel on the buckle or clip, as this makes the attachments heavy for a young horse. When a horse is jumping on the lunge it is cumbersome and can bang his nose.

Lunge Whip

This should be chosen carefully. Most whips are now made of fibreglass, with a thin plaited thong about 2.4m (8ft) long, with a lash at the end. The whip must be well balanced, and not so heavy that it will be tiring and difficult to manipulate. It must be long enough for the lunger to influence the horse and, when necessary, to touch him with the lash. To give extra length, a short lash can be replaced by a long leather bootlace.

Many cheap lunge whips used when teaching people to lunge are not long enough. This means that the lunger either has to walk with the horse or tends to lunge on too small a circle. It is preferable if the whip can reach the horse when he is out on a 20m circle.

Crupper

The use of a crupper when lungeing is optional. It can be a helpful extra discipline for an obstreperous young horse. It should be of leather, with a well-padded dock piece and a separate buckle for fastening round the dock.

Long Reining

Equipment for this is similar to that for lungeing, but it includes two reins which are often lighter and shorter than a full lunge rein. It is often easier to carry a long dressage whip rather than a lunge whip.

NB: When lungeing or long reining it is essential for the lunger to wear gloves and stout, sensible footwear. A hat is advisable.

GADGETS

Gadgets are auxiliary aids which, by positive action, increase the control and activity of the horse. In experienced hands they have their uses in the retraining of spoilt or 'nappy' horses. They can also be used, on veterinary advice, in the building up of back and hindquarter muscles after injury. In the hands of inexperienced riders they may produce more problems than they cure and can result in severe muscle strain. They have only a very limited place in the classical and systematic schooling of the horse.

Running and Draw Reins

These are the simplest and most commonly used auxiliary aids. They consist of a double-length rein made of leather, webbing or nylon, with a loop at either end. They may or may not have a buckle in the middle.

When fitted as running reins, the loops are fitted over the girth on either side of the saddle. The rein then passes through the bit ring from the outside to the inside and back to the rider's hands.

The lower the loops are fitted down the sides of the horse, the more severe the action and the strain on the horse.

When fitted as draw reins, both loops are fitted to the centre of the girth under the belly, pass together between the front legs and then divide, passing through the bit rings from inside to outside and back to the rider's hands.

When using either method it is very easy to force the horse into an artificial head carriage with a short neck. It can appear 'broken' at the fourth vertebra. This can be very difficult to correct later.

The BHS does not recommend their use.

The de Gogue: (a) fitted for use on the lunge; (b) fitted for use with a rider.

FURTHER TRAINING DEVICES

There are any number of training devices on the market and more are being devised and older ones adapted all the time. It is not within the remit of this book to analyse their uses in any detail. But before they are used the following points need to be considered:

- Is the device necessary?

- Is its use going to harm the horse in any way?

- Is the operator experienced in its use?

Some of the better known are:

- The Chambon

- The de Gogue

- The Pessoa

- The Abbot-Davies balancing rein

- The Schoolmasta

- The Market Harborough

The first four of these could more correctly be called systems. They are designed to be used progressively over a period of time. The basic idea is to encourage the horse to work with a lowered head carriage and rounded outline and to work through from behind. All the first four are designed to be used on the lunge. The Chambon can also be used when loose schooling and the de Gogue can also be used when the horse is being ridden.

The Schoolmasta and the Market Harborough are designed to be used on the ridden horse and their main function is to stop a strong horse from pulling. When using any of them remember the following:

- Read the instructions carefully before use.

- Preferably watch them being used by an experienced operator and receive instruction prior to using.

- Consider carefully if your chosen 'gadget' is appropriate for the situation.

- Horses with less than perfect conformation can be put under too much strain and damaged physically.

- All horses should be introduced to them very slowly and carefully so as to allow the muscles time to develop.

- Their inappropriate use can lead to the horse becoming mentally sour and uncooperative.

- They should never be used as a 'quick fix'. Young horses need time to develop naturally both mentally and physically and older horses who are set in their ways will also need time to alter their way of going. If they have adapted their movement to cope with an old injury or wear and tear, forcing them to change may cause them to become unsound.

The Chambon, as used on the lunge.

Market Harborough

This is a type of running martingale, and is the least severe of the auxiliary aids. The divided pieces of the martingale go through the rings of the bit. They either clip back on to 'Ds' stitched on the reins, or are attached by an adjustable buckle. When the horse's head is in a normal position it has no restrictive influence, but it comes into use if the horse raises or throws up his head. It can therefore be effective on headstrong horses. It is seldom seen today.

Chambon

This is used for lungeing. It consists of a divided rein which goes from the girth through rings on a special fitting attached to the headpiece behind the horse's ears, and from there to the bit where it is attached by clips.

A horse wearing a Chambon is worked on the lunge in a circle of 20m in a slow trot, and with the equipment loosely fitting until the horse is familiar with it. It is gradually tightened, so that the horse moves with a lowered head. He will then accept the restriction without worrying.

Schooling time should start with two to three minutes on each rein, and should never exceed a total of 20 minutes.

The horse should never be ridden in a Chambon.

In the hands of an expert, lungeing with the Chambon can be beneficial, but unskilled use can easily cause damage.

There are various other types of 'gadget' on the market, most of which, working on some form of lever principle, persuade the horse to lower his head and go in a rounder outline. Some gadgets can be attached to the tail, but it is worth remembering that the tail is an extension of the horse's spine. If the horse is not permitted to carry his tail in a natural manner, the use of the back muscles can be adversely affected and the muscles of the tail may suffer permanent damage.

One gadget, the **Balancing Rein**, introduced by Peter Abbott-Davies, can be placed in three positions:

(1) mouth to girth;

(2) mouth to tail, with a rope passed through a soft sheepskin sleeve; or

(3) mouth to behind the ears by means of a soft rubber connection.

To summarise: all 'gadgets' need understanding and experience for correct use. In most cases the value of a schooling aid is in the retraining of a spoilt horse. Muscles must always be allowed time to work hard and develop. Force will never achieve results and a stressed, overtired horse will resist and work will be wasted. In general, gadgets are not a replacement for correct classical training.

CHAPTER 30

BITS

The purpose of a bit is to enable a rider to control and guide his horse. The success of this control also depends on the effectiveness of the rider's seat and leg aids. The bit functions by bringing pressure to bear on the horse's mouth and head, either by direct action of the bit or by the indirect action of the bridle. This action will be affected by the horse's mouth, the angle at which he carries his head, the height of the rider's hands, and the design and fit of the bit. At no time should it inflict pain on the horse.

It is more important to be able to assess the action and suitability of a bit than to know its name. Try to identify the following:

• The family to which it belongs.

• The material from which it is made.

• How it will act on the horse.

• Its size and fit for a particular horse.

• The quality of the workmanship and any wear and tear.

STRUCTURE OF THE MOUTH

The horse has an upper and lower jaw, the comparative length of which varies in different breeds and can affect both the action of the bit and that of the curb chain.

The parts of the lower jaw bone lying between the incisor teeth in the front and the molars at the back of the mouth are called '**the bars**'. They are covered with a layer of skin and flesh containing nerves. In a young horse, this area is very sensitive, but can become deadened by rough use of the bit.

The top of the mouth is formed by the **palate** – a very sensitive area.

In stallions and geldings, **tushes** grow on either side of the jaw between the incisors and the molars. If present in mares they are usually rudimentary and barely visible. **Wolf teeth** may grow at the front and to the side of the first molars. They can cause bitting problems and should be removed.

The areas on which the bit and/or bridle act are:

• The corners of the mouth and lips.

• The bars of the mouth.

• The tongue.

• The roof of the mouth.

• The side of the face.

• The chin groove.

• The nose.

• The poll.

PROBLEMS IN THE MOUTH

CAUSES

• Sharp molars.

• Wolf teeth.

- Sensitivity of the skin covering the bars of the mouth.

- The length of the jaw, or the position and size of the tushes.

- The shape of the jaw relative to the size of the tongue.

- A badly fitting or badly fitted bit.

If, after inspection, the problem does not appear to lie in the mouth, other possible causes are:

- Physical discomfort and/or pain caused by ill-fitting tack other than the bit.

- Pain from unsoundness in the back or legs.

- The hands of an insensitive or unbalanced rider.

If the horse has discomfort or pain in his mouth he may try to ease this by altering his head position and opening his mouth, which brings pressure to bear on a less sensitive surface, e.g. the corners of the mouth rather than the bars. If the latter become deadened because of insensitive treatment, then all too often the rider will seek a stronger bit and a more severe method of control. If mouth problems are encountered, the cause should first be investigated. In many cases, a change of bit to a milder type often solves the problem.

Types of Problem

- A too narrow bit pinches and rubs the corners of the mouth. A too wide bit runs through the mouth when one rein is pulled, and a joint may even go across the mouth and rest on the bars. If jointed, it may press on the roof of the mouth, when the rider has a less direct feel of the mouth.

- A horse with a shallow mouth space between the upper and lower jaws, or a thick tongue, may find a thick bit uncomfortable because of tongue pressure. The joint of the bit may press up into the roof of the mouth, and a bit which is too wide aggravates the problem. With such horses, make sure that the bit fits the mouth, i.e. that it only extends just to the outside of the lips. Use a tapered mouthpiece, i.e. thick at the ends and thinner towards the centre. Try a double-jointed or French snaffle, as the smooth centre plate should lie comfortably on top of the tongue.

- A horse with a normal mouth space and sensitive bars may find a thin mouthpiece sharp to the tongue, and uncomfortable on the bars. Use a thick-jointed or double-jointed mouthpiece. This can be of the German hollow mouth type – which is light – or it can be covered in rubber or leather or made of plastic.

- A horse can double back his tongue and try to put it over the bit. This may be because of discomfort, especially if the bit is relatively low in the mouth, when there will be excessive tongue pressure. A mullen mouth snaffle can be more comfortable, and if fixed high in the mouth it may also discourage or check the habit of tongue over bit. Alternatively try a single-or double-jointed snaffle fixed high in the mouth.

- A dry mouth is the sign of an insensitive mouth, and the horse is often very strong. He must be encouraged to salivate. There are many types of alloy bits and synthetic materials, designed to encourage salivation, on the market. Ones with a high copper content are especially effective.

- A horse often tries to avoid the action or message from the bit by opening his mouth and/or crossing his jaw. Various nosebands can help this problem (see pages 229–30). Before resorting to forcing the mouth shut with a noseband, consider the cause. A milder bit used in conjunction with an Irish martingale will often help whilst the rider develops a more secure and balanced seat and therefore quieter hands.

CONSTRUCTION OF THE BIT

The mouthpiece of a bit can be made of a variety of materials. Stainless steel, various metal alloys, often containing copper, vulcanite rubber and various artificial nylon/plastic materials are the ones most commonly met with. It is still possible to find old nickel or rubber bits in some yards but they are likely to be very worn and must be inspected carefully before use. Nickel is not recommended.

Types of Material

STAINLESS STEEL is the safest and best-looking metal. The second choice is one of the named composition alloys.

ALUMINIUM can be used if a light but strong bit is required, as in racing.

COPPER is a soft metal. It is very popular in many of the modern bits, especially those designed on the Continent, as part of the various alloys and is used to encourage salivation. Sections of almost pure copper are introduced into some bits for the same reason.

VULCANITE is rubber hardened by heat. It makes a thick, heavy mouthpiece, which is kind in action. It is still sometimes found in some Pelhams.

NYLON is very light but strong.

RUBBER makes a very soft but kind bit. It should always have an internal mouthpiece of linked steel. It is seldom found nowadays. It should be wetted before being placed in the horse's mouth.

'HAPPY MOUTH' or 'NATHE' bits are mild, and made of a synthetic but hard-wearing material.

'SWEET IRON' bits are also popular and much used. They encourage the horse to salivate.

Bit Fittings

At each end of the mouthpiece are the fittings to which the headpiece and reins are attached. They can be of various designs. Loose-and flat-ring snaffles allow a certain amount of movement of the bit within the rings. Eggbutt, D-shape and cheeked snaffles limit this movement. Some rings are designed to move completely independently of the mouthpiece. Some bits have cheeks. This is the piece that lies against the side of the horse's jaw and to which the ring is attached. It is sometimes there to prevent the bit from slipping through the mouth and to encourage the horse to turn. Sometimes it provides poll pressure. Examples of the different types are found in the following text.

To Measure a Bit

Lay the bit flat and measure the distance between the inner sides of the bit rings or cheeks.

Bits are made in sizes ranging from 9cm (3½ins) to 15cm (6ins), and go up in 0.5cm (¼in.) to 1cm (½in.) stages.

To Measure a Horse's Mouth

Hold up a piece of thick string in the mouth. Mark with your fingers where the sides of the corners of the lip occur. Remove the string and measure between the marks. It can often be difficult to buy the exact width of bit required, particularly in the smaller sizes, and it may be necessary to approach several suppliers. Remember that the height of the horse will not reflect the size of the required bit. This will be governed by type and breeding. Bits that are not of correct width can be very uncomfortable and damaging to the horse.

TYPES OF BIT

There are five main types of bit or bridle, sometimes called 'families', all of which have many variations. These are:

- the snaffle;
- the double;
- the pelham;

- the gag snaffle;

- the hackamore/bitless bridle.

NOTE: There are restrictions on bits used in competitions governed by the FEI and the relevant competitive discipline's rules. Illustrations of permitted bits can be found in the relevant rule books and should always be referred to before competing.

THE ACTION OF THE SNAFFLE BIT

There are many variations of the snaffle, but the main ones are:

- Solid mouthpiece with no joint.

- One joint with two arms.

- Two joints with two arms and a middle link, which encourages more play in the mouth and has no nutcracker action.

- A straight bar or curved (mullen mouth) mouthpiece with no joint works on the lips and directly on to the bars of the mouth. If the tongue is large there is also considerable tongue pressure. If the tongue is small the bars will take more pressure. It is difficult to use the reins independently, as when one rein is pulled the other side of the bit will move forwards in the mouth.

- With a single joint mouthpiece there is much more movement within the mouth. If the bit is too wide the joint within the mouth will close and cause pressure on either the tongue or the roof of the mouth. This is often called 'nutcracker action' but in reality it is not so. The horse will always try to hold the bit to the width of his mouth. If the bit is the correct width, it should lie almost straight across the mouth. It acts on the bars of the mouth and the corners of the lips, depending on how the horse is carrying his head.

- A snaffle with two joints acts on the bars of the mouth and the lips. It has no nutcracker action. It may drop down on the tongue.

- A thick mouthpiece is milder than a thin one, but care must be taken that the horse can accommodate it.

- Eggbutt rings are less likely to pinch the lips or corners of the mouth than are loose, flat-ring or some cheek snaffles.

- A loose-ring snaffle allows more movement in the mouthpiece and encourages a horse to champ the bit.

- The severity of the bit is increased by any uneven or squared-off bearing surface, i.e. twisted, plated, roller.

TYPES OF SNAFFLE

Single Joint

FLAT RING There is some risk of pinching the lips.

EGGBUTT Prevents rubbing at the corners of the lips.

GERMAN LOOSE-RING HOLLOW MOUTH The mouthpiece has a broad, thick design. The hollow mouthpiece makes it light in weight. The cylindrical loose ring reduces pinching.

D-RING RACE SNAFFLE This is less likely to be pulled through the mouth.

LARGE RING RACING Will not pull through the mouth.

A FULMER OR AUSTRALIAN snaffle is a full-cheeked snaffle with the cheeks fixed to the corners of the bit; the loose ring is set outside the cheek. This bit should always be used with keepers attaching it to the cheek pieces. It is a very quiet, still bit, good for young horses, horses with fussy mouths or those ridden by beginners. When used with a drop noseband it works well. See diagram right.

CHEEK A cheek snaffle has the cheek jointed at the side of the mouthpiece and is one with the ring. It does not always need to be used with keepers but if the cheeks fall forwards across the horse's muzzle they should be used. It is often used for strong and uneducated horses and will also help to keep the horse straight.

SPOON This can have full cheeks or half cheeks, which can be either above or below the mouthpiece. The latter type is used for driving.

HANGING CHEEK This suspends the bit in the mouth and gives more room for the tongue. It can be useful for horses who put their tongue over the bit.

TWISTED This is severe because of the ridged surface.

Full cheek snaffle, with a flash noseband.

Fulmer or Australian snaffle, with keepers onto the cheek pieces.

Double Joint

FRENCH BRIDOON This has a rounded plate which joins the two parts of the snaffle. The plate lies flat on the tongue. There is no nutcracker action from this bit, and many horses – particularly if a little set in the jaw – relax and go better. If this bit has square arms, or a sharp-edged plate, it is not allowed in dressage tests.

DICK CHRISTIAN This has a small ring joining the two arms which removes the nutcracker action and gives room for the tongue. It prevents the horse taking hold of the bit and can help control a hard puller.

DR BRISTOL This has a plate with squared edges fixed between the two arms. The bit is severe, but when the flat plate is on the tongue it is less sharp than when the bit is turned the other way, and the plate goes across the tongue. It should not be used reversed.

Straight Bar

The following four bits are more comfortable for the horse, and have a milder action if they are of half-moon or mullen design:

- VULCANITE LOOSE RING.
- NYLON This has a half-moon or mullen mouthpiece.
- RUBBER This is a very mild bit, but not durable.
- METAL LOOSE RING.

New Designs

There are many new designs of snaffles being introduced to the market at the present time. Most of them are made from artificial materials or some form of 'sweet metal', German silver or similar alloys. Some of them have tongue grooves or ports. These can be bulky and if too high can cause discomfort or even damage to the roof of the mouth. Some are very precisely engineered with shaped mouthpieces and/or rotating sections in the mouth. Their action and design should be assessed very carefully to ensure the bit is suitable for the horse in question.

It is sometimes possible to hire or borrow bits for a period of time to see how the horse gets on with it before purchase. This is a good idea as some are extremely expensive.

Severe Snaffles

The bits below have a severe action, and none is permitted in dressage tests. Before resorting to such bits, expert advice should be sought. These bits should only be used when other methods of control have failed.

WILSON This has four rings, the two attached to the mouthpiece take the reins, the other two take the headpiece. A severe squeezing on the face results when the reins are pulled.

MAGENIS This has set-in squared-off arms with a small set of rollers set horizontally within the arms. It prevents the horse from taking hold of the bit and running away.

CHERRY ROLLER This prevents the horse from catching hold of the bit and running away. The uneven surface is sharp to the tongue and bars.

'Y' or 'W' The two mouthpieces can give a pinching action to the lips and tongue.

SCORRIER This has a square-section mouthpiece with grooves on one side, and two rings which act as 'Wilson rings' (see above).

CONTINENTAL SNAFFLE/DUTCH GAG or BUBBLE BIT This may have a single- or double-jointed mouthpiece. The rein can be attached to any of the three rings – the lowest gives greatest leverage with the first ring giving only a direct snaffle action.

AMERICAN GAG This has a slightly different cheek design from the Dutch gag and a very precise rein action. It should only be used by experienced riders.

ROCKWELL, NORTON, NEWMARKET These are forms of snaffle bridle which by various means produce pressure on the nose as well as on the mouth. They can be of some use on strong horses with uneducated mouths who have not been taught to obey, or who fight against more usual methods of control.

SPRING MOUTH This attachment is clipped to the rings of a snaffle giving a double bit action.

CHAIN SNAFFLE The mouthpiece is made of chain links.

TWISTED WIRE This has two mouthpieces of twisted wire.

THE GAG SNAFFLE A gag snaffle has two holes in the bit rings or cheeks, through which run roundings attached to the headpiece and ending in the reins. The mouthpiece is jointed and can be smooth, twisted or with rollers. It is generally used on its own, but can be operated as the bridoon part of a double bridle if greater control is required. Its action brings considerable pressure on the corners of the mouth and the poll. It can be effective on horses who put their heads down and pull, as its leverage action makes it possible for the rider to raise the horse's head. It should always have a second rein attached to the rings of the bit, which allows it to be used as a normal snaffle when the gag action is not required.

Used in the wrong hands this bridle can prove dangerous, making some horses rear. It should never be used by inexperienced children or novice adults.

The use of such bits may indicate failure in the correct training of the horse. Frequently the bits create more confusion in the horse's mind, thus compounding the problem.

Snaffles for Use on Young Horses

KEY-RING MOUTHING BIT This is still used by some trainers. The keys encourage the horse to play with the bit, but may also encourage him to put his tongue over the bit. Modern training methods require that the horse should learn to hold the bit quietly in his mouth with a relaxed jaw. For this purpose, a jointed or mullen mouth snaffle is now more acceptable.

TATTERSALL YEARLING BIT This is a circular bit sometimes used on yearlings to give greater control when being shown. The bit is attached to a show headcollar by short straps, and encircles the lower jaw with the key section in the mouth. The lead rein is attached to the back ring and when used the bit rises up in the mouth.

Special Bits

CHIFNEY ANTI-REARING This acts in a similar way to the normal ring bit, but if the horse should attempt to rear, the 'U' shape puts greater pressure on his tongue; therefore discouraging the habit. It is made of thin metal and is severe.

HORSESHOE CHEEK STALLION BIT This is a showing bit and is buckled to a show headcollar. It has horseshoe-shaped cheeks, and a straight-bar or mullen-mouth bit which acts on the corners of the mouth, the tongue, and then the bars.

Fitting a Snaffle Bit

As already explained the width is crucial, about 0.6cm (¼in) should protrude on either side. When fitting for height, pull the bit down gently in the mouth with even pressure on either side. An unjointed bit should not wrinkle the corners of the lips; a jointed snaffle should do so very slightly.

THE DOUBLE BRIDLE

This has two metal bits. The bridoon is a snaffle bit with small rings. The curb bit has no joint, and comes in a variety of designs, but it must have a curb chain. The curb bit should either be referred to as 'the curb bit' or more correctly as 'the bit'. Some types do not have 'Ds' for the lip strap.

The double bridle is used:

- On horses who, having been trained in a snaffle, are ready to understand and accept a lighter and more refined aid from the rider's hand.

- In the showing ring, where its purpose is not only to add to the horse's turnout but also to increase control.

- In the hunting field and competitive jumping. It helps keep the horse in better balance, and gives more control than the snaffle bridle.

- The double bridle is required wear in some levels of dressage competition.

Action of double bridle bits on horses trained in a snaffle:

- The bridoon acts in a similar way to the snaffle. It asks the horse to work on the bit, going forward with an even contact on both hands. It can raise the head.

- The curb bit gives a lighter and more refined aid. It helps to position the head as collection is developed through the horse's progressive training. It also helps balance and control. It should lie immediately below the bridoon, but not so low that it touches the tushes. Both bits must be able to act independently.

The mouthpiece of the bit acts on the tongue and the bars of the mouth, and as a fulcrum for the upper and lower cheeks of the bit. When the curb rein is used, the curb chain tightens and applies pressure in the chin groove. As this occurs, the upper cheek piece moves

A curb bit with double-link curb chain and lip strap.

Poorly fitted curb chain – the hook is behind the bridoon.

forward (its position governed by the tightness of the curb chain, and the size and shape of the rings attaching it to the cheek pieces) and brings slight pressure to bear on the poll. The longer the lower cheek, the greater the pressure and severity of the action, both on the chin groove and the poll. A shallow tongue groove or port gives added room for the tongue; a high port presses on the roof of the mouth, and in the wrong hands can cause discomfort and pain.

The curb chain should be adjusted to ensure that the chain comes into action when the cheeks of the bit are at an angle of 45° to the mouth. When fitted, but not in use, the bottom of the curb chain should lie in the chin groove and the top at an angle of 45° away from it. When the rein is applied the chain lies flat in the groove and pressure is applied. If it is always flat in the chin groove the pressure when the rein is applied is too extreme and can cause damage to the jaw in the long term.

Incorrect fit – the loose links left dangling.

Types of Bridoon

These can be loose ring or eggbutt. They can have hanging cheeks and either one or two joints. Eggbutt rings can be too bulky for some mouths and make it difficult to fit the chain correctly. The usual variations are:

- Ordinary bridoon with loose rings or eggbutt rings.

- Double-jointed bridoon with eggbutt rings.

- Hanging cheeked bridoon with one joint.

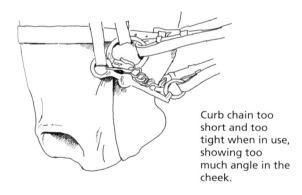

Curb chain too short and too tight when in use, showing too much angle in the cheek.

Correctly fitted curb chain.

incorrectly fitted curb bit. The angle of the cheek is too
extreme, therefore the curb chain has been fitted too long, and it is twisted. Also, there is no lip strap and

Correctly fitted double bridle with curb chain in play.

Types of Bit

These may have a tongue groove or port of variable height. The cheeks may also vary in length.

FIXED CHEEK with a low port and medium-length cheeks. This has a more immediate and precise action than the sliding mouthpiece. It is often considered more suitable for dressage competition.

WEYMOUTH SLIDING MOUTHPIECE with a low port and longer cheeks. The mouthpiece moves up and down. The cheeks go through the mouthpiece, so that increased contact on one will bring the other into play. More often seen on show horses.

THICK MOUTH GERMAN This has a thick, fixed mouthpiece which tapers in the centre to allow room for the tongue. The mouthpiece can be hollow. The cheeks can be straight or curve forward. Many Thoroughbred horses are uncomfortable in this bit owing to its thickness.

HALF-MOON OR MULLEN MOUTH This has short, fixed cheeks and a half-moon mouthpiece which allows some room for the tongue; though when the curb rein is used, pressure falls more on the tongue than on the bars.

BANBURY The mouthpiece is a round bar which is slotted through the cheeks. It has no port. It can revolve to give an independent action to each cheek, and to the corresponding curb rein. It may also be made to move up and down. It is now rarely used.

There are a number of variations on these basic designs. Many of them are from the Continent and are designed mainly for use on warmblood dressage horses. They do not always suit TBs with their narrow jaws and should be chosen carefully.

The **ELEVATOR BRIDLE** is designed with a padded headpiece and noseband in order to spread the pressure.

They vary somewhat in design with the sliphead and noseband sometimes going on top of the headpiece and sometimes underneath depending on the amount of poll and/or nose pressure required.

It is very easy to cause extreme discomfort or long term damage when using equipment that applies pressure to the bones. This is especially so with inexperienced riders or inadequately trained horses. Research at autopsy has shown horses with considerable bone damage caused by too tight equipment.

No noseband should prevent the horse from moving his jaw or opening his mouth a small amount. Nor should it restrict his breathing by being fitted too low.

Ideally, only a cavesson noseband should be used with a double bridle. Any other suggests the horse it not yet ready to use a double.

Always ensure that the design and style of the double chosen is suitable for the type of horse and the type of competition or event. Also ensure that its falls within the rules.

Curb Chains

These can be of metal, with either single or double links. They can also be of leather or elastic. Rubber or leather curb guards can be fixed to metal chains. For fitting see pages 228–9.

THE PELHAM

This bit is trying to combine the action of a snaffle and a double bridle in one bit. The mouthpiece can be jointed, straight or half-moon (mullen), either with or without a port. It has a lower cheek, which takes the curb chain. It usually has two reins: one attached to the rings on the mouthpiece and the other to the rings on the lower cheeks. It may be fitted with roundings on the bit and one rein. Some Pelhams do not have a lip strap. The longer the cheek, the greater the leverage.

The Pelham has a rather indefinite action, but many horses, and particularly ponies, appear to work happily

in it. It cannot be considered as a bit likely to improve a horse's mouth, but its use by an uneducated or heavy-handed rider probably does less harm to the horse's mouth. With a long-jawed horse it can be difficult to get the curb chain pressure in the chin groove.

Types of Pelham

MULLEN MOUTH This is widely used. The mouthpiece can be made of metal, vulcanite, nylon or rubber.

JOINTED This can be smooth or twisted, and has a more severe action than the mullen or vulcanite.

VULCANITE This refers to the material from which the mouthpiece is made. It can be seen in any design of Pelham and makes the bit quite bulky but kind in the mouth. Many cobs and ponies seem very happy in them.

FITTING THE CURB CHAIN It is often difficult to fit a curb chain correctly with a Pelham. This is because the bit's height in the mouth varies depending on whether one or both reins are being used.

Care must be taken that when the rein is applied the hook is not pressed against the horse's cheek. To this end, most Pelhams require the hook to be placed outside the top rein ring and the chain threaded through before being twisted flat and fitted in the usual way.

See diagram on page 229.

OTHER BIT TYPES

KIMBLEWICK A single-rein bit with a curb chain – neither a pelham nor a snaffle. The mouthpiece can be of metal or vulcanite. It is a strong bit, which some sensitive horses resent. The strength and severity of the Kimblewick is sometimes underestimated. It is sometimes used on ponies who are too strong for their child riders in a snaffle. As with all strong bits, its continual use soon deadens a horse's mouth. The child rider may be better using a Pelham, which is square attachment for cheek piece increases severity of poll pressure

A Kimblewick bit showing the curb chain fitted through the bit ring to prevent pinching.

less severe. (See also page 229.)

SHOW HACK or **GLOBE CHEEK** These are curb bits used without the bridoon, and only have one rein attached. They are seen on show ponies and occasionally show hacks. They are severe, and need to be used with a light hand.

ARMY REVERSIBLE OR UNIVERSAL This was designed for army use to suit as many different types of horses as possible. It is reversible, allowing either the smooth or the twisted side of the bit to be in action. The top rein is attached to 'D'-shaped rings; the lower rein can be used in either of two slots according to need. It does not have a lip strap.

THREE-IN-ONE or **SWALES** This is a very severe bit. It acts without poll pressure, the headpiece being supported by rings on the mouthpiece. When the curb rein is used, very severe pressure is put on the chin groove. If the top rein only is used, it is much less severe and many horses go well in it.

THE BITLESS BRIDLE OR HACKAMORE

This bridle is designed to control the horse by applying pressure on the nose without the use of a bit. It can be effective on horses with damaged mouths, or on those who through bad handling resent and fight a normal bridle. It gives good control, but steering can be difficult.

It consists of a bridle head, cheeks, and padded noseband held in place by a strap or chain. Reins are attached to rings on the noseband, and these apply pressure via the strap or chain. Considerable leverage is obtained on the nose, and to a lesser degree on the poll, the chin groove and the lower jaw. The precise action depends on the design of the bridle. Some hackamores can be very severe and should only be used by riders aware of their action and capable of using them with tact and discretion. They should not be used on ponies or by uneducated riders.

Bitless bridles are not permitted in dressage competitions.

BIT ATTACHMENTS

RUBBER BIT GUARDS fit on each side of the bit, and protect the face and corners of the lips of a sensitive horse.

TONGUE GUARDS are made of metal, and are held in place by a separate head strap. They are fitted into the horse's mouth above the normal bit to prevent a horse putting his tongue over the bit.

RUBBER TONGUE GRIDS fit on to a narrow straight-bar snaffle and may help to prevent a horse putting his tongue over the bit. It is important to check that they cannot be easily dislodged, as they may either be spat out by the horse or swallowed.

AUSTRALIAN CHEEKER This is a rubber device running from the headpiece down the front of the horse's face. Attached to each side of the bit, it helps to keep the bit high in the mouth, and prevents a horse getting his tongue over the bit. It is most often used on racehorses.

CHAPTER

31 BOOTS AND BANDAGES

BOOTS

Boots are used to protect a horse's legs and joints from injury, either self-inflicted or from an outside source. Self-inflicted injuries are the result of:

- Faulty conformation.
- Faulty action.
- Poor shoeing.
- Lack of balance in a young horse.
- Poor condition and lack of muscle.
- Fatigue.
- Careless riding.
- Galloping in deep going.
- Pecking over a fence.

Types of Injury

BRUSHING This occurs on the inside of the leg below the knee or hock. It is inflicted by the opposite foot, usually in the area of the fetlock joint.

SPEEDICUT This occurs when a horse is galloping and cuts into the leg just below the knee or hock with the opposite front or hind foot.

LOW OVER-REACH This is a bruise or cut on the heel of a front foot. The front foot stays on the ground too long,

and the inside edge of the hind shoe strikes down into the heel. It usually occurs over a jump, when an extra effort has been made and the jump was unbalanced, or the landing in deep going. However, big-moving horses can lose their balance on the flat and over-reach.

HIGH OVER-REACH This is an injury to the back tendon caused by the horse when over-jumping or losing balance when galloping. The front of the hind foot strikes into the back of the front leg below the knee. It is always serious, even if there is no cut. When caused by another horse it is referred to as 'struck into'. It is most likely to occur when racing.

All over-reaches must be treated seriously as they entail internal bruising and a possible seat of infection.

TREAD This can be self-inflicted, when a horse treads on the inner coronet of one front foot with the other front foot. It can occur during travelling or when a horse is weaving. Injury from another horse treading on the outside of the coronet can occur:

- When travelling with another horse if there is no partition.
- During a game of polo.
- Among a restless group of horses, e.g. out hunting.
- When riding one horse and leading another.
- Riding too close behind another horse.
- When racing, one horse can land on the heels of

another, causing severe damage.

Treads can be serious if they cause internal bruising.

BRUISED SHINS These are caused by rapping either front or hind shins on a jump.

POLO KNOCKS These can occur anywhere on the legs; but they happen more usually on the front legs below the knee. They are caused by a blow from a polo mallet or from the ball.

USE OF BOOTS

When schooling horses of any age it is a sensible precaution to fit protective boots according to the work to be done. This often saves an unnecessary injury, which could lay the horse off work. On a straight-moving horse during simple work or exercise they should not be necessary.

Boots are not advisable when out hunting or on long-distance rides, as mud works up under the boot. Pressures and friction over several hours will cause a sore place, which can quickly become infected and cause acute lameness. Many owners now use turnout boots to try to prevent damage when out at grass. They should only be used when the horse is out for a limited time and be removed when he is stabled.

Boots are designed to give protection to a specified area of the horse's leg. The range of designs and materials available is enormous and with care it is possible to find the most suitable for any given problem. In many types of competition, such as showing and dressage, boots are not permitted. Always check the rule book.

MATERIALS

* Boots are made of a wide range of synthetic materials, leather (usually lined with sheepskin or foam rubber), rubber or heavy cloth such as Kersey or box cloth (a lighter material) and neoprene.

* Regardless of material, it is important that after use, boots are either brushed clean, or if wet, washed.

* Leather boots and fastenings must be kept supple.

* Leather or cloth boots, if not well cleaned, become hard and cause pressure sores on a horse's leg. These can quickly become infected, resulting in a lame horse.

* Neoprene or another synthetic material is less likely to cause this problem, but cleaning after use is still essential. Synthetics are lighter and more comfortable for the horse, and easier to clean or wash. They are generally preferable to boots made of traditional materials and are extensively and predominantly used today.

* Some tendon and exercise boots are made with flexible polycarbonate shields and Kevlar inserts around the fetlock to guard against injury.

* Some boots have a removable washable lining which absorbs sweat more readily than the more solid outer covering.

FASTENINGS

Boots should always fasten on the outside of the leg, with the end of the strap usually pointing towards the rear. Fastenings can be buckles, clips or Velcro – sometimes more than one type. Front leg boots will have fewer fastenings than hind leg boots, which are usually longer. A short type of boot may have only one fastening.

Leather boots always have sewn-on leather straps and buckles. These are secure, but are time-consuming to fasten, and the stitching needs regular inspection. Kersey, box cloth and synthetic material have buckles, clips or self-holding Velcro fastenings.

Fastenings are often set on strong elastic, which makes the boots more comfortable for the horse. The elastic must be inspected regularly. If it becomes stretched and loses its strength it must be renewed.

If Velcro is used, make sure that the straps are wide enough and long enough, so that the boot is held securely. The Velcro must always be kept clean. The most common cause of Velcro losing its ability to grip is because of careless practice, putting the boots down on dirty surfaces and getting bedding, hair and school surface in them. If it wears smooth it must be renewed. As Velcro fastenings are easily dislodged in rough conditions, they are not suitable for hacking through mud or for cross-country work. They can be made more secure for these purposes by wrapping adhesive tape several times around the Velcro fastening. Care must be taken, however, not to pull the tape tighter around the fastening and so exert uneven pressure. Some boots have elasticated straps that fasten with a quick-release stud or tab mechanism.

APPLICATION

Consider the following:

- Are they necessary? If not, do not use just to follow a trend.

- Are they the correct design and material for the designated purpose?

- Do they fit the horse?

When applying:

- Fasten from the top down. Unfasten from the bottom up. That way the horse is less likely to tread on them if startled.

- Apply slightly high and slide down the leg. Never pull up.

- Ensure that they are a pair and free from sand, grit, straw or shavings before applying.

- After fitting always test that they are firm but not too tight.

- Always remove after use and rub the leg to improve circulation and remove any debris.

- Clean and dry boots and store in pairs.

TYPES OF PROTECTIVE BOOT

BRUSHING BOOT This is full size and protects the whole of the inside of the leg below the knee, including the fetlock joint. The boot should be placed on the leg rather higher than in its final position. It should be fastened firmly, starting from the top, and then eased a little down the leg so that it protects the fetlock joint. The boots should then be checked to see that they are firm, cannot move about, but are not too tight.

FETLOCK BOOT A short boot, usually with one strap. It gives protection to the fetlock joint only and often slips around during use.

YORKSHIRE BOOT This is used to cover the fetlock joint. It is a piece of heavy cloth about 30cm (12ins) long and 20cm (8ins) broad, with wide tape or Velcro stitched about two-thirds down its length. It is then wound round the leg, fastened on the outside above the fetlock joint and eased down over the joint. The cloth above the tape is then folded over to form a double

Yorkshire boot.

thickness. Note that in deep going the boot can be sucked off. Yorkshire boots are rarely seen today, having been superseded by synthetic fetlock boots.

They can be very useful when lungeing, especially horses who do not like the sound of Velcro being unfastened or to cover a wound where a more closely fitting boot might cause discomfort.

RUBBER RING This is a hollow ring with a leather or metal fastening running through its centre. It can be used round the horse's pastern or above the fetlock joint, and protects either area.

SAUSAGE BOOT This is a large, leather-covered, padded ring. It is fastened round the pastern, and prevents a horse bruising an elbow with the heel of the same front foot when lying down.

SPEEDICUTTING BOOT This is similar to a full-length brushing boot, but is cut to come higher up the leg and to give greater protection to the inner, lower part of the knee or hock.

OVER-REACH BOOT There are a number of different types of over-reach boot including the well-known bell-shaped boot made of rubber. This type is pulled on and off over the foot, which can be difficult. Care should be taken not to twist the foot when applying or removing these boots otherwise damage to the pastern joint can result. Over-reach boots made of individual rubber 'petals' are fastened round the pastern, making them easier to put on. Movement through the individual 'petals' prevents the boots from turning inside out and also allows replacement of damaged or missing 'petals'.

Over-reach boots can also be made to fasten with a leather tab that runs down through two metal loops set into the rubber boot or from Neoprene with Velcro fastenings.

TENDON BOOT This is shaped like a brushing boot, but has extra padding down the back of the leg to protect the tendon from being struck. Open-fronted tendon

boots leave the cannon bone area exposed and unprotected and are often used for show jumping.

CORONET BOOT This is a small, semi-circular covering, usually of leather or Neoprene. It fastens round the pastern, and protects the coronet. It is used for polo or travelling. Horses can easily tread on themselves or one another if travelling without a partition. The bruising may be invisible, but can be quite severe. Bandages and Gamgee give some protection if they are put on to reach down over the coronet, but coronet boots can be a wise precaution.

POLO BOOT This is similar to a brushing boot, but is longer – coming well down the fetlock. Some are designed with quite a 'flair' or 'skirt' below the fetlock to allow for the extreme extension of the joint required when playing. Some types which cover the coronet also strap round the pastern. The boots are put on in the usual way, or they may be secured with firm bandages, the latter being fastened with cotton or self-adhesive tape and the ends sewn for extra security.

MEDICINE BOOTS These reach from below the knee to below the fetlock joint. They fit closely around the whole of the joint and are fastened with strongly elasticated straps. They are sometimes claimed to help support the fetlock joint and they certainly protect it from treads and impact with the ground when running or jumping at speed.

EQUIBOOT This is a patented boot made in varying sizes to fit over a horse's foot. It is used:

- To protect the foot if for any reason the horse cannot be shod and is required for work.

- In the stable, to keep a foot poultice in place, especially for a horse who chews at bandages and sacking.

Its exact fit is very important. A boot which is too tight can bruise the heels and set up an infection. If it is too loose, it will come off. The fit can be adjusted by tightening or loosening the heel pads at the back of the boot.

POULTICE BOOT This is made of synthetic material or leather. Its purpose is to hold foot dressings in place. It fits over the foot and is fastened up the leg.

TREATMENT BOOT This is similar to a wellington boot, and reaches from the foot to well above the knee. It is used for cold-water treatment to an injured leg.

TRAVELLING BOOT Many people use a well-applied stable bandage with a generous lining of Gamgee or similar material. Bandaging, however, takes time, and labour-saving alternatives are leg guards or travelling boots. These are made from synthetic materials, and may have a thick, padded lining. They are fastened with several wide Velcro straps. They should be long enough to reach from above the knee and hock down over the coronet. It is then not necessary to use knee caps and hock boots. Young or nervous horses need to be familiarised with the feeling of having the whole leg enclosed in a fairly inflexible casing; they can also be

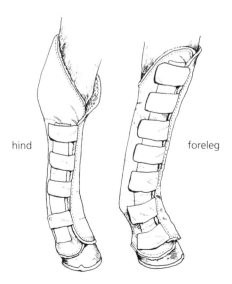

hind   foreleg

Travelling boots.

alarmed by the noise of the Velcro being pulled apart, and accidents have been known to be caused by their use. Using cheap and insubstantial materials can result in the boots slipping down, especially if the horse slips and loses his footing, or treads on the bottom. The boot then provides little or no protection.

KNEE CAPS These are used for travelling or exercising on roads, and sometimes by show jumpers, especially in puissance-type competitions, and are made of leather, heavy cloth or synthetic material. To be smart, the material should match the rest of the travelling equipment.

The front of the knee cap is covered with a reinforced pad of leather. The straps are leather. The top strap should be set in strong elastic to allow it to be firmly fixed without causing the horse discomfort. It should be fastened well above the knee on the outside. The spare end of strap will then be forwards. The knee cap can then be eased down and tested to make sure it cannot slip over the knee.

The bottom strap must be fastened very loosely, usually in the first hole, so that it cannot interfere with the action of the joint.

For long journeys pad the back of the top strap to prevent a pressure injury.

SKELETON KNEE CAPS These are lightweight knee boots consisting of a top strap and a reinforced leather pad to cover the knee. When hacking out on roads, skeleton knee caps can be a wise protection. For general use they should have two straps. For jumping, to prevent further bruising or to protect an old injury, they may have top straps only but sometimes flip up in use.

HOCK BOOTS OR CAPS Hock boots are designed to protect the point of the hock when travelling. They are of similar construction to knee caps. The top holding strap is usually set in strong elastic so that it can be firmly buckled without cramping the joint. It is fastened on the outside, quite close to the front of the hock. The bottom strap should be fastened more firmly than that of

Hock boot.

the knee cap but not too tightly. The spare end of strap should be towards the rear. The horse should be familiar with the feeling of the hock boots before they are first used for travelling. They can be especially useful when travelling a big horse in a trailer or rather cramped space where he may be otherwise cap his hocks.

BANDAGES

Use of Bandages

Modern research has found that tendons are best kept cool in order to minimise strain whilst working. The quicker legs return to their optimum temperature after exercise, the better. This means we need to reconsider how and when to apply boots and bandages.

Bandaging the Legs

Whichever type of bandage is used, it is essential for them to be correctly and skilfully applied. Badly or carelessly applied bandages can cause untold damage to a horse's legs.

Various methods of bandaging are acceptable, but the essential requirements are:

• The bandage must be correctly and firmly rolled. First, roll the tapes or fastenings in the position where they are stitched. Then roll the bandage round them.

• The bandage should be applied only as firmly as is needed to keep it in place and to prevent it slipping.

• It should be applied without wrinkles. The pressure should be minimal but even. The fastenings should not be any tighter than the bandage.

• Fastenings should be on the outside and, if tapes, the loose ends should be tucked away.

• Bandages should not be fastened over a joint.

CAUSES OF DAMAGE

• Fastenings and/or bandages which are too tight, or a twisted bandage, can cause marks on the leg and possible tendon damage.

• Fastenings at the back or front of the leg may cause pressure and injury to the tendons. Fastenings tied at the front are likely to bruise the cannon bone. Those fastened on the inside may be interfered with by the other leg, be less secure and less accessible.

• A poorly applied stable bandage can slip down and become dislodged when the horse stands up after resting. It may then be stepped on and torn. Poorly applied work bandages could cause injury to horse and/or rider if they loosen during exercise.

Types of Bandage

STABLE BANDAGES are used:

• For warmth and to keep the circulation active.

• To assist in the drying-off of wet legs.

• For keeping poultices in position. Crepe bandage can also be used for this.

• To protect the legs whilst travelling.

• To prevent the legs from 'filling'.

• Often used when the horse is on box rest or on the sound leg when the other is being treated for injury.

EXERCISE BANDAGES are used as a protection against injury during work.

SURGICAL BANDAGES are used to cover and protect wounds, for poulticing of the leg when there is a likelihood of swelling, and for wounds on joints. They are usually made of a synthetic stretch material.

VETRAP is a bandage that sticks to itself and is excellent for keeping dressings in place or for securing bandages on an awkward place such as a joint. It is seldom reusable.

POLO OR DRESSING WRAPS are wide, soft bandages designed to be used without under-bandage protection, when schooling horses or playing polo. They are relatively quick and easy to apply and remove.

TAIL BANDAGES are used:

- In the stable to help keep a tail tidy.

- When travelling, as a protection, both for the tail hair and the dock.

Under-bandage Protection

When worn under bandages the following give added protection and warmth:

GAMGEE is cotton wool in a muslin cover. It gives the best protection, but is expensive and easily soiled. If the edges of the Gamgee are machine stitched, it is easier to wash and will last longer.

PROLITE is an artificial material that is designed to prevent injury and damage from impact. It forms to the shape of the specific leg. It is wrinkle-free and non-absorbent.

LEG WRAPS are thick felt pads cut to fit the leg. They are more expensive, but are quick to put on, easy to wash, and durable. Long term they are very economical.

FYBAGEE is a synthetic cloth, similar to thick felt. It is easily washed and durable.

PORTER BOOTS are pre-formed synthetic shells designed to protect the leg and prevent the bandage from being applied too tightly.

FOAM RUBBER is cheap and easy to wash, but can draw the leg, and some horses are allergic to it.

HAY OR STRAW can be used for drying off wet, muddy legs. Pummel it well, then wrap it round the leg before bandaging. This is known as 'thatching'. After half an hour the bandage can be removed and the leg brushed off.

Bandage Fastenings

TAPE This should be wide and flat. When the bandage is washed, the tape should be smoothed out and, if necessary, ironed flat.

VELCRO This is a rough synthetic material, and is self-holding. It is efficient and easy to use as long as it is kept clean. In a shavings bed it can become impregnated with dirt, and then will not hold securely. It must also be long enough to secure the bandage.

CLIPS These are satisfactory for stable bandages, but their shape can cause unnecessary pressure.

SELF-ADHESIVE TAPES These are separate from the bandage; they add security to existing tapes. For extra security during competition, racing, or strenuous work, the end of the tapes can be sewn to the bandage. Surgical and crepe bandages are usually fastened with adhesive tape but the tape must not be tighter than the bandage itself.

Stable Bandages

These can be made of wool, stockinette or synthetic fibre. Thermal bandages are also available: one type keeps the leg warm, and the other, cold; the latter can be useful after an injury. Full-size bandages should be

10–12cm (4–5ins) wide by 2.1–2.4m (7–8ft) long. They usually have little stretch to them and are used when the horse is not working, so may be applied right down to the coronary band. They are usually used with padding underneath but it is not obligatory.

Additional Requirements

- **POULTICING THE LEG** A double thickness of Gamgee is often used for extra protection should there be a tendency for the leg to swell.

- **TRAVELLING** The Gamgee or other lining should extend well up over the knee and well down over the coronet. The bandage is applied as described below.

- **SUPPORT BANDAGES** This is the name given to a bandage applied to the uninjured leg when a horse is injured or on box rest. They do not support unless they cover a joint and even then it is minimal. They do, however, help to prevent filled legs. They should be applied as a stable bandage, with padding, and should be removed, the leg massaged, and then re-applied at least twice a day.

To Put on Stable Bandages

- Place the lining around the leg. It should show 1.2cm (½in) above and below the finished bandage.

- Start bandaging in the same direction as the overlap of the lining, just below the knee or hock.

- If the bandage is too short, start just above the joint, apply down to the coronet, and then back up the leg to the knee or hock.

- Many people prefer the latter method of bandaging as it is more likely to discourage filled legs: the bandage being put on upwards towards the heart.

- Place 10cm (4ins) of the bandage at an angle above the first round, which should be pulled firm, and should hold the flap of the bandage in place. This flap can now be folded down, so that the rest of the rounds of bandage help to secure it.

- Roll the bandage down the leg. About half the width of the bandage should be left exposed on each circuit. It should not be necessary to alter the angle or to pull the bandage.

- When nearing the coronet, unroll the bandage in a similar upwards direction, finishing just below the knee or hock.

- The tapes or fastenings should finish on the outside of the leg. The tapes should be tied in a neat bow with the ends tucked in.

The legs of a stabled horse can fill as a result of:

- Strenuous exercise.

- Standing in for a day.

- An old injury.

- A stomach upset.

- Old age.

- When first brought up from grass and making the change to living in the stable.

Such 'legs' usually walk down, but well-applied stable bandages at night help to keep the legs warm and the circulation active, which alleviates the problem.

Putting on a stable bandage.

Exercise Bandages

These should be made of stretch material: stockinette, crepe or elastic material. They should be 8cm (3ins) wide and 1.8–2.1m (6–7ft) long.

To Put on Exercise Bandages

- It is usual to put Gamgee, Fybagee or Porter boots under the bandage to give added protection, and to ensure that the bandage and tapes do not mark or injure the leg.

- The requirements and likely faults are similar to those of stable bandages, except that, being more elastic, and being used for work, these bandages need to be put on more firmly. There is more risk of them being too tight.

- The flap over at the top should be longer. When folded down under the rest of the bandage, this helps to keep it firm.

- The bandage should extend from below the knee to the centre of the fetlock joint. Stockinette or crepe bandages should not extend over the whole of the joint, as this may cause interference. Vetrap bandages, expertly applied, can be fitted over the joint for extra support and protection. Exercise bandages should be sewn or taped for extra security when going across country. Elastic bandages when worn for any length of time will contract if they get wet and then dry. This can cause serious discomfort and possible injury to the horse, by restricting circulation. It is therefore essential to use Gamgee or similar lining. They should be removed and the leg massaged as soon as possible after the work is finished.

The Purpose of Exercise Bandages

Exercise bandages are often used to ease the strain on tendons and ligaments in the front leg, but there is little evidence to indicate that they do. Their main purpose is to protect the leg from bruising when hitting a jump,

Putting on an exercise bandage.

and to avoid cutting and bruising the back of the front leg by an over-reach or blow on the inner surface of the opposite front leg. If the bandages are used in muddy conditions for several hours, the mud is likely to work up underneath the bandage, leading to friction and possibly infection.

Various new types of reinforced lining (e.g. Porter boots) are now produced which can be cut to fit the leg. Used under an exercise bandage they give good protection from tendon injury for competition horses.

Polo wraps or exercise wraps are soft, stretchy bandages designed to be used without further padding. They start just below the knee and extend over the fetlock joint before finishing where they started. They should be used in pairs, not on one leg only.

Removing Leg Bandages

- Undo the fastening and, using both hands, unwind the bandage and remove the lining.

- Shake out the linings and bandages.

- If they are dirty, wash them. If they are damp, hang them up to dry.

- When the bandages are dry, roll up the tapes. Position them where they are sewn. Roll the bandages as firmly as possible over them, and tuck in the ends.

Bandages should be put away in twos or fours. Unroll

enough of one bandage to wrap it around one or three other bandages, and secure by tucking in the flap.

Never use dirty bandages. Soiled material is stiff and hard, and is not suitable for either legs or tail. Elastic bandages should be washed frequently to retain their elasticity. Their correct application is then made easier.

When the bandages have been removed and before they are rolled, the horse's legs should be given a brisk rub in an upwards direction to stimulate circulation.

Tail Bandages

These are made of stockinette, crepe or elastic. They should be 6–8cm (2½–3ins) wide, and about 1.5–1.8m (5–6ft) long.

Correctly applied they will improve the appearance of the tail, especially if it has been pulled. They should only be left on for a few hours in the day after grooming, and should be removed at night. Left on too long they can cause discomfort and restrict circulation, leading to a sore under the tail and in extreme cases to death of the bone and loss of the tail.

When applying the bandage it is important to ensure that it is firm but not pulled too tight, and that the tapes are not tied tighter than the bandage itself. It should be applied from the base of the tail to just above the last tail bone.

To Put on a Tail Bandage

- Hold the bandage in one hand and lift up the tail. Put it over the shoulder or hold it up with the other hand. Slightly damp the hair with a water brush.

- Place the spare end of the bandage under the tail and out at an angle at the top of the tail.

- Hold this spare end, and put one or two rounds of bandage as high up as possible round the tail.

- Turn down the flap and roll the bandage firmly down the tail. Tie it firmly, but not too tight. If the horse is being travelled, ensure that the fastening is not on the top of the tail where it might rub. It should be on the side and rather lower down than usual.

- To give extra security, when bandaging an unpulled tail, take a small wisp of hair and put it over the first twist of the bandage and under the second.

- Some people put the tail inside a stocking or something similar to keep it clean. Always ensure that the hairs are smoothed down. Some of the German warmblood breeders like to have a wavy tail. To achieve this divide the tail into three and then plait each third into a pigtail. When the three pigtails are brushed out, the tail appears thick and bushy.

To Remove a Tail Bandage

Undo the tapes, and with both hands pull the bandage down from the top. It should come away complete.

Putting on a tail bandage. In the final picture, the overlap of the bandage is yet to be turned down over the ties.

Shake it out and roll it up.

If a tail has been plaited, the bandage must be unwound, not pulled off.

Dirty bandages should always be washed before they are put away.

When travelling, it is advisable to provide a fresh bandage for the homeward journey as they are often soiled on the outward one.

Some people prefer to use a tail cover or guard when travelling. This needs to be attached to a roller and breastplate to keep it in place. It can be used with a tail bandage or instead of one.

32 CLOTHING

Clothing includes the various rugs, blankets and sheets worn by the stabled horse. He requires rugs in winter to keep him warm, and in summer to protect him from flies and to keep his coat clean. All stable and day rugs are secured by a front fastening. A leather roller or webbing surcingle can then be fixed round the body. The roller may or may not have a breast girth. Modern rugs have cross-over surcingles and fastenings under the belly, or just leg straps.

Stable or Night Rug

This can be made of synthetic material, jute, canvas or hemp.

- JUTE, CANVAS or HEMP RUGS are seldom seen nowadays. They are sometimes called dealer's rugs. They are not as warm as synthetic materials. They usually need to be used with one or more blankets.

- SYNTHETIC RUGS, made of polyester and other man-made fibres, are light, warm, comfortable, easily washed, and easily kept in place. They usually have a polyester filling. They offer improved temperature control and better air flow to provide insulation. Synthetic rugs have taken over extensively from those made of traditional, natural fibres.

   They come in a wide range of designs and weights to suit different circumstances. Under-rugs are also available if extra warmth is required. It is important that the material next to the horse's skin is absorbent. Some horses, especially when they are clipped, object to the static electricity generated when the rug is removed and replaced. In this case the rug provided needs to have a cotton lining.

Most of these rugs are easy to wash although they may be too bulky for a domestic washing machine.

   They usually have integral straps to fasten: a chest strap and cross-over belly straps that should not fit too tightly so long as the horse cannot get a foot caught in them as he gets up.

   Some rugs also have leg straps but these are not usually necessary for stable rugs.

Blankets

These are rectangular in shape. They are worn under the stable rug for extra warmth. They are usually made from thick woollen cloth. Blankets are sold in different sizes, by weight. They are expensive but last many years and repay the outlay. Lightweight blankets are a cheap alternative, but are not as warm, and they tear more easily. They are seldom used nowadays.

Sweat Rug

There are many different types available. The large cotton-mesh type is used to help cool off a horse. It works on the same principle as a string vest – by forming air pockets – and effectively insulates the horse against chill. For it to work efficiently, it is essential to put a top rug or sheet over it. Worn on its own, it helps to keep flies away, but it has little other value. Sweat rugs made of cotton towelling do not need a top rug to work efficiently.

Many modern rugs work by 'wicking' moisture away from the skin and allowing the horse to cool down and dry without risk of catching a chill. They are excellent value, although quite expensive. They are good for travelling the horse, if he is likely to break out, and for sick animals. They are light and warm.

Day Rug

This rug is worn for a special occasion, such as for competition work. It is made of wool, and is available in a variety of colours. It is buckled in front. The hems are braided, and it usually has the initials of the stable or owner on the bottom corner. It usually has a matching roller and breastplate.

Summer Sheet

This comes in a variety of colours or checks, and is made of cotton, linen or synthetic material. In hot weather it protects the horse against flies and keeps the coat tidy and clean. In warm weather it is used instead of a day rug for horses travelling to competitions and for special occasions. It can be put over a sweat sheet in summer. As it is light in weight, it has a fillet string, which lies round the quarters and under the tail. The string is attached to both edges of the sheet about halfway down.

A summer sheet can be used to provide an extra insulating layer under a winter rug, and as it is easily washable it can be regularly laundered, thus helping to keep the weightier winter rugs clean.

It also often comes with a matching roller and breastplate.

Exercise Sheet or Paddock Sheet

This is usually made of lightweight wool, and matches the day rug in colour. It can be used under the saddle for exercise in dry, cold winter weather. For racing, it is worn in the paddock over the saddle. It reaches from the horse's withers and shoulders to the top of the dock, and is kept in place by a lightweight, matching roller or surcingle. Fillet strings are essential to prevent the rug from blowing up and frightening the horse. When used under the saddle, the sheet should have tape loops through which the girth runs, to prevent it from slipping back.

They also come in waterproof material and/or with fluorescent strips or bands for work in wet weather or road exercise.

Waterproof Rug

This is made from waterproof fabric, and can be lined or unlined. A lining helps to absorb any sweat and allows the skin to breathe. Waterproof rugs are used at competitions, to cover the horse and tack whilst waiting for competition. Sometimes they are designed to fasten to the day rug. A fillet string is essential.

Hoods, Caps, Neck Covers and 'Vests'

Racehorses are often exercised in cold weather wearing a hood, or a cap, which is a shortened version of the hood. They are made of lightweight, coloured cloth, and are of value to well-bred horses on walking exercise in very cold weather. They can be of waterproof fabric, and used in conjunction with a waterproof rug.

Hoods and neck covers are widely available in a variety of materials for warmth and protection from the weather and mud. They are also used extensively in the stable, for exercise and turnout. They are often an integral part of modern turnout rugs.

Close-fitting vests, usually of Lycra-type or silky materials, can be worn as undergarments. These cover the forehand of the horse and offer protection from rugs which tend to rub with continued wear, if they don't fit properly or are badly applied.

New Zealand Rug, Turnout Rug

This is worn:

• By horses and ponies living out in the winter, to protect them from wind and rain. It also helps to keep the horses clean.

• To protect stabled horses and ponies who are turned out during the day. The rug keeps them warm and comparatively clean.

The rugs are made of lined waterproof canvas or man-made fibre. Investigation into materials continues, and improved types are constantly coming onto the market. The canvas type is heavier and stands up to harder use, but the lighter nylon rug is less likely to rub or rip, and is easier to keep in place. Canvas rugs in the original design have no roller and are self-righting when the horse rolls. Other makes have a stitched surcingle, which is eased over the backbone to avoid pressure. Both ends pass through the side of the rug. Nylon rugs are either buckled under the girth, or have cross-over surcingles or leg straps. There is now a lightweight material on the market which is waterproof and allows the skin to breathe. The extra expense is justified by the well-being of the animal.

It is essential for a New Zealand rug to fit correctly. It should lie snugly round the neck, so that it cannot work back and rub the top of the withers. It should reach to the top of the tail. Many have an additional piece that covers the tail to give extra protection. Leg straps can either be passed round the upper thigh and clipped on to the rug on the same side, or crossed to the opposite side. They should fit neither tightly nor too loosely. They must allow room for the horse to move. The clips should fasten outwards away from the horse's body.

When animals are living out all the time in New Zealand rugs two rugs should be available so that a wet one can be dried.

Always put a New Zealand rug on in the stable. Although it is not intended for wear in the stable, allow the horse to get used to it before turning him out. If he has never worn a New Zealand rug before, he may need to be walked and trotted with the rug on before letting him loose. The following day, the horse should have settled and can be turned out wearing the rug. Even if the rug is dry it should be removed at least once a day and then replaced after the horse has been checked over.

Turnout rugs may be similar in design to New Zealand rugs but are of lighter weight material and are more prone to damage.

Rollers

A roller is is a padded belt. It has a number of uses:

• To keep a rug in place. Used with day rugs or jute night rugs.

• To prevent a horse from getting cast.

• For use when lungeing or long reining.

A standard roller is made from leather or webbing or cloth. It should be well padded to fit either side of the spine just behind the withers. A wide roller should have two buckles or fastenings to prevent it rocking. They are frequently used with an integral breastplate, this prevents the roller from sliding back and is especially needed with day rugs or when lungeing or long reining.

If the padding is not sufficient to protect the spine, extra sponge can be placed underneath it.

AN ANTI-CAST OR ARCH ROLLER is used for horses who habitually roll over in their stable and get cast. It can have a fixed or adjustable iron arch, and comes in a normal size, a small arch, or a giant-size arch. The giant size is more likely to prevent the horse getting cast. The small arch can be useless if the horse has a thick straw bed.

The main drawback to an arched roller is that although it removes all pressure from the spine, it concentrates it on either side of the withers. Even if a thick pad is used, it can have a severe pinching effect. An arch roller should have buckles on both sides, so that if a horse gets cast, it is possible to release the roller and then right the horse.

Rollers used over a day rug, summer or paddock sheet are usually made of matching woollen or cotton web.

Breast Girth or Breast Strap

This is a strap made of leather or webbing. It has a buckle at each end, which is fastened to a leather strap threaded through the 'Ds' placed on either side of the roller. The purpose of the breast girth is to prevent the roller from sliding back, which can easily happen with a fit or thin horse. The breast girth should rest close to, but not tightly, around the chest and just above the point of the shoulder.

Surcingles

Webbing surcingles are stitched on to a night rug, and take the place of rollers. They should not be stitched over the top of the back, as the surcingle should be loose in this area. If two surcingles are used, one should be stitched about 46–60cm (18ins–2ft) behind the other. This provides a very secure arrangement for holding a rug in place. The second surcingle need not be fastened tightly.

A most effective alternative is to use two surcingles stitched at an angle on the sides of the rug and crossed under the belly. They are usually referred to as 'cross-over surcingles' and are fastened with a flat metal clasp. This type of surcingle removes all pressure from the spine and holds rugs in place efficiently. Cross-over surcingles are seen extensively in modern rugs.

Surcingle is also the name given to an unpadded webbing belt. This can be elasticated or with an elastic inset. They are sometimes used to keep sweat rugs in place and should not be mistaken for an overgirth, which is usually longer and narrower and which fits over the top of the saddle.

This type of surcingle is not recommended unless padding is placed on either side of the spine.

Belly Straps

These are wide pieces of matching material used to hold in place a polyester or nylon quilted rug. They may be crossed straps, as previously described. They are attached to the bottom edge of the rug, about 15cm (6ins) behind the elbow, and are fastened under the belly.

Leg Straps

Leg straps, as used for New Zealand rugs, can hold a lightweight man-made fibre rug in place. A roller should not be necessary. For fitting, see page 267.

MEASURING AND PUTTING ON RUGS/BLANKETS

Measuring for a Rug

To find the correct size of rug, measure the horse from the centre of the breastbone along the side to the point of the quarters. Alternatively, measure from a point just in front of the withers to just above the top of the tail.

Putting on a Rug

A correctly fitted rug is comfortable for the horse, stays in place better, and lasts longer – as the material will be less subject to wear and tear. It should fit snugly, not loosely, round the neck. If it is too large in the neck, it may slip back, tighten over the withers, and eventually cause a sore. Also, when the horse gets up he can catch a foot in the neck, and in struggling he may hurt himself and tear the rug. If it is too tight, it will cause discomfort through pressure on the windpipe. It should cover the body down to the elbows and extend as far back as the dock. Sheepskin pads on the top inside part of the neck aid comfort, particularly for horses with high withers.

There are a number of methods of rugging up a horse.

One commonly used is:

- Tie the horse up.

- Make sure he is clean and dry.

- Fold the rug in half across its width so it is inside out.

- Place the side with the two edges just in front of the withers with the neck edge underneath.

- Holding the neck edge with your left hand, unfold the rug towards the quarters.

- Do up the chest strap.

- Do up the belly straps.

- Straighten it, if necessary, across the quarters.

- Do up the leg straps, if present.

It is a great temptation to stand behind the horse and give the rug a tug backwards. Try to avoid it! It usually makes the rug too tight across the chest.

Some horses may object to having the chest buckle done up and try to bite it. This is usually because of bad rugging in the past and can be avoided if the rug is placed on quietly. If needed, the belly straps can be fastened first but it is a little more difficult to adjust the fit.

To Put on a Rug and Blanket

Use either a surcingle or roller with attached breast girth:

- Tie up the horse.

- Collect up the blanket – the left side in the left hand and the right side in the right hand.

- Speak to the horse and then gently throw the blanket on to his neck and withers. Alternatively, fold the blanked in half and place it over the withers with the fold facing forwards. Unfold half the blanket up the neck and slide the whole blanket back (with the lie of the hair) into place.

- Repeat this procedure with the rug, being careful not to displace the blanket by needing to pull the rug too far back into place.

- The front part of the blanket should lie well up the neck. If it does not, remove it and start again.

- A rug or blanket must never be pulled forward, as this ruffles the hairs of the coat and causes discomfort.

- The blanket can be turned back on itself. Approximately 15cm (6ins) should show in front of the stable rug. Alternatively, it can be turned back over the front of the stable rug. This helps to stop it slipping back at the withers.

- Ideally the blanket should not show behind the rug on the quarters.

- If using a roller and pad, fit these after doing up the front buckle of the rug. Alternatively, fasten the cross surcingles to secure the rug, making sure that they are not twisted on the off side.

Removing Rugs etc.

The basic rule when fastening and unfastening a modern rug is:

- Do it up from the front to the rear: chest, belly and legs; undo it from the rear to the chest: legs, belly and chest.

This ensures that the rug remains secure for the longest period of time.

- To take off the rug, fold the rug, front to rear and slide it off. Fold in half again and place in a safe place, not on the stable floor as the rug will collect dirt and bedding. Alternatively, take hold of it at the withers and the centre seam at the quarters and pull it off sideways. It will then be folded in half lengthwise and the lining will be protected from dirt and damp.

- Remove the roller separately.

- Next, fold both rugs back and then draw them off backwards and over the nearside hip and buttock area.

- Fold up the rugs and put away, along with the roller.

When saddling up in cold weather, the rugs may be turned back sufficiently to allow the saddle to be put on, and then turned back over the saddle. If they have slipped back, do not pull them forward. Take them off and replace them separately. If the horse is left with his saddle on, he must be tied up.

The blanket or rug worn next to the skin should be taken out and brushed regularly, but well away from the horse. As mentioned earlier, a summer sheet next to the skin keeps rugs clean and is easy to wash.

CHAPTER

33 CARE AND CLEANING

CLEANING AND STORAGE OF CLOTHING

- Before clothing is put away in store, it must be washed or cleaned and, if necessary, sent for repair. If it is put away dirty, the ingrained manure rots the material, so the rugs and blankets tear more easily and the rollers and surcingles break.

- Woollen day rugs and blankets should be well brushed, and then sent to be cleaned.

- Badly stained blankets may need laundering.

- Stable or night rugs and New Zealand rugs can either be sent to a laundry, washed in a launderette or at home.

- Webbing rollers and surcingles should be washed at home, so that the leather fittings can be kept oiled. If they are soaked in hot water, they will become brittle and will break.

- Leather rollers should be washed clean and then treated with Kocholine, or some similar leather preservative.

Washing Rugs, Rollers and Surcingles

- Before starting the washing, all leatherwork should be oiled. Alternatively, fittings can be removed and sewn on later.

- The rugs should be soaked in cold water in a dustbin or yard water trough. A small amount of detergent can be added and/or a small amount of disinfectant. After soaking they can be laid out on clean concrete and scrubbed with a stiff broom. Do not be tempted to add more detergent as it will be very difficult to remove. After scrubbing use a hose to rinse, pushing the water off with the broom until no white froth or foam is present. Fold the rug up and stamp on it to squeeze out as much water as possible and hang up to dry on something substantial as a wet rug is very heavy. Timing should be 3–4 hours for soaking and 8–10 minutes of scrubbing and rinsing.

- Put more preservative on the leatherwork and buckles.

- Hang them up to dry.

- With rollers and surcingles, it is necessary only to soak the dirty section and then wash it. Hang up to dry, and oil leatherwork and buckles.

- Most rugs are too bulky to be washed in a domestic washing machine. With smaller items, take them outside and brush or beat them thoroughly to remove as much dirt and dust as possible before washing. Tie any metal buckles, etc. in a piece of rag to stop them banging about in the machine and do not fill the machine too full or use too much detergent. Many horses are very sensitive to chemicals on their skins.

Some laundries are very obliging and will take a batch of rugs and clean them professionally. However, it is not difficult to wash rugs manually and far too many horses are left in filthy rugs that contribute to a smelly stable and are very unpleasant to handle.

Storage

- It is essential that rugs are thoroughly dry before being stored. Two or three days in front of an Aga or boiler is ideal. It is then better to store them in paper sacks rather than plastic.

- Rugs should be stored in rug boxes or on shelves.

- Moth preventatives should be put with them if they are wool. (Modern materials will not be attacked by moths.)

- The storage area must be vermin-proof.

CARE AND CLEANING OF LEATHER

For safety, appearance and durability, it is essential that all leather is kept clean and supple. Water, heat, sweat and neglect are its greatest enemies. During use, leather loses a certain amount of oil and fat, which are drawn out by the heat from the horse. These must be replaced. Water – e.g. from rain or saturation during cleaning – also causes leather to become hard and brittle. An overheated atmosphere or drying by direct heat have a similar effect.

Leatherwork should be wiped free from mud and old saddle soap, with a fairly warm damp cloth. If it is not warm enough the soap will not be removed. Sponges, although generally used, are not ideal. An old towelling face flannel or lint-free cloth does a better job. Whatever is used, it should be rinsed out regularly in clean, warm water and squeezed out well. Allow the leather to dry and breathe for a while. The time taken to wash the other items of tack should be sufficient. If the tack is very wet, such as after hunting or competing in the rain, wash it, wipe it dry and leave overnight before soaping. Only in the case of heavy mud should it be necessary to use a wet cloth and more water. A chamois leather or dry cloth should then be used to dry off the leather. Never dry it by placing it near direct heat, or in a drying cupboard, as this destroys the natural oils.

Using a slightly damp sponge the saddle soap should be well rubbed in, particularly on the fleshy or rough side of the leather where it is best absorbed. If the soap appears white and frothy the sponge is too wet and the leather will be left sticky. In an ideal world the leather is wiped over before use with a tightly woven cloth or chamois leather to remove any remaining soap.

If a thumb nail is scraped gently against the leather and comes away with grease on it, the leather has not been cleaned correctly. If leather has been very wet, a suitable leather dressing oil should be applied to the flesh side when the leather is still damp and the pores are open. It will then be more thoroughly absorbed, will replace the oil and fat which has been lost, and will reduce the risk of any stiffening or cracking of the skin. When dry, it can be soaped.

The outer surface of a saddle should not be greased or oiled, as it will stain the rider's breeches when it is next used. Similarly, unless a numnah is used, too much dressing or oil on the lining of a saddle can stain a horse's back, and a sensitive skin can become blistered.

Leather which is stored often sweats, and becomes covered with mould spores. To prevent this, before putting it away apply Vaseline or leather dressing and store in newspaper and/or cover with cotton or natural fibre. This will also prevent the drying out which can occur when leather is not in use.

Care should be taken not to use excessive amounts of leather dressing or oil, as this can result in the leather becoming spongy and lacking in substance. Neatsfoot oil is no longer recommended for treating old or stiff leather as in some cases the leather becomes more brittle. There are many other, better products available.

Equipment for Cleaning Saddlery

- Saddle horse on which to rest the saddle.

- Bridle hook, preferably adjustable and with four hooks.

- Hooks for leathers and girths.
- Bucket, half full of warm water.
- Rough cloth for washing.
- Foam rubber sponge for soaping.
- Sponge or small brush for applying oil or leather dressing. The latter can also be applied with the fingers.
- Bar of glycerine or tin of saddle soap.
- Tin of oil or other leather dressing.
- Metal polish and cloth, or Duraglit.
- Duster for polishing metalwork.
- Chamois leather. This is only necessary if the leather has been very wet. To use, wet the chamois then wring it out. Do not try to use it dry.
- Clean stable rubber or saddle cover to place over the saddle when finished.
- Horse hair from mane or tail.
- Matchstick.

Cleaning Saddles and Their Fittings

The following notes apply to saddles with leather linings, Balding or Atherstone girths, leathers, irons and treads.

- Place the saddle on the saddle horse.
- Strip the saddle. Place the girth, leathers and stirrup irons including treads, on hooks. If the irons and treads are muddy, separate them and place them in the bucket of water.
- Up-end the saddle and, using a damp washing cloth, rub the underneath of the saddle clean. Put a clean stable rubber on the saddle horse and place the saddle on it.
- After rinsing the cloth, clean the rest of the

leatherwork, particularly any part which has been in contact with the horse's skin. Clean leather – usually the seat of the saddle – will not need washing.

- Wash the leathers and girth – especially the inside of any interleaving parts – the stirrup irons, and the treads.
- If the tack is not cleaned regularly, small lumps of grease called 'jockeys' can occur where two pieces of leather rub together, such as on flaps and panels and inside stirrup leathers. They can be removed by making a small, firm pad with some hair from the mane or tail and rubbing them away. This does not damage the leather as using a knife or something similar might do.
- If the punched holes get blocked with soap or grease it can be pushed out using a spent matchstick or a round nail.
- With brisk circular movements, using a very slightly dampened sponge, rub the soap into all parts of the saddle flaps, the girth, and the leathers. Take care to move the buckle guards, so that the girth straps receive full attention.
- Stainless-steel irons can be rubbed over with a dry cloth and the treads replaced. They need regular but not daily cleaning with metal polish. Nickel irons, if they are to look bright, require polishing each day.

Linings of saddles which have been on clean horses with numnahs should be washed only infrequently; this way they will last longer. Girths and leathers, however, should be cleaned carefully after use.

Top surfaces of doeskin, suede or reversed cowhide should never be treated with soap or leather dressing. They can be cleaned – i.e. the mud removed – by brushing with a soft clothes brush or by wiping with a damp cloth. Should the surface wear smooth, it can be scuffed up with a wire shoe-brush or sandpaper; this, in time, will reduce durability.

A lot of saddlery is available that is made entirely from synthetic materials. Much of this is considerably cheaper than the equivalent made from leather and can be a very practical solution for children's ponies, riding schools and trekking centres. This equipment will not need soaping but will need washing in the usual way to prevent a build-up of grease and dirt.

Girths

Many MODERN GIRTHS come in soft, durable synthetic materials that are easy to clean with just a wipe over.

NYLON, STRING, WEBBING, 'COTTAGE CRAFT' TYPE OR LAMPWICK GIRTHS If they are dry, brush them clean. If muddy, and/or stained, soak them in warm detergent (making sure that any leather parts are not submerged), scrub them clean and rinse them thoroughly to remove detergent. If a horse is allergic to detergent, pure soap flakes should be used. Hang them up to dry by both buckle ends to prevent any rusting of the buckle tongues. Leather parts should be soaped or oiled. These girths can all be washed in a 'cool' cycle in a washing machine. It is advisable to put them in an old pillowcase to prevent buckles causing excess noise and possible damage to the drum of the machine. Girth buckles, and the metal studs and stirrup bars on saddles should be cleaned regularly with metal polish.

Apply and remove the metal polish after washing but before soaping the leather. This will prevent the leather appearing cloudy or dull.

Pad Saddle and Felt Numnah

• Brush the felt with a dandy brush.

• When necessary, wash the underneath part with soap and a scrubbing-brush. Rinse thoroughly, and dry in a warm atmosphere.

• Keep free from hard knots of felt.

• Beware of moth damage and worn stitching.

• Clean leather and metal as already described.

Numnahs and Wither Pads

There are many different types. They must be kept clean, soft (no lumps), well aired, and in good repair. Clean them according to maker's instructions, or as detailed for washing numnahs.

Washing Numnahs

SHEEPSKIN Wash by hand in soap flakes. Thoroughly rinse and immediately apply warm glycerine or neatsfoot oil to the skin side. This prevents it becoming out of shape and hard.

SYNTHETIC SHEEPSKIN, QUILTED COTTON AND LINEN-COVERED FOAM Wash either by hand or by machine. Thorough rinsing is essential. It is best to wash numnahs etc. in a machine as the rinsing process is much more efficient than by hand. Use a detergent designed for people with allergies and if at all in doubt use half the recommended amount. Horse's skin is very sensitive to chemicals.

PLAIN FOAM RUBBER must be washed by hand.

Leather fittings are likely to become dry and brittle. They should be well oiled and regularly tested.

Putting up a Saddle

For saddles in regular use:

• Match the leathers to check that the holes are level and replace, putting the shorter one on the left side of the saddle so that they can stretch evenly.

• Put the irons on the leathers and put the stirrups back on the saddle. Run the irons up the leathers, and put the leathers through and under the irons.

• Place the girth flat on top of the saddle. With a three-ply girth the rounded edge should face towards the pommel.

• Place a cloth or cover on top of the saddle, and put

the saddle up on its rack. For saddles not in regular use, the girth, leathers and irons should be hung separately on adjacent hooks, and the saddle should be put up without its fittings.

Cleaning Bridles

1. If Taking the Bridle to Pieces

- Hang the bridle on the cleaning hook.

- Remove the bits and curb chain. Put them in a bucket after removing the lip strap.

- Hang the reins over a hook.

- Take the bridle apart, memorising the buckle holes and the order in which the various headpieces are put together.

- Hang the leatherwork on a hook, or put it on a convenient work surface where it will not be likely to slip down to the floor.

- Thoroughly clean all leatherwork with a damp cloth.

- Wash and dry the bits and curb chain, and put them on a hook or on the work surface.

- Polish the bits, the curb chain, and then the bridle buckles and billet studs. The mouthpiece can be washed in hot water and dried, to remove any taste of metal polish. Finish with a dry, clean cloth. Bits that are not made from stainless steel or nickel may not require polishing.

- Soap all leatherwork, paying particular attention to folds and bends, which are all too easily missed in the daily cleaning.

- If the bridle has been wet, it may require an oil or leather dressing. Having treated the straps, fasten them at the bottom holes and runners. When the dressing has been absorbed, the bridle should be soaped and then put up correctly.

- When cleaning the headpiece, hold it firmly with one

hand and use the cloth in the other hand.

- When cleaning the reins, step back from the bridle and hold the reins taut. Wrap the cloth round each rein in turn, and clean them or apply soap by rubbing to and fro.

- When cleaning a bridle with stitched-on bits, do not put the bits in the water, to avoid wetting the sewn ends of the leatherwork. Where the leather is folded over the bit rings, insert oil or leather dressing to help preserve the leather and keep it supple.

Re-assemble the bridle in the following order:

1. Thread the short side of the headpiece through the off side of the browband and then the near side, making sure the throatlash is to the rear.

2. Place the headpiece on the hook.

3. For a double bridle, first thread the bridoon headpiece (sliphead) through the near side of the browband. It should go under the main headpiece and buckle on the off side. Attach its cheek piece. Check all three cheek pieces as they are not always the same length. The odd one is for the sliphead.

4. Next thread the noseband headpiece through from the off side of the browband and buckle it on the near side. It should be on the underside of the headpiece.

5. Attach the two bit cheek pieces. On a double bridle, there should now be two buckles on each side of the headpiece.

6. Attach the bit and the bridoon to their respective headpieces. Make sure that the bit is not upside down or the wrong way round. Attach the lip strap.

7. Place all straps in their keepers and runners.

8. Place the noseband round the bridle, and secure by a keeper and runner.

9. Replace the reins. On a double bridle they should be

of different widths. The wider rein fixes on the bridoon. The narrower rein goes on the bit. The bridoon rein lies behind the bit rein.

10. The bridoon bit should lie a little above and over the front of the bit.

11. The lip strap on a double bridle should be pushed through the 'Ds' on the bit – from the inner side towards the outer side – and buckled on the near side. For neatness it should be threaded through the runner.

12. The curb chain can be hooked on, and should hang round the front of the bit with the lip strap ring hanging down.

13. Many people fasten the lip strap through the loose ring of the curb chain to avoid the latter being lost.

When putting a bridle together, buckle fastenings should be on the outside, and billeted fastenings on the inside of the headpiece and reins. The flesh side of the leather should be nearest to the horse's skin.

ELEVATOR BRIDLES – With some of these bridles the straps are put through the headpiece in a different order. This is to spread the pressure over the poll more specifically.

2. If Not Taking the Bridle to Pieces

• Hang the bridle on the cleaning hook. The buckle at the back of the noseband should be unfastened.

• Wash and dry the bit. A nickel bit needs polishing.

• Unfasten all buckles and put them in the bottom holes.

• Wash and soap all leatherwork, starting with the headpiece.

• Replace the buckles in the correct holes, with spare strap ends in their runners and keepers. If the double bridle is not specific to one horse do not thread the ends of the straps through the keepers, just through

the runners in order to save time when fitting it.

• Put the noseband round the outside of the bridle and thread it through the keepers.

A bridle in daily use can be cleaned as above. However, **at least once a week** it should be taken to pieces and given more thorough attention as already described.

Putting Up a Bridle

If the bridle holder is high enough, it is better for the leather if the reins are allowed to hang down. The noseband should be put round the outside of the bridle and secured by the keeper and runner. The throatlash can be put round in a figure-of-eight, secured by a keeper and runner, but not buckled as this causes delay in using the bridle.

Alternative Methods

• Double up the reins at the back of the bridle. Put the throatlash through them, and then buckle or thread it through its keepers at the back.

• Double up the reins and wind the throatlash round them in a figure-of-eight. Put the throatlash round the front of the bridle and through the reins at the back. Then buckle or thread it through the keepers at the front.

Cleaning tips

• Never balance the saddle on a narrow or unsteady surface – e.g. a pole or the back of a chair. The gullet may get damaged, and if the saddle falls, a broken or cracked tree and/or marked leather may result. If greater pressure is needed, place the saddle pommel down on top of your feet – never on the ground or on a hard surface – and work downwards.

• When undoing billet studs leave the end of the leather in the keeper and push it with the thumbs, so that the stud comes out of the leather. Then remove the leather from the keeper. When replacing it, put the end of the strap in the keepers and push the leather over the billet stud.

- If the buckles are stiff, it is easier to push the leather piece below the buckle upwards and through the buckle, rather than pulling the end of the strap up.

- During cleaning, inspect all leatherwork, stitching and metalwork for wear. The tongues of all buckles should be regularly greased; they are the most likely parts of the buckles to become worn and rusty.

- If more than one set of tack is being cleaned at a time, take care to mark all items in order to keep each set separate.

- Reins with the buckle on should be fastened to the left-hand bit ring, reins with the tongue should be on the right.

- Martingale neck straps should be buckled on the left side of the neck with the tongue hanging down.

- If the horse is clean it should only take six to eight minutes to clean a bridle and eight to ten to clean a saddle. If the set is being stripped and the bright work polished it may take about half an hour.

- All bits should be rinsed off immediately after each ride, before the bridle is put away.

CHECKING TACK FOR SOUNDNESS

The Saddle

The **tree** can be damaged or broken:

- If it is dropped on the ground.

- If it falls from a doorway or similarly unsafe position.

- If it slips off a horse's back before it is secured with a girth.

- If the girth is pulled to reach the girth straps, and the

saddle is not held with the left hand, it can slip over the off side.

- If it is left on the ground in the stable, and the horse steps on it.

- If a horse in the stable gets free, or is left free when saddled up, and rolls.

- If the horse falls and rolls over.

- If a heavy rider catches hold of the cantle of a spring-tree saddle when mounting and frequently exerts a twist and strain on the tree.

- If it is placed on top of a narrow stable door or gate when tacking up. The saddle must be supported on its pads, not in the gullet.

A saddle with a narrow or medium tree can be strained by being used on a horse with flat or wide withers.

Damage can occur in four places: the pommel or front arch, the waist, and at one or both points of the continuations of the front arch.

If damage to the tree is suspected or confirmed, the saddle should not be used but should be sent for immediate repair. A damaged tree can seriously injure a horse's back. A fracture of the front arch or to the points can be mended. Damage to the waist or cantle is more serious.

Other Areas Which Need Regular Checks

- The stitching of the girth straps.

- The stitching round the pocket.

- The girth straps and the holes in them, especially with synthetic materials.

- The saddle lining. If this is made of leather and is well looked after it should wear and stay smooth for many years. In all cases, the stitching requires checking as does the padding, which must be kept even so that there are no lumps to give the horse a sore back.

The stitching on other parts of the saddle may give way,

and look untidy, but the safety of the rider and the comfort of the horse should not be affected.

Parts of the Girth Which Need Regular Checks

- The suppleness and strength of the leather holding the buckles.

- The stitching of the leather round the buckles.

- The buckles and the wear of the buckle tongues. These must close firmly on the top part of the buckle. The buckles should be made of stainless steel.

- The strength of fabrics such as webbing, string and nylon, particularly in the buckle area. If Cottage Craft type girths are put in the washing machine the padding inside the cover can become twisted and difficult to straighten out.

- The front surface of a leather three-fold. This can crack and split, causing discomfort to the horse.

- The elastic inserts. These can become slack and unsafe.

Parts of the Leathers Which Need Checking

- The stitching round the buckle.

- The buckle itself, and the buckle tongues. Steel buckles are unlikely to break. Nickel is suspect and should not be used.

- The strength of the leather, and any stretching or signs of wear in the buckle holes. To avoid continual wear to the same areas, leathers can be shortened at the buckle end. This will bring the pressure on to a fresh piece of leather.

Stirrup Irons

STAINLESS-STEEL IRONS are preferable. They are strong and sufficiently heavy, so rarely cause trouble – although if treads are not used, they will in time wear smooth on the base. All irons require careful checking for cracks.

NICKEL IRONS are not recommended, as they: (1) crack and pull apart and (2) bend easily, lose shape and then break. When subjected to pressure, they can close and imprison the rider's foot – e.g. if a horse falls on his side, or if they are banged against a jump or gate.

If PEACOCK IRONS are used, ensure that the rubber band is not perished and the small piece of leather used at the base of the iron is not worn.

The Bridle

- All stitching should be regularly examined and tested by stretching and pulling the leather.

- Buckles and buckle tongues should be checked for wear. Buckles should be of stainless steel.

- Reins should be checked for wear. Reins which have been broken and then repaired should be examined closely. Unless the break was in the buckle area, the reins are only suitable for light work, as the stitching will be subjected to friction and strain.

- Re-covered rubber reins are also suspect, as the re-stitching of the new rubber can weaken the rein.

- Webbing, plaited cotton and linen-corded reins all wear more quickly than leather. They should not be patched, but must be replaced.

Bits

Particular points of wear are:

- The centre joints or joints of the mouthpiece.

- Where the rings or cheeks join the mouthpiece.

Nickel mouthpieces, rings and cheeks can become rough and/or sharp. Jointed snaffles can come apart at the joint. Rubber and leather mouthpieces must be regularly checked for wear, as they have a limited life.

Other Equipment

MARTINGALES, BREASTPLATES, and other leather or webbing equipment should all be checked for wear.

Particular attention should be paid to any buckle areas.

LUNGEING TACK The centre ring of the cavesson receives constant pressure, and is subject to strain. It should be checked regularly. The lunge rein can deteriorate, and should be checked for weak places. Side reins can stretch unevenly and be difficult to adjust if the rubber inserts lose their elasticity unequally.

SADDLING UP AND UNSADDLING

SADDLING-UP PROCEDURE

Before Saddling up

If the horse is stabled:

- Tie up the horse.

- Brush him off if necessary.

- Wipe eyes, nose and dock.

- Pick out feet.

- Oil feet, if needed.

- Replace one rug if cold.

Collect the Bridle (which is assumed to be a snaffle)

- Undo the throatlash and noseband. If necessary, double up the reins to keep them clear of the ground. Carry the bridle on the shoulder. Collect the martingale (if used) and the boots.

Collect the Saddle

- Check that it is complete, including buckle guards. If a numnah is to be worn, it should be put under the saddle and the straps fastened. Either:

- Place it on the lower arm with the pommel towards the elbow, or

- Place the cantle under the upper arm and hold the pommel with the same hand. Take the required tack to the stable. On a wet day, cover the top of the saddle with a stable rubber.

Putting on the Saddle

- Enter stable talking to horse. With free hand, undo rug and fold it back, leaving it on loins.

- With the saddle on the left arm, and the girth attached on the off side and folded over the saddle, approach the near side of the horse. Pat the saddle area and then, using both hands, place the saddle up on the withers, and slide it back to its correct position. Never move a saddle against the lie of the coat. Check the numnah to ensure that the surface next to the horse's skin is smooth. Pull the numnah well up into the arch of the saddle. Move round quietly under the horse's neck. (If the horse is unknown or headshy, unclip the headcollar and hold the headcollar whilst going underneath, then re-fasten.) Check the saddle on the off side and unfold the girth. Return to the near side and fasten the girth. This should be secure, but not tight. Make sure that skin is not wrinkled or caught up under the girth. Replace the rugs, but do not buckle them up, as if the rugs slip, it is better they fall clear than hang suspended round the horse's neck where they can frighten him and get torn. If restless horses are left, the rugs should be fastened and the roller, if used, replaced.

- If a martingale or breastplate is used, it may be put on

before the saddle. Untie the horse. Put the neck strap over his head with the buckle on the near side. Re-tie the horse. Alternatively, put it on after the saddle but before the bridle. Unbuckle the martingale, adjust it to the approximate length, and when doing up the girth, put it through the loop of the martingale. If two girths are used, fasten the one nearer the horse's elbow first. The second girth is placed on top and then buckled.

By putting the saddle on first, the horse's back has time to warm up before being ridden. It is also not necessary to put the saddle on top of the door or on the ground and the horse remains secure.

It is convenient and saves time if horses become accustomed to being saddled from either side.

After girthing up, before mounting, pull the horse's foot and leg forward to stretch the skin and ease any wrinkling.

When saddling up a young or nervous horse, it is advisable to untie the headcollar rope, but leave it through the loop. Should the horse resent the saddle or play up, there will be less chance of his pulling back and getting frightened. It is advisable that such an animal, once he is saddled, is not left unattended.

Putting on the Bridle

(For bridle fitting, see page 227)

- The bridle and reins should be over the left arm, with the browband nearest to the elbow.

- Go up to the horse, talk to him, and stand behind his eye on the near side. Unfasten the headcollar and put it round his neck. Undo the rope but leave it through the string. Put the reins over the horse's head. At this stage, either of the two following methods can be used:

1. Take hold of the headpiece of the bridle with the right hand. Put the left hand under the bit and move the first finger around to the off side of the horse's mouth. Persuade him to open his mouth by inserting

Putting on a snaffle bridle.

your first finger in the gap behind his front teeth. As the horse opens his mouth, guide the bit into the mouth with your left hand and at the same time lift the bridle up towards the horse's ears with your right hand. Once the bit is in his mouth, use your left hand to help the right hand move the bridle carefully over the horse's ears. The ears should always be pushed forwards through the headpiece not flattened back by it. Ease out the mane and make it tidy, and put the forelock over the browband. Check that the browband, noseband and bit are level.

Adjust if necessary. Try to keep it even on both sides or only one hole difference on one side. Fasten the throatlash and noseband. Put all the keepers into place and replace the headcollar.

2. This method can be used with horses who resist or raise their head when being bridled. Hold the top of the bridle in the left hand. Place the right hand under the horse's jaw and round to the front of his face. Take hold of both cheek pieces of the bridle just below the browband. Move the left hand to hold the

bit. Open the mouth with the left thumb, and continue the procedure as for 1.

• When doing up a bridle, fasten it from the top down. Throatlash, noseband, curb chain, lip strap. When removing, reverse the procedure: this way the bridle is secure for longer and there is less likelihood of forgetting a buckle.

• Finally, thread the reins through any martingale rings and check the fit. Put on any boots and bandages.

To Put on a Double Bridle

Undo the throatlash, noseband, curb chain and lip strap. Make sure the bridoon is on top and in front of the bit. Proceed as when putting on a snaffle bridle. When checking the bridle for fit, hold the bridle up against the side of the horse's head and then make approximate adjustments before putting it on. Ensure that any alteration to the noseband or the bridoon does not make the bridle crooked. If this happens, hold the browband and pull the leather through it. Fasten the curb chain and lip strap.

See also page 228, Fitting a Double Bridle.

Leaving a Saddled Horse

• If a saddled and bridled horse is to be left, put the headcollar back over the top of the bridle. Double the reins twice round his neck, tie them in a knot on his withers or twist and loop them through the throatlash. If the reins are put behind the stirrups they may upset a sensitive horse and cause an accident.

• A saddled horse should always be left tied up. If loose in the stable, he may get down and roll.

• It is inadvisable to leave a horse tied up in the stable wearing a double bridle. The bridle should be left outside until just before the horse is required. The bridle should then be put on and the horse taken straight out to work.

When Saddling in a Field

If it is not possible to tie the horse up, it is sometimes advisable to put the bridle on first in order to have more control.

UNSADDLING

There are several accepted methods of unsaddling. The following is the normal procedure:

1. On dismounting, run up the irons on the leathers and ease the girth one or two holes.

2. Take the reins over the horse's head, lead him into his stable, and close the door.

3. Take up the headcollar and place it round the horse's neck with the rope untied.

4. Unfasten the curb chain (if there is one), the noseband and the throatlash. If there is a running martingale, unfasten the reins, and release it. Remove boots and bandages and rub legs. Place boots, etc. outside the door.

5. With your right hand, ease the bridle over the horse's head, at the same time steadying his face and then taking the bridle with your left hand. The horse must be allowed time to quietly let go of the bit.

6. Place the bridle over your left arm so that both hands are free to put on the headcollar and to tie up the horse.

7. Place the bridle over your shoulder.

8. Unfasten the girth. If there is a martingale, take it out of the loop. Lift the saddle, draw it over the horse's shoulder and place it on your left arm. The girth can be put over the top of the saddle, but if the girth is wet or muddy, leave it down. The martingale neck strap should be undone, and the martingale should be placed, with the bridle, on your shoulder.

9. Put the saddle and bridle outside the stable. If you put the saddle on the ground, place the pommel down first, with the girth between the wall and the

cantle; this prevents the leather from being marked or scratched. Avoid putting the saddle on the door where it could be knocked off. It is ideal to have a folding saddle horse outside each stable.

10. Return to the horse, and pat the saddle area briskly to restore circulation.

11. Replace the rugs.

12. If the horse is wet, or is likely to break out, put either a sweat rug or straw underneath the rugs.

13. Take the saddle and bridle to the tack room ready for cleaning. Mud will come off easily if it is sponged when still wet.

14. Always wash off the bit immediately after each use.

An alternative procedure is to take the saddle off first, as detailed in 8, 9 and 10 above. Then remove the bridle as in 3, 4, 5 and 6 above. This method can be useful for restless horses, who are better controlled in a bridle, and obviates the necessity of separating a martingale.

Procedure after Unsaddling

1. Pick out the feet.

2. If the feet are muddy, wash them. Take care not to wet the heels.

3. Check the legs.

4. Sponge off any sweat marks. On a hot day, the horse can be washed off outdoors.

5. Check for any signs of rubbing in the saddle, girth and mouth areas.

6. If the horse is wet and cold, rub him briskly with a handful of hay or straw to increase circulation and rug him with a wicking rug under his day rug. If he is hot and wet, sponge him off, use a sweat scraper and walk him around until dry.

7. Tie up the haynet.

8. Groom horse – or at least brush off sweat marks.

9. Replace all the rugs.

10. Refill the water bucket.

SPECIALIST CARE OF THE COMPETITION HORSE

GUIDELINES FOR COMPETITION HORSES

The success and well-being of a horse who is in training for a stressful activity is very much dependent on his stable environment and the care and expert attention that he receives from his groom. As well as being given the specialist care outlined in the following chapters, the horse should be accorded the normal day-to-day care already detailed in Chapters 9–25.

Worming

An appropriate worming programme should be planned. Worming should be carried out when the horse comes in from grass, and regularly thereafter, but avoiding major competition dates.

Flu/Tetanus Vaccinations

These should be given as necessary, starting when the horse is first brought in, then according to current veterinary practice and as required by competition rules.

Teeth

Teeth should be inspected every six months, and attended to as necessary; some horses require attention more often.

Passport

It is required by law that all horses and donkeys have a valid passport. The only animals exempt are Dartmoor and New Forest ponies whilst they are living on the moor. Once they are sold off the moor or forest they also need passports. This must be completed by a veterinary surgeon who is not the owner of the horse. It is a proof of identity. It must be correctly completed according to the regulations laid down for the current year. It must give an exact description of the animal, with details and dates of equine influenza and tetanus inoculations. For horses travelling abroad, it should contain details of immunisation programmes and blood tests.

In the UK all horses competing in any affiliated discipline need to be registered with the British Horse Database.

Definition of Fitness

A horse is fit when he is able to perform his normal work without undue strain and effort. This state is achieved by an ongoing process of good stable management, good feeding and a progressive exercise regime.

A basic fittening programme will probably take between six and eight weeks. It will then become more specific to each competitive discipline.

It takes longer with a young horse who has not been fittened before.

Schooling for a specific discipline will be ongoing and the schooling programme will run alongside the fittening one. It is unlikely, on its own, to achieve the optimum state of fitness required to compete successfully.

General Notes on Fittening the Horse

These will obviously vary according to the competition for which the horse is being prepared, but many points will apply to all disciplines.

It is important to have a fitness programme. This should be worked out well in advance of the main competition of the season. There may be interim competitions along the way. One of the most common causes of breakdown in horses is not being fit enough for the task. The programme needs to be sufficiently flexible to cope with any minor problems that might arise and it is advisable to keep notes, and monitor the level of fitness and stage of training. Always allow enough time. It takes at least six weeks for any significant development to take place.

- It is important to ensure that horses are given plenty of variety in their work. If hacking out, the route should be varied as far as possible. Loose jumping in the school may be of benefit. Drag hunting can provide a good opportunity for schooling over fences. A half-day out with hounds can add extra interest for an older horse who has become stale, or to educate a young horse.
  Some horses find fast work more interesting if accompanied. This often improves the stride of the stuffy horse, but will not benefit an excitable one.

- Fitness work should aim to improve the overall performance of the horse through correct work and feed. It is essential to start with a healthy, sound horse. Fitter horses are less liable to suffer lameness problems. Fatigue is a common cause of breakdowns.

- Make the horse work into the bridle; he should not slop along on a loose rein.

- Discretion must be used as to the type of terrain. For example, sand is very heavy going, and artificial surfaces often slide under the horse. Grass may be uneven or slippery. Roads are hard but even.

- Strenuous work should not be undertaken the day before or the day after a competition or fast work.

- Fast work must be supported by rest periods, to allow the heart rate to return to normal.

- Extra care must be taken in humid conditions.

- If the horse is balanced he will suffer less strain: therefore, training should be over a large area and should avoid sharp turns.

- Fast work must not be in sudden bursts, as this puts strain on tendons and lungs. Horses must be well warmed up before starting any strenuous work, and speed should be decreased gradually to avoid strain to the limbs.

- In fittening work, go faster uphill to increase the length of stride. Take it easy downhill. In a competition, allow the horse to flow on downhill. Do not put on pressure uphill.

- After fast work the horse should be kept walking to allow the build-up of lactic acid in the muscles to disperse.

- In bad weather, slow canters on a prepared surface make it possible to continue fittening work. This also applies when there is hard ground in summer. If a horse is not used to the prepared, artificial surface of a gallop, this work should be introduced carefully, as he may well feel insecure and might slip.

- If canter work has to be in a school, the rein should be changed, through trot, every three circuits. Continual cornering makes for increased effort, and can also put greater strain on the legs. It is important to ensure that the surface is not dusty.

- It is important to remember that the rider should also be fit.

Checks on the Horse During Training

Check the horse's legs after work and again in the evening, to ensure that any signs of strain are noted in good time. This is particularly important after fast work. If there is any heat in one or more legs, work should be reduced and cantering should be discontinued until the legs are normal. Concentrate diet should also be reduced.

Any change in the horse's attitude to work, appetite or stable habits may be a sign of stress. The workload may have to be reduced and possibly the competition schedule altered. It is better to under-train rather than to over-train. Once the horse attains peak fitness he will then stay fit longer, with less risk of being overstressed, or, as it is more generally described, 'going over the top'.

Blood Tests

Many owners arrange to have their horses blood-tested when first brought up from grass, and repeat the testing after eight to ten weeks. Should there be any incipient problems they can be recognised and dealt with in good time. It is sensible to have a blood test done when the horse is well and healthy so that a comparison may be made if problems arise. Blood tests for monitoring condition should be made when the horse is in regular work and eating his normal diet.

Feeding

It is important to feed the horse according to the work he is doing. As he becomes fitter he will need more energy feed and less forage but when the ratio gets to 50:50 in the case of the average horse or 60:40 concentrates to forage in the case of the horse in very hard work, it is better to increase the carbohydrate/protein value of the concentrates, rather than the amount. This will vary between different disciplines but the principles remain the same.

Daily consumption of feed varies enormously between different horses. Some fit horses get and stay fit on as little as 4.5kg (10lbs) of concentrates, while others may eat more. Many horses will eat their greatest quantity of food before they are fully fit and start competing. However, so long as they stay healthy and eager for work, there is no need for anxiety. The diet of 'good doers' may have to be restricted: unnecessary weight puts additional strain on heart, lungs and legs. Daily in-hand grazing, or a short daily spell in a suitable small paddock, helps to keep a horse happy and relaxed.

For more detailed instructions, see Chapters 20–24.

Planning for an Overnight Stay Away

Forward planning is essential when staying away overnight. When booking the stable find out what is included in the price and whether suitable bedding is available. It is always advisable to take your own feed and forage as many horses will not eat strange food even if it appears to be the same as they have at home. Some animals will not drink strange water either, in which case that also has to be taken.

Many lorries now have built-in storage and secure tack areas. Always put heavy, bulky items low down and only light items in high lockers. Make sure nothing can move or fall on top of the horses if you have to brake suddenly or go up and down steep hills.

When making lists of equipment to be taken, make two, one can then be stuck on the trunk/locker door – this will help ensure that all the equipment comes home again.

Equipment to be Taken to a Competition when Staying Overnight

- Stable tools, skip and muck sack.
- Sacks of shavings or paper bedding (if required).
- Two haynets.
- Two water buckets and water carrier.
- Feed bowl.
- Concentrate feed, which should be pre-packed and labelled.
- Hay or hay alternative, e.g. haylage.
- Supplements and electrolytes.
- Grooming kit, including extra sponges, towels, sweat

scraper, hoof oil.

• Plaiting kit, fly spray.

• Spare sets of shoes, studs and fitting kit.

• Tack-cleaning kit.

• Spare rugs and blankets.

• Two sweat sheets or coolers.

• Waterproof rug.

• Stable bandages, Gamgee and/or liners.

• Passport/vaccination certificate.

• Lorry passes and operator's licence if required to enter the show ground and to show that the journey is legitimate. In some instances travel documents are required to show details of the journey. These are usually not needed unless the journey is part of a business enterprise.

Other Essential Items

• Tack – depending on horse and competition.

• Bandages and/or brushing boots, over-reach boots, plus spares.

• Spare girths, stirrup leathers, irons, rubber-covered reins.

• Spare headcollar and rope.

• Lungeing equipment.

• Travelling equipment for the horse.

• First-aid kit for rider.

• First-aid kit for horse: to include scissors, cotton wool, crepe bandages, Gamgee, salt, wound dressings and wound spray, kaolin and/or Animalintex, ice-packs.

NB: No forbidden substances may be taken to a competition. Even being in possession of illegal drugs or syringes is an offence.

Packing the Lorry (see also Chapter 45)

• Equipment should be listed and ticked off as it is loaded. In this way vital equipment will not be overlooked.

• Use containers for horse equipment. This will help efficiency in loading and unloading. They should not be too large or too heavy as this will make handling difficult.

• Feed is best packed in plastic sacks. If the journey is long, the horse will need to be fed en route. These feeds should be individually packed and labelled: e.g. Monday am, Monday pm, etc.

• Filled water containers should be available for en route refreshment.

• Plan to arrive at your destination with plenty of time to spare so that the horse can settle in and recover from the stress of the journey.

• It is extremely poor practice to muck out the lorry onto the showground.

• Leave hired stables tidy. When staying in private yards it is always best to leave the stable spotless.

CHAPTER

36 THE EVENT HORSE

FITNESS

The following guidelines should help to plan a fittening programme, but schedules need to be adjusted to meet the requirements of individual horses. A chart of the intended work programme should be made and used to monitor the horse's progress. This should show diet, exercise (specifying fittening work, fast work and schooling), shoeing, worming, flu/tetanus inoculations, veterinary checks and competition dates. Ten to twelve weeks should be allowed for a horse to reach one-day event fitness, from grass.

The event season is now almost continuous from mid-March to mid-October. Schedules must be carefully planned, so that the horse can be given a rest. He cannot be expected to compete throughout the season. Bear in mind that it is not advisable for a horse to reach peak fitness by his first one-day event. If he is brought on steadily he will stay fit longer, with less risk of being overstressed and losing form.

Fittening must be a gradual process, so work must be increased progressively. Each horse must be treated as an individual and carefully observed, with note taken of his pulse and respiration rates and type of breathing. Body weight and condition of limbs must be carefully monitored and the programme adjusted accordingly.

Weeks 1–4: the horse requires walking exercise starting with ¾hr on the flat and gradually building up to 1½–2hrs with a progressive increase of hill work. Trotting can be introduced, initially on the flat, between the second and fourth week.

From **week 5**, trotting can be gradually increased. The aim of this fitness programme is gradually to work the heart harder, to demand greater effort and thus to build up stamina. Hill work is highly recommended for this purpose, and as the horse's fitness improves the hill work can be developed from walk into trot.

From **week 6** dressage training may be included together with hacking. From **week 7** jumping training can start. From **week 8** – depending on the individual horse and how long his lay-off has been – it should be possible to take part in small dressage and show jumping competitions.

By **week 9** some fast work can be introduced. Begin with a 3-minute steady canter (15mph/400m/min), followed by a walking period during which the horse's breathing returns to normal. Follow this with another 3-minute canter. This canter work can be gradually increased in duration, building up to 15 minutes in total (5 minutes x 3) during weeks 9 to 12. After a 5-minute half-speed canter (15mph/ 400m/min) the breathing rate of a fit horse should return to normal in 5 minutes.

In **weeks 10 and 11**, the horse can do some cross-country schooling to give him additional fast work and jumping practice before his first event in **week 12**. The cross-country schooling replaces the canter work.

A horse who is already in work could start the specific fittening programme at about **week 6**. Bear in mind that fittening and schooling do not achieve the same end and a nice balance between the two is needed to achieve a successful result.

A horse who has had a long lay off or a youngster who

has not been fit before will need longer to build and tone muscles.

With most horses it is better if they are not let down completely. Turning them out in an undulating or sloping field will help them retain a residual level of fitness.

Extra Fittening Programme for the Two-or Three-Day Event Horse

A horse can be expected to tackle a three-day event four months after coming up from grass. The first part of the programme is the same as when preparing for a one-day event.

During **weeks 9–12** canter work can be built up to 20 minutes in total (5 minutes x 4), thus developing the horse's stamina. Two sessions a week is sufficient for this, each session followed by an easy day for recovery. If a good all-weather gallop is available on a hill, then the length of the canter work can be decreased.

To avoid pounding the legs, increase the workload without increasing the speed. If any hills can be used, the heart will be worked much harder.

In **weeks 12–14**, build up the half-speed cantering at this pace to 6-minute sessions by four repetitions; if the horse is recovering easily the rest periods can be reduced from 3 minutes to 2 minutes, and, in some cases, to 1 minute. The main criterion is the ease and speed of recovery.

During the weeks before a three-day event, one-day events provide additional fast work. If there are no such competitions, then Wednesday can continue as a cantering day and Saturday can become a day for faster work at cross-country speed, approximately 570m (625yds) per minute for 1 mile, then rest, then repeat once more.

With the introduction of short-format three-day events there is no longer a need to teach the horse to steeplechase as this phase and the roads and tracks have been removed.

Occasionally three-day novice events are run which include steeplechase, in which case some training in

jumping at speed will be needed.

All fast work must have a good warm-up period of at least 30 minutes, and also a warming-down, cooling-off period.

During **week 15** work can be eased off. Keep the horse healthy and relaxed, and not overtaxed or overtired. The horse must stick to an exercise pattern and not lack schooling, but it should not be stressful. The horse will require a sharp burst on the Wednesday and Saturday.

Week 16 is the week of the three-day event. The horse should be given a short canter on the Tuesday, and another on the Friday after the dressage.

NB: Stuffy horses who take longer to get fit may require three short, sharp gallops a week at about 600m (656yds)/min for ½ mile in the last two weeks of fittening.

Interval Training

This is an alternative to galloping as a means of getting a mature eventer fit. Several short periods of work are alternated with brief recovery periods (the intervals). The principles are:

- The body will adapt itself to the stress of demands made upon it, as long as it is given time. Therefore repeatedly small but increased demands are made upon it.

- The intervals are timed so that the recovery is not quite achieved before the next period of work.

- The work periods are designed to avoid maximum stress, so that the respiratory, cardiovascular and muscular systems are all gradually developed.

- Used not more than once every three or four days as it takes this long for the metabolism to return to normal.

Interval training is only suitable for:

- A mature horse.

- A sound horse.

- A horse who has completed 4 to 8 weeks of basic fittening and conditioning work (i.e. capable of hacking for one and a half to two hours).

Six to twelve weeks of interval training are needed before a three-day event.

The programme

A programme is devised so that the distance and speeds are gradually increased. A number of competitions can be integrated into the interval-training programme to prepare for a three-day event.

Before cantering, the horse should be warmed-up with 30 minutes of walking and trotting.

After cantering he should be cooled down by gentle work for up to an hour. This is essential to help the vascular system remove waste products accumulated during exercise.

All work must be carried out with the horse going into the bridle and on the aids.

It is vital for the programme to be adjusted to suit the needs of the individual horse. The aspects which can be varied are:

- The **rest intervals**. Range of one to four minutes. Four minutes may be needed for the horse to 'almost' recover at the beginning of training, but only one minute if the horse is very fit.

Work periods

- **Duration**. Range 3 to 12 minutes, but in total a training session should not be more than 35 minutes.

- **Number**. A maximum of three work periods.

- **Frequency**. Interval training may be used once to twice a week. With a young horse, once a week might be sufficient, but it is usual to progress to twice a week (every four days).

- **Speeds**. These range from trot, through canter to a gallop at about 600 metres per minute. Young horses might begin their interval training with trot periods, but the major part of the work is done at 'half speed' –

a canter of approximately 400m/min. As the horse becomes fitter it can be increased to 500m/min and eventually for $\frac{1}{2}$ mile or 1 mile periods at 600m/min.

NB: Horses competing in one- or two-day events before the three-day event need not do faster work until the last two or three weeks. Horses with a history of leg problems should work up hills instead of doing the faster work, and depending on their 'wind' may need one or two pipe-openers, going at close to maximum speed for 500m uphill 10 days before the event.

- **Terrain**. If hilly, canter distances can be reduced by up to 25%. Varied terrain helps to keep the horse fresh.

- **Work on non-cantering days**. If the horse works strongly for $1\frac{1}{2}$ hours on these days, less cantering may be needed. If he does not do much, more may be needed. Work on non-cantering days depends on the particular trainer and is a major cause of differences in cantering programmes. NB: After a competition a horse will need usually a minimum of seven days before cantering again.

- **The horse**. The type of horse and how recently he has been fit affects the programme. A small Thoroughbred which has been very fit recently needs less work than a cold-blooded horse which has never been really fit.

TACK

A **SNAFFLE BRIDLE** should be used in basic training. The simpler the equipment used, the better. If gadgets, special nosebands, martingales, etc. are considered necessary, try to gradually wean the horse off them with effective schooling. It may be that more specific bits are needed in the actual competition but not at home. A double bridle is no longer a requirement for three-day event dressage.

An **ALL-PURPOSE SADDLE**, suitable for all disciplines, is the basic necessity. A straighter-cut saddle for dressage is useful, but not essential. A forward-cut saddle for the cross-country is essential, as it enables the rider to get his weight forward over the centre of gravity.

A **BREASTPLATE** and a **SURCINGLE** or overgirth are necessary for the cross-country. Holding straps on the girth prevent the surcingle from sliding back. Rawhide or buffalo hide leathers and stainless steel irons are also necessary.

REINS for the cross-country must prevent the hands from slipping, so rubber ones are best. For the cross-country a bootlace can be used to secure the headpiece of the bridle to a plait just behind the horse's ears.

BOOTS or **BANDAGES** are advisable for protection in the cross-country phase. Tendon and over-reach boots are often used for the show jumping phase. Boots must be strong enough to protect the legs, and supple enough to prevent sores, but not too heavy and absorbent, particularly on a wet day or if there are water obstacles. Care must be taken that the boots allow for movement of the joints and do not only fit when the horse is standing still.

Bandages must be applied with great care and with even tension. They must always be worn with Gamgee or other similar protection underneath. If Porter boots are used under bandages, the boots must be carefully trimmed to fit the horse when the leg is bent. Bandages must be secured by tape, as cotton tie-tapes and/or Velcro fastenings are not sufficiently secure.

However, research has shown that the cooler a horse's legs are kept, the better. Tendons and ligaments are far less prone to damage when kept cool therefore the balance between protection from knocks and legs being too warm needs to be weighed up. Removing protection and cooling legs as soon as possible after work or competition is good practice.

Protective boots should be worn when schooling, both on the flat and jumping, to prevent injury. For hacking on roads, it is sensible to fit exercise knee caps.

CARE OF THE HORSE AT A THREE-DAY EVENT

Much of the following advice also applies to one-day event horses.

Care Before Cross-Country Day

• Clipping will help the horse in hot weather.

• The night before the cross-country, give the horse his usual evening meal, and hay ration.

• It is preferable not to bed the horse on straw. If there is no choice, then use a muzzle.

Care on the Morning of Cross-Country Day

• For a one-or two-day event feed the horse at least four hours before the start of the cross-country. In short-format three-day events, if the horse is going early in the day a small concentrate feed is necessary to keep the digestive juices working, and thus to prevent the possibility of colic. Horses going late in the day may have their normal early morning feed, plus 0.5–0.9kg (1–2lbs) of hay. Research has shown that either chaff in the feed or a small haynet four hours before exercise is beneficial.

• Water should be available for the horse at all times. However, do not suddenly offer water in the last hour before the start.

• Everything should be left ready for the return of the horse after cross-country.

Care of the Horse Before the Start of the Cross-Country

The following items should be readily available:

• Water containers.

• Two water buckets.

• Two sponges – one for washing down, one for rinsing the horse's mouth.

- Sweat scraper.
- Towels.
- Waterproof rug.
- Sweat rug.
- Thick rug.
- Spare set of shoes with studs already in place.
- Stud equipment and hoof pick.
- Scissors.
- Spare bridle, reins, saddle, stirrup, leathers and girth.
- Spare boots.
- Hole punch.
- Grease.
- Jacket, gloves, whip and drink for rider.

In short-format horse trials the warm-up period before cross-country is much longer as the long-format phases A, B and C are not included. Whatever form the warm-up takes, the horse needs to be relaxed, supple and ready to gallop and jump, whatever the conditions. Approximately ten minutes before he is due to set off, go through as much of the following procedure as is considered appropriate.

- The rider must now be free to talk to the trainer, and to prepare mentally for cross-country.
- It is useful to have someone to hold the horse and one or two assistants to prepare him for cross-country.
- Check shoes, boots/bandages.
- Cover the horse with a rug suitable for the conditions. However, if the weather is very hot do not use a rug as it will trap air and slow cooling. Lead the horse around. All this should take approximately three minutes.
- Keep an eye on the horse.
- Start to prepare the horse for cross-country four

minutes before he is due to start.

- Check the saddle, tighten the girths.
- Help the rider to mount. It may be necessary to alter the stirrups.
- Make sure reins are clean and dry. Using rubber gloves, grease the fronts of all four legs to protect knees and stifles from bangs and bruises. (See also notes on grease application in hot weather, page 297.) Do not touch the reins or tack with greasy hands.
- Check the surcingle or overgirth.
- Use a piece of rope, minus the clip, to lead the horse into the starting box, if necessary.

Care of the Horse After the Cross-Country in Normal Weather Conditions

- In two-or three-day events, after inspection by the vet, the groom can attend to the horse.
- Remove the tack. Cover the horse with a sweat rug, and a light blanket if the weather is cold; do not use any rugs if the weather is hot. Offer the horse a small drink of about a litre (¼ gallon) of water with chill taken off. Walk the horse slowly for about five minutes, or until the horse appears to be breathing normally. This allows the build-up of lactic acid in the muscles formed during work to disperse.
- The horse, particularly in hot or very humid weather, recovers more quickly if electrolyte salts are added to his drinking water. If he is used to being given these after strenuous exertion at home, he will be more likely to accept them at a competition. For advice on type and quantity, consult your veterinary surgeon.
- Take the horse to the stable area or to his box and remove the boots and bandages. Apply cooling wraps, if used, or hose legs or sponge off.
- Check the horse for injury.
- Remove the studs.

- Wash off the horse. Remove any surplus water with a sweat scraper. Cover the horse with a sweat rug and a light blanket if the weather is cool (in hot or humid weather dispense with the rugs), and walk the horse again. Re-apply leg cooling treatment.

- Give the horse another drink of about 2 litres (½ gallon). From this time on he may have 2 litres (½ gallon) of water every 15 minutes.

- Put the horse in the stable and encourage him to stale.

- Some competitors give the horse a small mash to get his digestive juices working. This may be bran and oats or sugar-beet feed and grass nuts, according to the horse's normal diet.

- Treat any injury as necessary, apply cooling lotion or cold kaolin or more cooling bandages. Do not use any cooling preparations that you have not used before as the horse may be allergic to them.

- Tie up a small haynet, give the horse a bucket of water and leave him to rest for a couple of hours.

- After two hours or so, lead the horse around to loosen his muscles.

- Give the horse another feed and more hay. At this stage, the horse should have water ad lib.

- Do not give the horse more feed than he is used to eating.

- Make a late-night check to see that the horse is resting and comfortable.

- If the horse is travelling home after the cross-country, walk him around on arrival and then give him a second feed and more hay.

Care in Extreme Heat

- Immediately after the horse has finished the cross-country lead him around for a few minutes.

- Wash the horse down, especially the large muscle masses, with large sponges and iced water. It is preferable if two people work together, one on each side. Scrape off surplus water and walk around. The cooling process is brought about by evaporation. Repeat the process until the horse is less distressed and the temperature, pulse and respiration have returned to normal. It is possible to sponge and walk at the same time. This speeds up the process.

When conditions are humid, evaporation is less efficient and it is even more important to keep applying iced water to bring the temperature down to normal.

- Keep a check on the horse's temperature.

- Small drinks of water can be given every fifteen minutes, to prevent dehydration, until the horse has drunk its fill.

- Add electrolytes to the water, but offer plain water as well.

Horses who are hot (above 40°C/104°F) and competing in hot environments (above 26.5°C/80°F) and who are cooled quickly during or after competition are less likely to suffer heat stress, will recover more quickly, will not become as dehydrated and are almost certain to perform better.

It is not necessary to scrape off excess water after each application; it is more important to continue to apply cold water. If you wish to scrape off the excess water, do so quickly at the end of each 30-second cooling period and while the horse is being walked between cooling periods.

The walking promotes skin blood flow and the movement of air aids evaporation. If possible, carry out the cooling and walking in the shade.

Check the horse's rectal temperature at intervals. It should be possible to reduce rectal temperature by around 1°C in 10 minutes.

There is no evidence to suggest that there is any harm in letting the horse drink small amounts of water (half a bucket) during a competition (e.g. whilst in the 10-minute box in three-day eventing), between rounds (e.g. show jumping) and during long warm-up periods (e.g. dressage), which will also help to cool the horse down and reduce the effects of dehydration.

When to stop

- When the horse's rectal temperature is less than 38°C–39°C.

- When the horse's skin feels cool to touch (over the quarters) after a walking period.

- If the respiratory rate is less than 30 breaths per minute.

- If the horse begins to shiver.

What not to do

1. Ice in the rectum does very little to lower body temperature. It makes it hard to assess body temperature and can hide a high temperature. Masking a high temperature from vets at events is unwise as it will prevent a horse receiving appropriate cooling and other necessary treatments, which may result in the development of heat exhaustion and death. The chances of injury will also increase if the horse is allowed to continue when overheated and dehydrated.

2. Don't hold small bags of ice over the head, neck, under the tail, on the quarters, etc. Instead, concentrate on cooling as much of the body surface as possible. Holding bags of ice is likely to reduce cooling by stopping skin blood flow to the area under the pack.

3. Do not place wet towels on the neck or quarters. Although at first the towel may be wet and cold, it soon warms, and hinders the loss of heat, acting as an insulator.

4. Excessive application of grease prior to the cross-country acts as an insulator, prevents sweating and limits sweat evaporation.

5. Do not let horses stand still for prolonged periods. If cold-water cooling is adopted, do so completely and not tentatively. The cold water on the skin will reduce the horse's sweating rate. This has the advantage that because the horse sweats less, he becomes less dehydrated.

6. As stated, there is no harm in allowing horses to drink small amounts (half a bucket) during competition. Water should also be left in the stable until 15–30 minutes before exercise. Water is emptied very rapidly from the stomach. Do NOT give the horse ice-cold water to drink. Recent research has also shown that it is important to feed hard feed and some hay together, at least four hours prior to exercise.

There is **no** evidence to suggest that cold-water cooling causes other problems such as 'tying-up'.

Care Before the Veterinary Inspection on the Final Day of a Three-Day Event

- Start early.

- Feed and water the horse.

- Remove bandages if used, wash off poultices, and hose legs.

- Lead the horse out at the walk, then jog him to check the state of soundness. If the horse is in good order, lead him out for half an hour to remove stiffness from the muscles. Massage is also beneficial if the groom is practised and the horse is accustomed to it.

- On return to the stables, groom the horse and plait up.

- Thirty minutes before the veterinary inspection, take the horse out again for further walking. In some cases the rider may prefer to give the horse a hack or a light school to loosen the muscles.

37 THE DRESSAGE HORSE

The dressage horse is the gymnast of the equine world. His training is a continuing process. For this reason, as soon as he is fit and working he is rarely given long rest periods. Any prolonged time without work allows his muscles to slacken, which will necessitate weeks of preparation before he is once more in hard condition and ready to continue his training. If it is decided that a horse needs a rest from intensive work, he can be turned out or hacked out daily.

The basic fittening work is described on pages 288 onwards. Once the horse is fit, his exercise programme will usually consist of lunge work, ridden work in the school, and hacking out. Most horses will benefit from a daily spell in the field to allow them to relax mentally. Jumping makes a refreshing change from work on the flat, and gymnastic jumping exercises in particular also improve athleticism. The horse's mental attitude to his work is of prime importance, and this is affected by his stable environment and daily care, as well as by the work itself. Every horse must be treated as an individual.

Feeding

The dressage horse needs to be fit, but not in the same way as the event horse. He must be muscle fit, but does not need the same reserves for endurance and galloping as an eventer or racehorse. He should look well covered, but should not be overweight, as this makes his work unnecessarily stressful.

Feeding must balance the energy requirements of his work, and he must approach this work with the right mental attitude, especially when at a competition. Time must be spent working out a suitable diet for the individual horse.

Grooming and Clipping

The dressage horse requires thorough daily grooming to keep him healthy. In warm weather, a wash-down after work ensures a clean coat.

He should be clipped as necessary. Most horses do not require clipping in summer, but those who grow a heavy summer coat should have it removed by a total clip. In winter, when competition is more limited, most horses are comfortable if given a blanket or chaser clip, but by February they could have a whole clip, so that they will grow an even summer coat. Horses should be kept neatly trimmed through the year. Tails are usually left long, well below the hock, unlike those of the hunter or event horse.

Plaiting

For competition, manes should be plaited. Some riders use Continental-type plaits, with white tape wound around the top of the plait. Tails can be either plaited or left full.

Shoeing

An experienced farrier should advise on the best type of shoes for the individual horse. It is usual to put on fullered and concave shoes of light iron, with stud holes in front and behind. Cushion pads may be used in front to lessen concussion. As slipping is less of a problem in dressage, flat, Continental-type shoes are now often used for dressage horses.

When competing on grass, the choice of stud depends on local conditions. It is usual to put studs in the hind shoes. Studs in front shoes can shorten a horse's action and sometimes they can cause unlevel steps. On the other hand, slippery conditions are just as likely to affect the stride. Studs are not necessary for competing on artificial arenas.

Tack

• A dressage saddle is an essential item.

• Use of a numnah is general practice. The square-shaped Continental ones are the most fashionable, but those shaped to fit the saddle are neater and less conspicuous.

• To stop the saddle slipping forward a foregirth can be worn.

• A snaffle or double bridle, depending on the test.

• For permitted saddlery and bits, see the current British Dressage rules.

• Boots or bandages are usually worn when working at home and riding in before a test. They must be removed before entering the arena. There are a number of designs available both in boots and bandages. Bandages called dressage or polo wraps, which can be applied without added padding, are popular. However, remember that legs need to be kept cool.

Cooling Down

In very hot weather, follow the guidelines set down for event horses in the previous chapter.

38 THE SHOW JUMPER

Show jumping is an all-year-round sport, but a horse cannot be expected to compete indefinitely. Careful forward planning is therefore necessary to ensure that there are rest periods so that the horse will be fresh and keen and will give of his best.

Fittening

- After a rest period of two or three months, a horse requires an eight-week fittening programme before competing in a major competition. The initial exercise should be organised as outlined in Chapter 35.

- Roadwork and hacking out should continue throughout the fittening period, but after the third or fourth week, lungeing, school work and gymnastic jumping may be introduced. Too much jumping at home once the horse has learned his job is not recommended as it can wear him out and/or make him stale.

- A show jumper needs to be fit to compete over present-day courses, and slow cantering, as detailed for one-day event horses, is needed.

- During the summer, if the ground becomes hard, it is essential to avoid unnecessary pounding of the legs.

- Road exercise should be restricted to active walking, preferably including some hills. School work and jumping should be carried out in a field with a thick, matt surface of grass, or on a non-skid prepared surface.

- A horse walker can be used instead of much of the road work.

- After a three- or four-day show, it is sensible to arrange for a few days' rest and daily grazing.

Feeding

The show jumper must feel and look well in himself, but should not carry any excess weight.

He requires plenty of energy food, but high protein feeds should be avoided. It is important to adjust feeding so that the horse will keep his condition. A daily spell at grass helps to ease any stress.

A horse may have a normal feed two hours before jumping. When at a show, arrange his feeds according to the time of his classes, but as close to his normal feed times as possible. If necessary, give a smaller feed during the day and make up for this at night.

He may have a small amount of hay (1kg/2lbs) after jumping, but he should not be allowed more if he is expected to jump again within three hours.

Grooming and General Care

For grooming details see Chapter 11. A horse should always be well turned out for a show.

Clipping

In winter, a blanket or chaser clip is recommended, so that the horse will not catch a chill when standing about at a competition.

In summer, a well-bred horse should only need tidying up. A more common-bred horse with a thicker coat may benefit from a full clip.

The show jumper should be kept well trimmed, with mane pulled short, and a tidy or pulled tail.

Plaiting

This improves the turnout of most horses. Although it is not a requirement, it is expected at the bigger shows. Pulled tails are quicker and easier to keep tidy.

Shoeing

Normal fullered and concave shoes are used. They can be fitted with road studs behind. The inner web of the hind shoes may be bevelled smooth to minimise the risk of an over-reach. Stud holes should be put in all four shoes, so that suitable studs can be used according to local conditions. A spare set of shoes should be taken to the show.

Tack

- Jumping saddle.

- Breastplate.

- Surcingle.

- Bridle and martingale to suit.

- Tendon boots and over-reach boots in front.

- Hind leg protection may be necessary for some horses.

- Horses who catch their girth area with their front feet when jumping big fences may need a leather guard fitted to the girth.

Care at the Show

It is important to warm up the horse before jumping. There will then be less risk of strain to muscles and tendons. After jumping, the horse should be kept warm and walking. Warm rugs should be put over him in winter, and a summer sheet and/or sweat sheet in summer.

When competing in very hot conditions, follow the cooling guidelines on page 296.

THE ENDURANCE HORSE

Endurance riding is a unique competitive challenge for horse and rider and a supreme sport for learning about equine fitness. It is not a long pony trek ambling through the lanes. Endurance requires dedication, good horsemanship and involves long hours in the saddle, but can be enjoyed by riders and horses of all types and abilities. Horses with a high proportion of Arab blood are generally more suitable for longer distances.

In England and Wales the sport is governed by Endurance GB which is affiliated to the FEI for international competitions. Rides of varying distances are held over all kinds of terrain and in all weathers between February and October. International competitions take part in many countries, and European and World Championships are held biennially.

Types of Competition

Rides run under EGB are of three types: Non Competitive Rides (NCR, including Social, Training and Pleasure Rides), Competitive Rides (CR) and Endurance Rides (ER). NCRs are normally up to 40km (25 miles) and generally do not have veterinary inspections, CRs can extend to 80km (50 miles) whilst ERs run between 80 and 160km (50–100 miles) normally in one day. Some rides can extend over more than one day. Horses can participate in NCRs at the age of 4 but may not compete in CRs until 5 years of age and ERs until 7 years old. Horses and riders compete at Novice, Open or Advanced level depending on qualification, and non-members can take part in shorter

rides as Temporary Day Members. Riders should have one or more helpers (crew) particularly at longer rides to assist with the care of the horse and his presentation to the vet, as well as recovery from the course if needed.

NCRs and CRs have to be ridden at or above certain speeds depending on the class and the experience of horse and rider in order to complete successfully. Competitors normally start in small groups at intervals. The minimum speed for Novices is above 8kph (5mph), whilst Advanced horses can travel at up to 18kph (11mph). Strict veterinary inspections are undertaken before, during and after the ride. Horses must have a heart rate (pulse) of 64 bpm or below, be sound metabolically and in a trot up, and be judged fit to continue in order to avoid elimination (spun). Heart rates after the finish determine the grade of completion.

Endurance Rides

Competitors in ERs all start at the same time and the first combination over the finishing line is the winner subject to passing the final veterinary inspection. The minimum speed for ERs is 10kph (just over 6mph) with no upper limit. Horses are met periodically en route by their crews and cooled with water (sloshed) and given feed and drink. There are compulsory veterinary checks (vet gates) followed by short rest periods (holds) approximately every 30–40km (18½–25 miles). Riders must assess their speed and the condition of their horses carefully as they approach the vet gate in order to avoid wasted time in presenting to the vet. Extensive cooling of the horse may be required in hot weather although care must be taken not to allow the horse to get cold or stiffen up. The clock continues to run until the horse is presented successfully to the vet and horses are spun if the horse is unsound for any reason. During holds, horses and riders need to be fed and watered to ensure they have sufficient energy to complete the ride and do not become dehydrated.

Fittening

Basic work for the first weeks after a rest is as for any discipline, with long periods of walking followed by slow trotting on good going. Later, faster trotting and canter work, particularly up hills, helps to develop the muscles, especially those of the heart and lungs. The horse must learn to trot down hills, but once he has learned to do so, downhill trotting is not recommended for fittening purposes as it puts a strain on the tendons.

After the first month, training can be varied by work on the lunge, in the school, over jumps, etc. The type of competition will determine how fit the horse should be. For a 30km (18½ mile) ride, an hour daily is sufficient with a three-hour ride once a week. For 80km (50 mile) or further in faster competitions, more hours of work are needed. These may include interval-training-type fittening work.

Whenever the horse is being exercised, it is important to make sure he is working. If he is just slopping along on a loose rein, he does not use his muscles, heart or lungs and cannot get fitter. A heart-rate monitor is often used to indicate the recovery rate and level of fitness in training.

If the ground is very hard or deep and unsuitable for interval training at the canter, work up long hills at a strong trot. This will raise the heart and breathing rates as in cantering, and will cause less strain on the legs.

Interval Training

This is a method of increasing a horse's fitness by using varying intervals of cantering and walking. For a horse competing in 30–50km (18½–31 mile) rides, the interval training system would be very similar to that for novice event horses. For the more demanding longer rides, more specialist stamina work will need to be undertaken to extend the endurance horse's fitness level.

The horse should be basic 'walk, trot and canter fit' (4–6 weeks) before commencing. Before the interval training it is important to warm up the horse at the trot and afterwards to walk him until he is cool. If the heart rate is checked immediately after cantering, and again after the 3 minutes walking, a fair idea of the horse's fitness can be gained from noting the speed with which the heart rate drops back to normal. When the heart rate fails to return to normal in less time than on the previous occasion after doing the same work in the same weather conditions, the horse is as fit as possible. The trainer should aim to achieve this condition shortly before the day of the competition.

A stethoscope can be used to check the heart rate at rest in the stable before starting, and also during and after interval training. The resting pulse rate for a fit horse, standing in the stable, can be as low as 25 up to 40 bpm. The warm-up pulse rate would be in the range 40–50 bpm. During trot work the pulse would rise to 80–100, and in canter would be between 100–120. The maximum rate should be limited to approximately 150–160. Recovery to 64 or below is required before presentation to the vet in competition.

Feeding and General Management

This is the same for any horse in hard work. All feedstuffs should be of the best quality obtainable. As training progresses, bulk feeds should be cut down and replaced by a series of short feeds – oats, barley, proprietary nuts, etc., supplemented by anything that the horse likes – e.g. soaked sugar beet pulp, carrots, boiled linseed – to encourage his appetite. When the horse is in hard work, salt should be added to the feeds, as this is lost in sweat and lack of it may cause muscle cramp (tying up). Most trainers also like to add a mineral supplement to supply any trace elements which may be lacking in the diet.

There are no hard-and-fast rules as to the quantity of feed required; it varies according to the horse's build and temperament. If, however, a large quantity of short feed is given, this should be divided into four feeds during the 24 hours to avoid putting the horse off his feed altogether.

Fibre is very important to the endurance horse. Good-quality hay or haylage is fed and alfalfa is often fed with the hard feed. This fibre is important when the horse is competing to help retain fluid in the gut and to provide a slow-release energy source. The horse can be kept in a paddock for part of the time, as long as there is shelter from cold winds and flies. This helps to keep him relaxed and to give him exercise.

Water should always be available for him to drink. On rides, he should be encouraged to drink freely from any source, whether a bucket, stream, cattle trough or even a clean puddle. This is particularly important in hot weather as, because of sweating, horses in work soon become dehydrated. No harm will come to the horse if he drinks when he is hot as long as he moves off immediately. When competing it is advantageous to add electrolytes to water given from buckets, as these replace the salts lost in sweat. If the horse will not drink water with electrolytes, plain or sugar beet water should be offered. At no time should the horse be put off drinking.

Grooming

The horse should be groomed thoroughly each day. Any sweat should be removed and particular attention should be paid to the saddle area. An endurance horse should become accustomed to being sponged down and having 'slosh bottles' of water poured on him – a vital process for cooling during competition. Fabric conditioner bottles are ideal because they have wide necks and strong handles. Take special care of his feet, and have him shod regularly by a skilled farrier. He should ideally be shod a few days before competition. Under some conditions hoof pads can be beneficial.

Worming and Vaccination

As well as regular worming, all endurance horses should be immunised against influenza and tetanus, as required by Jockey Club regulations. Many rides are based at racecourses and any horse not immunised will not be allowed on racecourse premises. See Appendix 4.

Saddlery

SADDLE English, general purpose, Western or special endurance type, worn with or without numnah or saddle blanket as required. Flex-type stirrups help to reduce concussion on the rider's knees and ankles.

BRIDLE All recognised forms of bit are acceptable including bitless bridles. Synthetic tack is popular as it can be cleaned easily and leather can be damaged by slosh water and sweat. Coloured tack is also popular as it can be easily spotted from a distance.

Preparation for the Competition

Each horse and rider should have a back-up crew, consisting of one or more people in a vehicle, one of whom should be a good navigator. This crew follows the horse, meeting up with him at points on the course and at the veterinary checks.

Before the day of the competition, the rider and crew should discuss the plan of campaign. The rider will have been sent a map of the route and possibly written instructions too. Notice should be taken of any instructions from the Ride Organiser – particularly any areas not suitable for crewing. They should outline the route on a local Ordnance Survey map, study it, and decide upon suitable meeting places. They must calculate the times the rider expects to pass each point, and check whether it is possible for the crew to get there by car in time to meet him. The crew often has to take a longer route, for example driving around a mountain and up the next valley, while the competitor travels straight over the top, so good timing is essential. Having settled the route to be taken, with meeting places and arrival times, the crew's next duty is to load the vehicle with all the equipment needed during the ride.

Equipment

Minimum equipment would include:

- At least one 25 litre (5 gallon) water container (full) or more depending on length of ride and weather conditions.

- Two buckets – one for drinking and one for washing down.

- Electrolytes, and measure, to add to drinking water if required.

- Funnel to pour unused clean water back into container.

- Sponges and 'slosh bottles' for washing down. Sweat scraper.

- Towels.

- Headcollar and rope (bridle may convert to a headcollar).

- Rugs, including sweat rugs and waterproof sheet.

- Surcingle.

- Spare set of shoes (ready shaped to fit the horse) plus protective hoof boot.

- Spare reins, leathers, girth and numnah (if worn), plus a leather bootlace or string for emergency tack repair.

- Crepe bandages and basic first aid kit for both horse and rider. Veterinary surgeons are always present at competitive rides and can deal with more serious problems.

- Isotonic drinks for rider in suitable container.

- Jacket and seat for rider at compulsory halts (with food for longer rides).

- Soaked sugar beet and water for horse.

- Feed and hay or haylage.

- Pocket knife.

- Grooming kit.

The above should be carefully packed in the vehicle, making sure that the essential items, such as water, are readily available and that the rider and crew know where everything is.

When competing the rider should carry:

- Folding hoof pick.

- Map of route, together with 'talk round' if supplied. Both should be in a plastic case to keep them dry. (Mark on map the times of meeting up with crew – this acts as a guide as to whether the rider is keeping up the correct speed).

- Compass and whistle in case of fog or getting lost.

- Safety pin and piece of string or leather bootlace (for emergency repairs).

- Small crepe bandage and wound powder for first aid en route.

- Mobile phone (charged!) with Ride Organiser's emergency number stored.

- Coins for telephone box.

- Energy-giving snack bar.

Veterinary Inspection

On the day of the ride the crew takes the horse to have his shoes inspected by the farrier and then to the preliminary vetting. The crew holds him while the vet checks his pulse and respiratory rates and examines him for lumps and bumps. The crew will then be expected to trot the horse up for soundness. This should have been practised beforehand so that he trots up freely and obeys the crew's spoken commands to stand, trot, walk, etc. The rider may attend the vetting in order to hold rugs, etc. and to answer any queries about the horse that the veterinary surgeon may ask. When the vetting has been completed, the rider then saddles up.

The Start

The crew assists the rider to mount, checks the girth, etc. and ensures that the rider has everything he needs. As soon as the timekeeper allows the horse to start, the crew makes sure that all the necessary equipment is in the car. They can then set off for the first meeting place.

Meeting Places

As the horse approaches, the crew should have ready a bucket of water for the horse and a drink for the rider. At later points on the ride, slosh bottles should be handed to the rider to pour on the horse's neck to cool him and a bucket of water for sponging down the horse should also be available.

- First the horse should be offered a drink, then a quick check should be made to see if all shoes are in order and that there are no cuts or scratches in need of attention.

- If the horse is very hot, slosh bottles should be poured on the neck, or sponging of the face and neck will freshen him (See also the guidelines on cooling horses on page 296.)

Compulsory Halt

When the horse arrives at the compulsory halt (vet gate) the horse must quickly be prepared for presentation to the vet (within 20 minutes or half an hour depending on the type of ride). The saddle must be removed and the pulse brought down by applying water (by pouring or sponges) to the neck and inner thighs. The feet should be checked for stones and when the pulse is satisfactory the horse should be taken by the crew for presentation to the vet. The rider should be in attendance.

After a successful presentation to the vet the crew should take the horse while the rider has something to eat and drink and takes a rest:

- The bridle should be changed for a headcollar (an endurance bridle may have a removable bit), and water should be offered.

- A rug may be needed to prevent the horse from stiffening up.

- The legs may be sponged down and any cuts dressed. The head and neck may also be sponged.

- The reins should be washed free of sweat, the girth and numnah changed and the girth area cleaned.

While this is being done the horse should be allowed to graze and given a short feed in preparation for the next leg of the route. The crew then repacks the vehicle.

The Finish

At the end of the ride the horse must be prepared for the final vetting, with particular attention being paid to lowering the pulse and checking the feet for stones. The horse should be presented by the crew to the vet within half an hour of finishing the ride. The rider should be in attendance.

- After the final vetting, surplus mud and sweat should be removed, any cuts should be dressed and the horse's legs should be well bandaged for travelling.

- The horse may then be offered more water, a small feed and some hay or allowed to graze and possibly have a roll.

- If rugs are worn, frequent checks should be made to see that he has not broken out in a sweat.

- He should not be loaded for the journey home until perfectly dry and cool.

Further information is available from Endurance GB, Stoneleigh Park, Kenilworth, Warwicks CV8 2RP Tel: 02476 697929 or www.endurancegb.co.uk

THE DRIVING HORSE OR PONY

Driving can be an all-year-round pursuit, although the outdoor competition season starts in April and ends in October. Activities range from showing classes and driving club meets, to horse driving trials.

Fittening

This depends on the type of activity, as driving trials horses require a much more intense fittening programme than show horses. The programme starts according to the date of the first competition; six to eight weeks should be sufficient fittening for show classes and competing in club driving trials.

When first starting work, horses may be lunged or long-reined, beginning with 5 minutes on either rein, building up to a total of 30–45 minutes according to the required degree of fitness. The work is carried out in trot, with boots or bandages on all four legs. In some yards the horses are not ridden, but in many cases – particularly with older horses already broken to harness – it is more practical to hack them out and they benefit from ridden schooling and variety in their work. If hill work can be included, it helps the fittening process.

Horses due to compete in marathons should, by the sixth week of their basic fittening programme, be doing at least 2 hours work a day. The week before a competition their work may then be eased off, so that they are fresh and eager for work on the competition day.

The suppling work on the lunge, long-reins and riding is a very important part of the preparation of any driving horse, especially for the dressage section of a three-day event.

In the first few weeks of driven work, care must be taken to see that the horse's shoulders and chest do not become tender from pressure by the collar or breast collar. The skin can be hardened with methylated spirits.

Horses working in pairs, as a tandem or particularly as a team, require extra time to get used to working together. Team wheelers need particular care in respect of fitness as they pull the vehicle.

Feeding

The show horse must look good and must be well covered,; but the driving trials horse must be – and must look – very fit, so he needs more energy feed than the show horse. However, the feed regime must ensure that it does not negatively affect controllability.

Health

Horses competing in driving trials in very hot weather may suffer from dehydration, and precautions must be taken against this.

Grooming

Details are given in Chapter 11.

Clipping

This should be carried out as required. See Chapter 12. A horse taking part in driving trials may benefit from a full clip in summer.

Trimming

No part of the mane should be clipped, nor should it be hogged: it is a protection against collar sores on the withers. For presentation showing and turnout classes manes should be pulled short and plaited. Driving horses do not have their tails plaited. Legs should be tidied. Mountain and moorland ponies should have their manes and tails tidied, but not pulled. Different styles of plaiting can be used to reflect the origin of the turnout.

Shoeing

Shoes can be fullered or of plain iron. The custom of putting very heavy shoes on a show horse to improve his action is now less popular and, in the extreme, illegal. The weight and type of shoe varies between different horses and according to intended work. If possible, obtain advice from a farrier experienced in shoeing horses for driving.

Road studs can be used behind for roadwork. Depending on conditions on the day, studs may also be used in the ring or on a marathon.

An alternative is the use of borium let into the steel. This provides a good non-slip surface, and unlike studs, it does not jar the legs.

Horses destined for driving trials should preferably be shod several days before a competition, so that the shoes are well bedded and sure. A spare set of shoes should be taken to the competition or show.

Harness

Driving harness is more complex than riding tack, and takes much longer to clean and maintain. Collars, breast collars and cruppers in particular should be kept clean and the leather supple, so that the risk of rubbing is minimised. All harness should be closely inspected for worn material, leather and stitching. The underside of leather show harness should be treated with saddle soap, and the top surface with boot polish or patent leather cream. Modern synthetic harness is appropriate for everyday driving and in driving trials. This is easy to clean (in the washing machine) and is readily available. All harness should be carefully adjusted to ensure a correct fit.

Vehicles

These must be kept in sound and safe condition. Show vehicles and those used for presentation should be kept immaculate. Wheels may need professional attention. All parts of the vehicle should have regular safety checks.

In presentation, show and turnout classes, it is essential for the turnout of horse, vehicle and groom to be correct and according to the requirements of the competition. The whole turnout – horse, vehicle, harness, driver and groom – should all match.

CHAPTER
41 THE HUNTER

Hunting, as it has been practised for centuries, has been banned in Britain by law in 2004.

However, many hunts have found various solutions to continue riding to hounds and staying within the law. Hound exercise, drag hunts and hunt rides are examples.

This means that the practice of fittening horses for winter work is still relevant and can be adapted to suit differing activities.

Fittening Work

Heavyweight hunters, particularly if in gross condition, should be brought in to work at the beginning of August. This gives them time to get fit before hunting starts in November.

Thoroughbreds and lightly built horses require less time to get fit, and their fittening programme may be left until the end of August. The value of plenty of walking exercise cannot be over-emphasised. It helps to develop muscles without strain.

Horses not going out with hounds until November require canter work twice a week in September–October. The actual speed and distance of the cantering depends on the individual horse and whether suitable going is available. Trotting up hills can be a good substitute if canter work is difficult to organise.

The aim is to have the horse fit to gallop by 1 November. See Basic Fittening, Chapter 16.

Work During Hunting

A fit horse hunting three full days a fortnight or two short days a week should only require about 1 to 1¼ hours' exercise a day to maintain his fitness. Should there be no hunting, he should have a minimum 1½ hours each day.

- During snow or freezing weather, if normal exercise is not possible, and if there is no indoor school, a large ring of shavings or mucked-out straw can be laid down. The horse should either be ridden, lunged, or led round on this surface.

- If the snow is dry and powdery it will not ball in the feet so riding in fields or woods is usually quite safe. Roads must be avoided because of the danger from and to traffic. Wet snow does ball in the feet, and may not be safe to ride on unless the feet are packed with grease or fitted with pads.

Feeding

For suitable diet, see Chapters 22 and 23.

The night before the horse's rest day he should be given less concentrates.

- Horses subject to azoturia or lymphangitis require special treatment, i.e. on the day off reduced concentrates and walking out.

- All horses benefit from some in-hand grazing or regular turnout to grass for at least an hour a day.

- For November hunting onwards, horses should have their normal hard feed at least two hours before leaving the stable. They can be given a small amount of hay at 7am, despite the fact that this takes longer to eat and to digest. Assuming that the meet is not before 11am, strenuous effort would not be required before 11.30am, allowing four hours for digestion.

On return from hunting the horse should be watered according to the method described later in this chapter, then given a small net of hay, and half an hour later a small feed. He requires a nourishing but an easily digested feed. Three hours later he should be able to digest his normal evening ration of a concentrate feed and hay.

The next day should normally be a rest day, and as long as the horse is well and sound, he can be given normal rations.

Preparing for Hunting

The Day Before

- Check the horse, particularly his shoes.

- He should be given a thorough grooming.

- Tack should be checked for damage to stitching and put ready for the morning.

- Bits and stirrup irons should be of stainless steel.

- Reins should be rubber-covered to give control when the horse sweats and/or when the weather is wet.

- Double bridles may have a laced or rubber-covered bridoon rein.

- The headcollar and roller should be cleaned.

- The day rug, sweat sheet, leg protectors or bandages with Gamgee and knee caps should be put ready.

- Plaiting should be left until the next morning.

Equipment for Hunting Day

- Grooming kit for tidying horse on arrival.

- Haynet for the return journey.

- Water carrier and bucket for giving the horse a small drink on his return to the box and also to enable any cuts to be washed clean.

- If a tail bandage is used, take a second to use on the return journey.

- First-aid kit consisting of small bowl, cotton wool, antiseptic spray, oiled lint dressing, crepe bandages and a bottle of saline solution.

The Morning of the Hunt

- The horse should be allowed to eat his feed undisturbed. If time allows, he can then be mucked out. If not, this can be left until later, provided that someone is available to do it. Otherwise, the box must be mucked out and bedded down before leaving.

- The horse should be groomed, tail bandage put on, mane plaited and feet oiled. If the bed is of shavings, his feet should not be oiled until he is ready to leave. If the going is likely to be very muddy, it is sensible to plait the bottom of the tail, turn it up, and stitch it. This makes it more comfortable for the horse. For horses who kick out when their tails are wet and muddy this should definitely be done. An unpulled tail looks smarter if plaited.

- Any small cuts or cracks should be protected from infection with antiseptic cream or spray. The horse's legs can be oiled (with neatsfoot, olive oil, liquid paraffin or glycerine – which is best) to prevent mud getting into the pores of the skin and to make cleaning easier.

- Horses are often transported to the meet saddled and bridled and without protective clothing, except for a tail bandage or tail guard. As long as the journey is short and the driver careful, this arrangement is quite satisfactory. Horses travelling on longer journeys should wear protective clothing and be saddled up on arrival.

- Rugging should be according to temperature. A sweat rug, though not worn on the way to the meet, should be taken and put on for the return journey. Roller or surcingle must be long enough to buckle over the saddle but must also fit if the saddle is removed for the journey home.

- Ideally, transport should be parked a minimum of one mile from the meet, and out of the way of passing traffic. A short hack to the meet helps to settle both horse and rider and makes tacking up on arrival easier.

- Transport should be left locked and any equipment or valuables put out of sight and made secure. Trailers can be padlocked to the towing vehicle to deter thieves, or a wheel clamp can be employed.

Return Journey by Horsebox or Trailer

On a dry day, horses should arrive back at the box cool and dry, having walked the last mile. On a wet day, they are better trotted for the last mile, so that they are warm before being loaded.

Procedure

- Loosen girths and ease the saddle. Put on sweat and top rug and fasten roller or surcingle. Alternatively, the saddle can be taken off and the back of the horse slapped to restore circulation. Considerate riders dismount and lead their horse for the last half mile.

- Take off the bridle and put on a headcollar. Tie the horse to a safety loop on the box. Anxious or excited horses should not have their bridle removed until they are safely loaded.

- Offer a small drink of water. Check and deal with any obvious injuries.

- Put on travelling gear, in particular a tail bandage or tail guard to prevent rubbing. Horses facing a long journey (over 1 hour) benefit from well applied stable bandages over Gamgee or similar, as these give support to a tired horse and keep him warm. Knee

caps are advisable.

- Load the horse. Tie up the haynet.

- If transport is parked on busy road or it is raining, it may be safer to load the horse first before putting on the travelling gear.

Hacking Home

On a **dry day,** walk for ½ mile, then intersperse slow, steady trotting with short walk periods. Always walk the last mile home and lead the horse for the last ½ mile. He will then return cool and dry.

On a wet day, proceed as above, but trot the last mile home so that the horse returns warm to his stable.

On Return to the Stable

- Unload the horse. His feet can either be washed and checked, or done later. Take the horse to his stable. Hay should be available. Remove the saddle. Check over the back and girth area and replace the rugs. Stand back, shake up the bed and whistle to encourage the horse to stale. Should he roll, watch to make sure that he does not get cast.

- Offer the horse a drink. In cold weather, take off the chill. Very tired and dehydrated horses may be offered water plus electrolytes, but plain water should be offered as well, as he may prefer this and it is important that he should drink. If he has had a drink before travelling home, he can be allowed 4.5 litres (1 gallon) of water at this stage, and then allowed his fill 15 minutes later. If he has not had any water, he should be rationed to 2.5 litres (½ gallon) every 15 minutes. This avoids too much chill to the stomach.

- Tie him up and allow the horse to eat his hay.

- Remove the travelling gear. Pick out and check feet. Check shoes, heels and legs for cuts and thorns. Treat any injuries. The knee, upper arm and front and inner thigh are likely places for thorns, which can usually be felt under the skin, and the horse will flinch under pressure. Thorns can sometimes be removed with tweezers. If they are deeply embedded, the area has to be poulticed or fomented to soften the skin. Blackthorns, in particular, often cause infection and should always be treated with care. Gorse scratches are hard to see and very prone to infection. Consider using boots whilst riding and wash off legs with a weak antiseptic wash on arrival home. Sponge the eyes, nostrils, dock and sweat marks behind the ears and around the nose. If dry, the legs should be brushed off.

- It is important that sweat and mud are removed from the horse as soon after arrival home as possible. If sweat is allowed to remain he may well 'break out', and be uncomfortable and unable to settle. If the horse is very muddy, especially in clay country, it is common practice to wash or hose it off immediately on arrival. If it is possible to hose with warm water, this is ideal. Putting a light oil on belly and legs before hunting can make the process even easier. The tail can either be hosed off or dunked in a bucket and then swung around in an arc to dry off.

  After washing, use a sweat scraper and towels to remove as much wet as possible. Use a 'wicking' rug or sweat rug under a lightweight night rug and walk him around until he is dry or place the horse under lamps until he is dry and then rug up.

- Turn back the rugs: first from the front and then from the quarters. Clean off sweat and mud. Sticky sweat in the saddle and girth area is often better removed with warm water and a sponge. Rub with a towel to dry. Replace the rugs. Make sure that they are dry. Unplait the mane.

- Give the horse a small feed and haynet.

- The tack can now be cleaned. It is best to do this the same evening. If very wet or muddy, wash off and leave overnight to dry. Do not apply soap to wet, soggy leather.

- After an hour, return and check that the horse has not broken out, i.e. in a cold sweat. This should not have

happened if he has been treated correctly, initially and was clean, warm and dry when left. Should this happen, first rub or towel-dry the ears until they are warm and dry. If the evening is suitable, walk the horse out. If it is not suitable he should be rubbed with straw or towel-dried – particularly in the loin area – or stand him under an infra-red lamp to warm and dry him. His rugs can now be changed for his normal night rugs although some people like to leave a wicking rug on underneath. He can now be fed his normal evening feed.

- He may then be left, but should be checked every half hour until he remains dry and is settled.

- Water buckets should be filled and more hay given.

- In all cases, hunters should be visited later in the evening to check that all is well. They can then have water buckets refilled and be given their late feed.

- Feeling the horse's ears is a useful indicator of how warm he is. If the ears are cold or wet the horse needs more care. If they are warm and dry the rest of him is likely to be so also.

- Very tired horses should not be worried by too much cleaning. They should be dried, kept warm, fed and left to rest.

Alternative Care After Hunting

If the horse is inclined to 'run up light' after hunting, if he has had a hard day or is wet or cold, he can be offered an oatmeal gruel (see Chapter 24), instead of water, on his arrival home. Some people give electrolytes, but plain water must also be offered as an alternative if this is done.

After his gruel, instead of his normal small feed he may be offered a bran and linseed or barley mash (see Chapter 24). If bran is not liked, some warm, cooked feed can be used instead of his usual concentrates.

For horses who return cold, wet and muddy

METHOD 1

- If the horse is wet and cold, rub his neck large muscle areas with handfuls of dry hay to increase circulation and encourage natural body heat.

- Thatching can be used. Put a small amount of dry, fluffy hay or straw under a sweat rug over the saddle and loin areas in order to allow air to circulate. Put a light rug over the top. If the thatch is too thick or not clean and dry it will have an adverse effect. It should be removed after an hour and fresh, dry rugs put on.

- Thatching legs by putting hay/straw loosely around them, kept in place by stable bandages, will dry off wet, hairy legs. This is especially useful in sandy areas when the mud can then be brushed off easily. The bandages should be removed and the legs brushed off when the night rugs are put on; they should never be left on overnight.

- The rugs should be turned back and the horse cleaned, as already detailed. Replaced rugs must be dry.

- Alternatively, the horse can be put under heat lamps until warm and dry and then brushed off and rugged in the normal way.

METHOD 2

- In some areas, particularly if the mud is likely to blister, it is better to wash the horse's legs, belly and inner thighs with cool water (not hot) and a horse shampoo.

- Remove all mud.

- Use a sweat scraper to remove any surplus water from the belly and upper arm. These areas can be towel-dried or rubbed with straw.

- Dry the heels and bandage the legs over a dry lining, or thatch them.

The Day After

- If the horse appears well and has eaten up, he should be given his normal feeds and hay.

- Remove the bandages if used and check the legs for heat and/or swelling. Check the shoes.

- Remove the rugs. Check the horse all over and give a thorough grooming.

- Check for soundness by having the horse walked and then trotted up. He may at first appear stiff, but this should walk off.

- Replace the rugs.

- The horse should be walked out for 45 minutes at a brisk pace to ease any stiffness. An exercise blanket (with a fillet string) could be used on a cold day. To check on his soundness, trot him up again.

- He should be left to rest.

- He may be turned out, weather permitting, or a horse walker used.

42 THE POINT-TO-POINTER

The point-to-point season now begins in December and at present continues until June. Many owners aim to have their horses fit for particular races in their own and neighbouring counties, others aim to race a whole season by choosing races over a wider area throughout the season and adjust fitness accordingly. Some National Hunt trainers use point-to-points to give their young horses experience, so the races have become very competitive over recent years, especially early in the season.

When choosing meetings take into account the soundness of the horse and the going. Some horses race better on soft going and cannot cope with hard ground, whereas others prefer to run on firm going. Horses who prefer soft going should be ready to run early in the season; those who prefer firmer going can be timed to appear later as the ground firms up. Knowing your horse is an advantage but if it's his first season aim to be fit for the beginning as adjustments can always be made for later races if necessary.

In order to qualify to point-to-point and to obtain a hunter certificate it is necessary for a horse to have a minimum of four days hunting, although this can vary with the hunt. The fittening programme for racing will begin with a horse who is hunting fit; depending on the horse it will take him six to eight weeks to become racing fit. Traditionally, point-to-pointers were hunted until Christmas then given a short break of ten days to a fortnight to freshen up before the fittening work began. Exercise during this period can be reduced to an hour's walking every day and if possible a couple of hours turned out, with a turnout rug; if this is not possible then grazing in hand every day is an alternative. Do not allow the horse access to excess grass as this will unbalance his rations and fill up his stomach with too much roughage. If he is able to graze during this period reduce his roughage accordingly. Many racehorses are turned out every day now for a couple of hours throughout the season, as it keeps them more settled and happier in themselves, leading to less display of the 'vices' such as crib biting and weaving often caused by boredom.

With the season now beginning earlier everything will need to be moved forward for horses to be fit in time, so horses will hunt earlier to qualify and need to be ready to begin their race fittening work early in October. If a horse has raced until June the previous season his rest period will be quite short as he will need to come into work again in August, so this is another consideration when choosing your races. Future seasons may be shortened but that is up to the Jockey Club.

Some horses may take longer to become racing fit, for instance those who have a wind problem, carry too much weight or are naturally lazy. With these horses it may be advisable to forgo the short break before beginning the fittening work.

Fittening Work

Fittening work for the first 3 to 4 weeks should consist of long, slow canter work. Traditionally horses were cantered between 3.2km (2 miles) and 4km (2½ miles) two or three times a week with road and hill work in between canter days. Now many trainers canter their horses almost daily but over a shorter distance, using either grass or an all-weather surface gallop and cantering up to 1.2km (¾ mile) then walking back to the beginning and repeating the process as many times as necessary. The amount of work and the speed can be varied to suit each horse's training requirements but if this method is used horses can become stale with the lack of variety so a couple of days each week could be spent doing hill and road work to prevent this. Whichever training method you adopt, when a horse is working in canter he should be on the bit and ridden in balance. All horses need one day off per week to rest and keep their interest; if possible turn the horse out for a couple of hours on rest days.

As the horse's fitness improves the speed can be gradually increased until in the last month before racing he is working at three-quarter speed over a reduced maximum distance of 2.4km (1½ miles). If cantering every day, do not work at this speed more than twice a week. A pipe-opener should be given over the last 400m (¼ mile) of fast work for the preceding two weeks before a race to help clear the wind. Should the horse not be as keen as you would expect, cut his work back a little and check that he is in good health. It is a fine line between getting a horse fit enough for the purpose and over-training him; when in doubt do a little less fast work except if you know the horse is naturally lazy.

A horse should be given his last gallop three days before he races, and not over-exercised the following days before the race. Some horses benefit from a day off before racing: others do not, but never leave a horse standing in the day before a race – he should at least be walked out for half an hour, either in a horse walker or ridden. If a horse is at all thick in the wind he should be given a pipe-opener the day before the race, and possibly the morning of the race if he needs it.

Horses vary enormously in their training requirements and this is only a guide to a fittening regime. It is essential to know what are the normal parameters for each horse (temperature, pulse at rest and respiration) to help you decide if anything is wrong during training. To avoid strains on muscles and joints horses must be warmed up before they start their canter work and cooled down afterwards. After cantering a horse should be walked for at least half an hour to disperse any lactic acid that has built up in the muscles during fast work – this can be done in a horse walker, ridden or in hand but is essential for the horse's well-being.

Between canter days work should consist of 1½ to 2 hours' walking exercise, with some trotting up hills. If no hill work is possible then a longer time should be spent exercising. If canter work is difficult to organise then more fittening hill work should be done. An occasional day's flat work or gymnastic jumping in a school helps keep a horse supple and adds variety to his routine.

It is essential to give horses the opportunity to jump fences at racing speed, in company, before they race as it is a skill they need to learn. A young horse should be taught to jump using poles and small fences, then progress to larger racing-type fences, usually behind an experienced horse. It is not fair on the horse or his jockey to expect him to learn on the racecourse; not only is he a danger to himself and his jockey but to others in the race and failure to school properly at home can lead to a serious accident.

During the week before the first race the horse's walking work can be reduced to 1 hour sessions and two short, sharp three-quarter speed canters. Care must be taken that he does not become overfresh or wound up. Stress can be quite a problem with some horses losing their races before the start! Regular turning out can be of great help, allowing the horse to relax mentally.

The Day of the Race

The horse should be transported to the race meeting in good time, preferably arriving 1½–2 hours before the race is due to start (Chapter 45). After a long journey the horse may benefit from a walk out in hand but should not be allowed to eat or drink in the last hour before racing. He must be declared to run 45 minutes before the start of the race.

He should be prepared in time to walk down to the paddock half an hour before his race. Point-to-pointers are saddled in the lorry or trailer and led down saddled with a paddock sheet and roller to the paddock. If it is very cold or wet, extra blankets or a waterproof sheet will be needed. A leather or webbing leading rein is used attached by a chain or leather rounding to the horse's bit for leading in. This is usually removed after the jockey has mounted and before the horse leaves the paddock. It is important that the girths are checked after mounting.

After the race, if the horse has been placed in the first four he has to go into the winner's enclosure; the jockey must weigh in with his saddle, which he removes himself. An unplaced horse can be walked straight back to his lorry. A sweat sheet or fleece cooler should be put on, unless the weather is extremely warm and the horse walked about until he is cool and his breathing normal. He may be offered a small drink (2 litres/½ gallon) with electrolytes to assist his recovery. His legs and feet should be checked for injury and if necessary treated. Weather permitting, the horse should be washed down, scraped off and a cooler rug put on, then he should be led around until dry. In cold or wet weather the horse should be loaded and then the worst of the mud and sweat sponged off and the eyes, nose and dock cleaned. He should then be rugged up and watered. Before leaving for home, bandage over Gamgee or thick leg wraps (this gives more support to his legs than travelling boots). Change his rug if it's damp and give him a haynet for the journey home. Encourage him to stale if he hasn't done so, although many horses will not stale until back in their own stables.

On arrival home check the horse has not broken out in a sweat on the journey home and if necessary change the damp rug. He should be given water, a small feed and some hay. Later in the evening if he has eaten up, he can be given his usual evening feed.

Post-race Treatment

The next day the horse should be trotted up and if all is well, put on normal rations and turned out for a couple of hours, weather permitting (if not, a walk out in hand will ease any stiffness in his muscles).

Horses usually race six to eight times a season and sometimes may race on succeeding weekends, so it is important they are kept fresh and keen to run. If a horse blows up (runs out of wind) in his first race or is very tired it is possible he was not fit enough. He should be given time to recover before being worked again (about a week), a couple of days being turned out for a short while before resuming slow work should be sufficient.

In between races he should have steady exercise of about 1½ hours per day and a couple of 1.2km (¾ mile) canters every week. Canter distances and speeds can vary between horses; some require more fast work than others. At this stage it is a mistake to do too much fast work as the horse may well get stale and go off his feed. If this does happen, reduce work and feed and do not race him until he is back to normal.

After the season is finished, the horse should be roughed off and turned out for a few weeks. From July, though, flies can be bad during the day so it might be better to bring horses in during the day and turn them out at night – this also prevents them from becoming too fat! Walking exercise can be started again in August to bring the horse back into work gradually with the minimum of strain. Long periods at grass are not recommended, unless it is necessary because of injury. Muscles get very slack, causing more risk of strain when the horse goes back into work.

Feeding

Getting the point-to-point horse fit for racing is different from getting other horses fit because the point-to-pointer will have been hunted and be fairly fit, but may be lean. If he is given a short break after hunting before his final training begins he will be on reduced rations during this time unless he is considered too lean.

Because he is now partly fit his feeding can start at the sixth week with a ratio of 50% roughage and 50% concentrate. The traditional method of feeding point-to-pointers was on good quality oats and hay. This is still practised but usually with haylage replacing the hay and a balancer fed with the oats. There are several good compound feeds for racehorses on the market, both in coarse mix form and cubed. These are designed to be fed with no additions as the ration is complete and balanced, so nothing is left to chance. They are widely used by professional trainers and fed together with haylage to form the roughage part of the diet. Recent veterinary findings indicate that high levels of starch in diets are not beneficial to horses and most manufacturers are adjusting their compound feeds in line with this. Diets designed for racehorses are free from any banned substances but if other compounds are used this needs to be checked.

Bedding

Horses are preferably bedded on shavings, paper, recycled cardboard or hemp, grown especially for bedding in this country. If bedded on straw they are likely to eat a certain amount, which may affect their wind and certainly unbalances their diet!

Grooming

Not many yards have time for the traditional strapping any more but it is important to brush a horse off daily and keep his coat clean. When possible, wash horses off after exercise to get rid of sweat, which can cause soreness in the saddle and girth area. A bucket and sponge can be used to sponge saddle, girth and bridle areas after exercise and the horse left in the stable with a cooler rug until dry, when his normal rug can be put on.

Shoeing

Most horses are shod with lightweight steel shoes, which stand up to normal exercise and are suitable for racing. Some horses are plated, which means fitting racing plates the day before the race and replacing with normal shoes a day or two later. This practice puts a lot of strain on the horse's feet and is not advisable unless he has a very strong growth of horn. Studs are not allowed because of risk of injury to horses and jockeys in case of a fall. Screw-in road studs can be used for exercise if necessary but must be removed before racing.

Racing Tack

Saddlery Requirements

- Steeplechasing saddle (4–4.5 kilos).

- Non-slip racepad.

- Stainless steel irons.

- Rawhide or buffalo hide leathers. As these can stretch, use well before racing in them.

- Point-to-point double girth (nylon webbing with two elastic-mounted buckles).

- Weight cloth.

- Overgirth with elastic mounted buckle.

- Breastgirth, elasticated.

- Snaffle bridle with stainless bit, cavesson noseband and rubber-covered reins.

During a race considerable strain is put on all tack. Everything must be in excellent condition and thoroughly checked.

Most jockeys use their own saddles. Though most race saddles fit most horses it is sensible to take your own saddle just in case.

Turnout

Manes and tails should be plaited, unless this causes the horse to sweat up. A loose mane is awkward for the jockey to handle and, for safety, the headpiece of the bridle should be plaited into the top plait. Tails may be plaited or tied up and secured with tapes.

Boots or bandages may be worn. Protective boots may be worn in front and behind, but should be as light as possible. Bandages are rarely seen now for racing but if used must be securely stitched.

Clothing on Race Day

- Travelling rug.

- Fleece cooler or sweat rug.

- Paddock sheet/roller.

- Waterproof sheet.

- Spare rug.

Paperwork

Hunter certificates must be obtained from the secretary of the hunt you have qualified with. These must be sent to Weatherbys at least two weeks before the first race you wish to enter. It is advisable to purchase from Weatherbys a *Point to Point & Hunter Chase Race Planner* which is a schedule of the season's point-to-points and hunter chases, giving all details of meetings and contacts. This allows you to plan the whole season, if you wish, and is an invaluable aid. Except for members' races, a horse is not eligible to run unless registered with Weatherbys. He must have a passport, which must be taken to each meeting the horse is to run at – there are fines for non-production of a passport when required at a race meeting. The passport shows the horse's breeding and provides an exact description with proof of up to date vaccinations, completed by a veterinary surgeon. On receipt of your hunter certificate, Weatherbys will send you a letter of confirmation and entry forms for racing. These are to be sent to the entry secretary of each race meeting, with the appropriate fee and by the closing date for entries.

43 THE SHOW HORSE OR PONY

The show horse is often rested during the winter months. He is usually stabled at night and turned out during the day.

Preparation for the next season begins in early February, to give a clear eight weeks before the early shows. Young horses are given a rest after the summer shows, and then continue their education and training throughout the winter. For animals who do not appear in the ring until May or June, preparation can begin later.

Some people prefer to give their horses a little hunting, to provide a change, but there is a risk of injury or acquiring a blemish.

Well-bred ponies who winter out need extra feed to ensure that they are in good condition. They are usually brought in during February, when they require careful rugging to encourage the summer coat to come through. Ponies who are known to be slow in losing their winter coats may need to be brought in by mid-January. They should then be clipped out so that their summer coat is well established by the early shows.

It is now acceptable for mountain and moorland ponies who are working under saddle to be clipped. All the native breed societies recognise that, during the winter months, working ponies need to be clipped on welfare grounds.

All animals should be regularly wormed, their teeth checked and their inoculation programme completed.

Feeding

- Feeding a show horse or pony needs thought and care. Show animals must look and feel well, but must accept discipline, and must display good manners. The show hack and pony must look well covered, and have an elegant movement, great presence and impeccable manners.

- A show hunter should carry more flesh than a competition horse, but must not be overweight or heavy-topped. Overweight animals – particularly young growing stock – suffer strain in joints, tendons and muscles, which can lead to soundness problems in later life. An experienced judge is quick to recognise any weak points in conformation, even if the owner has hoped to disguise them with excess flesh. The show hunter must be sufficiently fit to gallop without undue strain on heart, legs and wind. His diet should have more energy content than that of a show pony or hack.

- The feeding of lead rein, first ridden and small ponies requires extra care. The pony must look well, but must be safe for a small child to ride. Such ponies require very little energy food. In the spring and summer, their grass intake needs to be carefully monitored to avoid obesity or laminitis, and they are often better kept in a small paddock. In winter good meadow hay is all that many of them will require.

- Food must be nourishing but not overheating. Flaked barley, sugar beet, horse and pony cubes, cool mixes and a good quality chaff provide a suitable diet. There is a plethora of special 'showing' mixes designed to give sparkle without making the horse over-exuberant. Meadow hay is generally preferable to seed hay, as it has more taste, and the variety of herbs and grasses is important if horses are stabled throughout the summer. A period of daily grazing gives a change of diet and helps to keep the horse happy and relaxed. If grazing is not possible, fresh-cut grass or sliced carrots make a welcome addition to the diet.

Grooming and General Care

Thorough daily grooming is essential for the horse's appearance. (See also Chapter 11, Grooming.)

If the horse is kept well rugged and well fed, his summer coat should come through in time for the spring shows. He should not be clipped after mid-January, or if this proves necessary he should be given a total clip so that his coat grows through without untidy saddle, leg or blanket lines.

Trimming

(See also Chapter 12, Clipping, Trimming, Pulling and Plaiting).

The correct trimming of show horses and ponies is of the utmost importance; well done it can enhance their appearance; badly done it detracts from their looks.

- The areas that will need attention include underneath the jaw, the edges of the ears, the bridlepath (underneath the headpiece of the bridle), the heels and the tail. The cutting of the tactile whiskers around the muzzle and eyes is controversial, and is banned by some breed societies.

- Mountain and moorland breeds have varying rules regarding trimming. Exmoors and Fells are never trimmed, whereas Dartmoors and Shetlands can have their jaws and ears tidied. You may trim the heels of a New Forest, but not a Connemara. It is therefore essential to consult breed profiles and showing rules before starting to snip. Mistakes cannot be rectified in a hurry.

Shoeing

- Regular attention from the farrier is essential. Show hacks and ponies are often shod with lightweight steel shoes or aluminium plates to encourage the sought-after floating and extravagant action. Toe-in horses should have the clip of the shoe to the outside of centre; toe-out horses the clip to the inside.

- Rolled toes in front or behind should not be used, as they may be taken as a sign of foot or joint problems.

- Screw-in road studs can be used on hind shoes. Front shoes should have prepared stud holes. The type of stud, and whether to use them all round or only behind, depends on conditions on the day. If the ground is hard, front studs can shorten the action.

- Youngsters are usually not shod until they are three years old, and some ponies are not shod at all. It depends on the work they are doing and the quality of their feet.

Exercise

- A show animal requires sufficient work to keep him cheerful, happy and well-mannered, and to get him supple, obedient and well-balanced. Daily hacking, with as much variety as possible, should be combined with regular lungeing and schooling. Systematic and skilful training enhances the muscular development of the horse and improves any weaknesses in conformation. At the same time, it is essential to keep the horse bright and cheerful in himself, so that he will give his best in the ring. Towards the end of the showing season many horses become stale and bored, which affects their performance.

- Horses unaccustomed to a double bridle often accept this more happily if it is put on for hacking.

- Over-fat ponies when brought up in the spring may need the fat sweating off, if they are to be ready for the early shows. They can be exercised in rugs and hoods, but on returning to the stable care must be taken that they do not catch a chill.

- All show animals must be trained to stand correctly when they are being looked at in hand. The traditional method is for the horse to stand with all four legs visible when viewed from the side. If the judge is viewing from the left side, the left fore should be in advance of the right fore, and the right hind in advance of the left hind. The horse must be obedient and active when trotted up. This should be practised at home. In hunter, hack, riding horse and show pony classes, they are required to walk away from the judge, turn (to the right) and trot back directly towards and past the judge. In mountain and moorland classes, this trot up is immediately followed by a lengthened trot down the long side of the ring to show off the pony's action.

- All young animals should be trained to load, and should be accustomed to travelling before the show season starts. This helps them to cope with the added stress of a show without undue worry. (See Chapter 45, Transportation.)

Tack

All tack should be of best-quality leather and must be looked after well. Bits and stirrups must be spotless, brass buckles polished and white girths and lead reins scrubbed and whitened.

RIDDEN CLASSES

Saddle
This must be comfortable for both horse and rider, must sit well on the horse and must show off the shoulder. A showing saddle with too straight a flap can be uncomfortable, both for the rider and judge. A modified version of the general purpose saddle with a less forward-cut flap and a longer and less deep seat is the most practical and does not spoil the line of the horse's back. A dressage-type saddle can also be suitable for hack classes. Stirrup irons and leathers must suit both the rider and the judge. A spare pair can be taken.

Girths in hunter classes are usually leather; in hack and pony classes they can be either leather, or white lampwick type. Bright colours should be avoided. Saddles should fit without the use of a numnah, but a horse with a sensitive back may go better if a numnah is worn. They should be plain white, black or brown, fit the line of the saddle, and not show more than 2.5cm (1in) beyond it at any point. Linen-lined saddles can be more comfortable for the horse.

Bridle
- Hunters, hacks, riding horses and cobs are normally shown in double bridles (see drawing on following page), but Pelhams are acceptable. The leather in hunter and cob bridles should not be too light or narrow. The bridoon rein can be plaited for more control in wet weather. Browbands for hunters and cobs should be plain.

- Hack, riding horse and show pony bridles should be of lightweight leather with stitching on the noseband and browband. Coloured browbands can be used. They should preferably be of plaited satin or velvet, not plastic.

- Working hunters are allowed any type of bridle, but are usually shown in a plain double or snaffle. They may wear a standing or running martingale. Brushing or tendon boots can be worn for the jumping phase, but must be removed before the showing section.

- Novice ponies should be shown in snaffles.

- Mountain and moorland ponies are usually shown in doubles or Pelhams, though snaffles are accepted. Some native ponies have short mouths and find a double bridle too much. A Rugby Pelham can be a good alternative. This gives the illusion of a double

headpiece

browband

slip head

cheek piece

noseband

loose-ring bridoon

leather curb chain

fly link

bridoon rein

hook

lip strap

sliding-mouth Weymouth bit

curb rein

Double bridle suitable for showing and its component parts.

bridle, especially if the 'bridoon' rings are supported by a sliphead, and many ponies go very well in them. They should have plain browbands and no stitching on the noseband.

IN-HAND CLASSES

Bridle

- All leather work should be of the best quality, and finely stitched.

- Buckles should be of brass, and neat in shape, unless a riding bridle is used. The buckles should then be of stainless steel and the browband plain. Brass buckles should be polished.

- Fancy browbands can be worn, except for hunters and mountain and moorland ponies. Brass link on leather, braided ribbon over leather, or plaited leather are the most acceptable.

- If in doubt as to suitable equipment, ask the advice of an experienced exhibitor.

Hunter Breeding Classes

Brood Mares

- Double bridle or snaffle bridle.

Foals

- Foal slip or brass-mounted foal headcollar with white lead rope or leather rein.

Yearlings, Two-or Three-Year-Olds

- Young horses are more easily and more safely controlled if shown with a bit in their mouths. This is usually a mullen-mouth snaffle, often rubber, and is buckled on to a brass-mounted headcollar. Well-behaved young horses or ponies may be shown without a bit. A 3.6m (12ft) leather or white lead rein with a coupling is fastened to the headcollar or bit. Alternatively, a brass-mounted bridle with a snaffle bit can be used. A ring bit such as a Tattersall is sometimes put on strong yearlings, as it gives more control. Some breed societies do not allow yearlings to be bitted, and others forbid Chifneys. Mouths should be treated with care, and if a coupling is used on the bit, it can also be linked through the noseband so the primary pressure is on the nose rather than the mouth. Some pony breeds have shallow mouths, and this method prevents the coupling from pulling forwards and becoming hooked up in the mouth.

Stallions

- A brass-mounted stallion bridle with a mullen mouth snaffle or a stallion bit should be used. It may have couplings to which the lead rein is fastened. The lead rein should be at least 3.6m (12ft) long. It may have a chain end to go through the bit rings or couplings. This will give greater control and safety to the handler if the horse should play up and rear.

Dress

- Exhibitors showing horses or ponies in hand should be suitably dressed. Jackets should be worn unless the breed society requires a different form of dress. Ideally the handler should wear smart trousers, leather shoes or boots, a hacking jacket with shirt and tie, a hat and gloves. Jodhpurs, or breeches and long boots, are not practical. A showing cane should be carried, and can be used to help keep the animal straight by holding it level with the side of the muzzle. A horse with his head and neck bent round to the left does not show

himself properly, and will be unbalanced in trot. When showing young stock or stallions, it is wise to wear a riding hat in case the animal rears.

The Day Before the Show

- After exercise, the horse should be thoroughly groomed. He can be washed all over with a suitable shampoo. Grey horses may need the addition of 'blue bag', and there are also colour-enhancing shampoos on the market. A chalk block can help to remove yellow stains, particularly on the tail. White socks should be washed and bandaged over clean Gamgee.

- Tack must be taken to pieces and cleaned thoroughly. It should be dressed with glycerine saddle soap. The outside surfaces of bridles can be treated with cream or tan boot polish to give a bright, hard sheen, though this is more usual with driving harness. The underside of the leather should be soaped to keep it supple. Saddles should be rubbed over with a duster to avoid the possibility of marking light breeches.

- Day rugs and protective clothing should be brushed and put ready.

- A list of necessary equipment should be drawn up. Some of this may be ticked off and loaded the day before.

EQUIPMENT

- Clean grooming kit. Two clean stable rubbers.

- Tack cleaning kit.

- Plaiting equipment: needles, thread, scissors and comb.

- Hair lacquer, mousse or gel.

- Hoof oil and brush.

- Vaseline.

- Chalk block.

- Fly repellent.

- Coat gloss.

- Baby oil.

- Studs and fitting tools.

- Waterproof rug.

- Exercise rug for use in the ring.

- Spare rug and sweat sheet.

- Headcollar and rope.

- Protective travelling gear.

- Show saddle and bridle complete with girths, irons and leathers.

- Exercise saddle complete with numnah and bridle.

- Lungeing cavesson and rein, side reins and whip.

- Exercise bandages or boots.

- Water container.

- Two buckets.

- Hard feed.

- Haynets and spare hay.

- First aid kits for humans and horses.

- Spare set of shoes.

- Spare headcollar and rope.

- Spare lengths of binder twine.

- Suitable boxes and chests, with a printed list of contents, so that the above items can be easily packed and located.

Additional items which can be listed include:

- Horse passports/registration documents.

- Show schedule/timetable.

- Entry passes/tickets/competitor numbers.

- Map.

- Mobile phone.

- Money.

The Day of the Show

- On some occasions it is necessary to plait before leaving for the show. If possible, leave the plaits on the withers and the forelock, and do them at the show. It is not recommended that plaits are done the night before as the horse may rub them overnight. Plaits can be protected from hay seeds and dust by lying a nylon stocking (or half a pair of tights) down the mane, and carefully putting an elastic band around each plait to hold the stocking in place.

- Unpulled tails can be plaited and then bandaged. To keep the bottom of the tail clean it can be bandaged all the way down or put in a stocking or bag. The bottom of the tail should not be plaited or turned up, as it will be difficult to straighten out.

- When undoing plaits, be sure that hairs in the mane are not snipped off with the thread, as these will give an untidy appearance when the horse is next plaited. Such hairs have to be continually trimmed back, resulting eventually in a thin mane and very small plaits.

- Travel arrangements should ensure that there is plenty of time to see to the horse on arrival at the showground. Allow extra time for horses who have to have more exercise than others.

- On arrival, get your bearings, check where your ring is and whether the show is running to time. Check the exercise area, then saddle up the horse with the spare tack and exercise him. A tail bandage should be worn, with either travelling bandages or fresh bandages put on to cover most of the pastern to help keep him clean. In some cases the horse will be lunged.

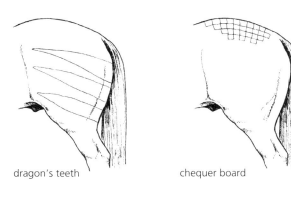

dragon's teeth   chequer board

Quarter marks.

- After exercise, box him or tie him up outside the horsebox. He must then be groomed, have his mane plaited (if not already done) and his tail bandaged to produce an immaculate turnout. White socks may require re-washing. Any whitening powder used must be well brushed out, so that it does not mark the opposite leg or hoof.

- Use the body brush and a small comb to make quarter-marks. Draw lines on the quarters against the lie of the hair, then draw it down the quarters in the lie of the hair to form a chequerboard pattern. The patterning shows off the quarters and proves that the coat is clean. Hair lacquer can be used to set the hair. 'Dragon's teeth' (sometimes called 'shark's teeth') can be made on the flanks by brushing the hair with alternate angled strokes. Quarter-mark templates are now available from most equestrian retail outlets.

- Studs should be fitted if required.

- On whole-coloured horses with dark feet, hoof oil can be used. Horses with white feet and/or legs should have their feet dressed with neatsfoot oil. If the show ring is not on grass, hooves are better polished with shoe cream rather than oiled, as most arena surfaces stick to oil.

- In hot weather, anti-fly dressing may be necessary. Some horses will not put up with being sprayed, in which case put the spray on a cloth and wipe it over the horse. Take care when doing this, as some fly dressings leave oily marks.

- Vaseline or baby oil can be applied around the eyes and nose to give a gloss.

- Saddle the horse up and walk him about to keep him warm. In wet weather, he can wear a waterproof sheet over his saddle and back whilst he is waiting to enter the ring. This can be removed quickly.

- Immediately before entering the ring, remove the tail bandage and wipe the horse over with a cloth. Sponge his eyes, nose and mouth if necessary. Hooves may need attention. The rider's boots may need dusting.

- During the class, after the individual show or the judge's ride, an attendant is required to help strip the horse and tidy him before he is trotted out for the judge. Attendants should be clean and neatly dressed. They should bring into the ring a rug or light sheet, depending on the weather, and a container or bucket with a body brush, a stable rubber, a damp sponge and hoof oil. It is also useful to include a hoof pick just in case the horse has picked up a stone in the ring.

- The attendant should take off the saddle and place it behind the horse, standing it on its pommel. They should then remove any sweat marks, sponge the horse's nose and mouth and check his feet.

CHAPTER 44

THE POLO PONY

The polo season lasts from May to September. Ponies usually winter out, but in a very cold or wet season they may be stabled or yarded at night. They require hay throughout the winter, and when the weather gets cold they should be fed concentrates to ensure that they will be in good condition when they are brought in to start work in early March. During the winter they should be regularly wormed and their feet should be trimmed as required.

Condition

Many ponies start the playing season carrying too much weight. This puts unnecessary strain on tendons and joints and limits their capacity for fast work. Ponies should look fit and well, but more like racehorses than show horses. They should be well muscled and round, with ribs covered but no excess tummy weight. This hard condition must not be mistaken for that of an animal receiving insufficient feed with poor muscle development and therefore no condition.

Fittening Work

Ponies need approximately eight weeks to get fit before playing their first match. A few practice sessions during the ten days before the first match provide the chance to check on their fitness and also to re-introduce them to stick and ball.

A suitable programme is:

Week 1: Half an hour's walking exercise, increasing to 1 hour by the end of the week. Ponies may be lunged or ridden in an arena for a few days if not sufficiently settled to hack out on the roads.

Weeks 2 and 3: Begin schooling in walk and trot to make the pony supple and obedient. This can be ridden work in an enclosed arena, lungeing and/or long-reining. Sessions should start with 5 minutes and increase over two weeks to 30 minutes. Cavalletti work and gymnastic jumping also develop balance and agility. Schooling sessions should be interspersed every other day with 1 hour of road exercise, but this will depend on individual ponies and circumstances.

After schooling, ponies should still have at least half an hour per day active walking exercise, or if weather is suitable they may be turned out in a field for a short time.

Week 4: Active walking exercise, together with some jogging. At first these slow trot periods should be of 10 minutes' duration, working up to 20 minutes, e.g. walk 10 minutes, jog 10 minutes, walk 3 minutes, jog 10 minutes, walk 3 minutes, jog 10–20 minutes, walk 20 minutes to finish. Total time: 1¼ hours. If it is possible, some hill work will improve fitness.

Weeks 5 and 6: Some cantering can be started with 3-minute sessions on alternate days. Canter work should develop progressively over the next two weeks, with the periods gradually extending to 4-and 5-minute canters, repeated twice and up to three times, to give a total canter work-out of 12–15 minutes. Ponies should have at least 15 minutes warming up before starting canter work. When cantering, they should be relaxed and on a very light contact. They must not be pressurised.

Weeks 7 and 8: To clear the wind in the last 10 days before a match, cantering can be done at half speed and then three-quarter speed. This can be done every other day and for short spells, i.e. 5 minutes followed by short road exercise. On alternate days, either schooling or road exercise may continue.

When hacking out, it is usual for one groom to ride one pony and lead another, but the pony to be ridden should be changed each day. If ponies are well behaved and traffic-proof, and if the hacking circuit is suitable, two ponies may be led out. Care should be taken to ensure that other road users are not hindered.

Playing Tack and Turnout

BRIDLES The most popular bits are doubles, Pelhams, or varying types of gags. Running/draw reins are often used with a gag bit. These keep the head straight when riding with the reins in one hand, thus assisting control of the quarters and quick turns. Rubber bit-guards can be used and may save a sore mouth, particularly with a Pelham. Curb chains should be adjusted with particular care. On a Pelham it is preferable to fit them through the ring, thus keeping the hook away from the face. A lip strap helps to keep the curb chain in the chin groove.

SADDLES Fixed-tree half-panel saddles with reinforced plates at the pommel are usual. They have no knee or thigh rolls. The girths should be of leather or webbing, the irons of stainless steel, and the leathers of buffalo hide. Rawhide leathers tend to stretch. A thin blanket or a lightweight numnah helps to prevent scalding of the back.

MARTINGALES A standing martingale is used.

BOOTS It is essential to protect both front and hind legs. Polo boots extend from just below the knee and hock to the coronet. Shorter boots or bandages can be used, together with coronet boots and/or over-reach boots.

TAILS These are plaited and tied up and secured either with Velcro straps or with a tail bandage.

MANES These should be hogged.

Match Days

- On match days, ponies should be warmed up before starting to play. Older ponies, or those likely to hot up, can either be walked or trotted about. Others may be ridden by their rider, who perhaps needs to get his eye in and have some practice with stick and ball.

- A polo match is divided into four or six 7-minute chukkas. Ponies usually begin by playing one 7-minute chukka an afternoon. When fully fit they may play two chukkas in an afternoon, with a rest in between.

- At the end of his first chukka, the pony should be unsaddled and sponged down, particularly around the eye, nose, dock, saddle and girth areas. He should be walked about, and in cool weather needs a sweat sheet and light rug.

- After the second chukka, or if not to play again, he should be unsaddled and his boots and/or bandages be taken off. He should then be washed down and surplus water scraped off. He may need a sweat sheet and light rug. He should be checked for injury. His tail should be unplaited, studs removed and he should be walked about to dry off.

Between Matches

- Ponies may be expected to play in two matches and one practice session a week. The day after a match, they should be trotted up to check on soundness. They should then be walked out for 15–30 minutes to relieve stiffness. Weather permitting, it is then usual to turn them out in a field for 2 hours or to graze them in hand.

- Between matches, exercise consists of 1 hour's active walking and jogging exercise. Because of the concussion which may be incurred from galloping on hard ground during matches, hard trotting on roads must be avoided. If there are enough spare days between matches, ponies may be schooled.

TYPICAL ROUTINE
Day 1: 15 minutes walk-out and/or spell in field.
Day 2: Road exercise.
Day 3: Gymnastic exercises.
Day 4: Work with stick and ball.

Roughing Off

This is done at the end of the season in September. If the pony has had daily grazing it takes up to two weeks.

- If the weather is warm and dry – particularly at night – it may be possible to turn the pony out after five or six days. Concentrate food is reduced, hay is increased and the pony is turned out to grass for increasingly longer periods each day.

- Rugs are gradually removed until none are needed. Grooming is restricted to spongeing eyes, nose, dock and attending to feet.

- Shoes should be removed and the pony may then be left out all the time.

- He must be well fed during the winter, so that he will be in good condition in the spring and ready for work.

Feeding and Watering

- Concentrate feed is built up steadily to a total of 4.5–6.4kg (10–14lbs), according to the requirements of the individual pony.

- It is important to ensure that a pony does not hot up. Cubes or coarse mix are often found more suitable than oats, particularly for Thoroughbred ponies.

- Amounts of hay should range from 3.6–5.4kg (8–12lbs) a day.

- Because of their playing timetable it has been found that ponies do better if fed their concentrate feed twice a day: in the morning and (the larger amount) at night. There is then the minimum alteration to feeding routine on match days. During tournaments, ponies may play several days in succession. On a match day, the normal feed is given in the morning.

- Hay, if given, should not exceed 0.9kg (2lbs). Food should be withheld for four hours before the match. Water should always be freely available but a large intake of water should be avoided within 30 minutes of the match. After the match, the pony may be allowed a quarter of a bucket of water and then his fill half an hour later. On a cold day he should be preferably kept walking for 10 minutes after watering.

On return to the stable, he may be given a small feed followed later by his normal feed and hay. During hot weather, it is essential to check late in the evening that the pony has access to plenty of water.

Bedding

Ponies who are bedded on straw and who eat their bedding must be muzzled after allowing them time to eat their feed and hay, e.g. at midday on non-polo days. The muzzle should be of the lightweight wire mesh type. This particular problem can be avoided if ponies are bedded on shavings or paper.

Health

Apart from specialised treatment, the health of polo ponies should be looked after in the same way as for other horses.

- It is preferable for all necessary flu and tetanus inoculations to be completed before the ponies start work in March.

- During the season, they should be wormed regularly according to the agreed programme.

- After any fast work – whether when fittening or playing – their legs should be checked for any indications of strain or bruising. If there is the slightest sign of heat or swelling, work should be discontinued until the leg is back to normal.

- Ice is the best immediate first-aid for a bruised or strained leg. Cold-water bandages may also be put on after work, should there be any question of strain.

- After a match, the pony's mouth should be checked carefully. If it is sore, it should be bathed twice daily with salt water. To allow his mouth to heal, the pony should be led out in a cavesson or ridden in a bitless bridle.

Teeth

A polo pony's teeth require attention from a 'polo dentist'. Teeth should be examined in the fifth or sixth week of the fittening work, and rasped down as necessary.

Many mouth injuries can be avoided by attention to teeth and by an examination of the mouth and shape of the jaw before deciding on which type of bit to use. Teeth should again be checked halfway through the season.

Grooming

A thorough daily groom helps to get the pony fit. After fast work or a match, it is essential for the pony to be cleaned thoroughly.

Clipping and Trimming

Usually it is unnecessary to clip ponies when they come in during March, as late clipping spoils their summer coat. The exception is a pony recently imported from the southern hemisphere, such as South America, who will not be accustomed to the change of season and will grow a thick coat.

Normal trimming of heels and chins can be carried out as required. Manes should be hogged, which may need to be done every week.

Shoeing

During fittening, fullered or concave shoes of normal weight should be put on. When fast work starts, lighter shoes should be used. These must be fixed securely, with pencilled heels in front and hind shoes well set back.

To save strain on joints when turning, feet should be kept as short as possible.

Ponies should be shod at least every four weeks and their shoes should be checked carefully before a match.

Screw-in road studs should be used for exercise in the outer web of both hind shoes. The rules allow two studs in each hind shoe, if required. Studs are not allowed in front shoes.

45 TRANSPORTATION

LEGAL REQUIREMENTS FOR ROAD TRANSPORT

There are strict regulations regarding the construction of vehicles intended for the transportation of horses. They have been drawn up to protect the horse's welfare, and can be found in the *Transit of Animals (Road and Rail)*, current edition available from HMSO. They apply to all horse transport, whether it is used for business or pleasure.

When first constructed, all chassis are plated and issued with a plating certificate. The plate gives the weights which each axle can carry, and above which it should not be loaded. To exceed these limits can be dangerous, and is an offence. The vehicles also have to have an annual Ministry of Transport test to make sure that the plating certificate is still correct.

Before deciding to buy a horsebox or trailer, especially if being ordered to personal specifications, it is advisable to check that its measurements and its weight-carrying capacity conform with EEC regulations. All vehicles with an unladen weight of 1,525kg (30cwt) must have an annual test at an HGV Ministry of Transport station. An MOT certificate, as issued by garages, is not valid for these heavier vehicles.

Drivers of vehicles over 7.5 metric tonnes gross weight must have an HGV (heavy goods vehicle) driving licence; they may also need an operator's licence.

The vehicle must be fitted with a tachograph.

There are regulations as to the weight of the towing vehicle in relation to the loaded trailer. These should be verified before you arrange to tow a horse trailer.

There are a number of regulations both national and EC generated which refer to how horses are transported. They refer not only to how the animals are treated but also to who is licensed to transport them.

These regulations should be checked out carefully by anyone running a horse business which involves transporting either their own or other people's horses for profit. They may well need an operator's licence.

People travelling their own horses for non-profit-making pleasure are exempt.

CONSTRUCTION

Horse transport must be strongly built and must fulfil legal requirements. Before buying your vehicle check with your local Department of Transport office for current regulations.

BODY WORK is usually steel framed, and may be constructed from aluminium, fibreglass, glassonite, steel, hardwood or wood. Wood is the heaviest and requires most maintenance.

FLOORS must be safe, sound, non-slip and easy to clean. Wood, rubber composition on wood, or rubber granulastic floors are all suitable, the last-named being the easiest to clean. Wood floors should have gripper treads, as they can be slippery. Horses travel better –

particularly over long distances – if the floor of the box is low to the ground.

RAMPS are made of wood or metal. They should be covered with a non-slip surface or heavy-duty matting. Gripper treads can be used. Ramps should all be fitted with efficient control springs to facilitate lowering and raising. Some vehicles have both side and rear ramps; others only one of these. Most modern lorries have hydraulically operated ramps.

Consider carefully before buying a lorry with only a side ramp. In the event of an accident it may not be possible to get the horses out.

PARTITIONS should be strong, well padded, and fitted so that they can be easily moved over or removed if a larger space is required.

THE GROOM'S DOOR is a small side door which enables an attendant to reach the horses without opening the ramp. Many boxes have an integral cab and therefore direct access to the horses.

VENTILATION is very important. It should be arranged by means of sliding windows (which should be of toughened glass and protected by bars), adjustable vents or roof ventilators. Provision should be made to keep the temperature reasonable when the vehicle is stationary for any length of time.

LIGHTING Skylights provide natural light and a more pleasant travelling environment, although in hot, sunny weather the box can become very warm. Internal lighting is required by law.

LIGHTWEIGHT GATES, when opened, act as sides to the ramp. They help to guide the horse up the ramp, and prevent him from slipping or stepping off the side. They can be quickly closed if the horse should try to back out.

All horse transport should display clear warning notices front and back, stating that horses are being carried. All vehicles and trailers should be given regular servicing and safety checks, both from the maintenance aspect and for the safety of the animal.

TYPES OF TRANSPORT

There are three main types of road transport:

The Horsebox

The modern purpose-built horsebox varies in quality from functional to very luxurious. Boxes for competition horses can be fitted out according to the customer's requirements. They can be made to take from two to eight horses, as well as providing storage areas, sleeping and sitting accommodation, and washing and cooking facilities. Even the least elaborate boxes are expensive, but they offer the safest and most comfortable transport for the horse, giving a smoother, quieter ride with less vibration than a lorry or trailer.

Partitions can be designed so that horses are divided off from each other to face forwards, backwards or diagonally.

Ventilation arrangements should always be checked. Whilst a stuffy atmosphere makes the horses more liable to respiratory problems, draughts increase the risk of chill.

The design of the box should allow horses to lower their heads to chest height at least. This is particularly important for horses with respiratory problems.

Care needs to be taken to ensure that not only is the laden weight of the lorry not exceeded, but that it is correctly distributed over both axles.

To find the unladen weight of the vehicle, take the empty lorry with a full fuel tank and the driver to a weighbridge. You will then be able to calculate how much load you can put on board. For example; if it is a 7.5 tonne lorry, the total laden weight must not exceed that amount. If in doubt, load the lorry with the horses and all the normal equipment you carry and take it back to the weighbridge.

The way the lorry is loaded is also important. If there is living accommodation up front and two big horses behind or a lot of equipment, including water which is very heavy, in the living quarters and two ponies behind, there may be too much weight on the back or front axle.

The Vehicle and Operators Service Agency (VOSA) is quite entitled to target horseboxes in spot checks at the roadside and if the vehicle is not within the law it can issue an enforcement order which prevents the vehicle from proceeding until the fault has been put right.

The Cattle Lorry

These lorries, if high enough, make suitable horse transport, but they are understandably less comfortable than a purpose-built vehicle. They lack padding and insulation, and can be draughty and noisy. Extra clothing may be needed in cold weather. Usually there is only a back ramp.

Horses may be divided by wood partitions or slotted-in rails. It is inadvisable to stand them parallel to the front of the box, as this makes balance difficult when the vehicle is moving. They should stand either facing forwards, backwards or diagonally.

The floor should be bedded down with clean straw or shavings. The ramp may be spread with straw to make it less slippery and to assist loading. This is particularly helpful when the ramp is uncovered metal.

If the animals are not partitioned separately the Welfare of Animals (Transport) Order 1997 states that they should not be shod.

NB: If a caravan or similar vehicle is towed behind a box it will then become a long vehicle, subject to HGV regulations.

Horse Trailers

These are built to carry one to four horses.

Most trailers are now built on a double axle, and have four wheels which makes for greater stability and a better allocation of weight.

Two-wheeled trailers, though they are light and manoeuvrable and can be towed by a smaller car, are far less stable. They are suitable only for small ponies.

The great advantage of a trailer is that it is low-loading, unlike a horsebox or lorry with its steep ramp, which can be off-putting for a nervous horse. Conversely, the roof of a trailer is lower than that of a horsebox, and the space is more confined. This can be inhibiting for a tall horse, both when loading and when travelling, and can often turn him into a bad traveller and make him difficult to load.

Trailers can be towed by Land Rovers or similar 4-wheel drive vehicles, or by a suitably powerful motor car. The 4-wheel drive type is preferable, as it tows a heavy load with less strain and copes better with rough or muddy going. Regulations about the weight ratio of towing vehicle to laden trailer need to be checked and adhered to.

It is essential for the towing-bar on the towing vehicle to be at the correct height, so that the trailer rides level and in line.

The joint lighting system has to be professionally installed, and the towing arrangements should be checked at the same time. Trailers have been known to break loose from their towing vehicle. The latest models have an automatic brake which prevents this from happening. A strong extra chain between vehicle and trailer is a useful safeguard.

THREE-AND FOUR-HORSE TRAILERS are heavy to handle and to tow. With the three-horse type, two horses travel facing the front; the third – and preferably smallest horse – is loaded from the front and travels in the middle, facing backwards. The horses are separated by partitions which swing across for easier loading and unloading.

TWO-HORSE TRAILERS are the most popular type. They have one partition, but if a horse travels better with more space, the partition may be removed (see Welfare of Animals (Transport) Order 1977). There are two models: a front unload, which has an angled front, a back ramp for loading and a front side ramp for unloading; and the shorter model which loads and unloads from the back. The front unload trailers are more expensive, but are worth the extra cost if young or valuable horses are to be carried. The horses are less worried when being unloaded from a front ramp, as they can see where they are going. Horses unloaded from the rear are more likely to rush backwards, and may be injured. Making some horses step back can be difficult; others learn to pull back when they are tied up in the trailer, although the back strap should control this. Difficult loaders may be more willing to enter the trailer if the front ramp is down and they can see out.

ONE-HORSE TRAILERS should be considered only if the horse is a good loader and travels well. The small space can be very off-putting, and many horses understandably refuse to go inside.

PONY TRAILERS are smaller in height and width, and are also cheaper.

Breeching straps should be fitted at the rear of each partition. When one horse has been loaded, the strap should be hooked on to the centre partition. It will help to keep him in place while the second horse is loaded. Remember that if a small horse or pony fights to get out he may end up under the breeching strap. If partitions are not used, the straps can be hooked together behind both horses.

All trailers are equipped with **breast bars** which fit across the front of the partitions. If the partitions are removed, a single long bar should be fixed in the same place. The bars give the horse support if there should be an abrupt stop, and prevent him from standing too close to the front of the trailer.

Adjustable legs should be positioned at all four corners of a two-wheel trailer. These should be lowered to help to steady the two-wheel trailer during loading and unloading. They are rarely needed with a four-wheel trailer. If it is necessary to remove the towing vehicle while the horses are on board (in an emergency only) the legs can be lowered. But note that it is very easy to forget to raise them again and to drive off with them dragging along the ground.

A **jockey wheel** on the front of the trailer is a worthwhile extra. It enables the front of the trailer to be raised or lowered, thus making for easy hitching on and off. It also makes the trailer easier to move when not attached. It is important to check before moving off that the wheel is well clear of the road surface.

For security, it is advisable to have a postcode or address painted clearly on the trailer roof and to have a wheel clamp or tow-lock in place when parked at home. This will reduce the trailer's vulnerability to thieves.

PROCEDURE BEFORE TRAVELLING

Home Transport

Regular servicing of all vehicles prevents unnecessary problems. All ramp and door fastenings should be kept well oiled, so that they can be easily undone and done up securely. It is possible for the back ramp of a horsebox to come undone when travelling, and for it to fall on top of a following car.

Horsebox

Check petrol/diesel, oil, water, battery, lights, indicators and tyre pressures.

Towing Vehicle and Trailer

- Check as for horsebox. Also, when the trailer is hitched on, check the coupling hitch and safety chain. If the towing attachment has been adjusted or moved for use on another vehicle, make sure that it is securely bolted and at the correct height. The trailer should ride level, so that the tow bar is in line with the ball hitch on the back of the towing vehicle.

Check that the following are working: trailer brakes, brake lights, indicators, side and back lights, internal light.

- Before moving off, make sure that the groom's door is closed, the jockey wheel and light cables clear of the ground, and the stability legs raised. If the top doors at the back of the trailer are to be left open, make sure that they are fastened back securely.

- To avoid theft, it is often advisable to carry the spare wheel of the trailer in the towing vehicle.

- The floor of all horse transport should be regularly checked for wear. This is very important. Wooden floors often get damp and in time will deteriorate and may break under the weight of a horse. When travelling, the box floor should be bedded down with straw or shavings to give protection from vibration and jar. It also encourages a horse to stale on a long journey. The floor should be swept clean immediately after each journey and allowed to dry out. Rubber matting makes an excellent floor covering but underneath it needs checking, at least on an annual basis.

- If you are planning a long journey, particularly if using a trailer and towing vehicle, it is advisable to have them both checked over by a garage experienced in this type of transport. Make sure that the trailer springs and tyre pressures are correct, as these affect the ease of towing and the horse's comfort.

Hired Transport

Before hiring a horsebox it is advisable to check its condition and to make sure that the driver is experienced.

As there is always a risk of infection and contagion, the box should have been washed out, and clean bedding should have been put down.

The Driver

Anyone who has passed their driving test since 1 Jan 1997 is required to take further tests before towing a trailer.

Basic details follow but anyone thinking of towing should apply to the DVLA for full details.

Category:

- B+E (minimum age 17) B class vehicle with large trailer where the Maximum Authorised Mass (MAM) of the combination is more than 3,500kg. All but the lightest single horse trailer will come into this category.

- CI (minimum age 18) Lorries between 3,500kg and 7,500kg with a trailer up to 750kg.

- C + E (minimum age 21) Lorries between 3,500kg and 4,500kg with a trailer over 750kg – total weight not more than 12,000kg.

- C (minimum age 21) Vehicles over 3,500kg (rigid) with a trailer up to 750kg.

- C + E (minimum age 21) Vehicles over 3,500kg with a trailer over 750kg (articulated lorry).

All but the B + E test also require a theory and a medical test to be passed.

- Pre-1997 licence-holders can drive vehicles with up to 16 seats and trucks up to 7.5 tonnes. They can also tow trailers with a large car.

- It is advised that anyone who has not towed before should take some lessons, especially in reversing, before taking animals out on the public highway.

- Drivers must always take extra care to avoid sudden braking, rapid acceleration and cornering too fast. They should pay particular attention when travelling over a rough or uneven surface. Though horseboxes can be driven safely at a greater speed than horse trailers, it should be remembered that horses may still become frightened and liable to injury when their driver is cornering at speed or driving too fast.

- Overhanging boughs and hedgerows along narrow lanes can hit the top and sides of the box and make frightening noises. Drivers should be aware that this often upsets horses.

- The driver of a horse trailer must be aware of the stability of the towed vehicle. Trailers, when towed too fast, soon start to sway and can easily turn over or jack-knife, with disastrous consequences. Drivers should also take extra care in high winds or on a slippery surface, as the vehicle and trailer can be difficult to control. No exact limits can be set under normal road conditions. A speed of 30–35mph (48–56km) is acceptable.

- In hilly districts drivers can expect excessive wear to the clutch and gear system, particularly on a car.

- Reversing or turning a horsebox or a towed vehicle takes considerable skill and practice. It is recommended that drivers practise with the vehicle unloaded. On some trailers, before reversing, the brake pin has to be put in to prevent operation of the automatic trailer brake. Before moving off, the pin must be taken out so that the brake functions correctly. Many modern trailers have an automatic reversing system.

PROCEDURE AFTER TRAVELLING

- The box or trailer should be skipped out and all damp bedding removed.

- The remaining bed should be placed at the front of the vehicle, and the floor should be thoroughly swept and allowed to dry.

- If necessary, remove and store dry bedding.

- Scrub down and hose out the vehicle regularly. Removable rubber matting should be lifted so that the floor can be aired and also checked for wear.

- Only muck out at competitions if there is a designated area for disposing of the muck. Do not muck out onto fields and parking areas.

LOADING

- Loading creates few problems if the handler is experienced and knows what he is doing. He will then give the horse confidence.

- Site the vehicle alongside a wall or solid fence. Avoid a slippery surface. If loading from a field or on a road, try to park by a fence or gateway. It is often helpful to site the vehicle so that a gate can be closed behind the horse so that he is surrounded on three sides. If in a yard, the gate should be closed.

- Inside the box or trailer, a short loop of string should be attached to each tie ring. The headcollar rope should be passed through the string and not tied directly onto the ring. This makes for greater safety – if the horse pulls back the string should break.

- Baler twine is not recommended as it may not break – use parcel string.

- Wooden flooring should be bedded down.

- To make loading easier, partitions may be swung across, secured, and then replaced when the horse is on board.

- A horse in a box without partitions can travel loose. A mare and foal are best travelled loose, with the partitions taken out.

- The ramp should be level and firm. To achieve this it may be necessary to use wedges.

- Some yards have a loading bay, i.e. a built-up bank with high, boarded sides. Park the box alongside the bank and let the ramp down on to it.

- If there is no unloading bay the ramp of the horsebox will be less steep and more inviting if the box is parked on a slight downward slope with the ramp opening up the slope.

- A covered school is a safe and convenient loading area. Lead the horses into the school and leave the doors open. Park the vehicle so that the ramp opens into the school. Fill any gaps with straw bales. Horses should associate the school with discipline, and the enclosed space encourages them to load without trouble. If a scuffle should develop, there is less risk of injury to the horse. Alternatively the vehicle can be backed into a corner of the school along one wall. The doors of the school can then be shut.

Training Horses to Load

Horses should be trained to load at an early age; if this is done there will then rarely be problems later. As long as the mare is a good loader, a foal will usually follow her. Young or inexperienced horses can be encouraged by loading an older stable companion first.

- A trailer should have the partition removed so that there is a visibly larger space.

- Front-unload trailers may have the front ramp let down or just the front top opened.

- A bowl of food should be at hand to encourage a shy loader and as a reward after loading. A worried animal can be given a feed in the horsebox or trailer, and then unloaded. This procedure should be followed several times before any travelling is done. For the first journey a short, smooth trip should be arranged. If you are using a box, an attendant should stay with the horse. This is illegal in a trailer.

Time spent training a horse to load is never wasted. A horse who is easy to load can save hours of frustration, worry and possible injury to both himself and his handlers.

Loading Procedure for Experienced Horse Handler with One Assistant

ASSISTANT

1. Check that everything is ready.

2. Be ready to carry out any instructions.

3. Stand quietly at the side of the ramp, making sure to be behind the horse's eye as he walks in.

4. When the horse is in the vehicle, secure the partitions or bar; in the case of a trailer, secure the breeching strap, then the ramp. When lifting a ramp, always stand at the side. If the breeching strap should break and the horse backs out, the ramp will drop down and can trap the lifter. A heavy ramp requires an assistant on either side to lift it.

HANDLER

1. Stand on the near side by the horse's shoulder. Look forward, not at the horse.

2. Start on a half-circle or well away from the vehicle and lead the horse straight up the ramp into the vehicle.

3. If the horse hangs back, do not pull him. Feed him a titbit, pat him on the neck, look ahead and persuade him forward. If he is inclined to pull back, allow him to do so, and move back with him. The horse will then not be upset and the loading process can be resumed without fuss.

4. When safe inside, as long as there is room, stand beside the horse without going under the front bar, as this is likely to make the horse pull back. Wait until the partition bar or back strap is in place.

5. Go under the bar and tie the horse to a loop of string placed through the ring. A single horse in a trailer without partitions should be tied on both sides so that he cannot swing round. He must have room to move his head and should not feel too restrained.

6. Go out through the groom's door.

Loading Procedure without an Assistant

SIDE-LOADING HORSEBOX

Tie a haynet to the tie-ring. Shut the yard gate. Lead the horse in as described above. Manoeuvre him into position. Thread the rope through the ring and hold the end while fixing the partition (or tie the horse to the string loop and then fix the partition).

BACK-LOADING BOX OR TRAILER

Lead the horse in. Put the rope through the rings. Do not tie him up. Quietly move to the back of the vehicle and secure the bar, the breeching strap or the gates. If the horse has a tendency to run back, use a lunge rein or long rope with which to lead him. Put it through the ring and take it back; this way the horse can be encouraged to stand. Should he pull back you can retake the rein as he comes down the ramp.

A good horse who travels well can often be persuaded to enter the vehicle ahead of the handler. Many horses prefer this. As the horse moves forward, the end of the rope can be put quietly over his neck. The bar, breeching strap or gates can then be secured behind him before he is tied up to the string loop.

If the haynet is not required it should be removed. Horses on a restricted diet, or before hunting, or fast or concentrated work, should not be given a haynet on the outward journey. Worried travellers, however, often stand more quietly if hay is available. If a haynet is used it is essential to tie it as high as possible and to make it very secure. Serious accidents have occurred when horses in transit have become entangled in empty or loose haynets.

Many horses load and travel more quietly if the centre partition of the trailer is taken out, or if it is swung across and secured. Horses rarely kick when travelling, but there can be real risks of a tread, so precautions should be taken – i.e. use protectors and coronet boots. (See Chapter 31.) Some horses panic in a restricted space, as they like to spread their legs to balance themselves. The Welfare of Animals

(Transport) Order 1997 stipulates that horses travelling without a partition should be unshod behind.

Loading a Reluctant Horse

Try to establish the cause of the problem.

- If the horse is unwilling to leave the others, a stable companion can be loaded first.

  - If the horse is frightened the causes can be:

  - Fear of the unknown.

  - Fear of a small enclosed space.

  - The memory of a frightening journey.

  - Fear of a steep ramp.

Some of these problems can be resolved by dealing with their causes and by not hurrying the horse. However, if he has had a fright when travelling, or has been upset by being loaded with unnecessary force, it is a more difficult problem to overcome.

Many horses and ponies are difficult and very obstinate to load because they have been handled by inexperienced and often nervous people who have given in to them. Such animals handled by experienced people often load with little argument.

Horses are very sensitive to atmosphere. Try to be calm and unhurried when loading and have a positive attitude.

PROCEDURE

- Make suitable arrangements for loading, as above. The handler should be experienced, strong enough to prevent the horse from whipping round and running off, and able to hold him straight, facing the ramp.

- The handler should wear suitable clothing – i.e. non-slip boots or shoes, gloves and a hard hat. Assistants should also be suitably dressed.

- Start loading in plenty of time so that there is no feeling of haste or worry. Enlist experienced helpers, and if possible choose a quiet time and place so that outside noises, unwanted onlookers, cars, horses, etc. do not prove a distraction.

• Put plenty of straw on the ramp and under the bottom edge. The ramp must be firm.

• Make sure that the horse is well protected by suitable clothing, bandages, knee caps, and hock caps. Make sure that he is not worried by the extra clothing. However, young horses may be better loaded without anything on their hind legs unless they are used to it.

• Have food available to encourage and to reward.

• Have at hand two spare lunge lines and lunge whip, in case you may need them. The horse should not wear a saddle.

• A cavesson with lunge line attached to the centre ring should be put on over the headcollar.

• If the horse is very headstrong, a snaffle bridle can be put on. The cavesson and lunge rein can be placed above it. The bridle gives greater control and ensures that the horse can be kept straight and looking where he is going.

• Remember that a firm attitude and a quiet, encouraging voice are the most important aids.

Other Loading Methods for Reluctant Horses

Handler with Two or Three Assistants

• Stand the horse by the ramp, facing forwards. Feed him from a bowl. Pat and encourage him to sniff the ramp. Encourage the horse to go forward. An assistant on either side can lift first one front leg and then the other, followed by the hind legs. Do not use force. If the horse draws back, follow him and start again.

• Buckle lunge lines on either side of the vehicle. Have two assistants holding the ends to make a passageway. As the horse walks forward, the assistants cross over and bring pressure to bear on the horse's quarters. A sensitive horse can rear up and may slip or fall backwards. The handler must instruct the assistants and be quick to forestall any such problem.

• It is important that the handler does not pull on the horse's head when pressure is being applied from behind. They should stand at the side of the horse and face forwards. Once the horse has loaded in this fashion he will often then load as soon as he sees the lines lying on the ground and he is asked to go up between them.

• If the horse is not a kicker, two assistants can link fingers (not hands) behind his quarters and push him

Loading a reluctant horse, with two assistants.

up the ramp. It is safer to do this with a short rope or strap. If a fourth assistant can be found he can lift one foot at a time. This is probably the most successful method of all, and most horses will accept and give in to it. Though there is some risk, an experienced person can usually assess the horse and his reactions. The closer the two assistants are to the hind legs, the less is the danger of injury should the horse try to kick. They may hold the side of the trailer or horsebox gate to apply more pressure.

Handler with One Assistant

- Lead the horse towards the ramp. An assistant walking behind with a lunge whip can swish or crack it, or touch the horse on the quarters, to encourage him forward. He can also flick the horse on the hocks, first on one side then the other. He must stand out of kicking distance.

- Apply a wet yard broom (gently) to the quarters.

- A blindfold can be used, but this may cause panic; some horses will not accept it.

The successful persuasion of an unwilling horse to enter a horsebox or trailer depends on the handler's
(a) experience and firmness;
(b) horse sense, quickness of reaction, skill in forestalling trouble, and ability to foresee if strong methods will succeed or are more likely to cause increased resistance and possible injury.

It can be comparatively easy to load an awkward horse if experienced help is available and if firm methods are used. If it is not, then inexperienced handlers must rely on kindness and patience. In time these should result in a more amenable and obedient horse.

There are a number of headcollars on the market which encourage the horse to move forwards and prevent him from either rearing or running backwards.

They can be excellent but should not be used for travelling. Always replace them with a regular headcollar once safely installed.

UNLOADING

If you are away from home, park in a safe and suitable place. Make sure that there is enough room for the horse to move safely down and off the ramp, and to keep straight for a few strides to avoid strain. Avoid unloading a side ramp horsebox or front-unload trailer towards the road unless help is available to warn traffic. When unloading horses, the safest method is always to untie the horse before removing the holding barrier, whether it is a partition, front bar or breeching strap.

Horsebox, Side Unload, Handler with One Assistant

- Handler enters by small door or through the cab, speaks to the horse, pats him and unties him.

- Assistant lets down the ramp and, when told, opens the gates and swings the partition across. Handler turns horse and leads him quietly down the ramp.

Trailer, Front Unload, Handler with One Assistant

- Begin as for horsebox.

- Assistant opens top door of front trailer ramp and, when told, lets down the ramp. Assistant and handler remove front bar from horse nearest to the door. Handler then leads horse out.

- Any attempt on the horse's part to hurry or jump off the bottom of the ramp should be restrained. If a second horse is being unloaded, and if help is available, keep the first horse close by so that the horses can see each other. When unloading the second horse after undoing the bar, move the partition across so that there is more room.

Horsebox, Side Unload, Handler without Assistant

- Speak to horse.

- Let down ramp.

• Untie horse but leave rope through the loop.

• Open gates and/or partition.

• Free rope and lead horse out as before.

Trailer, Front Unload, Handler without Assistant

• Speak to horse.

• Open top door and let down front ramp.

• Untie horse nearest to door and remove bar.

• Lead horse out. Put the horse in a loose box. If away from home, tie him to a string loop on the back of the trailer.

• The second horse can then be unloaded in a similar manner.

Trailer, Rear Unload, Handler with One Assistant

• Handler speaks to horse and enters by small door.

• Handler unties horse.

• Assistant lowers ramp and, standing to the side, removes bar or breeching strap.

• Handler stands at first to side and then in front of horse and allows him to step back. Assistant stands beside ramp and helps to keep the horse straight with a hand on his quarters.

• If quarters swing to the right, the horse's head should be moved to the right, which helps to straighten him. If the horse rushes back, he should not be restrained but followed, keeping hold of the rope (use a lunge line if he is big and strong).

Trailer, Rear Unload, Handler without Assistant

• Speak to horse and enter by small door.

• Untie horse.

• Climb out of the small door. Move round to the rear.

Let down the ramp and unfasten the breeching strap.

• Allow the horse to step back. Take hold of the rope as he moves back. Alternatively, if there is room, move in alongside the horse and persuade him back. A lunge line or longer rope put through the tie-ring and attached to his headcollar can be of help should he rush back.

Horses travelling on their own in a trailer without partitions should not be allowed to turn round. Ponies and animals under 15hh are usually able to turn and walk out forwards without strain.

IMPORTANT: When unloading two horses it is advisable to have someone to help.

CARE OF THE HORSE WHEN TRAVELLING

The requirements of the horse when travelling are similar to those in his normal loosebox. He should be warm in winter, cool in summer, with a plentiful supply of fresh air, but no draughts, have a resilient, non-skid surface to stand on, and the minimum amount of noise and disturbance. These points are covered in detail by the Welfare of Animals (Transport) Order 1997. The Order requires that a suitably competent person travels with the animals at all times, to care for them on the journey.

Most horses travel well, provided that they are driven with consideration, that they have sufficient space, and that the vehicle has suitable suspension.

Many of the problems and ills associated with travelling can be traced to overheated or draughty transport and inappropriate clothing. These can be avoided if the person in charge of the horses is thoughtful and conscientious about their welfare.

Many horses sweat when travelling. Common sense should be used as to suitable clothing.

Regular checks should be made, especially on long

journeys. Bear in mind the type of vehicle that you are using. A fully enclosed horsebox containing three or more horses is very much warmer than a cattle lorry containing one horse. Check the front and roof ventilators, as these can cause draughts.

Two horses in a trailer may generate considerable heat. The back top doors of trailers can be left open except in very cold weather or if on motorways, in tunnels, or in heavy traffic when horses become disturbed by vehicles coming up close behind them. In these conditions they travel better if the top doors are closed.

Food and water are not usually required on a short journey of under 2 hours. On a long journey of 6–8 hours, regular watering, feeding and hay are necessary. If feasible, the opportunity to stretch legs adds to their comfort.

Clothing for Travelling

The following factors should be taken into consideration:

- Time of year.

- Temperature on the day of travelling.

- Length of journey; whether travelling alone or in company.

- Whether a good traveller, or likely to get upset and sweat.

- Type of horse.

- Type of vehicle.

Stabled Horse in Winter – Journey 1–4 Hours

- Headcollar and clip-on rope (poll guard is optional).

- Sweat rug plus normal stable rugs or their equivalent in day rugs.

- Bandages with Gamgee or Fybagee, or leg protectors that cover the knees and hocks and won't fall down if trodden on.

- Knee caps and hock boots if no leg protectors.

- Tail bandage.

- Tail guard – preferable to a tail bandage for a long journey.

- Surcingle or roller with pad and breast girth.

- If thought advisable: coronet boots and hock boots.

- In very cold weather, a hood is often put on a clipped Thoroughbred.

Spare rugs should be available during and at the end of the journey, in case the travelling rugs get wet or the horse has sweated.

A sweat rug helps to ensure an even temperature, and keeps the horse from getting a chill should he sweat. If needed, the sweat rug can be fastened round the horse's chest, the other rugs may be folded back and buckled over the withers. They should be secured by the roller.

Thermatex rugs are light but warm and make good travel rugs.

Stabled Horse in Summer
Summer sheet with sweat rug or sweat rug only. Protective clothing as detailed above.

Long Journeys
Horses should be checked regularly to see that they are comfortable. They may require an extra rug or, if too hot, a blanket removed or turned back at the shoulders.

Short Journeys
When travelling hunters to a meet, or horses and ponies to a rally, they can often be fully tacked up. This can save worry and hassle on arrival, and is a safe procedure if the animals are good travellers. Protective clothing is often not used except for a tail bandage and knee caps.

The bridle reins can be twisted up as for lungeing, or crossed and doubled round the neck, or tied in a knot. The headcollar should be put on top of the bridle. Running martingales should not be attached to the reins. The ends of the martingale should be tied up and then fitted on arrival.

Rugs should be used as already described. The roller or surcingle must be sufficiently long to fit over the saddle. Rugs must always be secure. Horses may be wet and/or hot when boxed up and their rugs can get damp. A sweat rug should be put on and dry rugs should be available when they arrive home.

It is advisable to carry an extra blanket or sweat rug.

If protective clothing is required, leg protectors are easier to put on.

Rugs are not necessary for grass-kept ponies, although in summer a sweat rug or summer sheet will help to keep them clean.

An unclipped pony in winter is best left without rugs, unless he is wet and cold, in which case a sweat rug and light blanket, with straw underneath, is recommended. This 'thatching' allows more air to circulate.

Make sure that the pony does not become overheated.

NB: It is dangerous for horses and ponies to travel with jump studs in their shoes.

Equipment for One or Two Horses

SHORT JOURNEY

- 13.6 litre (3 gallon) water-carrier (filled).

- Bucket. Haynet for return journey.

- Suitable grooming kit and hoof pick.

- Horse first-aid kit.

- Spare rope.

LONG JOURNEY

- Spare headcollar and rope.

- 13.6 litre (3 gallon) water-carrier (filled).

- 2 buckets.

- 2 haynets.

- Feeds.

- Removable manger.

- Grooming kit.

- Horse first-aid kit.

- Spare rugs.

- Skip and tools.

LOADING EQUIPMENT

This will vary considerably depending on the type of transport and the reason for travel.

Many horseboxes have designated secure areas for tack and equipment. A lockable trunk is useful as long as it is not too heavy to move and can be accessed in situ when full.

Always load equipment before horses
Put heavy objects at floor level. Overhead lockers should only be used for lightweight objects. They should not move or rattle when the vehicle brakes or goes up or down hill and they must be secure when on the move.

Underfloor lockers sometimes get quite hot.

If haynets and forage are carried outside the vehicle they should be covered or put in a bin bag to prevent contamination.

Make sure nothing can slide forwards or backwards and become a hazard to the horses when braking or on hills.

TRAVELLING ABROAD

- Research is necessary to find out about the various injections and blood tests necessary for foreign travel. These must be carried out in good time. The bloodstock agency arranging your transport will provide all necessary information. If the horses are travelling as part of a team, this is the responsibility of the team manager.

- The necessary documents for the countries to be visited or travelled through must be obtained. This applies to horses, people and vehicles.

- Check that all dates and descriptions on the horse's passport are correct.

- Have all the necessary documents for returning home.

- Check that any medicines carried are permitted in the countries which you are visiting.

- Arrange for the horsebox to be serviced and supplied with any small spare parts which might be difficult to obtain overseas and which could cause delay.

- Careful driving will diminish the stress of travelling.

- Air conditioning in long-distance horseboxes is a great advantage, as humidity in the box can cause respiratory problems. When a horse becomes affected in this way it lowers his resistance to infection.

- The EU is contemplating under what circumstances air conditioning in horse transport should become mandatory.

- When loading the horsebox it is healthier for the horses if hay and straw are stored separately and partitioned off.

Feeding

Before a long journey, give a laxative, low-energy diet and continue this throughout the journey to avoid the risk of azoturia and/or colic. If the horses need to be fed during the journey, make up small individual feeds beforehand and use when required. Check if it is possible to import horse feed to your destination. If so, carry as much as space allows in the horsebox. If there are restrictions, it will be necessary to find out what feed is available.

Keep a supply of apples and carrots to help encourage the horses to eat up and to calm and distract them during moments of stress.

Watering

Horses should be watered every 2 hours. Filled water containers should be carried. Horses who travel regularly soon learn to drink to order.

Horse Clothing

Use rugs which are easy to alter, so that layers can be removed or added as the temperature and climate dictate. Tail bandages can tighten and rub, so it is better to use a tail guard. Knee caps and hock boot straps should be protected with Gamgee. Leg protectors are easier to fit and more comfortable. If necessary bandages and Gamgee may be fitted under them. With leg protectors, knee and hock boots are unnecessary. A poll guard is advisable.

Keep a simple bridle within reach at all times. It may be necessary to restrain the horse, and a bridle will give greater control. This applies particularly when loading and unloading.

Regular exercise is essential. Try to walk the horse in hand in a bridle for at least 30 minutes at every morning and evening stopover. If possible, a short trot on the lunge allows the horse to lower his head and encourages him to cough up any mucus. It is important to allow him to drop his head. Horses should be allowed to lower their heads to chest level at least every two hours or whenever the vehicle stops. Untying them and offering water and a few slices of carrot will encourage them to do this.

Bandages or leg protectors should be removed twice daily, and the horse's legs should be given a brisk rub by hand, upwards towards the heart. Bandages may become tight on long journeys, so it is preferable to fit leg protectors.

After a long journey, the horse requires a day to recover – with very quiet exercise – and then a gradual build-up to the competition. It is therefore very important to leave plenty of time, both for the journey and for recovery. Anyone travelling abroad for the first time should consider using a professional horse carrier who knows the ropes and is up to date with all EU regulations.

AIR TRAVEL

- As well as being the speediest method of transport, this has the least effect on the horse's fitness.

- There is usually a baggage restriction, which should be checked with the agency or airline.

- Various methods are used for travelling horses by air. The most usual, and the best, method is the loading of two horses into a crate (similar to a horse trailer) which is fork-lifted into the aircraft and then secured.

The actual loading of the horses is carried out by expert handlers, who are employed either by the airport authority or by the company arranging the transport. The groom or owner should always be at hand so that the horse can be reassured.

During the inevitable wait before customs clearance, and during loading and unloading, the unaccustomed activity and noise may well alarm the horse. A supply of carrots will help to keep him occupied and to allay fear.

At no time on the journey – whether it is by air or by ship – should the horse be left unattended. It may be possible to arrange a rota system with other grooms, so that a rest period is possible. Once the aircraft is airborne, the journey is usually smooth, and most horses relax and travel well.

Sedating a horse, either before or during transit, is not usually advisable. He needs to be fully conscious in order to balance himself. Most airlines prefer a horse to travel in a bridle.

On rare occasions, it has been known for a horse to react adversely when travelling by air, by trying to kick himself out of his crate. For the safety of all concerned, the captain of the aircraft may demand, under such circumstances, that the horse should be destroyed.

SEA TRAVEL

It is now customary for horses to travel in their horsebox, which is driven into the hold of the ship.

Try to organise sufficient space for the ramp to be let down or opened slightly at the top. This allows the horses more air in the hold, which can be very stuffy and hot. All vents in the horsebox should be open and clothing should be adjusted as necessary. Someone should stay with the horses throughout the journey if this is allowed by the shipping line.

Partitions in the horsebox should be arranged to allow horses to spread their feet and thus help their balance.

Horses can suffer badly from seasickness – although, of course, they are unable to be sick. The effects can last for several days.

Although it is not supposed to happen, some lorry drivers will turn on their truck engines well in advance of moving off from the hold. This is very bad for the horses and should be prevented if possible.

When passing through customs and frontier posts there may be considerable delays. Make sure to allow for this when planning the journey.

THE HORSE AT GRASS

46 GRASSLAND MANAGEMENT

Constant use of the land for grazing by horses will always present problems.

Horses are very selective in their grazing habits. Unlike ruminants, who spend much of their day resting and chewing their cud, horses graze more or less continuously – except for short periods of rest or when sheltering from hot sun and flies. Fields grazed only by horses, even with a low number on a large acreage, develop 'roughs' where they dung (also called 'camp areas') and 'lawns' where they graze. Only if very short of food will horses graze on these 'roughs', and unless good management is practised, the 'roughs' increase in size and so reduce the grazing area. They also become reservoirs of infection for internal parasites and a home for infective larvae. In wet weather, the latter are able to migrate to the 'lawns', with a corresponding greater risk of infection to the grazing horse. Thus fields grazed entirely by horses are likely to deteriorate, unless given knowledgeable and experienced management.

Objectives of Good Management

1. To provide grazing over a long period of time by the establishment and/or maintenance of a dense, vigorous sward of suitable variety.
2. To minimise infection from worm larvae. If rigorous grassland hygiene is practised it can greatly reduce anthelmintic strategy but should never replace it entirely.
3. To provide suitable working areas: e.g. for jumping and schooling. Using fields for jumping even if only

show jumping and putting the jumps away after each use, may have cost implications. More and more councils are classing this as 'change of use'. It may require planning permission and there may be tax implications. This can apply to paddocks for personal use only as as well as those that are part of a commercial establishment.

4. To maintain the land as a visual amenity, thus avoiding complaints from neighbours and possible action by local authorities. Well-kept fields and fencing are a good advertisement for any commercial establishment, and a source of satisfaction to the private owner.

Management must be geared to provide conditions which encourage the most productive and palatable grasses and discourage weeds and less productive species. Palatability tends to be a reflection of good management rather than of species.

The following procedures are recommended.

Soil Analysis

This should be carried out every four or five years, and when moving into a new establishment, particularly if the grassland appears to have been neglected.

DEFRA through their local Agricultural Development Advisory Service Office (ADAS) advise on local seed and fertiliser merchants qualified to carry out soil analysis. Results are in accordance with the ADAS index. In fields grazed only by horses, soil samples should be taken both from the 'lawn' and the 'rough' areas. The latter are likely to be high in potash as a result of horses urinating in the area. According to the results of the analysis, lime, phosphate and potash can then be applied.

Beware of expensive 'trace element' fertilisers and sprays. If horses are found to be deficient in particular trace elements, it is usually more effective to feed or inject these, rather than to make up the deficiency in the soil. Breeding establishments may need to take specialist advice.

Drainage

Signs of poor drainage are:

• Surface water.

• Plants such as rushes, tussock grass, buttercups and couch grass, though the appearance of these plants may also indicate poor management.

Any drainage scheme is expensive and may be beyond the finances of a small establishment, but if the field is part of an agricultural holding it may be possible to obtain a grant.

Before embarking on a drainage scheme, make sure that all boundary ditches and outlets are cleared, as these can be one of the main causes of surface water in a field if they are blocked. Drainage problems can also result from damage to soil structure, by the use of heavy machinery when the ground is wet, or by 'poaching' from animals left out in the winter. If damage to soil structure is suspected, advice should be sought from ADAS. Improvement can usually be achieved by subsoiling and pan bursting (to break up the top layer of heavily compacted soil). Such work has to be carried out by a specialist firm.

If a drainage system has to be installed, its design depends on soil structure, the lie of the land, and other natural features. In areas of clay soil, underground channels – preferably in a herringbone design and connected to piped major drains – can be successful. It is possible to install drainage pipes by machines without disturbing the top surface. In all cases, professional advice from a reputable firm should be sought.

Harrowing

Before allowing tractors on to a field, the surface should be sufficiently firm to take the weight without damaging soil structure.

Harrowing should begin as soon as the land is dry enough. Depending on the season and the soil, this may range from late February to early April. A spiked or pitch-pole type harrow is the most efficient, as it removes the dead grass and moss, aerates the soil, and encourages new growth. Chain harrowing to spread the dung and tidy the paddock may be carried out through the summer, when paddocks are rested, and preferably during hot, dry weather. In a dry season, the hot sun helps to desiccate the manure and kill off worm eggs and larvae. In a wet season, both eggs and larvae tend to thrive, so there is a danger in spreading the droppings over a wide area. They could increase the area of tainted pasture, especially in fields which do not drain well.

Rolling

Rolling is beneficial:

• If a severely poached field is to be used for riding. Rolling, followed by harrowing (to aerate the soil), will provide a level surface.

• If the field is to be cut for hay. Rolling can reduce the risk of damage by hay-making machinery when it is travelling over a rough surface.

• In early spring, when it can encourage early growth by raising soil temperature.

A light-ribbed Cambridge roller is most suitable. With certain soils – particularly clay and heavy loam – there is a risk that rolling may damage the soil structure and assist in the formation of an impervious pan. This inhibits growth and causes drainage problems. Such areas should not be rolled unless this is absolutely essential.

Fertilisers

In areas where soil fertility is good (usually a sign of careful management over many years), the application of fertiliser may not be essential. Lush grass is not required for horses, and unless other stock is available to graze off the first growth, the application of fertiliser can be unnecessary and indeed unwise. Ponies are quick to gorge on new grass, with resultant digestive upsets and risk of laminitis. Establishments with a limited acreage find that the application of suitable fertiliser is essential if grass is to be encouraged and weeds kept in check.

The four major substances necessary for healthy plant growth are lime, phosphate, potash and nitrogen. Magnesium is included in the soil analysis. Nitrogen is not included, as amounts vary according to the season and rainfall.

Following the soil analysis, local fertiliser firms who know about the soil features in the district can be consulted. Representatives may need to be reminded that horses have different grazing requirements from milking cows, beef cattle and sheep. A steady growth over a longer period is needed, not a lush growth of grass.

LIME Levels are measured on a 'pH' scale, 7.0 being neutral. A 'pH' level of 6.5 is suitable for grass – below this level the soil is acid, leading to the growth of poorer grass – above pH7 the soil is alkaline and the large amount of calcium results in the locking up of certain minerals. A high pH (excess lime) can seriously affect the growth of young stock. A level above pH7 is inevitable on chalk soil.

A deficiency of lime is usually adjusted by a dressing of limestone or chalk, both of which contain the calcium which is so important for healthy bone growth in the young horse. This dressing can be applied at any time of the year, but preferably in autumn or spring and on a calm day to avoid drift loss by the wind. In the past, basic slag was used, but it is now difficult to obtain.

Calcified seaweed is an excellent, organic fertiliser and it is not necessary to remove horses from the field for any length of time after it has been applied. However, it is not widely available.

PHOSPHORUS (P_2O_5 is phosphate) DEFRA have drawn up an ADAS index from 0–8. For horses, a suitable index should be 1–2. This allows for the phosphate level to be below the calcium level. This correct balance is essential for good bone development in young stock and general health. A low phosphate level, e.g. index 0, hinders grass growth.

ROCK PHOSPHATE This should not be applied unless the soil is very acid (below pH5), but experiments are continuing to make rock phosphate more soluble and thus more readily available to plants. Super-phosphate can cause sudden bone failure and should not be used.

POTASSIUM (K_2O_1 is potash) Potash is necessary for plant growth. An index level of ADAS 1–2 is suitable for grazing land. If hay is to be cut, then a dressing of potash after the hay has been taken corrects any loss. In general, if land is grazed by horses, potash levels once established remain constant. Little is known about the ingestion of this mineral by horses.

NITROGEN (N) Nitrogen is the key to grass growth, although success also depends on the correct balance of the lime, phosphate and potash. Nitrogen is leached out of the soil by rain, so it is best applied during the spring and summer months. Swards containing large amounts of clover manufacture their own organic nitrogen from bacteria on the clover root. It can make them self-supporting in nitrogen, but the amount of clover needed to achieve this is too much for horses. It can lead to digestive upsets and laminitis.

Too much nitrogen on grazing land, with resultant over-fast growth, can produce unsuitable grasses and a lack of balanced nutrients. This can affect the bone growth of young horses.

Application of Fertilisers

These are best applied in the spring when the field is not being grazed. If the grasses are to take full advantage of the treatment, a period of rest is advisable. Should this not be possible, the fields should be safe to graze once a liquid fertiliser has been washed in by a light shower or heavy dew, or the dry granules are not visible on the surface.

To save expense, a suitable mix of required fertilisers in either granulated or liquid form may be put on in one operation as a compound. Since grass growth for horses is required over a long period, it may be advisable to apply a small amount of nitrogen in the spring and some more later when the fields or paddocks are being rested.

Some people object to the continual use of chemical (inorganic) fertilisers. Owners of breeding stock often prefer to use organic fertilisers (such as farmyard manure or seaweed). These are slower-acting and more expensive but provide minerals which may otherwise be lacking. Adult horses, other than brood mares, are unlikely to be affected by the use of chemical fertilisers. There is normally a second natural growth of grass in September, and fertiliser applied in mid-August promotes this.

Manures

FARMYARD MANURE (FYM) If available, FYM is a complete fertiliser. It also sweetens those parts of a field which have been soured and made 'horse sick'. It provides material to improve soil texture, corrects any tendency for the soil to be alkaline, and supplies the main plant nutrients of phosphate, potash and nitrogen. It is best used on fields intended for hay and should be applied in the autumn when the weather and earthworm population can work it into the soil. If applied on grazing fields it should be stored for at least six weeks before use and the field should not be grazed for six weeks after spreading, to ensure that any infection is eliminated.

Unless linked to a farm or smallholding, the average horse establishment is unlikely to have any opportunity of obtaining FYM. It is sometimes possible to obtain cattle or pig slurry and also human sewage sludge from council sewage farms. The latter is treated and sterilised. All of these make excellent fertilisers, but are strong and therefore they should only be used in small quantities and not on grazing fields. They are suitable for hay fields, encouraging strong growth.

Once spread, the strong smell of any FYM or slurry can linger for days, which is a consideration for establishments dealing with the general public.

HORSE MANURE This is not as valuable as FYM and is generally inadvisable for fields grazed by horses, as it may increase the area of tainted grass. There is also a risk of worm infection, as it requires considerable heat over several weeks to kill worm eggs and larvae. Manure must be left to heat and rot well before applying. It can also increase the acidity of the soil.

Early Grazing

Grass starts to grow as soon as (a) soil temperature rises and (b) there is sufficient rainfall. If the sward is to profit from the treatment already outlined, it must not be grazed until the grasses are well established, i.e. approximately 10cm (4ins) tall. Earlier grazing is to the detriment of the better-quality grasses, which need to develop strong roots and invariably grow more slowly than the poorer grasses and weeds.

Rotation

Where there is sufficient acreage, a system of rotational grazing should be practised. This involves dividing large fields into smaller paddocks. An area of 3 acres is a useful grazing size. The divisions can be achieved either with permanent fencing or by the use of electric fencing (see Fences, later in this chapter). In early summer – i.e. May or June – the stocking rate could be as high as ten horses or fifteen ponies per paddock for periods from ten to fourteen days. The paddock may then need top-cutting, usually referred to as 'topping' (see below), and should be rested for three weeks before being grazed again. In July and August grass growth slows down and the paddocks take longer to recover. If more growth is required, they may benefit from some nitrogen. Growth accelerates again in September, but the first frosts check it until the following spring. In June, the grass which is surplus to grazing requirements may be cut for hay. An alternative is to cut grass daily and use it for fresh green feed for stabled horses. If possible, the paddocks chosen to be cut for hay or green feed should be rotated each year.

Top-Cutting

From June onwards, it may be necessary to mow over lightly or top-cut all paddocks. If horses stay in the field and if the weather is fine, much of this taller grass may be eaten as the sun helps to sweeten it. Any heavy patches of grass which remain should be forked up and burned. If left, they check the re-growth of the underneath grasses.

This topping is necessary to prevent weeds and uneaten coarse grasses from seeding and to encourage growth from the better grasses.

When you are topping, a careful watch should be kept for ragwort. It is sensible to have the paddocks searched before cutting is started. Any ragwort plants should be pulled up and burned. This task is most easily carried out after rain, when the ground is soft.

Over-Grazing

Fields which are over-grazed, and the sward not allowed time to recover and establish new growth, are bound to deteriorate. Such treatment can result only in the encouragement of weeds and coarse, unpalatable grasses, an increase in worm infestation, and the loss of what could be valuable grazing. Where the amount of land is limited, it is sensible to try to obtain alternative grazing, and certainly to avoid grazing any damp fields between October and May.

It should also be noted that the sward deteriorates if under-grazed and the grass allowed to seed.

Cattle as Alternative Grazers

Cattle make excellent followers-on for paddocks grazed by horses. They eat the coarse grasses rejected by horses, and ingest and kill the worm larvae deposited on the soil from the horse's dung. Sheep and goats can also help to free grass from worm larvae, but may require special fencing. Sheep in particular prefer short, sweet grass, similar to that enjoyed by horses. To buy cattle or sheep for the above purpose can be a considerable capital expense with no guarantee of a cash profit at the end of the summer. As an alternative, it may be possible to arrange for a neighbouring farmer to graze his cattle in return for hay or help with upkeep and field cultivation.

Picking up of Droppings

If time and labour are available, the daily picking up of droppings in small paddocks is extremely worthwhile. It decreases the worm infestation, improves the appearance of the field, and encourages the growth of more palatable grass. A vacuum machine, which collects droppings and can be attached to a tractor, is now on the market and is strongly recommended.

Horses usually drop mainly in one area of the field, so if the droppings are collected regularly the task is not so onerous.

Poaching

If animals are kept out during the winter months considerable damage can be done to a sward. Low-lying or clay soil areas are likely to be worst affected. Damage is caused by deep hoof prints in the sward, which in a wet season often remain full of water, adversely affecting the root system of the grasses. Exposure to frost causes further damage. If wintering out animals, it is sensible to use only one or two paddocks, preferably the best drained. Shelter, water and access must also be considered. In low-lying areas, in a wet season it is sensible for fields to be shut up in October and not grazed again until April or May. The decision to close the field depends on the season. Well-drained and/or hill fields may be safely grazed through the winter.

Fields on sandy soil are also less adversely affected.

Stocking Rate

This varies according to the following factors:

• Soil type and fertility.

• Length of grazing season.

• Rainfall.

• Period of daily grazing.

• Area of land available and whether divided into separate paddocks.

• Parasite control.

• Quality of management.

Given good soil fertility, an approximate stocking rate throughout the year would be one horse or two ponies per acre, or two horses or five ponies per hectare (possibly more during the summer months if grazing is very good). From October until the following May, supplementary feeding will be necessary. On land with poor fertility, this rate of stocking could be halved: one horse or two ponies per two acres. Supplementary feeding may be necessary from July onwards, particularly if the animals are working.

If rotational grazing is practised from May to October, three 3–acre paddocks with periods of rest should accommodate ten horses or fifteen ponies. The period of daily grazing affects the consumption of grass. Many private and riding school animals stand in during the day. Others, if working, may need to have their grazing time limited so that they will not become overweight.

IMPROVEMENT OF GRASSLAND

Reduction of 'Camp' Areas or 'Roughs'

These are areas of the field contaminated by the horse passing dung and urinating. The grass becomes coarse, horses refuse to graze it, and the sward rapidly deteriorates. The situation is worse on poorly drained soil.

Procedure

• Daily removal of droppings.

• Alternate grazing with cattle or sheep. Cattle and sheep eat down the coarse grass and also ingest and kill the worm larvae and eggs. Special attention to the fencing may be necessary to contain the animals.

• Regular top-cutting and resting of the field. This allows the grasses and plants to establish a healthy root system, which leads to increased growth.

• Use of farmyard manure.

Control of Weeds

• Good management encourages the better grasses, and discourages weeds: buttercups in particular. They are also a sign of acid soil.

• Some weeds, such as nettles, thistles and bracken, can be controlled or eradicated by regular cutting, i.e. six times in the growing season. This method may have to be repeated for a second year before success is achieved.

• Clumps of weeds, i.e. nettles, thistles and docks, can be treated by using a suitable herbicide applied directly on the clumps by a knapsack sprayer. Strict regulations exist concerning the use of sprays by untrained personnel. Unless used by the land owner a NPTC (National Proficiency Test Certificate) of competence must be held. This necessitates attendance by the individual at a one-day training course to ensure competence and gain a certificate in use and management of sprays.

If the weeds are widespread, total spraying of the field may be necessary. A weed-killer can often be combined with a fertiliser to give a boost to the fine-leaved grasses. It should be remembered that some selective weed-killers are effective against all broad-leaved species, and thus many other beneficial and appetising herbs will be destroyed. More sophisticated weed-killers are now available which may avoid this problem. There is specific legislation covering the spraying of weed-killers. This should be checked before any spraying is done. Professional advice should be sought.

Weed-killers should be applied in late spring when the plants are growing vigorously. In some cases, a second application will be necessary later in the summer when regrowth has occurred. Spraying should take place in calm weather to avoid drift and when rain is not expected for 24 hours. Some sprays are toxic to stock, so fields should not be grazed for some time after spraying. If poisonous plants are present – e.g. ragwort – they must have withered and crumbled before stock can return to the field. The residue of ragwort or bracken is still poisonous and should be removed.

Agricultural merchants can usually be trusted to give some advice as to the necessary type and quantity of weed-killer to use. For some species – e.g. docks and bracken – this has to be applied later in the summer. They will also advise as to which weed-killers are toxic to stock. It is important to remember that horses are much more sensitive to weed-killers than other stock.

Improving Pasture

Small areas of badly poached ground should be harrowed or, if necessary, raked over by hand. Suitable horse paddock mixture should then be broadcast, and the area should be rolled. For small areas a grass 'hand seeder' (on sale in specialist shops) can be used to introduce herbs into a pasture which is deficient in them. It is then advisable to treat a narrow strip of the field.

Whole fields can be improved by direct drilling or slot seeding. This work is usually undertaken by contractors. Advice should be taken as to whether (a) the soil is suitable and (b) the process is likely to succeed. The best times of year are spring or late summer, when the soil is warm and there is sufficient rain to germinate the seed. It may be advisable to kill off the poor-quality turf and weeds with herbicide. This will not affect the new seed and will ensure that the new grass has a good start and is not smothered by already established seeds. A special drill is used which cuts into the ground, making channels into which the grass seed and fertiliser are directed. The field is then rolled.

This process does not disturb the top layer of soil and encourages the rapid establishment of a dense sward, which can be grazed by horses at a much earlier date. It is of particular value in fields where stones and flints are close to the surface. If such fields are ploughed, the surface can be unsuitable for riding and schooling horses for several years.

Ploughing and Re-Seeding

It is now considered more sensible to improve pasture by good management and perhaps by direct drilling, rather than by ploughing up and re-seeding. Ploughing should only be resorted to in urgent cases where the sward appears to have gone beyond reclaim. Advice should be sought from the local ADAS office.

Ploughing and re-seeding are usually undertaken by local contractors in late summer. The old poor-quality, weed-infested turf can be killed off by herbicide. The field is then ploughed, and then scarified to make a suitable seed bed. Seed and fertiliser are drilled together and the field is rolled. The following summer, the field is best grazed by sheep to consolidate and encourage a dense sward. In the first year it should not be ridden on, but a hay crop may be taken. It can be grazed by horses in late summer, but in a wet season care should be taken to ensure that it does not get poached. If the new grasses are to thrive it will require careful management. There will be competition from indigenous plants, which may have been germinated with the ploughing.

Special seed mixtures are now available for horse pasture. Advice should be taken as to whether they are suitable for the particular area. They contain appropriate quantities of grasses palatable to horses and some clover and selected herbs. Hardy grasses which will withstand being ridden on should also be a consideration when choosing the seed mix if the grassland is to be all-purpose.

GRASSES

The requirements for horse pasture are prostrate growing grasses with a good bottom growth and the ability to produce a dense sward. The following grasses are of value:

- Perennial rye grass. There are several varieties, which are all of value.

- Smooth meadow grass, known in the USA as 'Kentucky blue grass'.

- Creeping red fescue.

- Chewing fescue.

- Sheep's fescue.

- Tall fescue.

- White clover in small quantities. Too high a percentage of clover will make the grass too nitrogen-rich. Clover can also be slippery to ride on.

- Timothy, cocksfoot and the tall, early rye grass (Lolium spp) are all suitable for hay, but do not make good grazing for horses or a hard-wearing sward.

Some grasses, which on fertile soil would be classed as weeds and therefore undesirable, have advantage where the soil is poor in natural fertility, e.g. hill areas. In such areas, some of the better grasses will not flourish. Crested dog's tail, sweet vernal and common bent grass all flourish on poor soil, but they only provide third-rate pasture (often suitable for ponies).

Comprehensive research is being carried out into the development of new strains of grasses, which may in time supersede the strains recommended above.

The altitude of the fields will also make a difference to the choice of grasses. Taking local expert advice is always recommended.

HERBS

Horses relish herbs, which provide nutrients often lacking in more shallow-rooted species. The following are of value:

- Narrow-leaved plantain.

- Yarrow.

- Dandelion.

- Chicory.

- Comfrey.

- Ribwort.

- Burnet.

HAYMAKING

Aspects of haymaking which need consideration are:

- The sward should be of a reasonable quality. Fields infested with weeds and growing inferior grasses with only a small proportion of good grasses are not suitable.

- When the fields are shut off for hay, sufficient grazing should be available. Depending on soil fertility, sward and rainfall, hay fields will not be ready for grazing for at least four to six weeks after cutting.

- It is not economical to buy haymaking machinery for small acreages, so a local contractor or a neighbouring farmer should be hired to do the work. Such arrangements often result in small acreages being left until last, which will mean the risk of deteriorating weather, a crop of poor quality, and grass past its best.

- Fertilisers cost money, but they are necessary if the crop is to be worth harvesting. Contractors charge per acre for cutting and turning. A poor crop of grass can often be just as costly to make as a heavy crop, although baling costs will be less.

The **advantages** of making your own hay are:

- The hay (subject to the factors mentioned above) will be of good quality and cost less to make and store than buying from a corn merchant.

- The fields should benefit from being cut for hay; good grasses will be encouraged and weeds and inferior grass cut before being allowed to seed. The sward, if well harrowed, improves by not being continually trodden.

- In May and June, establishments with ample grazing have an over-abundance of grass. Unless this is (a) set aside for hay, (b) cut as green fodder for stabled horses, or (c) efficiently grazed, the sward deteriorates. Grasses are likely to be swamped by stronger-growing varieties and weeds. Cattle can be bought in to eat off this grass. This is an expensive capital outlay and not necessarily profitable.

The **disadvantage** is that it is very likely that horses and ponies will dislike and not eat hay that has been made from pastures that have been grazed only by horses.

Preparation of Hay Fields

Meadow hay is made from fields of permanent grass specially 'shut up' (not grazed). Low-lying fields should not be grazed during the winter, in order to avoid poaching of the ground. In early spring, fields should be harrowed and fertiliser should be spread; rolling is not usually necessary, and can be detrimental by increasing panning. The grass can then be left to grow. Before cutting it must be checked for ragwort.

On dry, well-drained fields it is possible to allow grazing during the winter and not to 'shut up' until mid-April. Harrowing and fertilising can then be carried out. Though the resultant crop will not be as heavy and will be late growing, it can provide a useful supply of hay.

Seed hay is made from fields specially sown, called leys. They may not have been grazed at all; the turf may not be established, and grazing – particularly if the ground is soft – would seriously damage the sward. The crop is much heavier than that from permanent pasture, and may take longer to 'make'. It should be of superior quality because of the specific choice of grasses sown, and also free from weeds.

Cutting and Baling the Hay

Hay is made by cutting the grass preferably just before flowering, but if the weather is uncertain it may have to be delayed. The grass is left lying in rows. After a few hours of hot sun the top surface begins to wilt. The grass is scattered by a machine, a process known as 'teddering', which scatters the rows of grass and allows wind and sun to penetrate and dry the crop. A heavy crop will need teddering at least twice; after rain it may need to be done several times. When the hay feels dry and crisp it can be 'rowed up' (two rows put into one) ready for baling.

The hay should then be baled. If the baling is not completed in a day, the hay must be turned again the following morning so that it will be dry and crisp. If the baler is drawing a sledge, the bales can be left in convenient stands of eight to twelve. This makes for quicker and more convenient carting. If there is no sledge, the bales should be stood up in groups of four. The knots of the baling strings should be at the bottom of the bale nearest to the ground. Hay stacked in this manner 'shoots' any rain.

It is usual to cart the bales as soon as possible. However, if the weather is settled, the bales improve by being left out in the field for a few days before carting, so that they can sweat and dry naturally. There will then be less risk of overheating.

The making of good hay is a skilled process. Fine weather is essential. In a wet summer, good hay can be difficult to make and find.

With fewer contractors and farmers making hay and the machinery used for making small bales becoming older, it can be difficult to make good, small bale hay.

Silage

Silage is cut from young grass (5–10cm/2–4ins) and carted at once, with no wilting. It is stored in a 'clamp'. Here the grass is piled up and covered tightly with polythene sheeting. Air is excluded. The grass then 'pickles' and preserves in its own juices. This method of grass preservation is primarily used for feeding cattle. As ruminants, cattle are able to further ferment and digest any bacterial contamination possibly associated with the close cutting of the grass to the soil surface (e.g. botulism). While some use is made of silage for horses and they thrive on and enjoy the rich nutritional forage, there is an element of risk when feeding it.

With the improved methods of making haylage in both big and small bales, especially for horses, the feeding of silage is not recommended.

Haylage/Big Bale Silage

This is harvested from grass older than that taken for silage but younger than grass to be taken for hay. The cut grass is left to wilt for 24 hours or even longer and is almost as dry as hay before being vacuum-packed in sealed polythene bags. Depending on the manufacturer the bags may be round or square and vary in size from 20kg (45lbs) up to large bales which can only be moved mechanically with a tractor or fork-lift truck.

Contractors who produce haylage especially for horses often cut the grass a little higher than they would for cattle. This helps to prevent contamination of the grass which can occur especially if there are mole hills in the pasture. Haylage contamination by earth can lead to botulism in horses. This is fatal.

Haylage is widely used as a dust-free forage for competition horses. It is nutritious but higher in water content than hay. It has less fibre than hay and horses tend to eat it quite quickly.

It is often useful to mix it with good quality oat or barley straw to prolong the chewing process and ensure the horse has enough fibre in his diet. Because of the nutritional value of haylage, it is usually possible to reduce the concentrate intake for the horse thus making an economic saving.

Storage of haylage is a major consideration. While it can be safely stored outside it must not be vulnerable to accidental puncture by vermin or machinery. If the vacuum is broken, contact with air will cause spoiling of the contents and there will be a risk of bacterial contamination if fed to horses. Once a bale is opened it should be fed in three to five days (depending on the weather – it will keep longer in winter). Some smaller yards would be unable to utilise the big bales satisfactorily (see also page 175).

One very satisfactory method of using haylage is for the bales to remain with the producer and be delivered on a regular basis, supplying only bales in perfect condition.

This is only practical if the producer is local. Less than perfect bales are often used for cattle, who have a more robust digestive system than horses.

MANAGEMENT OF HORSES AND PONIES AT GRASS

In most parts of Britain, ponies and cobs can be kept out throughout the year. It is their natural lifestyle, especially if they are part of a herd. If suitably fed and properly looked after, they keep healthy and sufficiently fit for hacking and light to medium work. Most of them can withstand dry cold and freezing temperatures. The worst possible conditions are cold, driving rain, inadequate shelter and a wet, poorly drained field. In such weather conditions, horses benefit from New Zealand rugs.

The better-quality animals with lighter coats do less well in winter, and will benefit from being stabled at night. Those turned out by day may wear a New Zealand rug (see Clothing, Chapter 32). If stabling is not available, quality animals need extra concentrate food to maintain body heat. This should maintain their health, but if they are to keep their condition they must be very well looked after.

FIELDS

Appropriate Fields

Though your choice may be limited, before buying or renting a field to be grazed by horses you should first consider the location, the type of land and the keep. The following factors should be considered:

- The field must be easily accessible in winter, so that the horses can be fed and the water supply checked.

- Well-managed, old-established ley or meadow field is

the best type of grazing. It provides a great variety of grasses and herbs, whereas a newly sown ley often lacks herbs in the sward. Old turf also provides the thick sward which is important for maintaining the soundness of young, growing stock and will stand up to poaching better than newer leys.

- Rich pasture makes most animals fat and more liable to laminitis; sudden access to lush growth can cause laminitis, even in thin ponies. A strict system of controlled grazing may have to be practised.

- If the fields are wet and marshy animals will not thrive on them in winter. In summer, however, as the grass is often of poor quality, it suits ponies likely to get over-fat.

- High, exposed fields lacking shelter are very cold in winter and provide no escape from sun and flies in summer.

- Gently sloping fields encourage horses and ponies to maintain some fitness.

- Very steep fields are only suitable for small ponies. Larger ponies and horses – particularly young stock – may develop back, hock and/or stifle strains.

- Small paddocks can be invaluable in providing limited grazing for small ponies, or a daily exercise area for a stabled horse. They can, however, become heavily poached in winter. In general, horses are happier and thrive better in larger fields where there is more room.

- Low-lying fields or those with a clay-based soil are not

suitable for winter grazing. The land becomes poached – i.e. cut up – with the roots of the grass exposed and often killed by frost. The quality of the pasture then deteriorates. Animals standing in mud are reluctant to lie down to rest and may develop skin problems such as mud fever and cracked heels. Much of the hay fed in the field is trampled in and lost.

WATER SUPPLY (SEE ALSO CHAPTER 19)

A regular water supply is essential for health. If piped water or a suitable unpolluted stream is not available, alternative arrangements have to be made. When grass is plentiful and rainfall normal, a horse may well drink less than 4.5 litres (1 gallon) a day, the extra water intake being provided in the grass. In hot weather, when the grass is dry, or in freezing weather when the horse's diet is hay or other dry food, his daily water consumption is much greater, up to 45–54 litres (10–12 gallons) a day.

Water Troughs

The best way to ensure a satisfactory supply of water is to pipe it to a carefully sited concrete or metal trough and control it with a covered ballcock system. As the horse drinks and the water level drops, the ballcock drops with it; this releases a valve and allows the water to flow. As the trough fills, the ballcock rises with the water level and the valve shuts off the supply. This system usually works without problems. However, on occasions, the valve can stick and restrict the water, or the ballcock can puncture, so that the water will not be cut off and will spill over, causing flooding. Daily inspection is advisable.

Troughs vary in size and can hold as much as 900 litres (200 gallons). They should relate to the size of field and the normal stocking rate, and should be large enough to allow several animals to drink at once.

Old baths and other metal and plastic containers are often used in small paddocks as a cheap alternative to purpose-built water troughs. These are suitable as long as there are no projecting edges likely to cause injury. Boxed-in baths are safer and less of an eyesore. If they are filled by piped water and a tap, the tap should be placed out of reach of the horses, so they cannot play with it or get caught up.

If they are close to a suitable supply, water troughs can be filled by means of a hosepipe. When the trough is full, the hose should be moved out of the way so that water will not syphon out. In freezing weather, the trough should be emptied. If water has to be transported, 25–45 litre (5½–10 gallon) plastic water containers can be used. A strong wooden broom put through the hand grips enables two people to carry the container more easily.

Siting of a Water Trough

The cost of piping may influence the siting of your trough.

It should preferably be sited in a well-drained area of the field, away from the corner and near enough to the gate for easy checking. Do not put it near trees, as their roots make pipe-laying difficult and in autumn their leaves foul the water.

Troughs can be placed lengthways along a fence line, so that there is the minimum of projection on which a horse can knock his legs. In this position they can be made available to an adjoining field. Rails or boards built above the trough will prevent horses jumping out or fighting above it.

If sited away from the fence line, troughs should be at least 10m (33ft) into the field and well away from the corner, so that there is less risk of a horse being trapped and kicked.

All troughs should be set on solid brick or concrete supports.

The ground surrounding a water trough may become poached. Horses' legs can get very muddy, with the consequent risk of mud fever and cracked heels. Thick mud may also discourage regular drinking. To avoid these problems, loads of rubble, stone or rammed chalk

Metal water trough with a covered ballcock system.

can be put down, or a roughened concrete apron (approximately 10m² (33ft²) can be placed up to or around the trough (but note that in freezing weather the surface can become slippery, in which case straw should be put down).

Water troughs must be kept clean, so they should be scrubbed out regularly. During the process, the ballcock should be tied up. Troughs which do not have a base outlet must be emptied by bucket. A plastic dustpan is useful to finish the job.

Precautions in Freezing Weather

All exposed piping should be lagged and then boarded. The cavity should be filled with fibreglass. This system also helps to prevent the pipe freezing in the ground.

If metal pipes should freeze, they can be thawed out by covering them with straw and then setting light to it, or by using a blow lamp. Remember that as ballcocks are usually made of plastic they will puncture if exposed to flame.

With plastic piping, hot water can be poured over the pipe, which may also thaw the ballcock. Frozen plastic piping should not be subjected to direct flame, e.g. a blow lamp or burning straw.

When water freezes in the pipes, they can split or loosen at the joints, causing floods when it thaws. It is then necessary to turn off the water at the mains. The location of all stop-cocks should be noted.

In freezing weather, ice on a water trough must be broken each morning. Horses drinking during the day help to keep the water from freezing, but in very cold weather it may be necessary to re-break the ice at night. These tasks must never be neglected.

It is not advisable to throw thick lumps of ice on the ground. They can stick to the frozen earth and make walking and standing difficult.

Sometimes adding buckets of hot water to the trough will melt the ice and not leave jagged edges.

If some salt is added to the water it will take longer to freeze.

Rivers and Streams

This water supply can be satisfactory as long as the watering place is safe and the water unpolluted. There must be a sound approach area, sufficiently wide for several animals to be able to drink at once. If the stream is a field boundary, fencing should be constructed to prevent horses crossing over or moving up or down the stream.

Streams with steep banks must have the approach area set well back so that the slope is less steep. Streams with a sandy bottom are not suitable, as a horse when drinking absorbs a certain amount of sand and this in time can cause sand colic. Streams adjoining or near buildings are often polluted by farm or stable drains, or by a neighbouring factory. If there is any doubt, a sample of water should be sent for testing. It is illegal to pollute any water source.

Stagnant ponds should be fenced off, as they are not suitable drinking places.

POISONOUS PLANTS

Ragwort, buttercup, bracken, cowbane, foxglove, deadly nightshade, horsetails, meadow saffron, water dropwort and leaves of most evergreen plants are all poisonous to horses. Fortunately, their bitter flavour ensures that as long as other grazing is available, they are rarely eaten. Occasionally an animal develops a taste for one of them and will suffer 'colic' or may even die.

When found in hay, poisonous plants are particularly dangerous – except buttercup, which when cut and dried loses its toxic properties. Old pasture which is about to be cut for hay should be closely examined, especially for ragwort.

After the use of weed-killer some of the plants listed above become palatable, so stock should not be allowed into a field which has been sprayed until all such plants have rotted down or been removed.

RAGWORT Of the above plants, ragwort is the most common, and the one most likely to be eaten. In winter and early spring, young plants can be recognised by their prostrate growth and distinctive leaf shape. They bloom in July, August and September, when the yellow flowers can be easily seen. Mature plants grow to a height of 90–120cm (3–4ft). Young plants may only be 10–15cm (4–6ins) in height. When cut, pulled, or poisoned by herbicides, they become palatable. If you are top-cutting fields in July and August, take particular care either to pull up the plants or to pick up the cut plants and burn them. This is even more important if the grass is cut for hay.

The poison from ragwort acts on the liver and has a cumulative and long-term effect, which is usually fatal. Grazing with sheep in the early spring may eliminate ragwort.

YEW All parts of a yew tree are poisonous, even when the tree is dead. It appears to be palatable. Twigs falling off a tree are easily eaten with a mouthful of grass. Even a small quantity can be lethal. If a horse snatches at yew tree branches when being ridden through woods, the rider should dismount and remove all of it from the animal's mouth.

DEADLY NIGHTSHADE The berries, although rarely eaten by horses, are poisonous. They are brown to purple in colour. The plant is found as a creeper on hedges only in very limited areas. The less toxic plant, woody nightshade, which has red berries and a purple flower, is more common. Hedges should be checked and any plants pulled out and burned.

WATER DROPWORT is only likely to be a problem after deep ditching.

Ornamental hedges and trees such as **LABURNUM, LAUREL, PRIVET** and **RHODODENDRON,** are more often found in the hedges or boundaries of fields adjoining parks and gardens. It is seldom possible to have them removed, so the area surrounding them should be fenced off. Laburnum seeds are particularly lethal. However, horses are unlikely to eat them unless very hungry.

ACORNS and **CRAB APPLES** Fields containing oak and crab apple trees should be carefully checked in the autumn when the ripe acorns and fruit have fallen. Horses eat both acorns and crab apples. A small quantity does no harm, but a large quantity of acorns causes poisoning, and of crab apples, severe colic.

Weeds such as **DAISIES, DOCKS, CHICKWEED** and **BROAD-LEAVED PLANTAIN** are of no food value. Their presence in a pasture reveals poor management. They are rarely eaten, unless cut with the hay. A large quantity of docks can then cause a digestive upset.

NETTLES, THISTLES and **DANDELIONS** are all relished by the horse when cut, but their presence signifies poor grass management.

GARDEN WASTE Pony paddocks in suburban areas may have grass mowings or weeds thrown into them in the mistaken belief that they are good for horses.

They must be removed immediately as they may contain poisonous plants, and grass mowings can cause colic or even death. Either fence off the area or try to educate the neighbours.

LITTER

Fields which have roadside hedges or which are crossed by a public footpath should be inspected regularly for tins, broken bottles and other litter. In some areas, such fields require daily checking.

Fields newly acquired should be checked for abandoned farm implements such as harrows, which can be covered with grass and go unnoticed. Binder twine from used hay bales, or on occasions from rotted-down old bales, can also be very dangerous and should be picked up as it can entangle an animal's legs.

RABBIT HOLES

Fields in which rabbits are known to live should be checked regularly for holes. This is particularly important if foals or young stock are grazing them. Unsafe areas may have to be fenced off.

SHELTER

This is essential to protect horses from cold winds, driving snow and rain and in summer from hot sun and flies. A field bounded by thick hedges, stone walls or banks provides shelter in winter. Any trees give shelter from the sun.

Field Shelter

The only effective escape from insects is a field shelter. This is more likely to be used as a refuge from flies in summer than from cold in winter. If well positioned, artificial wind breaks made from stone, sleeper walls or heavy plastic mesh, give welcome shelter in winter.

A field shelter should be placed either against the fence or well away from it, with the back of the shed to the prevailing wind. If placed well out in the field it gives some shelter from several directions. Open-fronted L-shaped sheds are the most practical, and they ensure

A good field shelter.

that no horse can get trapped inside by another horse.

In poor draining areas, a concrete floor may be laid, with an apron extending well beyond the shed. A cheaper alternative is to put down loads of stone, rubble or rammed chalk, according to availability. The floor area should always be kept well strawed down. Concrete can be slippery in freezing weather. On well-draining soil, with the shed on a slight slope, a base may not be necessary.

Shelter sizes vary from a pony-type structure 3m x 3m (10ft x 10ft) to buildings of 12m x 18m (40ft x 60ft) which hold a number of animals. They must be strongly constructed to withstand horses rubbing against them. Some field-shelter manufacturers insist on a concrete base. In certain districts, planning permission is necessary.

Shelters should be kept regularly free of droppings and once or twice a year they should be thoroughly hosed out and disinfected.

FENCES

It is the responsibility of the stock keeper to ensure that his fields are securely fenced. Animals who get out on a road can cause accidents, damage to life and property, and often fatal injury to themselves. They can also damage crops and gardens. It is possible to insure against these risks, but insurance companies rightly expect suitable care to be taken. An habitual escaper who causes damage may be responsible for his owner being taken to court. Subsequent insurance may be difficult to obtain and expensive. Animals who make a habit of getting out can rarely be contained against their will. A 1.5–1.8m (5–6ft) gate or fence is no deterrent; however, electric fencing will usually contain them.

If cattle or sheep are kept, either to run with horses or to provide alternate grazing, fencing must be strong enough to contain 'gadding cattle' (when pestered by flies in summer), and with the rails sufficiently close to contain sheep.

Owners of valuable stud and competition horses should take greater care with the choice of fencing. It must be secure and safe. If the animals are kept in adjoining fields it is best to separate them with a double line of fencing approximately 1.8m (6ft) apart, which prevents squealing and playing over the fence. An electric fence alongside the permanent fence will safely separate animals.

Hedges

A well-trimmed, thick hedge is the best type of field fencing. It should be kept at a height of 1.2–1.5m (4–5ft) and should be cut back annually to encourage growth at the bottom. This work can be carried out by arrangement with a neighbouring farmer or a contractor. If it is done regularly by mechanical means the hedge trimmings will be chopped up by the machine and can be left to rot. Older, overgrown hedges have to be cut by a large circular-saw type of machine, and the large hedge trimmings should be collected and burned. Weak, long and straggly parts of a thorn hedge can be cut and laid. Elder should be dug out or cut down, as it weakens the other parts of the hedge line; its only use is as a protection from flies, and for this purpose two or three large bushes can be left. Holly should be encouraged, as it gives good winter shelter. Yew, because it is poisonous, should be completely cut out.

Hedges under trees are often weak. Any gaps or weak parts should be filled with solid, treated posts and rails.

Plain wire is inadvisable. Barbed wire should not be used.

It is natural for horses to browse. They may well take great pleasure in barking any trees left unprotected. Plastic mesh laced round the trunks, or a protective guard of posts and rails, will keep horses away from trees: note that link fencing or wire netting can be dangerous if horses strike or stamp at flies.

Walls

In certain parts of the country, stone walls are used as field boundaries. If they are of a suitable height and are kept in good repair they are stock-proof and safe, and provide good shelter. A low wall may need a rail above it to prevent animals jumping out. In the case of cobs and ponies, a cheaper alternative is one or two strands of well-tightened, plain wire or an electric fence.

All wire fences should have strainers at intervals to keep the wire taut.

Banks

Banks are found in Ireland, the west of England, and in some other areas. They give good shelter, but to be stock-proof low banks require topping with a hedge, rails or wire. Some banks have a deep drainage ditch on one side, which can be a danger to young stock and should be fenced off. Steep banks can present a hazard, particularly to foaling mares and young stock, and it is often safer to fence them off. It may also be necessary to fence across a ditch or stream at the field boundary.

Post and Rail

If in good repair, these make safe, stock-proof fences. Though expensive, they have a life expectancy of over twenty years, but can be damaged by chewing, rubbing and leaning. They should be regularly treated or painted if the rails were not tanalised before being used. Broken rails must be replaced promptly as the split timber and any exposed nails can be a danger; morticed rails, though less easy to replace, are safer, as no nails are

Post and rail fencing with safe corner.

used. If the rails are nailed, they should be set on the inside of the posts. This way they will not be pushed out if an animal leans on them.

Fence posts should be sawn off at an angle, flush with the top rail. If horses try to jump out, projecting posts can cause damage.

Stud Rails

These make a safe, secure fence: they are more durable than wood, will not split, will not be chewed, and require less upkeep. In many cases they are also cheaper. From an environmental aspect, however, some people consider them to be less attractive.

Stud rails consist of plastic strips 10cm (4ins) wide, incorporating high-tensile wire. The strips come in rolls and are erected either on wooden or plastic posts. Three or more lines of rail strips are used. A cheaper but less substantial alternative is a plastic rail at the top with two or three lines of plain wire below. This fence requires very exact straining. It stands up to considerable impact and also has some resilience. In time it stretches and requires tightening.

High-Tensile Wire Mesh Fencing

This is a heavy-duty wire mesh, preferably topped with a wooden or plastic rail to give clear visibility. It is cheaper than stud rail, and is escape-proof against any stock, but it presents the risk that animals – particularly foals or small ponies – may put their feet through the

mesh and get caught. Small, diamond-shaped mesh will considerably lessen the risk, but horse owners should be aware of dangers. Mesh fencing must be well maintained and checked for any holes and tears.

Plain Wire

If well erected and firmly strained, this can be the economic answer to many fencing problems. Topped with a rail, it makes a more solid, clearly sighted fence without too much expense. The drawback is that horses may loosen the wire by putting their heads through and leaning on it; this can be prevented by using electrified wire. High-tensile steel wire is more expensive than ordinary wire; it is less easy to work with and requires greater skill to erect, but it lasts twice as long. However, if horses cut themselves on it the wounds tend to be very severe.

Plain wire can be seen more easily by animals if pieces of coloured cloth are tied between posts.

Barbed Wire

Barbed wire is not recommended but it is cheap and effective, and if it is well maintained and regularly inspected the risk is diminished. If barbed wire must be used, the safest place to put it is as the second line of wire with a single strand of plain wire above and two strands of plain wire below.

Electric Fencing

This is cheap and easily erected. Its main uses are:

- To keep horses away from a weakened hedge-line, fence or boundary.

- To provide safe separation from horses in adjoining fields.

- To permit strip-grazing of a field.

- To divide fields temporarily so that areas can be rested.

Electric fencing.

• To help prevent horses/ponies jumping out of their field.

It should be placed 1.5–1.8m (5–6ft) from the boundary fence.

The fencing usually runs off a portable unit containing a 6-volt battery. However, if it is close to a mains electricity supply, it can be wired to this, with a transformer which will reduce the voltage to approximately 6 volts.

The fencing material consists of:

• Iron or plastic-coated posts with insulators at the top. These can be heeled into the ground. The latter are less likely to cause injury.

• Wooden posts with insulators attached. This type is preferred for permanent fencing. Iron or plastic posts are easier to erect if the fence is temporary, or has to be moved each day as in strip-grazing.

• Plain round wire or tape strips stretched between the posts and attached to insulators at either end. The latter can be seen more easily. It is essential to cut back any long grass or overhanging hedge so that there is no risk of earthing the current, which – particularly in wet weather – will very quickly run down the battery. It is important to check the wire each day and to test the strength of the current with a fence tester. Horses are quick to take advantage of a weak or dead battery.

Electric fencing should not be placed underneath or parallel to overhead electric cables, as there can be some risk of the current being diverted down the wire. When moving a fence it is important to ensure that all posts are well heeled in, that insulators are sound, and that attachments to hedges and gate posts have an insulator to break the current.

If netting-type electric fencing is used (which is excellent if sheep are being contained) it must be set above the grass height.

When first introducing animals to an electric fence, it helps to make them respect it if they are given a shock by feeding them close to the wire. Some horses never gain that respect, and happily jump out. Ponies with thick manes often run underneath. Such animals can sometimes be controlled by putting up two parallel lines of electric fencing. If this fails, they should not be turned out in a field with electric fencing, as they will encourage others in the field to imitate their bad habits.

ERECTION OF FENCES

Post and Rail and Wire

Posts should be at a minimum height of 105cm (3ft 6ins), but preferably 120cm (4ft) above the ground and 46cm (18ins) below the ground. Posts may be of timber or concrete. All timber should be treated with preservative. Droppers (lightweight wood or steel slats) can be used between posts to keep wire taut. Posts should face outwards with the rails inwards towards the field.

When erecting a fence, sharp corners and angles should be avoided, unless the posts can be stayed efficiently.

Heavy strainer posts should be placed at all corners, at changes of direction, and/or at intervals of 50m (54yds). They should be dug 75cm (2ft 6ins) into the ground. Stud rails and stud fences can usually be erected by the suppliers.

When renewing a fence, all old wire must be taken up and removed. To reduce the danger of a horse or pony getting a foot over the wire, the bottom strand should be of plain wire and never be lower than 38cm (15ins) from the ground. Another hazard is that if shod horses

Two strands of plain wire safely fitted below a plastic rail.

in adjoining fields start squealing and pawing through the fence, the bottom wire can get caught between the heel of the shoes and the heel of the horse as he pulls his foot back.

This usually entails cutting the horse free so wire cutters must always be readily available if this type of fencing is used.

If a lot of fencing needs doing it may well be cheaper in the long run to call in a contractor who has all the right machinery and expertise.

UNSUITABLE FENCING

For safety reasons, the following fencing cannot be recommended, as there can be a risk of horses getting caught up:

- Wire netting.

- Sheep or pig wire.

- Chestnut fencing.

- Old iron rails. These are likely to spring out of line, and the iron spikes can cause nasty injuries to horses.

- Barbed wire.

GATES

Wooden Gates

Oak is the most suitable type of wood. It is expensive, but it does not warp, and it lasts for forty years or more.

Softwood gates, though much cheaper, are inclined to warp, and the timber breaks more easily.

Gate-posts should be of oak, set 90cm (3ft) in the ground. They should be hard-rammed with stone filling, or set in concrete. Old railway sleepers make a suitable alternative.

All timber should be treated with preservative. Hinges should be of galvanised steel and of a strength suitable for the gate.

Fastenings should be of a secure type, with no sharp projecting edges on which a horse can get caught. When fastened, they should help to take the weight of the gate, preventing it from dropping.

Metal Gates

If of heavy-duty construction, metal gates are satisfactory. Lightweight metal has a limited life; it is easily bent and the spars can fracture or come apart from the framework, exposing dangerous edges. Posts are usually of metal set in concrete, but wooden posts can be used. All metalwork should be treated with rust-resistant solution and kept regularly painted. The hinges and fastenings used for wooden gates are suitable.

Hanging Gates

If gates are to last, they must be well hung, so that when opened they clear the ground and do not have to be lifted or dragged. If farm machinery has to go through the gateway it may be preferable to have double gates with a removable post at the centre. However, gates must be made absolutely secure against thieves and rustlers.

Padlocks

Owing to the increase in horse thefts, it is advisable to padlock any gates opening on to roads. The hinge end of the gate should be secured by a chain and padlock, or by a metal bolt driven in above the top hinge so that it cannot be opened by lifting it off its hinges.

Gateways

Gateways can become very muddy in winter. They can be improved with loads of stone, chalk or rubble, or by a roughened concrete apron. Surface water should be directed off the surrounding area by drains or ditches.

FEEDING

Summer

In summer, many horses and ponies at grass become too fat. If they are resting or only in light work (four hours a week), they are unlikely to require extra food. If they are on good grass, their grazing time may need to be restricted. If they are in heavier work and if the grazing is poor or limited, they may need a daily or twice-daily ration of hard feed. For amounts to feed, see Chapter 23.

Winter

In winter, supplementary feeding is essential. Hay should start being fed as soon as the horse shows interest when it is put out in the field. As long as there is grass to eat, they prefer this to hay. At first, they may only require hay at night, but as the grass diminishes, hay should be fed in the morning as well. If good hay is fed and not cleared up, this means that too much is being fed, and the ration should be cut down until all is cleared up.

If the hay is of inferior quality, it will often be left. This should not be taken as a sign that too much is being put out, but rather that the quality of the hay needs improving.

In wet weather, some hay is bound to get spoiled and to be trodden into the mud. In frosty weather, when the ground is hard, the horses should clear up all hay put down.

Methods of Feeding Hay

If one or two animals are kept, hay may be fed in haynets, which must be securely tied to a fence or tree and placed at least 3.5m (12ft) apart. In wet weather all animals prefer to eat with their heads down and their backs to the wind, so haynets may then be unwelcome.

If more than two animals are turned out together, hay should be fed on the ground. It should be placed in the most sheltered part and on the least muddy area, even if this involves taking it to the far end of the field. Hay should be put out in slices, according to weight, and not shaken up as it will then be less likely to be spoiled. Heaps should be at least 3.5m (12ft) apart, and there should be two or three more heaps than horses to allow for them moving about. If there are ten or more animals and if the weather permits, it is better to put the hay out in a larger circle. To check any fighting or bullying, wait and watch until all horses are settled and eating.

Herds of horses and ponies who live permanently together will usually feed amicably together from the types of hay racks supplied to farmers.

Choose the design most suitable for your stock and type of forage and shape of bale. They can be easier to refill and prevent a lot of waste. If they are placed on a hard standing there will be less likelihood of the animals getting cracked heels or mud fever.

Quantities

Good-quality meadow hay is suitable for feeding in the field.

If there is little or no grass, the following feed scale is suggested:

Small ponies	4.5–5.4kg (10–12lbs) hay
Medium ponies	4.5–6.8kg (12–15lbs) hay
Large ponies and cobs	6.8–9kg (15–20lbs) hay
Large cobs and horses	11.3–13.6kg (25–30lbs) hay

When the horses and ponies are of mixed sizes the hay ration at the beginning of winter should be about 4.5kg (10lbs) per animal. As winter progresses, this ration can be increased to 6.8–9kg (15–20lbs) per animal, depending on the weather and if it is being cleared.

In snow or freezing weather, extra hay must be given; it will not be wasted. Animals require extra food for warmth, and the process of eating and digestion helps to keep them warm and content. Their daily ration cannot be equated with that of a similar-sized horse kept in a warm stable. More food is necessary.

If hay supplies are short, oat or barley straw can be fed on its own, or the straw can be fed mixed with hay. Well-bred animals will then require a high protein supplement.

Concentrates (see also Chapter 22)

Healthy, resting ponies or those in light work (two to four hours per week) do not necessarily need a daily feed.

Ponies under 12.2hh rarely require extra feed.

Ponies and cobs in heavier work require a twice-daily ration of hard food suitable for their size.

Horses wintered out should receive a twice-daily feed.

All animals in light or poor conditions should receive as much food as they will consume.

When feeding concentrates, if only two or three animals are kept they may be fed in the field, provided an attendant stays to prevent bullying and fighting. This is not safe with a large number, and they should be brought in and fed separately.

Feed Blocks

These are manufactured specifically for feeding to horses and ponies wintered out. Together with rough grazing and/or hay, they provide a balanced and nutritious diet. They are weather-resistant and can be placed on the ground in a container or suspended from a fence post or tree. They should be placed well away from the water supply.

For groups of horses, allow one block per four to five horses and follow the maker's instructions. Generally speaking, horses only take up as much as they need and there should be no problem. However, certain horses develop a craving and finish a block in a day or within

days. This makes it an expensive feed, and in some cases it has been known to cause severe colic.

COMPANY

Horses are by nature herd animals and they are much happier if part of a group. In summer, by standing head to tail they are able to ward off flies. If it is not possible to find another horse for company, then a donkey or even a goat can be a successful substitute.

To avoid fighting and possible injury, it is important that groups of horses turned out together should agree. It is often arranged that mares and geldings are kept in separate fields. For this reason, many riding schools only keep either mares or geldings. If groups are mixed, be sure that you do not put two aggressive leader-type animals in the same field. Generally speaking, once animals know each other and have sufficient room they sort themselves out and there should be no trouble. However, care must be taken when adding a new animal to an established group.

Consider removing hind shoes. This reduces the risk of damage. Ponies and cobs in light work or who do little or no road work can work very satisfactorily without shoes. This also saves on farrier's bills.

DAILY CARE

Horses should preferably be visited twice a day, and on one of these visits they should be checked at close quarters. An observant person quickly notices if all is not well, particularly if the same person checks the horses each day. Any unusual behaviour or stance will then be noticed. A horse who is standing away on his own, or who is unusually slow or unwilling to come up when food or hay is put out, should be examined more closely. In areas where horses have been vandalised, a daily check of the whole horse, especially the dock area, is advisable.

Horses should look well and healthy with:

- A bright, alert expression.

- Weight evenly taken on all four feet, or a hind leg only rested. Well-bred horses and young stock sometimes flex a knee when grazing. This is normal.

- No discharge from eyes or nose.

- No stiffness or unevenness of stride when moving off.

- In summer, the coat lying smoothly and showing a gloss. In winter the coat may be rough, but it should not be dull and staring. A horse with a tight staring or standing-up coat is cold and may be ill. He should be caught, stabled and his temperature taken.

Resting horses or young stock should be caught up at least twice a week and their feet, eyes, nose, skin and coat checked.

When observing a group of horses, a tit-bit may be handed out from a pocket, but a feed or catching bowl encourages competitive aggression, with a risk of injury to all concerned.

Water troughs and fencing should be checked daily.

New Zealand Rugs

These are designed to keep the horse warm and dry when turned out or living out.

Two rugs are necessary for a horse living out all the time, so that one is on the horse and one is drying. Even in dry weather the rug should be removed daily, the horse's back massaged to restore circulation, and the shoulders and legs inspected for rubbing.

HEALTH

All horses should be immunised against tetanus, and a regular worming programme should be carried out. A careful worming strategy is essential if horses are to remain healthy and the level of larvae on the pastures kept to a minimum. The tactics are to use a suitable (veterinary advised) anthelmintic at correct intervals and according to the time of the year (see Chapter 17).

Teeth should be checked.

In **summer** many horses and ponies become grossly fat, with a consequent risk of laminitis, and if they are ridden the extra weight puts strain on the legs, heart and lungs. In many cases it is necessary to restrict their diet. Unless the paddock is bare of grass, one or two hours' daily grazing is ample. The animals may be stabled at night, bedded on shavings, and turned out in the day; sun and flies will then often deter them from eating. A small amount of hay can be given at night: a pony 1–1.4kg (2–3lbs); a cob 1.8–2.7kg (4–6lbs). If a secure yard is available, it can be used instead of, or in conjunction with, a stable.

In **winter** a pony's thick coat can disguise poor condition. However, if the crest, backbone and rib areas are felt, any lack of flesh will be apparent. The crest in particular is a reserve of fat and it should feel firm and solid. Well cared for, healthy ponies should look plump and well throughout the winter, whatever the weather. Ponies with staring coats and bony outlines are a sign of poor management, inadequate worming and insufficient food (see also Chapter 23). Horses who suffer from respiratory problems can be kept very satisfactorily out at grass permanently. With proper care, a field shelter, sufficient food and the right rugs they can often do much better than when stabled.

SEASONAL PROBLEMS

In Summer

LAMINITIS Ponies subject to laminitis must be kept on a strict diet. If there is any sign of 'footiness', heat in the foot, or standing with weight on the heels of the front feet, take the pony off grass and consult your veterinary surgeon immediately.

SWEET ITCH The signs are continual rubbing of the mane and tail until they become raw. Only certain horses – usually ponies – appear to react to the saliva of the midge which causes the allergy. The condition is improved if the horse is stabled before dusk and until well after dawn. Fly repellent should be used in the stable and in the field. It has been found that if the wind is over 3kph (3mph) midges will not appear. There are a number of rugs on the market designed to prevent midge attack.

BLISTERED MUZZLE Horses with white muzzles are particularly prone to sun-blistered mouths and noses, a condition which can be caused by an allergy to a particular plant. To prevent this, apply barrier cream. If blistering occurs, antiseptic ointment should be used. It may be necessary to stable the animal.

RUNNING EYES Flies settle round a horse's eye to feed on 'the tear'. Sensitive horses can wear a headcollar with a fly guard (browband with a string fringe). More sophisticated protectors, such as browbands impregnated with fly repellent, are now available from tack shops. Some fly repellents are safe to use round the eyes, and can be applied with a small sponge. Horses can be kept in during the day. The eyes should be sponged clean twice daily. If eyes become infected, veterinary advice may be necessary. Light-skinned horses are more subject to this problem.

BOT OR GADFLY From June to September the bot fly lays its eggs on a horse's front legs, particularly just below the knee. These hatch to larvae, which the horse licks. The larvae then penetrate the skin and the mucous membrane around and inside the lips, resulting in the start of the bot fly cycle. The flies cause great irritation, and although they do not land on the skin, horses will gallop about and kick to get away from them. They may then injure themselves and others. The eggs should be removed. They can be scraped off carefully with a blunt knife.

WARBLE FLY These flies are becoming much less common, but any swelling on the horse's back in spring and early summer should be suspect. When the larva hatches out it must be killed. Some modern wormers kill bots and warble larvae before they reach their final sites.

Various **fly repellents** are now available, which in warm weather help to make horses more comfortable. Many repellents have to be applied twice daily, but some are longer-acting and in dry weather are effective for several days. A paraffin rag wiped on the legs can be effective against bots, but should not be used on horses with sensitive skins as it may cause blistering.

In Winter

The following problems are likely to occur, particularly with fine-coated horses in a very wet season. Horses should be closely observed each day and preventive measures taken. At any sign of lameness, obtain veterinary advice.

RAIN SCALD The skin of the back, loins and/or quarters is softened by incessant rain, thus weakening the natural defence mechanism against skin germs. Inflammation and dermatitis follow; the hairs clump together and fall out in patches.

Prevention: Sensitive-skinned horses should wear New Zealand rugs. In autumn, liquid paraffin or barrier cream can be applied to the horses' backs when the coat is free from mud and clean and dry. In severe cases, consult your veterinary surgeon.

MUD FEVER This is similar to rain scald, but occurs on the legs and sometimes the heels. If on the latter, continual exposure to mud increases the infection. Severe cases may spread to the belly and inner thigh.

Prevention: In the autumn and during the winter months apply barrier cream regularly to the legs, after they have been cleaned and dried. Wet, muddy legs should not be brushed, but thatched and left to dry (see Bandaging, Chapter 31). Then they can be brushed clean.

CRACKED HEELS These are inflamed sore horizontal cracks occurring in the heel region. Cracks in the heel and pastern area become intermittently infected, which can cause acute lameness, particularly after the animal has been standing still.

Prevention: As for mud fever.

THRUSH This is a disease of the frog. Most cases are associated with poor foot hygiene or even foot disease. However, some horses will contract a mild form of thrush in winter through standing in mud.

Prevention and treatment: As soon as the ground becomes muddy, apply Stockholm tar in and around the frog area. Repeat it as necessary. The foot and frog must first be thoroughly washed clean and dried. The veterinary surgeon may recommend a spray treatment.

LICE These insects can be found in the coat at any time in the winter, but usually in early spring. Any horse rubbing his mane and tail should be suspect.

Prevention: Apply louse powder regularly, as directed by the manufacturer. If this proves ineffective, obtain veterinary advice, as more sophisticated treatment may be necessary.

RINGWORM AND OTHER FUNGAL INFECTIONS These can appear at any time of the year, but in winter the fungus in its early stages can go undetected, as the long coat covers the scabby area.

Horses at grass, or those brought in from grass to be stabled, should be examined closely for any raised area of hair or circular scabs. The fungus can appear anywhere on the body, but it is more likely to be in places where the horse has rubbed against a gate or fence post, i.e. head, shoulders and quarters.

Prevention: Particularly if cattle have been in the field, all gates and fences should be thoroughly scrubbed with disinfectant. Ironwork should be washed with a strong solution of soda, or repainted.

SUDDEN ACUTE LAMENESS This can usually be attributed to a punctured foot, gravel penetrating a sole softened by rain, or a small flesh wound, which has gone septic. It may be necessary to transport the animal to the stables. The foot and leg should first be thoroughly cleaned and the leg examined for injury. Veterinary help should be obtained.

WORKING THE GRASS-KEPT HORSE OR PONY

Grass-kept horses and ponies can be used for hacking and light to medium work. Highly strung or 'gassy' animals may then be more amenable.

Horses needed for hard work can be kept at grass in the summer, as long as they are given regular exercise and increased concentrates. If the horse starts to get too fat, grass intake on a good pasture may have to be restricted. In winter, if hard, fast work is required, the horse should be stabled at night and exercised regularly each day.

Summer

- Horses and ponies on good grazing should preferably be brought in two hours before being ridden, so that their stomachs are not gorged with grass.

- For grooming and care after work, see Chapter 11.

On a wet morning, the horse's back should be scraped with a sweat scraper and semi-dried with a stable rubber or straw. If a dry stable rubber or numnah is put on and secured by a surcingle or saddle, the back will quickly dry. The horse will not be harmed if ridden with a wet back, although this is not recommended. He will probably react by first hollowing under the weight of the rider; a sharp horse may even buck.

Winter

- If on hard food, the horse should be fed early in the field, or caught about 1½ hours before being ridden and given his feed.

- For grooming, see Chapter 11.

Wet and muddy backs should be scraped with a sweat scraper, dried as above, then brushed clean. All lumps of mud must be removed from the saddle and girth area, and a fresh numnah or stable rubber should be placed under the saddle.

If, on returning from work, the horse/pony is warm, any resulting sweat patches should be wiped clean or sponged off. Feet should be picked out and the animal should be turned out as soon as possible, so that he can roll and be less likely to catch a chill. If he is wearing a New Zealand rug, straw can be put under it to allow more air to circulate, and he can be given hay. He should be caught up again later and re-rugged as normal. His hard feed can be given in the field, or he can be caught later and fed in the stable.

If it is essential to keep the horse or pony in after work, put on either (a) a sweat rug and roller with straw underneath, or (b) a sweat rug and light blanket and roller, or (c) a wicking rug. The horse/pony may then be fed. It is important that ponies with thick coats are not allowed to sweat profusely.

THE COMBINED SYSTEM

This is a system whereby in winter the horse is stabled at night and put out in the day. In summer, the process is reversed: the horse is in during the day and out at night, thus obtaining protection from hot sun and flies. If time and labour are short the advantages are:

- Daily exercise is not necessary.

- If only ridden at weekends, the horse will be quieter and more manageable.

- Daily grooming is reduced.

- Less bedding is used and, at times, less hay.

- Mucking-out time is reduced.

- The horse can be clipped and turned out in a New Zealand rug.

- The horse can be made ready for work quickly, as he will be dry and comparatively clean.

- In winter, less food is wasted in the field, and the food ration can be reduced, as the horse will be in a warm, dry stable at night.

- In summer, if necessary, grazing time can be more easily controlled.

YARDING PONIES

This is a system whereby ponies are wintered in a covered yard or large barn, which may or may not have an adjoining railed exercise area. It is a system very suitable for riding schools. Pony mares and foals can also be kept in this way. Young stock are increasingly kept in this way during their first winter after weaning and often as two-and three-year-olds.

The yard is kept strawed down on the deep litter system and is cleared out at the end of the winter. Hind shoes should be taken off and, if feasible, front shoes also. Mares and geldings may have to be separated, or only a single sex kept or accepted for winter keep.

An area of 20m x 20m (65ft x 65ft) is sufficient for ten ponies. A hay and feed manger should run along two sides. Preferably there should be two separate water troughs.

ADVANTAGES

- Ponies will be clean, dry and warm.

- Less time will be needed to groom before being ridden.

- They will be available when required.

- They will need less feed and there will be less waste. (See The Combined System, page 371.)

- If access is suitable, the yard can be cleared by machine.

- Grassland can be spared unnecessary damage through winter poaching.

DISADVANTAGES

- Certain ponies do not settle and may fight and upset the group. Fights may occur, resulting in injuries. At feed time, it is sensible for someone to be present to prevent squabbling.

- Labour and suitable equipment will be needed in the spring to clear the yard.

CATCHING HORSES/PONIES

- Do not be in a hurry. Careless procedure can easily upset a horse, spoil him, and make him difficult to catch.

- The headcollar should be placed over the left arm. Difficult horses may be encouraged to come to a handful of food.

- With the rope in the right hand, approach the horse from an angle towards the shoulder so he can see you, and as he accepts the food, move closer towards his left shoulder, placing your right hand with the rope on and then over his neck.

- Avoid any sudden or jerky movements, and talk quietly to the horse throughout the procedure.

- Put on the headcollar quietly.

Procedure with Difficult Horses/Ponies

- Take a large feed bowl, half fill it with food of a type that will rattle when the bowl is shaken. Tuck the headcollar and rope under your left arm, or alternatively hold a rope under your arm or inside your coat.

- Always allow the horse to see you approach.

- If he moves away, make a big circle and again approach from the front.

- Talk to him as you approach.

- Shake the bowl, and then lower it to the ground, which may gain his attention.

- Walk up to him with the bowl in the left hand.

- As he takes the food, the right hand can quietly move up his jaw and towards his neck.

- If he moves away, do not try to hold him but try to go with him, but if he shoots off, do not follow. Reorganise your approach as from the start. When he stands and eats, move quietly round to his shoulder, taking hold of the rope with your right hand.

- Place the rope under and then up or over and down his neck. When the horse is held by the rope, you should be able to put on the headcollar. On some occasions, a length of string or thin rope may be less obvious.

If difficult horses are caught and fed each day, it becomes a routine, and when the animals are wanted for riding, they will be easier to catch.

Difficult horses are usually caught more easily if only one person makes the attempt and any onlookers are sent away. Other horses in the field should be caught and held at the gate or in the corner of the field. At first do not take them out of the field, as a horse left on his own will be encouraged to gallop about. However, if there is a convenient passageway or track to the stable yard, then the horse will probably follow the others along it, or he may walk in amongst the group and allow himself to be caught. If this occurs, it may be more sensible to move quietly alongside him from the rear. Talk to the horse and place a hand on his quarters (taking care he does not kick you), moving it up his back and neck as you walk alongside him. Secure him by placing a rope round his neck, and then quietly put on the headcollar. Horses must not be allowed to escape on to roads.

If the horse will still not be caught, leave a quiet horse or pony in the field with him and return in half an hour.

Horses are usually easier to catch in hot weather and more difficult in wet and/or windy weather, or when there is spring grass.

The catcher can often put horses off by wearing an unusual hat or raincoat, particularly if it is plastic.

A better contact is made with the horse if gloves are not worn, but put them on to lead him.

Horses who are difficult to catch are best turned out wearing a well-fitting leather or nylon headcollar. If of nylon, it should have a 'panic snap', which will give way if the horse catches the headcollar on a post, etc. A 16cm to a maximum of 20cm (6–8ins) length of knotted string can be attached to the centre 'D' and used when catching the animal; the string should never be in a loop. The horse's head should be checked regularly for sores and rubs.

Staff (e.g. an instructor or groom) catching a horse and riding him to the stables should first put a headcollar on the animal and then fit the bridle on top of it. If catching the horse with only a bridle, do not put the reins over first in case the horse pulls away and takes the bridle with him.

Occasionally it may be necessary to drive or corral animals before catching them, i.e. if they are wild or unbroken. Always use plenty of sensible helpers who will obey instructions and not get excited. They should form a line abreast behind the animals and walk slowly towards them, if necessary moving to the right or the left but keeping the forward line even. If they stretch lunge-lines or sturdy rope between them it may help discourage the animals from turning back.

Once the animals are in a confined space it should be possible for an experienced handler to catch them up.

This method can work well with unruly ponies but great care would be needed with highly strung horses or young stock.

Sometimes if the catcher sits down on a log or jump and has a bucket, the horse/pony will come up to investigate. Someone sitting down presents less of a threat.

This method is best used if only one or two animals are present. Any more and they may fight over the bucket.

Many horses/ponies who live in well-established communities can be trained to come to call. This can save a lot of time traipsing around a field.

Remember that the 'boss' is responsible for the safety of any helpers. Although horses and ponies are usually less upset by children and will accept them if they move near, fear of being caught may alter this attitude.

Unaccompanied small children should not be allowed to catch ponies, particularly if there are several ponies in the field.

TURNING OUT HORSES AND PONIES

It is important that safe procedures are followed. Horses will often kick out when first released, and can injure people or other animals.

When leading a horse through a gateway you must be on the side nearest the gate, to control and stop it swinging back and hitting the horse.

Procedure for One Horse

• Bring the horse through the gate.

• Turn his head towards the swinging end of the gate.

• Shut the gate.

• Take the horse several metres into the field and once again turn his head towards the gate and yourself.

• Pat him, take off his headcollar, and step back.

• Watch the horse as he moves off. Do not turn away.

• Never slap him on the neck or quarters, as this may encourage him to gallop.

• Try to proceed quietly and avoid any fuss. If he is wearing a bridle, follow the methods listed above, then undo the curb chain, if used, then noseband then throatlash, in that order. This ensures that the bridle is secure until the last moment. Many horses try to pull away as soon as the throatlash is undone and can be left with the bridle hanging from their teeth.

• Slide the reins up to the headpiece and ease the whole bridle off, staying close to the horse so that he releases the bit without pulling away. Give him a pat on the neck and move away from him so that he realises he is free.

Procedure for Several Horses

• All horses should be brought into the field, taken well away from the gate, with at least 3m (10ft) between each horse, and turned to face the gate.

• Shut the gate and proceed as directed above.

• Finally, release all horses together.

Horses who are unfamiliar with one another or who are likely to gallop off, should be taken to the field in pairs. When the first pair have settled, the next pair can be taken out and released.

ROUGHING OFF A FIT HORSE

This is the preparation of a fit horse for a holiday and a rest out at grass. The rest is important both from the physical point of view and to relieve mental stress. Rests are given to:

• Hunters at the end of the season.

• Competition horses.

• Injured horses, to allow the repair processes time to work.

The roughing-off process takes about two weeks and the procedure is:

1. Remove one blanket. After seven to ten days remove the top rug, or change to a lighter one.

2. Thorough grooming should be discontinued and the natural grease should be allowed to accumulate in the coat, forming a protection against cold and wet.

3. Diet should gradually be adjusted, reducing the hard feed and increasing the hay.

4. The horse should be allowed out daily in a small field or led out to graze.

5. Exercise should gradually be reduced and should now consist mainly of hacking out at the walk.

6. Veterinary checks should be made, and any recommended treatment should be completed.

7. Shoes should only be removed if the horse is to have a long rest of more than four weeks. Feet should then be rasped to prevent the horn splitting. Horses with brittle feet who are to be turned out on flinty or very hard fields may need to have their front shoes left on. (**NB:** Feet should be rasped or shoes should be removed every four to six weeks.)

8. In cold weather, the horse will be more comfortable if a New Zealand rug is used. For fitting and procedure, see pages 267–70.

Hunters are often turned out at the end of the season. This can be as early as the end of March, when they will need a New Zealand rug, a well-sheltered field, and hard feed and hay to help keep them warm until the weather improves.

Preparation for Turning Out

1. Check the field.

2. If you are turning out a horse on to rich pasture, he must be given short periods of grazing for several days beforehand.

3. Choose a mild day.

4. Make sure the horse has suitable company – preferably not a highly strung galloping type of horse.

5. Do not give a breakfast feed. If the horse is hungry he is more likely to graze than to gallop.

6. Turn the horse out early in the day, so that he will have time to settle in the field before night. He should be watched until he is quiet, and checked again during the day.

It is preferable to allow the horse several short 'holidays' in a year rather than one major let-down of several months. Where a complete reduction of muscle tone is allowed the horse may revert to very soft condition and carrying excess weight. This total let-down is now recognised as not being in the interests of the long-term welfare of the working horse.

BRINGING A HORSE UP FROM GRASS

It is better for the horse if the change is made gradually over a period of about ten days, as this will allow his microbial digestion time to adjust itself to the change of diet (see also Chapter 23).

Depending on the time of year and quality of grazing, some horses may be receiving hard feed and hay in the field. In this case, a sudden change of diet will present no problems.

Procedure

• Bring the horse into the stable for several hours a day. Give a small feed of 0.5–1.4kg (1–3lbs) of horse and pony cubes or equivalent foodstuff plus a 1.8–2.3kg (4lbs) net of dampened hay. Allergic horses should be given soaked hay or haylage (see also Chapter 25).

• If the horse is turned out on his own or with one or two others, it is possible to feed them in the field. Always stay to watch the feeding, so that there is no bullying or kicking. (There is no need to feed hay.) This practice is not recommended if there are more than two or three horses in the field, because of the risk of kicking. If the horse has not been receiving hard feed whilst turned out introduce the chosen product carefully and only increase the amounts in line with the exercise or fittening programme.

• The horse may have to be brought in and kept stabled. In this case, try to arrange for him to be turned out in a paddock for a few hours each day, or, alternatively, graze him in hand for 20 minutes or so.

Feed ration should be two or three 0.5kg (1 lb) feeds of 'horse and pony' cubes or their equivalent, and plenty of haylage or dampened hay – about 9–11kg (20–25lbs). Do not feed any grain for a week; grain fed too soon can be the cause of filled legs. If you are planning to use grain, change over to it gradually.

Often, if a horse comes in after a summer at grass, weight will need to be lost. Gradually accustom him to a smaller total quantity of feed, but one which includes more concentrates. As more concentrates are fed, hay can be reduced. If the diet is restricted to encourage weight loss, it is essential to put the horse on shavings or a similar bed, and not straw. For amounts of feed, see Chapter 23.

Recommended Treatments

WORMING A suitable dose should be administered. (See also Chapter 17, Internal Parasites.)

FLU AND TETANUS INOCULATIONS If due, these should be arranged. (See Appendix 4.)

TEETH The teeth should be checked by the veterinary surgeon or dentist and rasped if necessary.

FEET Arrangements should be made with the farrier to have the horse shod as soon as he is permanently stabled and starts exercise. Four weeks before he is due to come in, depending on the condition of his feet, have him shod with light front shoes. This allows some growth of horn and makes it easier to shoe him for work. Valuable horses should never be turned out in company with hind shoes on, as a kick from a shod foot can cause severe injury.

Precautions

With careful feeding and regular walking exercise, the problem of filled legs should not arise. Coughs and colds develop easily during this period, so ensure a plentiful supply of fresh air and take care if the horse sweats when exercised.

If it is possible, start the fittening process whilst the horse is able to be out either by day, or night, depending on the time of year. Many problems can be avoided if the first four weeks of the following exercise programme are done in this way.

Dangers From and Precautions Against Gaining Weight

Turning horses out for long periods in the spring/ summer may result in their putting on too much weight. The increase in weight puts strain on a horse's legs and must be reduced before he is fit for active work. Often the time allowed for fittening is insufficient, and horses are asked to work too early, which strains the tendons, joints, heart and wind, with the possibility of permanent harm.

Horses can be turned out for a shorter period of six to eight weeks. They can then be either yarded or stabled at night. In very hot weather, when there are many flies, they can be brought in during the day and turned out at night.

Suggested Exercise for an Unfit, Overweight Horse After Several Months at Grass

1ST WEEK
Walking exercise on the level. Half an hour on the first day, increasing to ¾ hour by the end of the first week.

2ND WEEK
Increase walking up to 1 hour by the end of the week.

3RD WEEK
Slow trotting, starting on the level, together with walking up and down slopes and slight hills.

4TH WEEK
As third week.

5TH WEEK
1½ hours exercise a day, to include some trotting up hills and short, slow cantering on good, level ground. Sweating will help to hasten weight loss. 20 minutes school work may be included.

6TH–8TH WEEK
1½–2 hours exercise a day, to include trotting up hills and longer cantering periods. School work may include jumping and canter circles.

7TH WEEK
If the ground is hard, cantering can be performed in a school. Start with 1 minute on either rein, building up gradually over successive weeks. As this can be very strenuous, care should be taken. Big, heavy horses unused to circle work should not be asked to do this type of work.

For the schooling, work boots should be worn all round. If, when hacking out, roads are slippery, or if the horse is fresh, knee caps and boots are advisable.

All exercise periods should include a good percentage of walking, as this helps to strengthen the legs and to develop muscle without unnecessary strain.

Some of the walking can be done using a horse walker or by ride and lead, if that is possible. However, a horse walker is very boring for the horse and he does need to have his back and skin conditioned by wearing tack and carrying weight.

Walking exercise, using hills, is probably the most beneficial exercise in the early stages.

Horses who are turned out for shorter periods – or in the winter, when grass is poor, who have received regular hard feed and hay – come in very much fitter. In these cases, preparation for active work may be shorter. The owner or stable manager must decide how fit a horse is and for what work he is ready.

Unfit, overweight horses should not be lunged, because working on a circle puts extra strain on muscles, tendons and joints. Lungeing may be included after two weeks of walking, but 5 minutes on each rein will be sufficient at first. This should have a beneficial and suppling effect on the horse, as long as a suitably prepared surface is used. Hard or slippery fields are not advisable.

Timetable for Fittening

If the horse is grossly fat the time taken over fittening must be increased.

- **RIDING CLUB** – after 6–8 weeks.

- **HUNTER** – can be brought up in August ready for gentle work by mid-September; more serious work in October, and hunting by November.

- **NOVICE EVENT HORSE/SHOW JUMPER** – 10–14 weeks.

- **ENDURANCE HORSE/SHOW JUMPER** – 8–12 weeks.

- **THREE-DAY EVENTER** – 14–16 weeks.

- **GOLDEN HORSESHOE HORSE** – 16–20 weeks.

Prevention of Sore Backs, Girth Galls and Sore Mouths

- Check the fit of the saddle. The horse may change shape considerably during the first four to eight weeks of regular work so keep checking the saddle for fit. Consider using a breastplate, especially when doing hill work.

- Ensure that the bit fits the horse's mouth.

- All leatherwork must be soft and supple.

- Tack should be cleaned each day.

- Use a numnah under the saddle. Natural cotton or sheepskin are preferable to man-made fibres. In hot weather, a padded cotton numnah helps to absorb sweat without overheating the saddle area.

- Numnahs and girths should be washed regularly – if necessary, each day.

- Use a 'Cottage Craft' type girth.

- Harden saddle and girth areas with salt and water or methylated spirit.

- The horse must be cleaned thoroughly each day; sweat marks quickly become sore if left. In warm weather, the horse should be sponged down; surplus water should be removed with a sweat scraper, then the horse should be walked in the sun until dry. In cold weather, sweat marks can be sponged off with warm water. In both cases the horse should be dried, and groomed thoroughly.

- During grooming the horse should be checked for any signs of saddle sores or girth galls. The first signs are rubbed hair, followed by tenderness and heat.

Treatment

- Harden the area with salt and water. Stop riding, and either lead the horse out in a cavesson or bridle alongside another horse, or, if he is fit enough, lunge him. If the saddle sore is damp, spread cold kaolin over the area and top it with a plastic covering. This will help to draw out the inflammation before hardening the skin with salt and water.

SECTION

7

THE STABLE YARD

50 CONSTRUCTION OF STABLES

Before constructing a new stable yard:

1. Consider your financial situation.
2. Obtain outline planning permission from the local authorities.
3. Consider security.

SITE

Any local byelaws relating to drainage and construction should be checked. If there is a choice of site, consider:

ACCESSIBILITY If an access road has to be built, this will increase the overall cost of the project. Installing services such as water, electricity and telephone, even over short distances, can be very expensive.

DRAINAGE Stabling requires a solid, dry, well-drained base. If the soil is sand, gravel or chalk, this should present no problem. With clay or a high water table, the sub-soil has to be removed, replaced, and built up with hardcore and gravel.

CONVENIENCE Ideally the stables should be sited so that they are visible from the house or staff living quarters. Regular checks can then be made easily.

If it is not possible for all construction work to be done at once, allow for future expansion from the start. This can save considerable money, long term.

Recommended Layout of Stable Yard and Surrounding Buildings

- Hay and straw barns should be well away from the stable area. Small amounts of hay and straw may be kept easily available for daily use in a convenient covered area.

- Tractor-sheds and horsebox garage should also be away from the stables and the hay barn.

- Petrol and diesel tanks are not in general use, but if you do have them on your premises they should be near the access road and away from all other buildings.

- If supplies of tractor fuel have to be stored, they should be in heavy-duty jerry cans. Not more than 50 litres (approx. 10 gallons) should be stored at a time.

  NB: Plastic containers are not safe for storing diesel fuel, petrol or paraffin.

SECURITY

Security needs to be an integral part of any new build or renovation project. It will take many forms. Some that need to be considered are:

- Safety and security of the horses.

- Safety of staff and clients.

- Security of the buildings.

- Prevention of theft by outsiders.
- Prevention of pilfering by staff and clients.
- Prevention of vandalism.
- Confidentiality of information.

General security

Always try to have someone living on site. If accommodation is situated beside the entrance it is easier to keep an eye on comings and goings.

If possible, have the yard ring-fenced. This prevents loose horses from going far. If there are separate stable complexes, have each one gated.

If there is more than one entrance, consider having the second gated and padlocked to deter thieves and only open it for deliveries, etc.

If gravel is used on drives or parking areas it can put off intruders if kept well raked. Consider the use of security lighting. There are many systems available. Some come on when it gets dark and some are activated by timers or movement. The latter will often be activated by animals and birds. Audible alarms are only useful if there is someone to hear them. Plan to have offices and client areas near the entrance. Consider having separate tack and feed rooms for self-livery clients. Site shops and tack rooms where they are easily visible day and night. Having a kennelled watch dog is sometimes useful.

Horses

In some areas it is no longer considered safe to keep horses out at night. When they are turned out, have them in fields away from roads and country lanes. Ensure that all fences are secure and not easily vandalised. All gates must be padlocked and also secure at the hinge end.

Horses who are freeze-marked are less likely to be stolen. Having notices to that effect or painting their number on New Zealand rugs acts as a deterrent. Do not leave headcollars hanging on the gate during turn out.

With stabled horses, especially racehorses and valuable competition animals, it is often safer not to identify them by name on the door.

Horses should not be padlocked in their stables because of the difficulty of rescuing them in the event of fire.

Staff and buildings

If staff are expected to live on site, they are entitled to feel safe, especially if they are required to do late-night checks or get up and go to bed in the dark on short winter days.

Adequate lighting needs to be provided in all areas. Getting in a lighting expert who can advise at an early stage in the planning process is strongly recommended.

Ensure there are working telephones, especially in areas where the mobile phone signal is poor. In large establishments staff may be issued with mobiles in order for contact to be maintained. This is especially recommended for trekking centres.

Staff should be briefed as to correct procedures to follow if they suspect intruders are present.

Siting of Buildings

Consider the siting of particular buildings carefully.

Feed rooms and feed stores need to be easily accessible for deliveries but also for feeding.

Tack rooms and shops need to be sited in full view of those who need to use them. They should also be built securely of brick or block and have roofs, windows and doors that are burglar-proof. Many insurance companies will specify what preventative measures they require in order to provide cover.

Theft and vandalism

Theft and vandalism are much greater problems in some areas than others. However, they are on the increase countrywide. Some methods have already been suggested. Others that may be considered are:

- Putting clamps on all trailers and vehicles not in regular use.

- Marking all tack and equipment with the postcode and publicising the fact.

- Doing regular inventory checks.

- Keeping all areas tidy and allocating specific areas for specific articles to be stored. It is then easier to notice when they are missing.

- Having a booking out and in system for expensive articles such as clippers.

- Putting firewalls between forage and bedding stores and stable areas.

- Only allowing people on the yard at specific times when staff are present.

- Liaising with your insurance company as to their requirements for tack room security.

- Keeping all flammable liquids in a secure area.

- Liaising with the local fire prevention officer to ensure an adequate water supply and easy access to all areas.

- Keeping all drugs, medicines and surgical equipment such as syringes and scalpels securely locked away.

- Having a system whereby strangers are always greeted and not allowed to wander around on their own.

- Ensuring that all children are supervised and not allowed to play in a working environment.

- Do not leave equipment such as ladders or wheelbarrows where they can be accessed to aid in a break-in or removal of equipment.

Clients

Yards have a duty of care to ensure that property and information belonging to clients is secure.

Provision needs to be made for all equipment, tack, rugs, trailers, as well as the horses, to be secure, not only from professional thieves but from petty pilfering between clients.

Depending on the type of yard, separate lockers, trunks or store rooms can be allocated, hired out or be a condition of the livery agreement. The fewer people who have access to a given area, the easier it is to secure.

Provision needs to be made for clients' belongings, such as handbags, keys and clothing, to be safe whilst they are on the yard.

Confidentiality

There needs to be a secure filing system in place for all records. Depending on the type of business the following need to be considered:

- Client records including livery agreements, invoicing, etc., training programmes, progress reports and inventories.

- Staff information, including contracts, payments, CVs, overtime, holidays, training and development, etc.

- Horse files, including purchase details, winnings, description with both summer and winter photos, passport and ongoing details of veterinary care, etc.

- Details of the business such as sales and purchases. All invoices, records of all dealings with suppliers, vets, farriers, studs, etc.

- All relevant insurance, both mandatory and voluntary.

This information may be kept on computer or in paper form. Always back it up with a secondary system. Ensure that any paper system is protected from fire. Ensure it is readily retrievable on a 'need to know' basis. If you want the records kept up to date, keep the system simple.

YARD AND ACCESS ROAD

Foundation

A good foundation is essential. If building a new stable yard, the access road may be put down first to give a firm base for lorries. It is usual to excavate down to the subsoil, but should it be an area of poor drainage and clay, it may be necessary to go deeper and remove the soil underneath. The whole area is back-filled with hardcore or similar material according to availability locally. It is compacted with a vibratory roller. This base should extend at least about 1m (3ft) beyond the area of the yard and 60cm (2ft) on either side of the access road.

The underground water main and electric cable which come from the public road or neighbouring buildings should be put in before the top surface is laid. They should emerge in the tack room or office area. If the water main is to cross an area used by lorries, it is likely to be fractured by pressure. To avoid this and to prevent the water freezing in winter, the main should be laid in a 60cm (2ft) deep trench to the side of the roadway.

The roadway should be edged with a concrete kerb, to prevent the sides from being undermined by surface water and giving way under pressure. The access road should have a width of 3.6m (12ft), and preferably should open out to a distance of 12m (40ft) as it reaches the road. This entrance should be surfaced to a width of 6m (20ft); to save expense the remainder may be left. The 12m (40ft) clear expanse should give good visibility for both riders and traffic.

Ensure that any form of entrance archway is not going to prevent the entry of emergency vehicles and delivery lorries.

Drainage

Surface water off the yard will collect at the lowest point, and should be directed off and away from the buildings. If the original area is flat, it must be arranged that the top surface should have a slight slope (approximately 1 in 60) towards an open shallow drain. This surface water can then be directed:

(a) away across the field by means of a 'French drain';
(b) to a soak-away; or
(c) if (a) and (b) are not possible, then to a septic-tank system installed to take the stable drains.

A **'French drain'** is a ditch dug to a suitable depth according to requirements, shallower at the yard and deeper as it gets to the field. It is filled with reject stone.

A **soak-away** is a large circular hole 3–6m (10–20ft) deep, filled with reject stone. This works successfully in a sand, gravel or chalk area, but should not be considered in a clay district.

If surface water is to join a drainage system, then one or more gullies will have to be constructed to collect surface mud and straw. They must have strong, removable steel covers, and be large enough to cope with heavy rainwater.

It is advisable to consult with experts and the local planning department to ensure that all environmental Health and Safety and local planning regulations are being adhered to. Redoing work later can lead to huge cost increases.

Run-off from large expanses of roadway or yard may overload the waste drainage system and need to be dealt with separately. Liquid waste from stables and muck heaps must not seep into local streams, rivers and ponds.

YARD AND ROAD SURFACES

Types

(a) Gravel, stones or chippings are attractive to look at and non-slippery, but are difficult to keep clean and tidy, and are not suitable for a yard with large numbers of horses.
(b) Concrete and tarmac are practical, although tarmac is inclined to be slippery. They are relatively easy to keep clean and tidy, and are of good appearance. If put down to a suitable thickness they will last for many years, provided they have good drainage. Frost

can be damaging to concrete and tarmac. Also, they are slippery in icy weather, and suitable precautions have to be taken, e.g. salt or sand put down, or straw tracks made.

(c) Rubber matting can also be laid.

The access road can be left untopped, but will then eventually break up. A top surface of concrete or tarmac makes a sound, long-lasting surface, and enhances the approach to the yard.

All yard and road surfaces need to be well maintained, and repaired as necessary. If cracked or broken surfaces are left, the deterioration becomes more rapid and more expensive to put right.

All yards must have a good gate and fences to prevent livestock getting on to the public highway. The gate must be wide enough for easy access, well hinged and have a sound fastening device. The yard gate should be kept shut at all times.

SHELTER

If a barn-type stable is selected (see Types of Stabling, page 387), shelter from cold winds need not be considered. If conventional lines of loose boxes are planned, try to select a sheltered area protected by other buildings, or by hills or trees. If building in a high, exposed position, an 'L'-shaped design, three sides of a square, or a rectangle, will give more protection.

When providing any form of shelter, ventilation must be the first consideration. 1,500–2,000 cubic feet of air per horse is the minimum requirement and this air should change completely every twenty minutes. This can be measured by using a smoke candle and measuring how long it takes for the smoke to clear.

New Ideas

Research is constantly being carried out with regard to flooring, ventilation, and labour saving. Anyone considering the building of new stables should study carefully all the various possibilities before going ahead with any plans.

Design Considerations

TACK ROOM AND FEED SHED These should be near the stable block, and preferably should be connected by an overhang. As the tack room is a security risk, it should be in view of the staff living quarters. In large yards it may be convenient to have more than one tack room in order to segregate types of tack and equipment or types of client.

This might also be a consideration for the feed room.

OFFICE, LAVATORIES, CHANGING ROOMS, STAFF AND LECTURE ROOMS should be adjacent to each other and with access to the car park.

MUCK HEAP This should be sited away from the car park and the yard entrance, but should be within easy reach of the stables. The road leading to it should have a surface firm enough to bear heavy lorries. The muck heap should cover an area which is practical for the size of the particular yard. It should have a concrete base and there should be a concrete path leading to the stables. The surrounds should slope so that the surface water will flow to an open drain and will be channelled away – but it should not be directed across fields because of the contamination. One side should be open and the other three sides built up to a height of 1.8m (6ft). Railway sleepers or concrete blocks can be used for this purpose. The path can be raised or the muck heap dug out so that manure can be thrown down rather than up. Good access for removal is an essential consideration.

Seepage from the muck heap must be safely controlled and the muck disposed of according to the law.

HAY BARN This should not be adjacent to the stabling because of the risk of fire. Preferably it should be connected to the yard by a hard surface wide enough to accommodate a large hay lorry.

If forage is bought in bulk and stored in a pole barn, it can be useful to have a small shed just large enough to store a week's supply adjacent to the stables.

POWER LINES If these are above ground, they must be high enough to give clearance for any muck and hay lorries.

YARD SURFACE This can be of tarmac or concrete – but remember that all surfaces other than gravel are slippery in icy weather. Gravel is not practical if there are large numbers of horses in the stables.

Tarmac will rot and break up if oil is regularly spilt on it as can happen when oiling hooves on a regular basis.

51   DESIGN OF STABLES

The design of stabling will be determined by:

- Planning authorities.

- Local conditions, e.g. lie of the land, shelter, drainage and other buildings.

- Personal preference.

- Cost.

TYPES OF STABLING

Individual Looseboxes

These are the most popular choice. Each stable is complete in itself and can stand alone or be built in

    (a) parallel lines,
    (b) an 'L' shape,
    (c) a square, or
    (d) U-shaped.

Types (c) and (d) are considered to be more liable to facilitate the spread of disease, as there is less circulation of fresh air. On the other hand, on exposed sites they give more protection. An overhang should be incorporated along the front of the boxes to give shelter to horses and grooms.

American Barn

Barn stabling consists of a large covered area containing two rows of looseboxes facing each other across a

2.5–3.6m (8–12ft) passageway.

ADVANTAGES

- Pleasant working conditions for the staff.

- Labour saving.

- Cost and space effective.

- In cold or exposed areas they provide more warmth and comfort for the horse.

- Less likelihood of water pipes freezing.

- Horses are happier when able to see one another, i.e. herd instinct.

- Horses, feed shed, hay store and tack rooms can be under one roof.

- Horses are more easily observed should anything be wrong.

- The work of student staff is more easily supervised.

Stables are sometimes designed to run along the long side of an indoor school. If this is done, try to ensure that dust from the school surface is not a health hazard to both horses and workers.

DISADVANTAGES AND PRECAUTIONS

- **Fire** This spreads more quickly and there will be greater problems from smoke. It is more difficult to get horses out of a barn-type building than out of individual looseboxes. To reduce the risk of horses being trapped, double doors should be placed at both ends of the building. These can be either sliding or hinged doors, and if the latter they should open outwards. The doorways must never be obstructed. In a very long building, doors should be placed halfway down each side to make it easier to lead horses out. Fire drills should be held regularly – see Prevention of Fire, page 490. A hay store inside the building, although convenient, is an added fire and dust risk.

- **Infection and contagion** These are always a problem where large numbers of horses are stabled together and there is a greater risk of this in barn stabling than in a yard of looseboxes. A design which gives good ventilation, large partitions and high roof, reduces the risk. Barn stabling with low ceilings, a warm, damp atmosphere and insufficient ventilation is more vulnerable to the spread of disease.

- **Ventilation** In all weathers and at all times there must be a sufficient supply of fresh air. The requirement for internal stabling is 56 cubic metres (2,000 cubic feet) of air space per horse.

A high roof gives ample air space and ventilation per horse and keeps the stables cool in hot weather. If a ceiling is installed, then the diminished air space necessitates the use of some form of mechanical ventilation. Double doors give a through-draught. Windows can be a source of fresh air, these should be set on the outside wall of each box and should open inwards, hinged at the bottom. If the horses are able to see out, it can help to prevent boredom. It is crucial that the free flow of fresh air is not impeded if doors and windows have to be closed for any reason. Louvre boards can be installed in the outer walls to assist the extraction of used air.

When deciding on the type of roof, cowls or continuous roof vents or ridge vents need to be incorporated.

- **Coughs and allergies** These can be a problem if some horses are bedded on straw, and other susceptible horses are on shavings or paper in the same building.

It is impossible to create a spore-and dust-free atmosphere under these conditions, and the susceptible horses are bound to be affected. Alternative outside accommodation must be available for these horses.

- **Boredom** This is rarely a problem as horses can see each other and watch work going on, but, if finance allows, windows or doors 90cm (3ft) square can be put in the back wall which, when opened, allow the horses to look out. They may be constructed of wood or unbreakable clear plastic and covered with a grid. When closed they must be draught-proof.

Conversion of an Existing Building

Most farm buildings can be converted into looseboxes or stalls, provided that the building is sound and the roof is of sufficient height. Low roofs are difficult and expensive to alter and roof height is important, both for ventilation and clearance for the horse's head. Few buildings provide sufficient space to incorporate feed and tack rooms. The ventilation may be more difficult to organise, as farm roofs are often tiled or slated. The other advantages and disadvantages are similar to American barn stabling.

Stalls

Stalls are individually partitioned stables in which the horse is permanently tied up, traditionally facing a blank wall. Water, feed and hay are placed in front of the horse.

Some horses do feel restricted and will not settle in stalls, but the majority are reasonably content. Although their movement is very limited, they can still lie down and get up without trouble.

The major advantage of stalls is that they allow more horses to be housed in a smaller space. They are warm, practical, save labour and bedding and are the cheapest type of stable to build. They are specially suitable as day standings for horses and ponies brought in from the field and can be very useful in riding schools.

The conventional design is one line of stalls positioned along the outside wall, with a passageway behind leading to either one or two outside doors. Given sufficient space, two parallel lines of stalls can be built and separated by a 3.6m (12ft) passageway. The more modern design for stalls is two parallel lines facing each other across a feeding passageway. Horses are tied up to the front of the stall, but can see each other through the rails. They are watered and fed from the central passageway. Two wider passageways running behind the horses give room for mucking out and bedding down.

SIZE OF STABLES

Considerations

- Cost – the larger the box, the higher the cost for ground, structure and bedding.

- Comfort of the horse – needs room to lie down.

- Ease of management.

- Larger stables can be used for smaller animals, but the reverse is not possible.

- Within limits, the larger the box, the more comfortable for both horse and groom.

- Looseboxes are preferably square, but if rectangular the longer distance should be from door to back wall.

Dimensions

- 3.6m x 3.1m (12ft x 10ft) is adequate for most horses of 16hh and under.

- 3.6m x 3.6m (12ft x 12ft) or 4.2m x 3.6m (14ft x 12ft) is a comfortable and suitable size for a horse over 16hh.

- 3.1m x 3.1m (10ft x 10ft) is adequate if under 15hh.

- 2.4m x 2.4m (8ft x 8ft) is suitable for small ponies.

- 4.6m x 4.6m (15ft x 15ft) is needed for foaling boxes.

- 1.8m x 3.3m (6ft x 11ft) for stalls for animals under 16hh.

- 1.3m x 2.4m (4½ft x 8ft) for stalls if under 14.2hh.

Roof Height

The roof must be high enough to provide sufficient air space, and to ensure that there is no danger of a horse hitting his head.

Horses in outside looseboxes require 42 cubic metres (1,600 cu ft), in barn stabling 56 cubic metres (2,000 cu ft) and in stalls 28 cubic metres (1,000 cu ft) each.

MATERIALS

Materials used in construction must be strong enough to withstand kicking or leaning against walls or attempting to chew accessible wood. Although ponies can be housed in a more lightly made building, it rarely lasts as long, and can be a false economy.

Types and Their Advantages

Bricks

- Pleasing appearance.

- Warmth.

- Longevity.

Using bricks is very expensive because, for a strong and weather-proof surface, the walls must be cavity built, i.e. double walls with a cavity between.

Concrete Solid Blocks

- Acceptable appearance.

- Hard-wearing and long-lasting.

- Minimal maintenance.

• Comparatively quick and easy to build.

• Cheaper than bricks.

Concrete Cavity Blocks

The advantages of these are the same as those for concrete solid blocks with the additional one of good insulation without extra expense. Although not as strong as solid concrete blocks, cavity blocks are of an acceptable strength for most stables. They can be reinforced with metal strips if they are likely to be subjected to unusual stress.

Concrete Breeze Blocks

These are of an acceptable appearance, are fairly hard-wearing and long-lasting, comparatively quick and easy to build and relatively cheap. These blocks are porous and only suitable for inner linings. For exterior use they need weather-proofing. They are not as strong as solid concrete or cavity blocks, and can sometimes fracture under stress.

Wooden Prefabricated Sectional Stables

• Pleasing appearance if well maintained.

• Readily available.

• Easily erected.

• Can be moved.

• Warm.

There is, however, an added fire risk. Also, wooden, prefabricated sections are more difficult to disinfect, the upkeep costs are higher and they have a comparatively short life compared to bricks or blocks.

Cedar wood is the most expensive material, but lasts longer. A foundation of two rows of bricks, to which the structure is bolted, is required. All wood should be pressure-treated with a wood preservative. Boxes should be lined with suitable hardwood or chipboard.

Whilst good-quality wooden boxes last thirty years and more, ones of inferior quality show wear very quickly. They can be damaged by horses kicking or chewing the wood, and the resulting cracked or splintered boards can be dangerous. Thus when selecting wooden stabling, it is advisable to buy the best that can be afforded, and even then to check on the quality of the timber used and the method of erection.

Concrete Prefabricated Sectional Stables

In recent years there has been some use of this material.

Composite Material Prefabricated Sectional Stables

Although not yet used as much as wood, composite materials may well grow in popularity as their design and structure become better known and proven. They are likely to be cheaper than wood.

Solid Wood

A log-cabin type construction is attractive to look at, strong and durable, but very expensive.

INTERNAL WALLS

Barns

The external structure of this type of stabling is a steel- or concrete-framed barn with a clear span of Onduline sheets. External walls can be made of Onduline, plastic sheeting or concrete blocks. The internal partitions making up the boxes or pens can be constructed of brick, blocks, wood or prefabricated sectional walls. The last are purpose-built, heavy wooden partitions topped with grilles or heavy galvanised mesh. Mesh is safer as there is no chance of a horse catching his foot when rolling and kicking. These partitions are usually 2.3m (7½ft) in height. Solid partitions between boxes can reduce the risk of infection and contagion. They will reduce draughts. The choice of internal partitions is a question of personal preference and cost. The range is from basic but sufficient, to very elaborate designs.

Partitions which are too low will encourage the horses to fight over the top or even climb in with each other.

Separate Boxes

These are usually of wood and may go up to the roof or to the eaves.

The more open and airy the stable is, the better. It is always better to go for more air and rug the horse to keep him warm.

LIGHT

Corrugated perspex roof panels can be placed in the roof above each loosebox. They will give ample daylight.

In hot sun the panels on the side of the roof exposed to the sun will increase the temperature in the stable. Those on a north-facing roof cause no problem.

More light can be provided with translucent panels in the outside walls, under the eaves, provided that the walls are high enough for the horses not to reach them.

DRAINAGE SYSTEMS

To install a drainage system, planning permission is required, and it must accord with local by-laws. Always find out about any existing drainage systems when planning for new build or change of use. Professional advice should be taken. The main systems are:

Mains Drainage

If this is available, it can be used only for lavatory and tack room drains. Other arrangements will have to be made for stable drains, roof and surface water.

Septic Tank

This consists of a system of tanks and can be used for the whole of the establishment's drainage. Bacteria present in the first tank work on the material entering it. The liquid then moves on and is eventually piped out under the surface, by which time it is clean.

On occasion it may be necessary to empty this system, by arrangement with a local firm specialising in drain cleaning. Some systems require emptying every six months, while others will function efficiently for many years.

Cess Pit

This is a system of one or more tanks which have to be emptied when they are full. A regular contract should be arranged for this.

Soak-away

If already installed, this system will probably be maintained as long as neighbours do not complain. Planning permission is unlikely to be granted for a new installation. The principle is a tank system with bacteria that work on the solids. The liquid is allowed to drain away across the field by means of a ditch running downhill away from the building.

This system works well in a chalk or gravel area, but not in a clay area. Lavatory and tack room drains must enter the drainage system via a system of sealed pipes.

Open Drains

Looseboxes and barn-type stables can be drained either to the front or to the back of the box. Drainage to the back results in less air contamination. This is particularly important in barns. Drains to the back of buildings may be more easily forgotten, whereas front drains are more visible and attract more regular maintenance.

Covered Drains

If possible, these should be avoided, as they are not practical, becoming easily obstructed with manure and straw. If already installed, they should have accessible drain traps, which should be fitted with a removable wire tray to catch any solid material. (See diagram page 121.) Alternatively, small-gauge wire netting can be used for small traps, but must be cleaned daily. It is essential that any lengths of covered drain can be cleaned easily with rods. If that is not possible, it should be easy to take up the top covering, e.g. in old-fashioned stalls. A covered drain often runs down the length of the building and must be cleaned out each day.

Traps and Gullies

The principle on which gully traps are designed is for water to separate the outside air from the sewer or main drain air, and so prevent the return of the latter. Stable yard and surface drains should have efficient traps between the drainage system and the stable yard, so that solids can be collected and removed. There must be a sufficient body of water between the main drain and the air to prevent sewer gas from emerging. Drains should be well ventilated on the sewer side with a long pipe going well above the building. This should act as a double insurance against unpleasant smells.

DRAINS

In Looseboxes and Barns

These should have a shallow slope of 1 in 60, towards either the front or the back of the box. A small opening at floor level in the centre of the wall can direct any liquid into a shallow open drain running along the outside of the stable wall. Traps for collecting straw and solids should be positioned so that no clogging material can reach the main drainage system, see diagram on page 121. The removable trays in the traps should be cleaned regularly. To avoid any draughts from the drain opening, straw should be bedded up the wall.

The **advantages** of drains at the back are:

• No smell of urine, so more opportunity for the horse to breathe fresh, untainted air.

• Drainage is out of sight but still easily checked.

• There is less chance of draughts, as bedding is always banked up.

• Most horses stand facing the front of their boxes so are less likely to stand in the drain.

The **disadvantages** are:

• Difficult to arrange if looseboxes are on a boundary line or attached to other buildings.

• If not easily accessible they are likely to be neglected.

• It is less easy to wash the box down and sweep out water because of smaller opening and no doorway.

Barn-type Stabling

There should be a shallow open drain, preferably along the outside wall to avoid contamination but, if this is not possible, along the inner walls of both lines of boxes. This should end in a sump to trap straw and manure.

All drains should be washed clean daily. In a very long building, drains should be of the hog-back type, sloping from the centre towards both ends.

Stalls

Stalls should have a shallow open drain 60cm (2ft) behind the back post of the stall.

Deep Litter

Horses bedded on deep litter or any form of solid bed should have any deep drains sealed off. Drainage is not required if this type of bedding is used, but it is convenient to have an outside shallow drain to take away the liquid after washing the floor and walls.

Yard

This should have a gentle slope (according to the natural lie of the land) towards one or more mud gullies or traps which allow surface water to join the drainage system. All drain covers should be of steel or reinforced concrete, capable where necessary of taking the weight of a heavy lorry.

GUTTERING

All stable buildings must have efficient guttering which is well maintained and regularly cleaned. The downpipes should be of a sufficient number and shaped to shoot the water away from the base of the building, to open or covered drains. Broken and leaking guttering gives a bad impression of a stable yard, makes buildings damp and shortens the life of any wooden structure.

In areas where water is short this rainwater can be diverted into covered water butts and used for washing down, etc. The butt should be covered to discourage algae growth and set 50cms (20ins) or so above the ground to allow a bucket to be set under the top.

FLOORS

For the comfort of the horse, and to save strain on the legs, stable floors should be as level as possible. To assist drainage, a slope of 1 in 60 is suitable, except for stalls, which should be slightly steeper. The necessary floor space is 11–14sq m (118–150sq ft).

Materials

CONCRETE is the most widely used surface and is very satisfactory. A minimum depth of 15cm (6ins) is placed on top of a well-drained prepared base of hardcore and shingle. A damp course must be included. It is easily put down, but it must be of an extra-hard mixture to withstand urine and the horse's weight, and 'roughed' to provide a non-slip surface.

CHALK AND CLAY FLOORS are non-slippery and quiet. They are cheap to put down if material is available locally, but they require more maintenance, having to be topped and rammed every year. A clay floor tends to be damp.

COMPOSITION FLOORING is very satisfactory, but very expensive.

RUBBER MATTING on concrete can be used and saves time mucking out. Rubber matting is now widely used and if the right type for the job is chosen and good management is practised, the cost of installation can soon be recouped. It must, however, be properly managed to ensure the horse's comfort and the absence of smells.

AISLES

The width of the aisles between rows of stables needs to be considered carefully. It will depend upon:

- Whether a number of horses are moved at the same time.

- Whether horses in the boxes can reach over their doors into the aisle.

- Whether vehicles will be used.

- The style of doors chosen.

When a number of horses are moving in and out of the barn at the same time (for example in a riding school or student training environment) the aisle needs to be wide enough for two horses and their leaders to pass safely. Horses passing down the aisle should not feel threatened by horses reaching out of their boxes on either side.

If vehicle access is required, personnel should still be able to pass down the aisle safely.

If outward-opening doors are chosen they should not clash in the middle if opposite doors are opened at the same time. There should be enough room for one horse and leader to pass safely if one door is opened.

Sliding doors are usually a better choice. They do not need to be full height.

WALLS

Height

RIDGE ROOFS The walls of most prefabricated looseboxes range in height from 2.1–2.3m (7–7½ft) at the eaves to 3.3m (11ft) at the ridge. This is adequate for a box with a ridge roof and which slopes up from both front and back walls to a ridge.

When building with brick or concrete blocks, it is advisable for the walls to be 2.4–2.7m (8–9ft). This will allow for a 2.4m (8ft) doorway.

PITCH ROOFS A roof sloping from the back down to the front is known as a lean-to or pitch roof, and stables with such roofs require a minimum wall height of 2.7m (9ft) at the front, and 3.3m (11ft) at the rear or vice versa. In areas likely to have heavy snow, a steeper pitch is recommended.

FLAT ROOFS Stables with a flat roof or a ceiling with store rooms or lofts above require walls at a minimum height of 3m (10ft), but the measurement is dependent on the ground area of the box. See Ventilation, pages 388 and 396.

Damp Course

All walls should have a damp course; tarred building paper or a strip of plastic paper is effective. This is laid on the foundations, at the base of prefabricated stabling, or a little above ground level for bricks or concrete blocks.

Insulation

The insulation of stable walls is not essential, but adds greatly to the warmth and comfort of the horse. It will also increase the ventilation rate. It is recommended that all prefabricated stabling should be fully lined, to increase the stability, strength and warmth. Effective wall insulation is then achieved by placing a sheet of foil-lined building paper between the outer cladding and the inner lining.

Cavity-wall blocks provide their own wall insulation. Brick buildings constructed with cavity walls, i.e. two layers thick, have full insulation.

Surfacing of Walls

WOOD STABLING To give sufficient strength and added warmth, all walls should be lined. Material should be exterior plywood, or board of similar strength. This is essential up to 1.5m (5ft) high because of the risk of kicking, and it is recommended that it is continued up to the eaves. Otherwise horses tend to chew it where it stops, bedding gets down between the two surfaces and the gap provides an ideal habitat for vermin.

Both exterior and interior surfaces of the wood should be treated with wood preservative. Regular painting of the outside keeps it in good order. If interior woodwork is painted with colourless preservative, the top half of the box can then be painted with white emulsion. The bottom 60cm (2ft) of the wall can be painted with black bitumastic paint.

PRE-CAST CONCRETE OR PREFABRICATED COMPOSITION Such stabling requires lining with wood or chipboard. The appearance of the exterior surface is improved by a coat of Snowcem or similar preparation and the wood treated as above.

SOLID CONCRETE BLOCKS AND CAVITY BLOCKS Exterior walls require weather-proofing with a proprietary plastic preparation.

BRICK Cavity walls of brick-built buildings are weather-proof.

The interior walls of both types of blocks and also brick walls are rough. If a horse gets cast, he may damage himself on the rough surface. The walls may be plastered and painted. Plastic paints are now available which can provide a smooth, washable surface.

Traditionally, plastered walls are painted with a

colour for the first 1.2–1.5m (4–5ft) and then cream or white above.

ANTI-CAST RIDGE This is a ridge standing out approximately 25mm (1in) from the wall surface and 1.5m (5ft) above the floor. For ponies, the height should be 1.1m (3½ft). The ridge enables a horse to right himself, should he get cast, by stopping the feet slipping up the wall. Wooden stabling can include a reinforced strip of wood fixed firmly to the wall with screws. Block or brick buildings can incorporate a row of blocks or bricks set out from the wall, or a metal strip set into the cement between the blocks and bricks. Whatever is used, it should be shaped so that a crib biter cannot seize it with his teeth. Alternatively, a groove can be made in the wall surface to give a foothold to a cast horse.

ROOFS

Roofs should be:

- Weatherproof.
- Durable.
- Noiseless.
- Non-flammable.
- Warm in winter, cool in summer.

Types

ONDULINE CORRUGATED SHEETING fulfils all the above requirements and is inexpensive. In winter it may need lining to prevent condensation, and for this, roof felting is suitable. Maintenance is nil, unless cracked by a falling bough or heavy blow, e.g. from the horse's head. Perspex roof panels can be placed on the north side to provide more light.

RUBBEROID, GLASS-FIBRE OR PLASTIC TILES AND SLATES have a pleasing appearance, are long-lasting, light in weight, suitable for wooden stabling, and inexpensive compared to conventional tiles and slates.

ROOFING FELT is the cheapest material available, but it does not last, and should only be considered if it is of high quality. Wooden strips should be fitted at frequent intervals to prevent it being torn by strong winds.

TILES AND SLATES are satisfactory, but expensive and heavy. They are not suitable for wooden buildings.

THATCH is not recommended because of the fire risk.

GALVANISED SHEETING is hot in summer and noisy in wet weather. It is satisfactory for day stalls if correctly ventilated. Although cheap to install, maintenance can make it as expensive as other roofing materials, as it requires regular tarring or painting to control rust.

RIGID PLASTIC ROOFING SHEETS are light to handle, reasonably long-lasting, require little maintenance, and compare favourably in price. They are noisy in rain and high winds. They become brittle in time and are then likely to split.

New materials are constantly being introduced for industrial or farming units and should be researched before a decision is reached.

Overhang

This is a short extension of the roof over the door and front wall area of outside looseboxes. It gives protection to both horse and groom, and is a great boon with no drawbacks.

With prefabricated stabling, the overhang is usually an extension of the roof and built of the same material. With brick or block stabling, its material depends on construction. It can be built as a continuation of the roof, or else as a separate structure. Translucent plastic sheets can be used, but these can raise the temperature in the box in hot, sunny weather.

CEILINGS

These can be installed:

• If storage space or living accommodation is required above stables.

• In a high building, to decrease air space and make stables less draughty.

The material used should be fire-resistant and, to avoid condensation, be capable of absorbing moisture. For living accommodation strict local authority building regulations regarding health, safety and fire will need to be adhered to. Professional advice is essential.

VENTILATION

To keep a stabled horse healthy requires a constant supply of fresh air, but without draughts. Except in very cold weather, the temperature in a stable should not be warmer than outside. Horses keep fit and healthy if well rugged. It is preferable to keep a horse warm with extra food, blankets and stable bandages rather than by restricting his supply of fresh air. At the same time, he must not be subjected to a draught, as this can easily give him a chill.

Ventilation is of prime importance when stables are being built or converted. Any deficiencies will adversely affect the health of the horses. Some prefabricated boxes and purpose-built modern barns are not designed with sufficient ventilation. As long as draughts are avoided, the supply of fresh air should never be restricted.

Ideally, horses should have a permanent opening of 0.3 sq m (3 sq ft) (inlets) per horse in the walls and 0.1 sq m (1.6 sq ft) in the roof (outlets). The acceptable air space per horse is 45.3 cu m (1,600 cu ft), and this must be borne in mind when deciding on area and height. It is not just the amount of air but the speed with which it is renewed that is crucial. It should be replaced every twenty minutes. To measure this, use a smoke candle.

In some barn stables mechanical fans are used to ensure good air circulation. Means of providing ventilation are as follows.

Open Top Doors

These are the main source of fresh air for individual outside looseboxes. Except in exceptional circumstances, e.g. driving snow or a very cold direct wind, they should be kept open. The lower door should be 1.4m (4½ft) to 1.5m (5ft) high, to give sufficient protection and discourage a horse from jumping over it.

If stables are in lines, then they are best positioned facing south. If the stables have to be built facing north or east, it may be necessary to shut top doors at times in winter. If so, other methods of ventilation must be used, such as opening the windows or fixing a short metal hook externally to keep the door just ajar. The hook must be short enough for the horse to be unable to insert his head between the door and the door post.

It is possible to purchase webbing 'gates' which can be used instead of the bottom door to provide extra air circulation. They should only be used when the yard is staffed. They are also excellent in preventing a horse from banging his bottom door.

Windows

Windows are necessary for light and ventilation. If two are installed, they should be placed in the front and rear walls. In very windy weather, if the top door has to be shut, the window at the rear can be left open. In very hot weather, a back window allows a through-draught of air. If only one window is to be installed, it is probably better to have it at the rear.

Windows should be hinged at the bottom or centre according to size, and preferably opening inwards. Cold air is then directed up and above the horse's body, before descending and mixing with the warmer air below. Windows should be fitted with unbreakable clear perspex and protected with a grid which opens with the window. Bars are not suitable as these can be dangerous, easily trapping a horse's foot should he kick up or rear. Glass, if already installed, should be replaced with perspex.

Windows fixed at too low a level and opening inwards can be a hazard for the horse. If opening outwards, they must, when fully open, lie flush with the wall.

Louvre Boards

These are broad, overlapping boards, set at an angle to prevent the entry of rain or snow, and with an air passage between. They should be fixed in outside walls at least 2m (6½ft) from the ground. They extract stale air, and if correctly fitted, will assist in preventing condensation on the roof and walls.

Yorkshire Boarding

This is narrow, wood boarding fitted vertically with 1.25–2.5cm (½–1in) between each board. It frequently forms the top half of walls of farm buildings. If the roof above has an overhang and the wall is reasonably sheltered from the weather it can provide useful extra ventilation.

Eave Vents and Ridge Vents

These are found in Onduline-sheet roofs, at the eaves where the sheets meet the walls, and at the ridge of the roof where the sheets are capped. They are efficient ventilators. They should also be installed in other types of roofs.

Ventilating Cowls

These are placed on the ridge of the roof. They are manufactured in several designs, and can be used for most roofing types. They allow the exit of stale, warm air and ingress of fresh air. It is usual to install one to a box or one to two boxes.

Air Bricks

Air bricks can be put just under the eaves in brick or concrete block stabling. They should not be placed lower down because of draughts.

Power-driven Air Extractors

These can be fitted on the roof and should be turned on when the air is very still and humid.

When buying prefabricated stabling, it is advisable to check on ventilation. Some firms make better provision for it than others.

In **summary**, it is reasonably easy to provide sufficient ventilation in individual boxes but much more difficult in barn stables.

DOORS

There are two types: conventional hinged doors and sliding doors.

Size of Doorway

The ideal size is 2.4m (8ft) high and a minimum of 1.2m (4ft) wide, although for mares, foals and high-class young stock, doors should be 1.4m (4½ft) wide. As an extra precaution against horses knocking their hips, rollers can be fitted on the inside of both door posts. The distance between the posts should then be 1.4–1.5m (4½ to 5ft). Many prefabricated stables have doors 2.1–2.3m (7–7½ft) high; 2.3m (7½ft) is acceptable, but 2.1m (7ft) is only suitable for smaller horses.

Conventional Hinged Doors

This is the usual type of door for outside loose boxes. They are divided into two, the bottom door being 1.4–1.5m (4½ to 5ft) in height for horses and lower for ponies. If the lower door is too high it encourages the development of the wrong neck muscles.

FITTING They should be positioned to the side of the box to reduce direct draughts. They should not adjoin the box next door, as this encourages biting and bullying. They should open outwards so that, should a horse get cast against the door, it is possible to open it. Outward-opening doors also reduce disturbance of the bed. The bottom door should fit firmly down to the floor, so that there are no draughts, and no danger of a horse getting his foot caught under the bottom of the door.

The top edge of the bottom door should be protected from chewing by the horse with a firmly fixed heavy metal strip, which is 8–10cm (3–4ins) deep on both sides. Some horses reach right out and down over the outside of the lower door and then draw their teeth across the wood. In this case the metal strip can be taken further down the door or an anti-weaving top grille fitted. If there is no overhang, then some protection is needed from the weather for the tops of both doors.

When the top door is open, ideally it should not cover the window.

Sliding Doors

Sliding doors suspended from an overhead gearing are usually made the same height as the partitions of the boxes or pens of interior stabling, and consist of solid wood to a height of 1.5m (5ft) with grilles above. A sliding door can also be used for outside looseboxes. Usually the horse cannot look out but the grille can be provided with a drop-down section so that he can. Half-height, sliding doors are difficult to source but are available. A light top door is sometimes fitted to seal the top half in case of need.

Sliding doors cause less obstruction than hinged doors, and are a great asset for interior stabling where horses and people are moving and standing in the central passageway.

FITTING Sliding doors are heavier than a hinged door, and require substantial posts, usually made of metal. They hang from an overhead gearing, and the door is guided at the bottom either in a groove or on a rail. As a groove easily becomes clogged with dirt, a round rail on which the door glides along a groove in the bottom of its lower edge is more efficient.

Doors at the ends of barn stables, because of their size (approximately 3m (10ft) wide and 3m(10ft) high) must be very heavy, so sliding doors are easier to handle than hinged doors.

Construction

Stable doors receive constant and often rough usage. To withstand this it is essential that they are constructed of strong material. They should be lined with exterior plywood, galvanised sheet metal, or a similar hard, smooth surface. This should also cover the 'stays' on the door, which easily damage a horse's leg or knee if left exposed. Inferior wood, particularly if left unlined, is unsuitable and will not last.

Hinges and **bolts** should be of heavy-duty galvanised iron. Door hinges should be capped to prevent the door being lifted off, and they must be long enough to support the weight of the door.

Ideally any fastening should be able to be opened and shut one-handed as the worker usually has tack or equipment to carry.

The bottom door requires a top bolt, and a lower fastening which can be of the kick-over type. Bolts should be of a simple design, and free from anything which could injure the horse or catch on a headcollar.

The ideal door fastenings are those built into the framework, as the horse cannot get caught on them or touch them with his teeth. There are also special horse-proof bolts on the market, which are excellent but expensive. Some horses are able to open doors, so if the bolt is not of the horse-proof type, it should be able to take a spring hook for extra security. The top door requires one bolt. Both doors should have the necessary catches to fasten them back, flush against the stable wall, securely. Because of the danger of fire, stable doors should never be locked.

Some stables have an iron bar with a universal joint at one end and a hook at the other set just inside the lower stable door. This can be lifted across the doorway and hooked into a ring set in the opening side of the door jamb. Once this is up the bottom door can be left open and the worker can walk in and out underneath it, or easily muck out into the barrow, etc.

It can be a very useful piece of equipment in a busy yard where a lot of time can be wasted opening and shutting stable doors.

Window latches must be out of reach of the horse and, if at a lower level, must be protected so that the horse cannot play with them.

STABLE FITTINGS

For safety reasons, stable fittings should be minimal, and in many yards, fixed feed and hay mangers, hay racks and automatic watering systems are not installed.

Tying Up

For tying up, the ring should be placed to the side of the back wall at a height of 1.5m (5ft) (lower for ponies) and adjacent to the haynet ring, which should be nearer the corner at a minimum height of 1.8m (6ft). A short piece of string may be looped through the tying-up ring, so the horse is tied to the string and not directly to the ring. The loop should be small and neat to discourage the horse from chewing it. Baler twine can be almost unbreakable and therefore defeats the object. Parcel string is a better option. A second tie-ring in the front by the manger can be useful.

A tie-ring should also be fixed outside the box so that the horse can be secured during mucking out and grooming. Care should be taken that adjoining horses are not tied up at the same time, as they may well kick at each other.

Rings should be of heavy galvanised steel. In brick or

block stabling, they should be bolted through the wall with a holding plate on both surfaces. In wooden stables, the ring should be on a metal plate secured by four heavy screws and fastened through on to the vertical cladding of the box.

Watering

There are a number of ways in which water can be supplied, and these are covered in detail in Chapter 19.

Feed Troughs or Mangers

There are a number of fittings/containers suitable for short feeds:

FIXED MANGERS

These should be solid, with a smooth surface and must be easy to clean. The lip should be broad enough to prevent a horse seizing it with his teeth in case he starts crib biting. An overhanging inner lip prevents food being spilt, but it is difficult to clean. Deep mangers conserve food but encourage a horse to take too large mouthfuls. Shallow mangers are easy to clean, but a horse can easily waste food by pushing it over the edge.

Mangers can be built at ground level. These are safe and create the natural angle for a horse to eat, but they are likely to get soiled with dung and need constant washing.

Mangers are usually positioned at a height of approximately 1m (3–3½ft). To prevent a horse catching his foot underneath or knocking his head as he gets up, they can be boxed in, down to and flush with the floor. Alternatively, they can be fixed across a corner with a sloped but solid boxing-in by boards. It is essential that there are no projecting edges or angles on which the horse could damage himself.

Mangers should be fixed on the same wall as the door to reduce the risk of anyone being kicked as they leave the box after giving the feed. In prefabricated partitions they can be fitted as an integral part of the partition and so designed that the ration can be fed from outside the stable.

In stalls, fixed mangers for food and hay are usually installed at breast height.

REMOVABLE MANGERS

These can be made of metal or plastic with hooks which fit either over a door or into metal fixtures. They can be fitted on the door or on to the walls of the front corner and can be fixed on to any type of wall. These removable mangers are easy to wash and cannot be knocked over. The problems are that if fixed on the door they are high, and at an unnatural angle for a horse to eat. Also, they can be lifted out and thrown round the box.

NOTE: Metal fixtures are available which run across a corner to hold the manger. These can be dangerous and are not recommended.

FEED BOWLS

• **Metal feed bowls** are heavy and less likely to be knocked over, but can bruise a horse's leg should he strike or paw at them. They are easily cleaned, but are heavy to carry when taking round feed.

• **Plastic feed bowls** are light and easy to clean and handle. They can get knocked over and thrown around the box, or stamped on by a playful horse. They are easily broken. Lightweight, shallow plastic bowls are comparatively cheap, but do not last, and should be removed when the horse has finished feeding. The heavier, deeper rubber feed bowls without handles are more expensive, but more worthwhile. Feed bowls with handles should not be used as a horse can trap a foot in the handle. This is particularly applicable to young or playful horses.

• Feed bowls fixed in a **rubber tyre** are safe, but should be removed from the box after the horse has finished eating. They are unlikely to be knocked over and cannot damage a horse's leg, but they are heavy to move about.

Feeding Forage

Forage can be fed in the following ways:

LOOSE HAY is a safe and natural method of feeding hay and is labour-saving. The disadvantages are that it can be wasteful if the horse is an untidy feeder, and does not clean up. Also, the yard is more likely to be untidy, and this method necessitates tying up the hay for weighing, which is difficult if the hay has to be soaked. If it is fed on the ground it can be contaminated by dung and/or urine. This will make it unpalatable and increase the worm burden.

HAYNETS are the most popular way of feeding hay as they are economical, tidy to handle, easy to weigh and easy to damp or soak. The disadvantages are that they are time-consuming to fill, tie up and take down and they can be a danger if not tied up correctly (some horses play with the cord, chew it and get caught up); and they are an expense to buy.

FIXED HAY MANGERS are built up from the floor to a height of about 1m (3ft). They must be boxed in, and wider at the top than at the bottom. They must be so designed that waste forage can be swept out of the bottom. It is more difficult to weigh loose hay.

FIXED HAY RACKS are made of galvanised steel rods or a lighter weight steel mesh. They can be fixed above head level, but dust and seeds tend to fall into the horse's eyes and eating is at an unnatural angle. These problems can be prevented if the rack is fixed breast high, but a horse can then catch his foot or knock his head or eye in the steel rods or mesh.

OPTIONAL STABLE FITTINGS

Grids and Grilles

These are fixed to the top door of looseboxes. They may be a permanent fixture or removable. They are made of steel rods or heavy mesh, and are made in several patterns:

- Covering the entire area of the top door, which will prevent horses biting at people or at other horses passing by, help to prevent banging of the door with the front feet, discourage weaving and prevent crib biting on the door. If there is no overhang, it allows horses to see out and yet keep dry.

- A V-shaped grid allows the horse to put his head and neck over the door, but prevents him weaving, unless he is the type who stands back in his box and weaves. It also helps to prevent crib biting. Care should be taken that the opening is large enough for the horse to draw back without catching his head.

Salt-lick Holders

These should be positioned in a corner. The danger is that a horse can knock his head or eye on one. Salt blocks can be used as a safer alternative, and placed in a corner where the horse is fed. Salt causes a wet or damp patch, which eventually rots through an unprotected metal or wood wall surface.

ADDITIONAL UNITS

Utility Box

In many yards one or more boxes are set aside as utility boxes. The number depends on the size of the yard. The box may be used for clipping, shoeing, washing or veterinary work.

REQUIREMENTS

- High ceiling, minimum of 3.6m (12ft), preferably 4.3m (14ft), to avoid the risk of the horse hitting his head if resisting when being clipped.

- Non-slip, well-drained floor. Rubber flooring is

excellent and gives added protection when using electrical equipment.

- Daylight from well-protected windows.

- Efficient electric light.

- Two power points.

- Water available nearby.

- Tie-rings on each wall.

- Haynet ring on one wall next to tie-ring.

- There should be no fixed mangers or other fittings.

If heavy clipping machinery is to be used, an overhead trackway is necessary at a height of 3.2m (10½ft) and running along the back and side walls. It is then out of the way, should a horse rear. A corrugated perspex roof panel can be installed to give added light. An infra-red light can be fixed and used to dry a horse after washing.

Isolation Box

To be effective, this box must be at least 100m (110 yds) away from the main stabling. It should face away from the stables, with the prevailing wind blowing away from the stables.

REQUIREMENTS

- Size: 4.3m x 4.3m (14ft x 14ft).

- Average height.

- Insulated walls and roof.

- Well-fitting, draught-proof windows and door.

- Electrics: 13-amp plug and fitting for heat lamp.

- Adjacent water supply.

- Adjacent weather-proof shed to store isolated horse's feed, mucking-out tools, grooming equipment, buckets, rugs, medical equipment, etc.

From a practical point of view, it is doubtful if an

isolation box is really either worthwhile or effective against infectious diseases, but a box that is quite a way from others is useful for ill horses. For this purpose it needs to be easily accessible from the house. A contagious condition (e.g. ringworm) can be contained successfully by a strict isolation procedure.

The box needs to be made from materials that are easy to clean and disinfect. It should be near staff quarters so that the horse can be managed through the night.

The path to it needs to be well lit. A surveillance system is often useful to monitor the horse's activity. The door should have an overhang.

Forge

Stables with a resident farrier require a forge. This should be sited away from the stables, hay and straw barn, because of fire risk. It must be on a hard surface and convenient to other buildings for supplies of electricity and water. In a large yard it is usually adjacent to the carpenter's shop (shed). Most yards now use travelling farriers, with a specially equipped van containing a portable forge. However, the farrier still prefers an area of hard standing, under cover in order to work comfortably in bad weather.

Useful Additions

A retractable hook outside each box is useful for hanging a headcollar or bridle. It should not be possible for the horse to reach it. A folding saddle bracket can also be an asset.

For looseboxes bedded with shavings, sawdust or paper a 0.90–1.2m (3–4ft) length of light chain fastened to the outside wall of the loosebox makes a convenient place on which to hang rugs and blankets.

Custom-made rug rails or folding brackets are useful.

ELECTRICITY

- A 'trip-switch' system is essential so that if there is any fault in wiring, fittings or machinery the electric current will immediately be cut off, and cannot be restored until the fault is located and repaired.

- It is required by law that all electric wiring and fittings must be installed by a qualified electrician, who should also attend to all servicing and repairs.

- It should be remembered that horses are much more susceptible to electricity than are humans. Quite a low voltage can kill them.

- All cabling should run through metal pipes and be fixed so that it cannot be chewed or pulled by a horse. Wherever possible, it should run outside the boxes and enter the stables from high in the roof.

- Switches should be of a water-tight design and positioned outside the box, where they are out of reach of the horse. Cabling should enter the switch or junction box from underneath to minimise the ingress of damp.

Lights

These can be fluorescent or bulb fixtures. Fluorescent lighting must be fixed high in the roof, out of reach of the horse. In adjoining stables, if walls do not reach the roof, one fixture gives good light to two boxes.

Fluorescent light is more expensive to buy and install than bulb fixtures, but is cheaper to use, lasts longer, and gives a better light. In very cold weather it may not be so efficient.

Lighting left on for any length of time presents a fire risk if the strip or lamp is not regularly cleaned. Cobwebs ignite, fall to the floor and ignite anything flammable they fall on, such as bedding or clothing. Environmentally 'green' light bulbs should be researched.

Bulb fixtures can also be placed high in the roof and

then need not be protected, but this height makes replacing and also cleaning difficult; encrusted dust affects their efficiency. If placed in storage areas, they can be a fire risk if they should come into contact with hay or straw.

A much safer but considerably more expensive fitting is the bulkhead type. If these are used, they can be placed at a more accessible height – 2.1–2.4m/7–8ft – which makes cleaning and replacing bulbs easier.

Low-wattage bulbs are long-lasting and economical to use. Light is not instant but progressively strengthens when switched on. This can be helpful in avoiding startling the horses.

Power Points

One 13-amp power point should be installed and available for approximately every six boxes. They must be out of reach or protected from the horse. They are used for clipping, grooming and heat lamps. They must never be used without a plug-in circuit breaker.

The utility and isolation boxes will need good lighting and an extra socket for the clipping machine, heat lamp, etc.

Yard Lights

Efficient yard lights are essential if work is to be carried out after dark. Good lighting will not only make work areas safer, but will save time and be cost-effective. High-intensity tungsten-halogen lamps or high-pressure sodium lamps give excellent light over a wide area. They are cheap to run, although expensive to install. They are very much more efficient than the traditional type of bulb fixture, and require less maintenance. The latter give limited light and are expensive to use.

Yard lights left on at night can be a deterrent to thieves. In this case low-wattage bulbs should be used for economy.

MAINTENANCE

Most manufacturers of prefabricated wooden stabling treat the wood used with a wood preservative, to make it weather-proof, and to protect it from attack by wood beetle and fungus. The woodwork will require regular treatment to ensure that it stays weather-proof and also to improve appearance.

Wooden doors and windows in brick or concrete block stables can either be treated in the same way, or painted. This is a matter of personal choice – painting requires more maintenance and is more expensive. The wood requires a primer, an undercoat and a top coat. Lead-based paint is poisonous and should not be used. Maintenance is important – cracked or peeling paint is a bad advertisement for any yard, commercial or private.

Metal doors and windows are now likely to be of a rust-proof metal and need no attention. Older fixtures require regular painting, with an anti-rust undercoat and a suitable top coat.

All door, window and stable fittings should be of galvanised iron or steel. These will not rust.

Efficient maintenance of buildings, equipment, facilities, fencing, yard and drive are an essential part of successful business management. This is why it is always better to buy the best that can be afforded. This does not mean that money should be wasted on non-essential buildings or equipment, or luxurious extras which are not necessary. The successful manager plans ahead, and knows what is essential and what is not.

Repairs to buildings and fencing, if carried out in good time, save further deterioration. Allowing surroundings to remain in bad repair invites accidents to animals and staff.

The impression gained on entering a stable yard is very important. It is possible to tell immediately whether the yard is efficient. Stable managers must be methodical and observant, to ensure that necessary repairs and regular maintenance work are carried out.

FEED SHED

REQUIREMENTS

- It is best constructed of brick or concrete blocks to discourage vermin. A wooden shed can be raised off the ground and the floor and walls lined inside with zinc sheets. This is not as expensive as it sounds. It is ideal if the feed is stored separately from the feed preparation area.

- A dry, light, secure room, convenient to the stables. A good door is essential, so that there is no danger of a loose horse getting into the feed shed.

- Large yards may have either a small feed shed for daily use, and a larger feed store next door for storing bulk supplies, or separate feed sheds for each area.

- The floor should be of concrete, level except in the door area, where it should have a slight slope and shallow drain to the side of the door.

- See also page 420, on feed storage.

THE TACK ROOM

Horse tack is a constant security risk. Insurance companies have individual rules about siting and structure of tack rooms. It is advisable to consult your own company before either building a new tack room or converting a building for use as a tack room.

Burglary Precautions

- Site to be in view of living quarters and adjacent to or part of the stable block.

- Structure to be of brick or concrete blocks with Onduline or tiled roof.

- Windows to be of glass, protected on the inside with steel bars.

- Doors to be of solid wood or steel, with a normal lock for use during the day and a Yale lock for security at night. Steel shutters for doors and windows, as used by inner city shops, can also be considered for use overnight.

- Communicating doors should have bolts on the inside.

- Yard lights should be left on at night.

- Burglar alarms can be fitted.

- Dogs have been proved to be the best deterrent, either sleeping in the tack room or loose in the yard. If the latter, they should have a well-insulated kennel and the yard must be secure so that they cannot wander.

- Have an inner windowless room for storage and an outer, working tack room for cleaning, etc.

- In a big yard with multiple activities, have a number of tack rooms: livery clients' tack, show tack, and seldom-used tack can all be stored separately to make thieves' task more difficult.

- Tack can now be marked with a registered number. This makes identification easier, and discourages theft. In conjunction with the British Horse Society, one scheme is run by Farm Key of Banbury, Oxfordshire, who supply the marking tools and keep a national register.

- Insurance companies often require to see security arrangements, and may give advice on further precautions.

- It is worth noting that many burglaries take place during the day.

If the yard is to be left, even for short periods of time such as over lunch, tack rooms should be locked.

In a yard with a high changeover rate of clients, such as a college, consider digital locks which can have the combination changed on a regular basis.

Try not to use the tack room as an office or changing

room. The fewer people who have legitimate access, the easier to keep track of property.

Layout of Tack Room

- Wash room for cleaning tack. Main tack room for putting tack up when clean.

- Combined wash and tack room.

- Two combined wash and tack rooms, one for school tack and one for livery.

Whichever system is chosen, the main requirements are:

- Floor: concrete is practical and should slope into one corner to drain. If covered with non-slip composition flooring, it is more comfortable for standing and working. The surface should be easy to both sweep and mop.

- Lighting: fluorescent strip lighting is the most efficient.

- Heating: there must be no direct heat to leather. All heating should be well away from any working areas to avoid any risk of fire and injury. The temperature suitable for working, and to keep tack in good condition, should be 13–16°C (55–60°F) in winter.

- Choose a heater that has a built-in thermostat. Ensure that it is not possible to drape or hang damp objects such as boots, numnahs, rugs or washing cloths directly on it.

- A sink with an extended draining board for scrubbing. A deep sink makes cleaning easier.

- Hot and cold water: electric water-heaters of the geyser type are suitable. It can sometimes be arranged for room heating and water heating to be on the same system, and connected to other areas requiring heat and hot water.

- Ensure it is possible to get a bucket under the tap.

- Hot water, soap and towels should be provided for staff use.

- Saddle-horses for cleaning saddles should be sufficient in quantity for the number of staff. They can be 3–4.2m (10–14ft) long and must be strongly built. When a large number of people have to clean tack at the same time, it can be preferable to have a number of short saddle horses 4–5 feet long with one worker at each end, as it is much easier to work.

- Telescopic bridle-cleaning hooks: these should be sited with care, as they can be a hazard if placed near a door or where others are working.

- Saddle racks: preferably of plastic or wood, as iron may mark the leather. Slip-in holders for horses' names make for efficiency.

- Bridle holders: preferably semi-circular in shape so that the top of the bridle is kept rounded. Slip-in holders for the horses' names are advisable.

- Although, for convenience, some people prefer the saddle and bridle to be stored together, more equipment can be stored if bridles are hung on one wall and saddles on another.

- Pony tack should be stored lower down to be readily available to smaller people.

- A safe stepping stool or short pair of steps must be provided for retrieving saddlery stored above head height.

- Hooks: for lungeing tack, spare girths, stirrup leathers, martingales, breastplates, etc. Name plates help to avoid disorder.

- Bit board for spare bits.

- Cupboard for tack-cleaning equipment.

- Cupboard with shelves or compartments for bandages, boots, shoeing tools, clipping machines, disinfectant, shampoo, hoof oil, Stockholm tar, etc. The top of the cupboard can be flat to provide a sound working surface.

- Human first aid equipment can be kept in the tack room.

- Medicine cupboard for first aid.

- Drugs, poisons and worm doses must be kept in a locked cupboard in the office.

- Storage for exercise boots and bandages.

- Several bar stools can make convenient and space-saving seats.

- A noticeboard showing what extra equipment each horse uses for specific tasks, such as boots for jumping and which size of double bridle or lunge cavesson if they are not owned individually.

- One or two roller towels.

- Battery clock.

- Dustbin.

- Fire appliance.

- Ideally personal lockers for staff or clients should not be housed in the tack room.

- Rugs should be kept in a rug room and, where individual horses or clients have a lot of equipment, they should have individual lockers or trunks for secure storage in an area specific to them.

- Grooming kits and other equipment that might be needed when the tack room is locked should be located in more accessible areas.

NB: The Health and Safety at Work Act (1974) should be checked and adhered to.

ADDITIONAL PREMISES

Wash Room

Large yards will benefit from an equipped wash room.

REQUIREMENTS

- Drying racks.

- Heavy duty, commercial washing machine and spin dryer.

- Heating to assist drying.

- Large sink with hot and cold water, and a draining board.

Rug Room

This is almost vital in any yard where a large number of rugs are used. Situated next to the wash room would be ideal.

REQUIREMENTS

- Nursery-style racks for hanging rugs and numnahs to dry.

- Individual rug racks for storing rugs in regular use.

- Storage trunks for storing rugs and equipment not in regular use, such as show rugs and travelling equipment.

- An efficient heating system.

Store Room

This should be a secure room or large cupboard, ideally situated near the office. Use for storing replacement equipment, soaps, disinfectants, cleaning materials. Also extra first aid equipment such as cotton wool, toilet rolls, towels and stationery.

Staff and Lecture Room

The need for separate staff and lecture rooms depends on the number of staff, and the size and the functions of the yard.

REQUIREMENTS

- Efficient heating.

- Floor covering, which is easily cleaned but provides some warmth.

- Sufficient upright chairs for students and working pupils.

- A noticeboard for daily staff timetables and duties, allocation of horses, etc. If this room is combined with the client rest room this board can also show times for clients' lesson/rides and allocation of horse and teacher/escort.

- One or more tables.

- Small easy chairs.

- Electric kettle, small serving table, power point.

- Blackboard and chalk or whiteboard.

- Wall charts to cover points of the horse, skeleton, muscles, main organs of the body, bits, etc.

- Specimen shoes.

- Specimen bones of the horse's leg below the knee.

- Noticeboard announcing coming events, competitions, etc.

- Battery clock.

- Long mirror by the door for use of staff.

- Fire extinguisher.

- Kitchen and small electric stove and sink with hot and cold water (not essential in a small yard).

- Staff and working pupils' individual shelves or lockers.

- Hot drinks machine (not essential in a small yard).

- Video camera and power point (not essential in a small yard).

- If combined with client rest room, ideally there should be personal lockers for clients, on the lines of those provided in public swimming pools. These could be provided free on an hourly basis or rented out for a weekly or monthly fee.

NB: The facilities must comply with the Health and Safety at Work Act (1974). The minimum requirements are stated in the Horse Riding Establishment's paper – 'Guidance on Promoting Safe Working Conditions' (HM Agricultural Inspectorate Health and Safety Executive 1988).

Changing Rooms and Lavatories

These must be sufficient for the size of the yard; and flush lavatories must be easily available for clients and staff.

REQUIREMENTS

- Changing room.

- Efficient heating.

- Floor covering which is easily cleaned.

- Basin with hot and cold water.

- Shower room, but this is not necessary in a small yard.

- Towels, soap and paper towels.

- Hooks and coat hangers for clothes.

- Boot jacks.

- Mirror.

- Secure storage for valuables such as keys and money.

- Equipment for cleaning basin, lavatories and floors, stored safely in an appropriate cupboard.

- Premises to comply with Health & Safety Regulations already stated.

NB: If areas requiring hot and cold water are close together, e.g. feed room, kitchen, changing rooms and lavatories, it is more economical as one water heater can be used.

OFFICE

In any but the smallest yard which deals with clients on a regular basis it is essential to have an office or at least a designated office space.

- Ideally it should be situated near the entrance and be easily identified from the car park.

- If it is not manned full time, information on office hours and whom to contact when it is closed should be posted on the door.

OUTSIDE REQUIREMENTS

- Specific fire regulations for the yard, to include nearest telephone, address of establishment, grid reference and what to do in the event of a fire.

- 'No smoking' notice and sand bucket for stubbing out cigarettes.

- Any notice about control of dogs or children or uninvited visitors relevant to specific yard.

INSIDE REQUIREMENTS

- Normal office equipment.

- Telephone and answering machine.

- Copies of relevant licences, qualifications and insurance details displayed as required by law.

- Copy of Safety Policy, also displayed.

- Noticeboard with information regarding type of services offered. Prices and details of staff members.

- Lists for the day detailing client names, activity, horse allocation, staff member responsible, start and finish time, etc.

- Filing cabinet for storing all confidential information.

- Desk and chairs for staff.

- Chairs for waiting clients.

- Cupboard for storing stationery, leaflets, etc.

- Lockable cash box and safe; possibly a till.

- Computer if most information is held in this way.

- All relevant books for sales and purchases.

- Files for relevant horse/client details.

- If boots, hats, etc. are hired out, an area specific for that provision.

- Daily diary – booking book.

- Wall charts – year planners.

- All relevant staff/clients/horse/service files. See Chapter 54, Organising and Running a Yard.

Tack and Clothes Shop

Many yards run a tack and clothing shop. This can be limited to a few items, or cover a large selection of goods. It can be a useful service for clients, and a source of extra income to the school.

REQUIREMENTS

- A trading licence.

- A suitable room, which is dry and essentially burglar-proof.

- A member of staff with sufficient time to cope with customers.

- Cupboards, shelves and counter.

- Cash box.

- Saddle racks.

- Bridle and tack hooks.

- Boot jack.

- Mirror.

- Tape measure.

However, such a shop may alienate local saddlers, who also do the yard's tack repairs. Thus it might be advisable to arrange for them to supply the goods at a discount rate.

INDOOR SCHOOLS

With the increase in the number of riders, the demand has grown for all-weather teaching areas and competition facilities, especially during the winter months. An indoor school has become a necessity for any progressive commercial establishment.

The construction will be governed by the amount of space and money available, and also the purposes for which the school is required.

Planning permission is necessary. If a large competition school is planned, understandably, local residents often object to the inevitable increase in horse traffic. The tactful canvassing of local support before applying to the planning authorities can possibly avert the refusal of a planning application.

There are now many well-established and experienced firms who will advise on construction, and also deal with the planning authorities. Before a decision is made, it is advisable to investigate a variety of types of schools. Owners are often happy to show their schools and discuss design and structure.

Size

20m wide x 30m long

This area is suitable for teaching small children, adult beginners, for lungeing horse and rider and training horses on the lunge. The minimum width should be 20m, both from a functional point of view and so that, if at a later date a school of the size of a dressage arena is required (20 x 40m, or 20 x 60m), extra bays can be added.

20m wide x 40m long

This size of school is suitable for general teaching, schooling of horses and small dressage and show-jumping competitions. It is the most convenient and economical size for practical work. It is also the minimum size acceptable to the British Horse Society if the school wishes to be recognised as an examination centre.

30m wide x 90m long

This size of school is suitable for all competition work, and also divides comfortably to accommodate two class lessons. The increase in width adds considerably to the expense, as the supports of a wider clear-span roof have to be so much stronger. There is also the inevitable increase in rateable value. A large school, fully enclosed with a seated gallery, has a much higher rateable value. A smaller school with semi-enclosed walls, small unfitted gallery and limited competition facilities should warrant a much lower rating.

A large indoor working area or two schools, side by side with a doorway between them will make the running of indoor shows much easier and more popular with clients, especially if warm-up areas are also under cover.

In very cold areas, consider being able to access all areas without going outside.

Having the office, changing rooms, tack and store

rooms, as well as the stables all adjacent to the school, makes working much easier.

However, this sort of planning concept is beyond the scope of this manual.

Construction

Most modern schools are of clear-span, steel-framed construction with a ridge roof. Translucent sheets are placed at regular intervals in the roof to provide light. The ridge of the roof is capped, and this should be ventilated. The height to the eaves is 4.3–5.5m (14–18ft) – 4.3m (14ft) may be taken as a safe minimum. When floor material is added, the actual roof height will be less. The outer cladding of the walls of the building can be breeze blocks, galvanised metal sheeting, rigid plastic sheeting, or brick. Brick is very expensive, but sometimes insisted upon by planning authorities.

If the walls are built up to the eaves, translucent sheets should be used on the top section to give light. These can be put on to frames that can be opened in hot weather to give essential ventilation. A fully enclosed school can become airless and an unpleasant place in which to work. A cheaper and more pleasant alternative is to have walls 2.4m (8ft) high with an open space to the eaves. The walls may then be of solid timber, and an outer cladding is not required. This system gives sufficient shelter in most winters, is lighter, and allows a greater feeling of freedom for both horse and rider. Yorkshire boarding for the top half of the walls is a cheap and successful method of introducing more light and better circulation of air. However, it can create a flickering effect for the rider if there is sunlight behind. (Note: it is not suitable for epileptics as it may cause a fit.)

Various forms of netting used in gardens to provide windbreaks have also been used successfully. In the summer, the school will be cool and pleasant to work in, even in hot weather. Schools used regularly for winter competitions, or situated in areas of heavy snow, may have to be fully enclosed, as do those where it is desirable to shut out external noise.

Kicking boards on the inner side of the wall cladding should be of solid timber, plywood or blockboard with a minimum of 1.5m (5ft) showing above the floor. They can be sloped from the top at an angle of 12–15° (wider at the top and sloping towards the floor), which will reduce the risk of a rider knocking a knee. To give added light they should be painted white. Dressage markers on the walls should be painted black.

If funds are limited, an alternative to solid walls is straw bales or woven fencing protected by a guard rail. Care must be taken when erecting these to ensure the rider cannot catch his foot, and a watch should be kept for any loose baling string. If a rider or horse falls against these they provide a more cushioned landing than a solid wall. The pillars supporting the roof must be padded up to a height of 1.8–2.4m (6–8ft) to prevent damage to horse and rider.

School doors should be a minimum of 3.6m (12ft) wide and at least 2.4m (8ft) high to avoid any danger of a horse jumping out. If regular topping up of the surface is envisaged, then doorways must be high enough to take the transporters. They should preferably be of the sliding door design, suspended from an overhead gearing and have guiding rails top and bottom. If the school has an apron of concrete outside the doors, the surface that will inevitably be tracked out can be swept back in on a daily basis. Hinged doors are heavy to handle and a problem in high winds. If used, they should open outwards, as inward-opening doors are a danger to horses working in the school.

Drainage

The roof needs efficient guttering and drainage. If other buildings allow, soak-aways can be dug at intervals round the outside of the building to take this roof water. The soak-away should be a minimum of 4.5m (15ft) deep and filled with stone or pebble. Alternatives are a 'French drain' along both walls or a shallow open drain to direct the water away, possibly to the yard drainage system. A 'French drain' starts at a minimum depth, and is dug out and sloped towards a deep soak-away. The drain and soak-away are filled with stone or pebble. Alternatively, a water collection system for roof water may allow the water accumulated to be re-used to irrigate the school surface or for cleaning or watering purposes.

The floor area, unless at a high water-table level, should only require levelling before being covered with the selected surface. It is necessary to take advice, but the extra expense of a prepared base and a plastic membrane is often avoidable. It should be checked that surface water from an upper level cannot seep under the school floor.

If the school has been cut into a surrounding bank, the drain-off from the slope must be channelled away from the school surface.

Galleries

These can be either at the end or along the side of the arena. For watching and judging jumping a side gallery gives better viewing. For dressage judging an end gallery or box is essential. For competition centres, a tiered gallery is recommended. For smaller centres where the gallery may be used for several purposes, a level floor is of more practical use. If used regularly in winter, some form of heat is needed. Fire regulations must be observed.

Lighting

This can be a very expensive item, and research is advisable as to the cheapest and most efficient system to install, maintain and use. Strip lighting has been the most popular, but improved alternatives have now become available. It is possible to install the lighting so that sufficient lighting can be switched on for normal use with extra being introduced for competition or night-time jumping. This can considerably reduce the day to day cost.

Lighting of pedestrian ways and the area in front of the doors may be needed for winter and night-time use.

Teaching Aids

A full-length mirror or mirrors in the corners and on the centre line and another, wider, mirror at the half marker on the long side are excellent instructional aids. They do not have to be made of glass but must not distort the image. Glass should not be used in arenas intended for serious jumping.

A video camera is an expensive but useful asset. A loud-speaker system is of assistance, for competition and instructional sessions where both the spectators in the gallery and the riders need to be able to hear what is being said.

Extra electric sockets for timing equipment and music equipment should be considered.

- Indoor schools are an extremely dusty environment and provision should be made for all electrical equipment to be locked away in a dust-and-damp-proof storage area.

- If much teaching is done, consider having a telephone.

Jump Store

It is convenient to have jumps readily available, and essential that they are stored in a secure, dry area. If space is available, the area underneath the gallery can be used, with a door in the school wall. For safety this should open inwards to the store and away from the school track.

If the area under the gallery is used for storage, care must be taken to ensure that no rubbish or flammable material from the seating above can fall through.

Surface

Choice depends on the proposed use of the school and the cost. Before deciding, it is advisable to visit other schools to inspect and ride on the surface they have chosen, to check on maintenance, and to consider whether it will stand up to the type of work required.

There are so many types of surface available that plenty of time should be used to research your choice carefully. Things to consider when choosing are:

• Cost.

• Ease of maintenance.

• Suitability for the purpose.

• Ease and type of going for the horses.

• Dust-free.

• Longevity.

• Ease of topping up or renewing.

Many surfaces come with a guarantee. A home-made surface of sand or sand mixed with shavings or wood chippings may be successful in a non-commercial enterprise, but will usually be false economy if needed for hard work. A surface used for jumping must not be 'dead' and must not move under the horse's feet or pan and become slippery if the horse needs to turn sharply.

It is usually best to employ an expert contractor to lay the surface and do any preparatory work needed.

Maintenance of Surfaces

All surfaces, given sufficient use, will require daily levelling. This can be done by hand, or by a tractor pulling a harrow and leveller. Specially designed machines for this are now available. The machine designed for the surface should be used. Particular attention should be paid to the outside track, the lungeing area and any part where jumping regularly takes place.

Some surfaces, particularly after several years of use, may become compacted and slippery. They will require scarifying and then levelling, and in damp weather this may have to be done regularly. They should also be topped up with fresh supplies. A scarifier is a deep type of harrow which digs up the under-surface. It should not be used if a membrane has been put down.

Control of Dust

In time, school surfaces break down into smaller particles, causing a constant dust problem in summer, and in dry, windy spells in winter. Neither staff nor horses should be required to work in a dusty atmosphere.

Preventative measures

• Surfaces made from wood will need regular dressings of agricultural salt, approximately 1 tonne per 20 x 40m arena. Salt is usually supplied in sacks of 50kg (110lbs) and can be most easily spread if carted on the back of the tractor and thrown out with a shovel. Care must be taken that not too much salt is applied as it can have a drying effect on horses' feet, with resultant problems. It may also affect the leather boots or shoes of anyone standing in the school for a length of time.

• Daily watering, picking up droppings as soon as they are produced. They break down to dust quickly and are then a health hazard.

• Install a header tank, save water from the roof, ensure the pressure is sufficient.

• Installation of an overhead watering system, which is expensive but efficient, quick and labour-saving, and will be a good long-term investment, if the system is carefully designed and the water pressure is sufficient. With water becoming scarcer and more expensive it may be cheaper in the long run to install a different type of floor.

• There are a number of waxed or treated surfaces on the market that need little or no watering. Other surfaces made from plastic or rubber waste material might be researched as new ones are coming on to the market all the time.

OUTDOOR SCHOOLS

Many firms now specialise in the construction and design of outdoor riding surfaces. If requested, they can provide a complete package deal, and some give a guarantee. It can be a short-sighted policy to cut costs, and finish up with a school only usable in dry weather.

Considerations When Choosing the Site

DRAINAGE Efficient drainage is essential. A site on a slight slope with natural drainage to a lower level can be a great asset. Sub-soils of chalk, gravel, sand or stone all drain well, which makes the site preparation cheaper.

Schools built at the bottom of a slope, or on a sub-soil of clay or other poorly draining material, need considerable work and extensive foundations if the final top surface is to be satisfactory and remain usable in wet weather.

Experienced advice should be taken, and no expense spared on this basic preparation of the site.

Consider building the surface up at the top of the site rather than cutting into a slope or bank lower down. It can be easier to provide shelter for the more exposed position, in the form of trees, than deal with the problem of run-off from the slope above.

ACCESS Preferably this should be convenient to the stable yard, with a hard or firm access to a roadway. A muddy track makes horses, staff and spectators unnecessarily dirty. Mud carried on and in the horses' hooves will not improve the school surface.

SHELTER In exposed areas, neighbouring buildings and/or barns can give welcome protection from high winds and driving rain, but they should not be so close as to interfere with drainage plans.

A tall hedge makes an excellent wind-break.

The surrounding fence can be built of wooden boards or plastic strips, and to a sufficient height to give shelter. As long as there are gaps between the boards, it will be unlikely to be blown down.

In summer, trees can give welcome shade, but if large they may interfere with drainage plans.

Consider the neighbours. Many will not object to a surface put down and used for a few hours a day, but will object to one where teaching takes place and perhaps which is lit until late into the evenings.

Fencing

The school must be safely and securely fenced according to its intended use. A suitable height for most purposes is 1.4m (4½ft).

Posts should be on the outside of the fence; the inside should have no protruding surface liable to cause injury. For economy, plain wire can be used below a top rail of wood or plastic. Barbed wire must never be used.

The entrance should be wide enough for a tractor and any maintenance equipment; slip rails or a gate can be used. The gate should open outwards, and have no protruding fastenings.

The school surface will need to be retained by a ground-level edging, possibly of railway sleepers or other strong timber.

Choice of Surface

This depends on intended use, and the amount of work done in the school. Suppliers of surfaces should be given full information, so that they are in a position to offer the most helpful advice. It is also sensible to see different surfaces under the working conditions similar to those envisaged. Most firms will supply a list of schools they have constructed, and owners are usually happy to discuss matters. It is a help either to ride on the surface or to see horses working on it. Jump training and lunge work are likely to cause the most problems, making greater demands on the security and durability of the surface.

It is essential that the correct type of foundation is laid to suit the top surface. This is one reason to arrange for the work to be done by a specialist firm, who will also have experience of blending different materials to produce surfaces suitable for particular work.

All surfaces must be put down on a properly prepared base, which should be built up to be well above the level of the surrounding ground surface.

Dust Prevention

Just as with the indoor surface provisions must be made to prevent dust. It is bad for the horses, especially if they work one behind the other, as in a riding school. It is also very unpleasant for riders and teachers and is a health hazard.

Dusty surfaces blow away. This is an expensive waste of the surface and spoils the surroundings. Options are as for the indoor school, or it may be possible if the area is big enough to use a water bowser pulled behind a tractor.

SAND

This has been the most widely used all-purpose surface. If laid too deep, it can be heavy to ride on and tiring for the horse. A starting depth of 8–10cm (3–4ins) is recommended, and this can be topped up as required.

In summer, it can be dusty without regular applications of salt and daily watering. In winter, if drainage is faulty, it may freeze, but salt helps to keep the school usable.

The sand used should be clean, and free from soil or debris which could make it compact under pressure.

Types of sand

- Sharp sand, double-washed, provides a workable surface.

- Silicon sand is the best. It is more expensive, and in some areas may be difficult to obtain. It is clean, dust-free, drains well and is therefore less likely to freeze.

- Grade 4 industrial sand is also recommended.

- Some grades of beach sand are used with success. Permission for its extraction must be obtained.

- Some forms of silica sand, such as the by-product from china clay extraction, are too sharp and abrade the horses' feet, so should not be used.

Mixtures of sand with shavings and plastic fibre are also workable surfaces, the shavings/fibre making the surface lighter to ride on and less likely to freeze.

SHAVINGS

These are put down on top of a solid base. They are then soaked by hose and compacted with a vibratory roller. The resulting surface is suitable for light work, but lungeing and constant jumping are likely to break it up, as is heavy commercial use of the school.

MANUFACTURED WOOD FIBRE AND WOOD CHIPS

Used on their own they are suitable for work on the flat. If mixed with sand, they form an improved all-purpose surface. In freezing conditions, shavings, wood fibre and chips, if well drained, will soften when ridden on and should not freeze.

All forms of wood-based surfaces will eventually break up and start to rot; they will then have to be removed and replaced – a costly operation.

PLASTIC

Various forms of plastic granules are obtainable. They form a clean, dust-free, long-lasting surface which drains well and is frost-resistant. They are not so suitable for jump training.

Some of the latest surfaces combine PVC granules, fibre and sand, and have a wax coating or water-retaining gel, thereby reducing the need to water in dry weather.

RUBBER

Shredded rubber products give a resilient non-skid surface requiring little topping up and are frost-resistant. The shredded rubber is laid on a base of washed stone aggregate which mixes with it to form the surface.

Membranes

A membrane has two distinct uses:

- **Non-porous type.** This is laid down before the foundation. It prevents water coming up, and on a clay soil stops the foundation and school surface from gradually being absorbed into the clay.

- **Porous type.** This is laid on top of the foundation and below the top surface. It allows surface water to drain through and prevents stones from working up. In time, porous membranes will clog and cease to drain effectively.

All membranes eventually disintegrate and their original function ceases.

Tarmac Base

Some surfaces are now laid on a prepared base of tarmac. This obviates the need for a graduated foundation, internal drains and a membrane. A site with good natural drainage is essential. Professional advice should be sought if considering this type of base.

MAINTENANCE

Depending on the amount of use, it is essential that the surface receives regular maintenance. Some very busy arenas may be harrowed twice a day.

- Pick up droppings regularly.

- Dig out tracks if material compacts.

- Rake sides onto tracks and rake corners back into school.

- Sweep in gateways and entrances.

- Water, harrow, level and smooth the surface, as needed, depending on its type.

- Ensure the right type of equipment is used. Many membranes are destroyed by being lifted with an incorrect type of harrow.

STORAGE OF EQUIPMENT

Both indoor and outdoor schools will need ancillary areas for the storage of jumps, poles, cones and other equipment depending on the type of yard.

- It is not good practice to store articles in the corners. This means the corners are not properly care for and riders cannot use the corners correctly.

- Poles can sometimes be stored on top of the kicking boards if they are not too high.

- Racks can be built just outside the school.

- Covered areas can be built just outside the school with a gate or door through to the surface.

- If there is a gallery, space can be allocated at the side for storage.

53 BUYING FODDER AND BEDDING

POSSIBLE ARRANGEMENTS

A contract can be arranged with a reputable corn merchant for regular deliveries throughout the year. This system is recommended for yards with limited storage space, or for inexperienced buyers. The latter have to rely on the good faith and reputation of the merchant to ensure that they receive goods of high quality. It should be agreed in advance that if any delivery falls below standard, the goods will be replaced at no extra expense to the buyer. This arrangement is likely to be more expensive than buying from a local farmer, but should ensure guaranteed good-quality supplies throughout the year.

A contract can be made with a local farmer to supply a given quality of fodder and straw throughout the year. Deliveries should be by arrangement, and as convenient. Prices are cheaper than when buying from a merchant. The quality of hay, straw and corn should be checked at harvest time, and then again before delivery, to make sure that there has been no deterioration.

Bulk buying can be arranged direct from the field, thus avoiding extra handling, transport and storage costs. The practice of buying from a neighbouring farmer has much to commend it. There will be many occasions during the year when goodwill on both sides is needed. It is important to be on friendly terms. As already discussed, wrapped haylage, especially if big-baled, can be stored by the farmer and supplied as required, only good quality bales being delivered.

Manufactured feedstuffs have to be bought either through a corn merchant or direct from the manufacturer. When bought by the tonne or tonnes, a considerable discount should be obtained. Bought by the sack, goods can be collected and paid for on a cash-and-carry basis.

Many feed merchants will give a discount to yards that order lesser amounts but on a regular, possibly weekly basis, if storage is a problem. It provides them with a regular income and also helps with organising delivery rounds.

Bulk Buying

It is always cheaper to buy in bulk, rather than in small quantities. Suitable storage facilities with a sound access surface are essential, as is the cash necessary to pay for the goods. If money is short, it is often possible to borrow from the bank; even with interest added, this may still make a considerable saving.

Always consider insuring bulk purchases.

Consider security. Petty pilfering – only 'borrowing' a bale of hay or bedding – can mean considerable loss to the yard if it happens on a regular basis.

Stealing in bulk is less likely if the hay/straw barn is within the ring fence and not tucked away out of sight.

BUYING OF HAY/HAYLAGE

- If hay is bought off the field at harvest time, extra handling, transport and storage costs are avoided. Even if it is bought at a later date, but in sufficiently large quantities, a favourable price can usually be negotiated.

- If bought in sufficient quantity, a continuing supply of good-quality hay is assured. There is no sudden change in quality and, with good management, enough old hay will be left to carry on until the new season's hay is ready for use.

- According to the condition of the hay when baled, a minimum weight loss of 25 per cent may have to be allowed for. This occurs as the hay dries out.

BUYING OF STRAW

The same points apply as with the buying of hay except that there is little weight loss as straw is dry when baled.

STORAGE OF PLASTIC-WRAPPED BEDDING

Many forms of bedding come plastic-wrapped. In theory they can be stored outside when storage is limited. They are usually quite costly and care should be taken that the wrapping is not perforated.

Any that are opened but not used immediately will obviously require shelter.

STORAGE OF HAY

Suitable storage is essential. Poor or inadequate facilities mean hay wasted and money lost.

Purpose-built Hay Barn

This is the most expensive but also the most satisfactory method. The necessary money can often be borrowed from the bank, and the yearly saving in hay costs should make it worthwhile.

The barn should have a ridged roof, with air vents to allow ventilation at the top of the stack and the escape of fumes from the new hay. If sufficient money is available, the north and west – or most exposed – sides of the barn should be filled in with slatted boards as a protection against snow and rain. The two most convenient sides should be left open to facilitate the unloading and stacking of the bales.

Conventional Barn of Brick or Stone Construction

This usually holds only a small quantity and is often more awkward to stack because of enclosing walls; however, the sides cannot fall out even if stacked by inexperienced workers. Although this type of building is useful if already in the yard, it may lack ventilation, and there will thus be more chance of the hay heating up if it has not been sufficiently 'made'.

Covering for an Open Stack

- Plastic sheeting.
- Canvas rick sheet.

Both of these can be used successfully to cover the stack, but there is more chance of hay and straw being wasted.

Building the Stack

BASE To avoid spoiling the bottom bales of a stack, it is usual to put down a base of old hay or straw. This can be loose or in bales, but must be thick enough to prevent any damp getting up into the new hay. Small amounts of hay (10 tonnes or less) can be stored on wooden pallets. These are not practical for the larger stacks because of the weight of hay.

BUILDING THE STACK IN A PURPOSE-BUILT HAY BARN If there are no outside walls, the stack must be built with great care. One bay should be filled at a time. The front should be filled first, and then the sides and back. The middle should be filled last. The bales should be positioned so that each layer locks the layer below and holds it steady. This requires experienced workers or careful supervision. Should there be any tendency for the side of the stack to bulge out, this can usually be checked by supporting the sides with long poles (jump poles will do). The same principles apply when loading hay or straw on to a lorry or trailer. If transporting it on a road, always rope the load for greater safety.

Heating in the Stack

If carted from the field immediately after it has been baled, hay heats in the stack. To avoid overheating, it is advisable to allow for air passages in each bay. Stand a bale upright at base level in the centre of the bay. As the layers of hay are stacked, pull up the bale with them, thus leaving a square ventilating shaft. At the top of the stack, leave a space between the top layer and the roof so that air can move freely. If the weather looks settled, hay often does better if stood up in the field for a few days before carting.

Before stacking at the end of a barn stable or indoor school consider the following:

- The risk of fire if the stack overheats.

- The contamination by dust.

Stack to be Covered by Plastic Sheet or Canvas Rick Sheet

Build the stack as described above, but with even greater care, as there are no uprights or boards to support the sides. The hay is stacked in a square or rectangle with a flat top. The sheet is put over the top,

and should be large enough to hang over the edge. If heating is likely to be a problem, build accordingly (see Heating in the Stack, above), but also put six bales on top of the last layer. When the sheet is placed over the bales, air can circulate underneath. When heating has finished (two or three weeks), the stack can be secured for the winter. Remove the six bales so that the sheet lies nearly flat; a very slight slope is a help to chute the rain. If using a plastic sheet, place spare bales or heavy-duty tyres on the top to hold it down. This is not necessary with a canvas sheet. The sides are tied down with rope or nylon string, or pegged to the lower bales. This arrangement should be weather-proof. Once it becomes necessary to start using the hay or straw, there is always the problem in re-securing the sheet – and wastage and spoiling of either hay or straw ensues.

Plastic sheets are cheap, and with a stack in a sheltered area and treated with care, they can be a success. If they are not well secured, or if the weather is very rough, they rip and tear very easily: so they are not suitable for windy districts. They usually last for only one year. Large-mesh nets can be bought or made out of baler twine. If these are put over the sheets they give added security and reduce the chance of tearing.

Heavy duty sheets are more expensive, last longer, and are easier to secure to the stack. When the stack is opened, they are easier to replace, and stand much more rough handling and rough weather.

Big Bale Silage/Haylage in Polythene Bales

These are easy to store outside, and will be weather-proof. The area must be vermin-proof and with no risk of puncture through horse interference (chewing over the fence!) or implement damage. Damage to bales will cause spoiling of the contents, rendering the feed useless.

Opening the Stack

This should be carried out by experienced staff, but if they are not available, the workers must be well briefed and supervised. When opening a stack, take hay from the top and work down. If individual bales are pulled out from the bottom this can unbalance the rest of the stack, which may fall and injure anyone standing below. It will also spoil many of the bales. When removed from the stack the bales should be stored in a hay shed adjacent to the stables where they will be ready for use.

Storage Areas and Quantities

Hay and straw can be bought either by the tonne or by the bale. When buying by the tonne:

- Each load can be weighed on a weighbridge. This is costly in time and fuel.

or

- 10–20 bales can be weighed, and from that an average weight per bale can be worked out.

A barn of dimensions 13m x 9m x 5m (45ft x 30ft x 18ft) houses approximately 100 tonnes of hay or 4,000 bales.

100 tonnes of hay is sufficient for approximately 50 stabled horses for a year.

65 tonnes of straw is sufficient for approximately 50 stabled horses for a year.

Hay bales can weigh 13–26kg (30–60lbs). Straw bales can weigh 13–18kg (30–40lbs). The weight of the bale depends on:

- The condition of the hay when baled.
- The setting of the baler. This can be altered to make light or heavy bales. An all-female staff will appreciate the lighter bales, even though there are more of them to the tonne.

BUYING LOOSE SAWDUST AND SHAVINGS

If you are in a wooded district, these (according to demand) can be:

1. Free. A verbal contract is agreed whereby all available supplies will be collected regularly.

2. Delivered by lorry. Transport has to be paid for.

3. Bought by the sack. Provide your own transport or pay for delivery.

Care must be taken that the product is not from poisonous trees, that there are no harmful objects or foreign bodies within the load and that the product is not damp.

BUYING BALED SHAVINGS AND PAPER BEDDING

These are both much cheaper when bought by the lorry-load. They can be stored outside without a cover, as they are packed in polythene bags. Choose a level site convenient to the stables.

BUYING AND STORAGE OF GRAIN

Bulk buying of grain presents more problems, and is not really practical for the small yard. The problems of good quality and an assured and regular supply can often be solved by contracting to buy an agreed amount from a local farmer. He will be responsible for storage and delivery as requested. Payment can be arranged monthly. Grain is often in short supply by July, and there can be a problem until the new grain is ready to feed. It is important to remember this when buying in bulk earlier in the year, or when making arrangements for regular deliveries. Make sure that the supplier knows the approximate total quantity needed for the year.

If keeping high-performance horses, this arrangement may not be satisfactory, as the necessary quality of grain may not be available locally. Under such circumstances, and if grain is being bought to last for the year, a silo capable of storing sufficient grain for twelve months can be the most practical proposition.

Quantities of up to 4 tonnes can be stored in purpose-built metal containers. Alternatively, a spare brick or concrete block loose box with a solid door can be used as a store. It must be made vermin-proof.

Whole corn can be bought in small quantities and stored in metal bins, or paper or jute sacks (not plastic). Living seed dries naturally, and will not deteriorate or diminish in food value. If losses are to be avoided, the storage area must be vermin-proof or well patrolled by cats.

Bruised, rolled, crushed or cut grain should not be bought in bulk. It is dead, the husk is broken, and its food value deteriorates within a week. Grain is often dampened during processing, which can cause it to heat and spoil if not fed within days.

BULK BUYING OF NUTS AND CUBES

In a large yard of similar animals the bulk purchase of processed feed can be a cheaper feeding method.

The considerations are:

- Processed feed deteriorates quickly so must be used up within 10 days of being opened.

- Loose nuts will need a silo for storage. The feed merchant will often provide this free if the contract to purchase is satisfactory.

- Enough horses need to be on a similar feeding regime to make it worthwhile.

- The processor of the product needs to be reputable and guarantee the ongoing quality of the product.

- The storage space must be available.

See also Compound Feeds, page 180.

CHAPTER 54
ORGANISING AND RUNNING A YARD

ORGANISING THE OFFICE

A well-organised and well-equipped office is essential for the efficient running of any equestrian establishment, whether it is a riding school, livery yard, training and competition yard or racing stable. It is needed to give a good impression to clients, and to facilitate the day-to-day running of the yard.

The Office

The basic requirements for the office have already been dealt with on page 408.

How the office is organised will depend in part on the type of enterprise being undertaken.

In an enterprise that deals directly with the public, such as a riding school or trekking centre, it is useful if the office can be manned at busy times such as the weekends.

The person in the office should be able to:

- take bookings

- receipt payments

- answer the telephone

- generally put clients at ease

The office should be the first port of call for anyone visiting the yard. If it is not manned full time consider how the telephone is going to be answered. Most people are now happy to use an answering machine.

It is possible to have portable phones that work over quite long distances. Mobile phones are an obvious answer but can be expensive to run, depending on the deal, and it may not be convenient to deal with the call at that time. Email and fax machines are other options that should be considered.

Make it a rule to answer every message within the day or the next twelve business hours.

The person in the office ideally needs to be able to communicate with other staff members without leaving the office.

Dealing with payments

Clients should be encouraged to pay for rides/lessons before they happen. In this way money is not lost if there is an accident or by a child losing it or spending it on something else!

- All monies received should be receipted and kept securely.

- A small cashbox kept in an unlocked drawer is very easy to remove. **ALWAYS** keep cash locked away.

- Cash up at the end of each day, and total up any payments by cards or cheques.

- Do not leave cash in the office overnight.

- Ensure that it is possible to identify who receipted it.

- If handling large amounts of cash, bank it regularly but do not have a regular routine that can be anticipated.

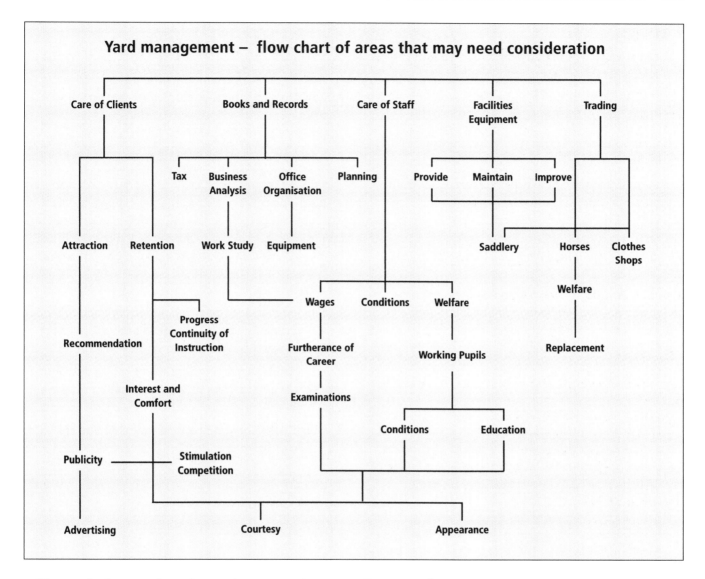

Yard management – flow chart of areas that may need consideration

- Clients who have paid in advance for a series of lessons or who have accounts should have each lesson/ride noted in the Daily Diary or booking book and that information should then be transferred to their personal file, ideally on a daily basis.

- The clearer and tidier the accounts are kept, the easier it will be for the bookkeeper or accountant to keep the finances in order.

Petty cash

Only a small amount of cash should be held in petty cash. An amount between £10 and £50 should be ample for most yards. Anyone removing cash should replace it with an IOU and that in turn should be replaced with a receipt for the goods bought.

Petty cash should only be used for small items such as milk, coffee or stamps. It should be cashed up daily.

Planning

A series of yearly planners displayed on the wall can be extremely useful for 'see at a glance' information on such things as:

- Deliveries of forage and bedding.

- Which horses are due for the farrier, worming or vaccinations.

- On a stud they can show when a mare comes in season and when she is due for covering.

- Staff holidays and days off.

- Exam dates, training days, local shows and competitions.

In many yards the human first aid box is kept in the office, along with the names of trained first-aiders on the yard and the name and number of the local doctor's surgery and hospital. This also helps to ensure that any use of the box, however small, is recorded in the incident book.

Security

The office needs to be secure. Clients and staff need to know that personal details are confidential and only available on a 'need to know' basis. See Keeping Records, page 427.

It has already been suggested that the office is situated near the main entrance of the yard, if it is commercial with many clients coming and going. The flow chart on page 423 indicates the areas which need consideration depending on the type of enterprise.

ACCOUNTS

Unless the proprietor or secretary has experience of accounting, it is advisable for all businesses to employ an accountant who can:

- Present a true record of the business to the Inland Revenue.

- Claim all available tax allowances.

- Advise as to the present state of the business, future prospects and trends, as well as providing essential information for constructive future planning.

The accountant may be asked to present the books monthly, three-monthly, half-yearly or annually, according to personal preference and the establishment's ability to maintain good records. As he will be paid by the hour, the more that can be done to keep the accounts in good order, the lower his bill will be. He will advise on the system that he wishes to use.

The accountant will require the following books and information:

- Main cash book. Receipts are noted on the left-hand page, payments on the right-hand page. All are totalled monthly.

- Petty cash book for recording small items paid for in cash. The total is transferred to the main cash book each month.

- VAT book. For recording inputs and outputs of VAT.

- Wages book.

- Bank statements for current and deposit accounts.

- Bank cheque stubs.

- Details of creditors.

- Details of debtors.

- Records of livestock, i.e. list of horses, with details of purchases, sales or deaths.

- Records of stock, i.e. machinery, tractors, cars, trailers and horseboxes, with details of purchase, sale and writing off.

- Stocks of hard feed, hay, straw and bedding.

- Details of equipment, e.g. saddlery, rugs, show jumps, clippers, etc.

INSURANCE

Riding is a hazardous sport, and accidents will occur in spite of every precaution taken by the riding school proprietors. Insurance policies are therefore a must.

Compulsory Insurance

Employer's Liability

This is a legal requirement for all businesses where staff are employed. See the Employer's Liability (Compulsory Insurance) Act 1969.

It covers legal claims by employees in relation to personal injuries or damage to their property whilst at work.

Public Liability

Sufficient public liability must be in place before applying for a riding school licence. It is essential to have it in any horse business where the general public are involved in any way, such as livery yards.

It covers death, injury or illness caused to a member of the public as a result of defects in the premises, the services offered, or negligence by either the proprietor or staff.

Motor Vehicle

A minimum of third party cover is needed on all vehicles. This covers other vehicles and people. Fully comprehensive insurance policies cover the replacement value of the insured vehicle as well. Vehicles used for hire or reward, such as horseboxes, will be subject to amendments to the policy.

- When seeking insurance it is sensible to shop around and get a number of quotes as it is a competitive market.

- However, it is also important to ensure that the company is reputable and has a record for prompt payment.

- Make absolutely sure that you get the cover you want.

- Make sure you give the company all relevant information.

- Insure for full replacement value and consequential loss.

- Read the small print very carefully.

- Get someone knowledgeable to clarify, if necessary.

- Make sure that all clauses for each policy are understood and conformed with.

- Some cover may only be valid when certain requirements are met, e.g. seat belts are worn or riders have correctly fitting headgear.

- Good practice can be encouraged by safety notices.

- Warning notices will not, on their own, preclude a charge of negligence.

- Disclaimers do not have a value in law.

- Active measures may need to be taken to prevent accidents.

Voluntary Insurance

Property

This becomes compulsory if there is a mortgage.

It is sensible to insure all buildings against damage by fire and adverse weather conditions such as floods and gales. Cover should be based on rebuilding costs and if the building is listed these can be considerably more than usual.

Contents

This will probably be considered in at least two parts – household contents and stable contents, particularly tack.

- All contents should be insured at replacement value.

- If large amounts of hay and straw are stored, consider insuring them.

Personal Accident

Anyone who is self-employed needs to be covered for financial security in the event of illness or injury.

- Employees involved in risky tasks (and all horses are unpredictable) would be advised to have personal accident cover.

- Employees are not always covered by their employer's liability policy, when working in their own time or when performing unauthorised tasks.

Business Interruption

This covers consequential loss of profits as a result of some interruption to the running of the business, such as flood damage, an outbreak of disease, or theft of saddlery.

Horses

There is a wide range of insurance policies available. Many of them are not economically viable for the small commercial enterprise, especially if the horses are of low value. They are worth considering for more valuable horses. They range from third party, through loss by theft or straying, to full cover, vet's fees and loss of use.

Clients' Personal Accident Insurance

In recent years there has been a considerable increase in injury claims by clients riding at riding schools. Many proprietors now recommend that clients should take out some form of personal accident policy before either learning to ride or continuing to ride as a hobby. This does not exonerate the school from legal action should an accident occur and negligence be proven.

Private Horse Owner's Liability

The private horse owner is advised to insure against third-party risks (at present this is included for BHS members, in the higher membership categories – Silver and Gold) and they should preferably insure themselves against personal accident.

Freelance Instructors

Independent freelance instructors are also advised to insure themselves against third-party risks and personal accident. As members of the BHS Instructors Register, freelance instructors enjoy comprehensive insurance and the benefit of automatic membership of the National Association of Sports Coaches.

INCIDENT OR ACCIDENT BOOK

It is essential for all types of yard to keep an Incident or Accident Book. This is a compulsory measure for BHS- and ABRS-approved schools. The book must record the time, place and date of any incidents or accidents, an account of what took place, and the name and address of any witnesses. It is often months – even years – before information on an accident is asked for. During this time, important details can be forgotten, staff may leave, and reliable information may thus be difficult to obtain. Suitable accident forms can be obtained from the BHS.

No riding establishment should be left in the charge of a person under sixteen years of age. It is the responsibility of the owner, proprietor or stable manager to decide when a person is sufficiently responsible and capable of being left in charge. The same responsibility applies when allowing riders to be escorted or pupils to be taught by young people without supervision.

At present, litigation is all too easy, and court cases and claims for damages are all too common, so it is essential for responsible proprietors or stable managers to take extra care. For example, a notice stating that: 'Although every care is taken, there can be no responsibility for accidents' gives no protection in law should a claim for accident and injury lead to litigation. The account of an accident should be signed by the person in charge, and, whenever possible, by the injured party and any witnesses. For legal requirements, see Chapter 55.

KEEPING RECORDS

One of the main tasks of the stable manager is to maintain records as necessary and ensure that the yard is run in an economical and efficient manner.

By keeping efficient records they will be able to provide information on a need to know basis. They will be able to keep track of all costings and equipment.

They will be able to provide the bookkeeper, accountant (and Customs and Excise if the business is VAT registered) with all the information necessary to keep the finances in order and the tax returns accurate.

The more accurate the initial record keeping, the more likely is the accountant to be able to save money – if only because his expenses will be less.

There are a number of systems available for use on the computer to help firms keep track of their business dealings. There are some specially adapted for use in riding schools or livery yards. Depending on their format, they can replace all or part of systems already in place. When deciding on which system to use, consider the following:

• What needs to be recorded?

• How often?

• By whom?

• How often does it need to be referred to?

• How often does it need updating?

• Who needs the information?

Any system or combination of systems chosen must be easy to use. Some information may need to be stored in a number of different files. For example, if some livery tack is repaired it would be recorded in the Repair Book, the horse's file and in the invoice sent to the owner asking for payment. By using a computer the entry only needs to be made once and then sent to the various files, whereas by hand it would need three entries.

All computer systems do need a backup in case of power or mechanical failure.

Other methods of recording are:

• Wall charts, very useful for seeing at a glance when things are due.

• Duplicate or triplicate books. These are useful for receipting payments or when sending equipment for repairs, hiring out articles or leaving instructions for staff.

• Diaries, essential for recording happenings on a daily basis.

• Account books will be required by the bookkeeper and accountant.

• Box files for storing paper copies.

• Loose-leaf folders for storing separate paper sheets such as inventories, treatment records, daily work sheets, invoices, horse and client records.

Confidentiality is essential. Consider carefully who needs to know, who must not know and how the information is going to be accessed.

Maintaining Records

The daily diary is an essential record. ALL incomings and outgoings should be recorded. The diary with a page to a day should be kept open in the office.

Only the basic information needs to be recorded in the daily diary. For instance 'vet visited'. Who he saw and what he did would be recorded in the appropriate files elsewhere.

• Make a note of all deliveries, store the delivery note.

• Make a note of all visitors, e.g. vet, farrier.

• Log all outgoings, payments, equipment going for repairs, horses to competition, etc.

• Receipt all monies.

• Maintain a file on each horse, client and member of staff.

• Work to a routine – try to find a regular slot on a weekly or daily basis to maintain records.

• Keep all receipts and file them according to item and date.

• Speak to your accountants and make sure you fulfil their demands. The less work they have to do, the more money they can save you.

• If you regularly have large sums of cash to pay in, do not advertise the fact. Make the payments at different times and on different days.

• Do not leave large sums of cash on the premises for longer than necessary.

ORDERING AND MONITORING STOCK

Ordering and monitoring stock is one of the major responsibilities of the stable manager.

You will need to identify what you need. You also need to identify when you need it.

CONSIDER:
Regular orders such as:

• Feed

• Forage

• Bedding

• Sundries such as saddle soap, cleaning materials, lavatory paper, etc.

Irregular orders such as:

• Medicines

• Tool replacement

• Haynets

• Wheelbarrows

• Rugs

• Saddlery

Major new orders such as:

• Jumps

• Vehicles

• Horses

With the regular orders you need to identify a reliable source of supply. Explain exactly what you require and then do a deal.

With small items like saddle soap, if you regularly deal with the same supplier, and they also do repairs or supply rugs, you should get a regular discount. Compare it with large companies and local agricultural merchants. You will only get discounts if you pay your bills promptly!

Compare at least three suppliers before making a decision and with something like forage make sure to agree a timescale for the deal, six months or one year, and then agree to review the arrangement.

All feed merchants will have differing price scales depending on the regularity and quantity being bought.

With irregular orders you need to research suppliers and again get the best deal you can. Always get at least three quotes.

Cheapest is not always best but in a student or trainee situation it sometimes makes sense. Articles like lunge whips that will quickly be damaged in inexperienced hands need to be bought quite cheaply. However you need to try to instil respect for equipment in the trainee and if articles are declared worn out, ALWAYS ask for the worn out one before handing over its replacement! This prevents fraud.

Articles such as wheelbarrows will always last longer if they are designed for commercial use and not just intermittent use in a suburban garden.

With a major new investment try to find out what aftercare is offered if it is relevant.

Check out the best loan/hire-purchase agreements if required. It is often cheaper to borrow from the bank than from the firm recommended by the dealer selling the article.

If the article is bought using a credit card this can offer extra protection in case the goods are faulty.

Note when goods are ordered and when they are due. Ensure they have arrived.

Always pay within the agreed time. It is not fair on small businesses for them to have to wait and no one will carry on making good deals with poor or erratic payers.

Deliveries

With all deliveries it is essential that they are checked in on arrival, both for quantity and for quality, and signed for. The delivery notes should be kept and checked against the invoice. Ensure that all stock, once delivered, is stored suitably and securely until needed.

Monitoring stock

Monitoring stock is quite time-consuming but it is a part of good yard management.

Any system you put in place must be as simple and practical as possible. If not, it will not be used.

Equipment/ stock which is used all the time needs to be checked on a weekly basis.

Feedstuffs and bedding need checking to ensure there is no waste or theft and tools to ensure that they are present and in a usable condition. Feedstuffs and bedding should be used in date order.

Saddlery, rugs and other equipment need to be checked against an inventory. Your accountant may require this once or twice a year in order to calculate depreciation. Otherwise you might want to do it termly if you have students. All equipment should be individually identifiable.

The inventory should include the identity, the description, the date of purchase, any repairs, inventory update dates and the date the article was declared obsolete.

Regular maintenance of machinery and items such as wheelbarrows will ensure a much longer life. Attention to detail can save considerable sums of money in the long run.

RECOMMENDED DRESS FOR RIDING CLIENTS

There should be strict rules as to suitable and safe dress for clients riding at any establishment. Correctly fitting BSI-standard hats to PAS 015 or BSEN 1384 should be worn, with attached chin-strap securely fastened. Under the Health and Safety at Work Act the wearing of a PAS 015 or BSEN 1384 standard hat is mandatory for all employees and students at Approved riding schools. **The casual loan or hire of hard hats is not recommended.** In establishments such as trekking yards where it is common practice to lend hats at least one member of staff should be professionally trained in fitting.

Care should be taken that the hats are not dropped – and check manufacturers' recommendations as to how often they should be replaced. This will probably be every two to three years if properly cared for. If, as the result of an accident, the hat should come off or be found faulty, the proprietor of the school could be claimed against for having provided it.

Shoes or boots should be worn with smooth soles and small heels, so that if the rider falls:

• The foot will not be caught up in the stirrup by ridges in the sole.

• The low heel will prevent the foot from slipping through the iron.

The following footwear should not be allowed:

• Any ridged Wellington boots or Muckers.

• Buckled shoes.

• Tennis, walking or game shoes with a solid sole and no heel.

• High-heeled boots or shoes.

Floppy plastic raincoats which, in a high wind, can blow about, making a sudden noise and frightening a horse, should also be forbidden.

When rain jackets are worn, attached rain hoods

should not be used. They make hearing more difficult and can prevent the wearer from seeing behind them. It is unsafe practice to wear earpieces when hacking or when it is important to have full hearing.

CATERING

Staff and students should have agreed meal breaks. They should have somewhere warm, dry and clean in which to take their breaks and there should be provision to make hot and cold drinks, to keep food fresh and to heat it if needed.

They should not be expected to share with clients.

Anyone contemplating supplying refreshments, whether they are made on the premises or bought in, must comply with all the relevant Environmental Health, Health & Safety and Food & Hygiene Act (1990) requirements.

These cover a number of areas such as:

- That the premises and equipment are suitable.

- Preparing the food according to present law.

- Ensuring that it is stored correctly, at the approved temperature and used within the proper time limits.

- Ensuring that all hygiene requirements are met.

- Ensuring that all personnel involved in preparation and serving have the required qualifications.

It is advisable to take qualified advice at the earliest opportunity in the planning stage, in order to avoid expensive mistakes.

ORGANISING THE TACK ROOM

Much has already been written about the tack room, see Chapter 51.

The reasons for having two tack rooms, one for cleaning and one for storage, have also been explained.

In a commercial yard where each horse may be ridden more than once, it is probably best if each set of tack is replaced on its own saddle and bridle peg after each use. In a small yard the dirty tack can be left in the cleaning room until cleaned.

The bit should be washed after each ride. The stirrup irons should be put up the leathers, the girth laid over the seat of the saddle and the numnah left underneath.

In order to tell at a glance which tack needs cleaning from that which does not, some yards have differing ways of putting up the tack. For example, once the bridle has been cleaned it can be put up with the reins hung through the throatlash, which is twisted around the front of the bridle before being fastened without doing up the buckle. The noseband is fastened round the outside of everything by the end being pushed through the keeper only. This means it is easy to undo the bridle and make it ready when next tacking up. The saddle has the girth unattached from the billet straps, put over the seat of the saddle and threaded through the stirrup irons. The numnah can be laid upside down over the top acting as a kind of saddle cover, or it can be stored separately. Martingales should be hung up by the neck strap and not left attached to the bridle.

By storing them differently when clean, it is easy to see at a glance which tack needs cleaning.

Each set of tack should be marked. In a private yard it may just be stamped discreetly with the owner's initials and postcode. In a commercial yard where many people may be required to tack up a horse, it is best if each set is clearly marked with the horse's name. This can be done with dog tags or the kind of tags used to identify farm animals. The latter can be much cheaper. Consider how many might be required per set of tack. If many people are cleaning tack together you may need to identify girths and leathers and even irons, separately.

Have a system of identifying boots, martingales, etc. that are not specific to one horse. This is useful if students or clients are required to tack up their horses and ensures that the equipment will fit. This can be done by colour or number coding to identify size and is used in conjunction with a chart which identifies which equipment is suitable for any specific animal. It can also identify when a particular horse needs certain equipment such as 'only boots for jumping', etc. A similar system can be used for double bridles and lunge equipment.

All equipment used frequently should have designated hooks for storage. This means that it is much easier to notice when something is missing.

Special equipment used only for shows etc. should be stored in locked cupboards or display cabinets. If possible do not use the tack room as an office or an area for storing hats and boots for hire. If there is nothing better, consider using a loose box or buying a garden shed.

Always lock tack rooms when unoccupied and discourage unauthorised people from entering. In a busy yard have combination locks and change the combinations on a regular basis.

All cleaning materials should be washed out and hung up to dry at the end of the day.

Sinks and buckets should be emptied and left clean. Saddle soap and leather treatments, depending on type, should be stored on a shelf. Metal polish and oils, if used, should be bought in large containers and decanted into small ones. In that way when they are spilt less is wasted.

The floors should be left clean and dry. Tack should be so arranged that tack for small ponies is stored at a lower level as it is likely to be used by smaller people.

Saddles that are seldom used can be stored on the higher racks. It is possible to buy a long-handled device to lift saddles on and off high racks. Another option is to have a proper footstool or short pair of steps. It is unsafe to stand on chairs etc. to reach equipment.

There should be a system in place for dealing with repairs.

Ensure that the tack room is dry but not too warm or the leather tack will dry out.

The cleaning room can be warmer, especially if it is also used to dry wet boots, etc. If all the equipment used is artificial, the tack room will benefit from being warmer so that it can dry out after washing.

It is not always advisable to keep the medicine cabinet in the tack room as it may not be quickly available if the room is locked.

Livery Tack

Each owner's saddles, bridles, martingales, etc. should be kept together, with the individual grooming kit below them, so that there is no muddle on a groom's day off. Livery owners should keep their spare tack and rugs at home, unless space is available for their own rug box. All livery tack and belongings should be clearly marked by the owner. It is preferable to have separate school and livery tack rooms.

ORGANISATION OF FEED ROOM

The design of the feedroom has already been discussed in Chapter 51.

In any but the smallest yard it is usually preferable to have the forage and hard feed stored separately from each other and the feed room.

Keep about enough feed for one week in the feed room.

Label all the feed bins clearly with their contents.

Brush out the bins before each refilling.

Keep the bins off the floor if it gets damp. Ensure that it is possible to move them in order to sweep underneath and behind them.

If the horses have individual rations, each horse needs his own easily identified feed bowl. This can either be named if the population seldom changes or can have the stable number if the horses change or move boxes.

It is important that each horse receives his own ration.

It is the responsibility of the yard manager to feed the horses but, on a training yard, consider allowing trainees to get hands-on experience in feeding, as long as they are supervised.

Feeds should not be made up hours before they are going to be fed. They are more likely to become contaminated by birds or vermin.

Damp feed should be added just before serving as it will quickly turn the rest sour.

In any but the smallest private yard it is advisable to have a feed chart. A large blackboard on the wall makes an excellent feed chart. Put the horses' names and box number down the left-hand side. Put the names of the various feedstuffs and forage across the top. (See diagram page 211.)

Divide each feed column into 3–4 smaller columns depending on the usual number of feeds each day. Write the amount of feedstuff fed in the appropriate square. The hard rations should be written in measures but elsewhere calculated in kilos. The forage can be written in kilos. The feed ration should be altered on the board immediately it is changed.

Once a week, ideally on the same day each week, the ration on the board is transferred to a paper record which can be stored. This allows calculations to be made such as how much feed is used monthly or annually or if one horse is more expensive to keep than another.

Any new feedstuff introduced should be weighed by measure so that the correct ration can be calculated.

Sometimes, if all horses are on the same feedstuff, it is easier if the ration is transported in one large container and dished straight into permanent feed mangers in the boxes. This cuts out the purchasing and cleaning of feed bowls.

Sometimes it is easier if the individual feed bowls are transported on a trolley. All feed bowls/mangers should be washed out after each feed and be left to drain, preferably without getting the feed room floor wet. If they have been on the stable floor, ensure that the outsides are also washed to prevent contamination.

All uneaten feed including forage should be thrown away. Take care that it does not go down and block drains.

All additives and medicines must be safely stored, strictly measured and only administered by trained staff.

Each additive or medicine must be identifiable and have legible instructions attached. It must be easy to identify which animals are to receive it.

The feed room should be secure to prevent equines, vermin and unauthorised people from entering.

All feedstuffs should be used in rotation and a record kept of when they were moved from store to feedroom.

The deliveries should be checked in on arrival and the delivery note signed and filed.

If a yard cat is kept, ensure that it has free access.

CHOOSING AND MANAGING THE MEDICINE CABINET

Have a basic code of practice that suits your yard. **Security and safety must be the first priorities.**

Label all medications:

- What is it?
- Who is it for?
- How is it used?
- Note the shelf life of medications.

Dispose of old drugs and syringes safely.

Some products are dangerous and should only be used by responsible people. Some people may try to abuse the contents.

It may be best to have two cabinets, one secure and the other available to all. In a shelved cabinet it can be useful to have a plan on the inside of the door, showing where everything is. This can save rummaging around in the dark.

The telephone number of the vet can be placed on the outside.

The person who empties or finishes any product needs to take the empty container to the yard manager for replacement.

Any medication prescribed or supplied by the vet needs to be carefully identified to the specific animal.

- Medicine should only be administered by personnel trained to do so.

- A record should be kept of when and how much was given.

- It must be used within the expiry date on the product.

- Any residue must be safely disposed of.

- It must be stored safely.

In some yards, qualified staff give injections.

- Unused syringes and needles must be stored safely.

- Used needles must be disposed of in a sharps box that must, itself, be stored safely.

- Most veterinary practices will dispose of the box when it is full.

- Used needles and syringes should never be disposed of in household rubbish.

Where should the cabinet be sited?
In a small yard it may well be kept in the house.

Sometimes it is sited in the tack room. This is not ideal if it is needed when the tack room is locked.

The same may apply if it is kept in the office, therefore give careful thought to who is likely to need access and at what times.

In a large yard with many workers, consider having two cabinets. One for everyday emergencies, housing safe things and the second for medicines and treatments that only trained staff should administer.

If two cabinets are used, consider housing the specialist one in somewhere like the office and the other in a more accessible area.

The type of yard run will govern, to a certain extent, the type of things needed.

It is wasteful and unwise to buy things 'on spec'. You will build up quite quickly a selection of products which are used regularly in your type of yard.

Listed below are many of the most usually kept products which you might consider initially:

Tools and Utensils
- Thermometer.

- Stethoscope.
- Scissors, both straight and curved.
- Tweezers.
- Palette knife.
- Measuring spoons.
- Drawing knife.
- Dishes of various sizes to hold swabs and poultices.
- Syringes, large for flushing out wounds. Small, only if the staff are trained to inject.
- Disposable gloves.
- Clean stable rubbers.
- Hoof testers.
- Kettle.

Dressings
- Bandages: crepe, elasticated, Vetrap, stable, cotton.
- Gauze pads.
- Clingfilm for poultices.
- Cotton wool, hospital quality.
- Lint.
- Wadding, Gamgee, etc.
- Sticky tape.

Medications
- A selection of wound treatments; creams, sprays, etc.
- Ointments for use on cracked heels, mud fever, etc. such as udder cream or zinc and castor oil.
- Vaseline/glycerine.
- Hydrogen peroxide, saline solution or a mild antiseptic solution as preferred by your vet.
- Ready-made poultices such as kaolin or Animalintex.
- Cough electuary.
- Vick.

Other
- Dettol or Savlon for cleaning utensils.
- Shampoo.
- Shoeing tools.
- Wire cutters.
- Torch.

- Twitch, cradle, muzzle.
- Surgical boots, including poultice boot.

The latter items may be kept separately but are useful to have readily available.

If saline solution is made up in double strength and stored in a 2 or 4 litre (3½–7pt) container, it can be dispensed as needed into a clean dish and a similar amount of newly boiled water added, when the need arises. This provides a warm and sterile solution almost immediately.

If cotton wool is bought in large rolls, it can be torn into small pieces that are stored in a clean plastic container (ice-cream containers are ideal): this prevents the whole roll being taken into the stable and contaminated when an emergency occurs.

Used dressings should be disposed of safely, preferably burnt.

A clean stable rubber is useful to put things on and keep them clean and easily seen when dealing with a wound, etc. They can also be used to dry areas after cleaning and are easily sterilised after use.

In the first cabinet should be stored everything that is used in emergencies.

In the second cabinet can be stored any medicines specific to a particular horse and also:

- Anything that can be abused.

- Anything used in treatments that must only be administered by trained staff.

- Any prescription products.

Ensure products are stored at the correct temperature. It is possible to buy small fridges. They are ideal if the yard is separate from the house.

When products such as wormers are bought in bulk, they can be stored in the secure cabinet to prevent accidental administration or pilfering.

A record should be kept of when products are bought; if possible it should be written on the packaging in permanent marker.

The cabinets should be checked by the yard manager on a weekly basis.

No out of date products should be used.

All usage should be logged.

All products should have their own space.

FEES

Fees for Rides and Lessons

The amount charged should depend upon:

(a) Keep of horse: feed, bedding, water, electricity.
(b) Labour – mucking out, grooming, tack cleaning.
(c) Instructor or escort time.
(d) Shoeing and veterinary expenses.
(e) Saddlery – upkeep and replacement.
(f) Horse replacement.
(g) Share of overheads – rent, rates, bank interest.
(h) Share of upkeep of box, yard, fields, fencing, water, cultivation.
(i) Share of insurance and office expenses.
(j) Local conditions.

It is a common problem in the less commercial riding schools for the fees charged to be uneconomic. If the service offered cannot be provided at an economic fee consider carefully whether it should be provided at all.

Livery Fees

Items to be taken into account:

- Items (a), (b), (g), (i) and (j) above.

- Exercising time if required.

- Profit should be a minimum of 10 per cent. Livery-only yards must take a bigger percentage if it is to be their main source of income.

Many livery yards charge a basic rate to cover general care and then have a list of charges for such things as training, clipping and preparing for shows. It should be made very clear what is included in the basic charge.

Such things as arranging for the farrier may well be done by the yard to fit in with their routine, but the invoice should be sent straight to the owner by the farrier. If it is passed on by the yard it may incur two sets of VAT and any non-payment may become the responsibility of the yard.

Veterinary fees should also be invoiced straight to the owner for the same reason.

Schooling Fees

These will be calculated on the time and expertise of the staff involved.

Working Liveries

The advantage of these is the use of an extra horse without additional capital expense, but before agreeing to this system it is essential to ensure that the horse will be really useful. Remember, too, that the box taken up by a horse could have been occupied by a full livery.

Clear arrangements must be made with the owner as to:

• Days and time when the horse will be available for use in the school. It is seldom useful if the owner wants to use his horse during the weekend, which is likely to be the time when the horse is most useful to the yard.

• The amount of notice given either side can also cause ill-feeling. If the horse has done a full day's work and the owner turns up to ride in the evening, it can lead to arguments.

• Responsibility for clipping, shoeing, veterinary expenses, tack repairs.

• Responsibility for livery if the horse is ill or off work.

Fees should depend on individual arrangements, but are usually half to three-quarters of the full livery fee. The livery owner's insurance company should be notified of the arrangement, as this may affect the terms of the policy. It is always advisable for owners of working liveries to insure their horses.

There should be a written agreement signed by both parties.

DIY Livery

Do-it-yourself livery can be an acceptable arrangement for the owner of the yard and the owner of a horse.

Arrangements from yard to yard can be hugely variable. Conditions must be clearly defined, agreed in writing and signed by both parties.

Part livery and DIY can be fraught with potential problems. The ongoing success of such arrangements depends to some degree on the mutual goodwill and endeavour of both parties to make it work.

It is proposed that livery yards will need a licence similar to the one required by riding schools. However, this is in abeyance until the definition of a livery has been agreed.

It is advisable that all livery yards keep up-to-date with new legislation.

STAFF

Staff Contracts

Within thirteen weeks of starting work, all staff should have a work contract. This should include:

• Job description.

• Date of commencement.

• Hours of work – but as the care of animals is involved these have to be flexible.

• Days off per week.

• Arrangements for holidays, including statutory holidays.

• Pay per week or month.

• Overtime.

• Sickness arrangements.

• Arrangements for termination of employment on

either side, and disciplinary and grievance procedures.

• Special arrangements: e.g. board and lodging, living-out allowance, keep of own horse, use of car or Land Rover and trailer, time off to compete, preparation for exams, and keeping of pets.

Employers are reminded that arrangements for terminating employment because of unsatisfactory work or behaviour should fulfil the guidelines laid down in the relevant pamphlets published by the Department of Employment.

Staff Duties

The following are the normal responsibilities of staff in a stable yard.

CHIEF INSTRUCTOR
Typical responsibilities:

• Interviewing prospective clients and students.

• Organising lessons and rides – checking daily ride-list in desk diary so that it is ready for the secretary to type. Allocation of suitable horses, instructors, riding areas and facilities.

• Providing private lessons.

• Preparation for exams.

• Schooling of horses.

• Liaising with stable manager regarding lecture and practical stable-management sessions, and allocation of yard duties, etc.

• Liaising with secretary to keep records and book of rides and lessons. Organising lectures and practical stable-management sessions for students and working pupils. These may be taken by a BHS Intermediate Instructor.

• Arranging and conducting regular staff meetings.

• Liaising with owners, managers and staff to arrange and organise courses, outside speakers, trainers and competitions.

• Ensuring that all Equal Rights and anti-discrimination laws are upheld.

STABLE MANAGER
Typical responsibilities:

• Overseeing the day-to-day organisation and running of the yard and the welfare and care of the horses.

• Feeding.

• Daily work lists.

• Supervision of stable management of staff, students and working pupils.

• Daily inspections of horses.

• Arranging clipping, trimming, shoeing and veterinary lists and saddlery repairs.

• Attendance at veterinary surgeon's visits.

• Feeding and checking of field horses.

• Buying and storage of fodder.

• Executing or arranging for necessary work in fields, e.g. harrowing, rolling, fertilising, topping, fencing, drainage, gates and water.

• Arranging and executing general upkeep of stable yard, fences, gates, drainage, school surfaces (indoor and outdoor), show jumps and cross-country fences.

• Liaising with livery owners about the welfare and care of their horses.

• Keeping up-to-date inventories of all equipment.

• Doing risk assessments of all working practices on the yard to conform with current Health and Safety recommendations and ensuring that all codes of practice are adhered to.

SECRETARY

Typical responsibilities:

- Answering telephone.

- Welcoming clients.

- Booking rides and taking ride money.

- Typing out daily ride sheets.

- Supervising petty cash.

- Dealing with correspondence.

- Keeping accounts: VAT, wages and record books.

- Liaising with chief instructor and stable manager with regard to record books and client problems or requests.

- Keeping livery and ride accounts.

- Sending out monthly bills.

- Paying accounts.

- Working out PAYE and employees' National Insurance contributions.

- Making up weekly wage packets or preparing wage cheques for signature.

- Making regular visits to bank to pay in cash and cheques, and collecting wages and petty cash money.

INTERMEDIATE INSTRUCTOR

Typical responsibilities:

- Looking after two horses.

- Supervising stable management of students and working pupils.

- Giving stable-management lectures.

- Teaching.

- Schooling.

- General yard work.

They may be given overall responsibility for one small area of the yard such as maintenance of riding areas, or day-to-day feeding. If there are a number of junior instructors these responsibilities can be rotated to give each one an insight into what is required to run the various areas.

NB: If preparing for BHSI, suitable help will be needed from the chief instructor.

ASSISTANT INSTRUCTOR

Typical responsibilities:

- Looking after two to four horses.

- Some teaching.

- Joining in general yard work.

- Helping to catch and groom field ponies.

NB: If preparing for an exam, lessons from the chief instructor and help from the stable manager will be needed.

WORKING PUPILS

Typical duties:

- Looking after three horses.

- Helping with beginner lessons.

- General yard work.

- Looking after and grooming field ponies.

Education should include:

- Set periods of stable management each week, theory and practical.

- Extra help as the examination date approaches.

- Four riding lessons a week plus teaching practice.

PAYING STUDENTS

Work and instruction according to individual arrangements, but typical duties and education might include:

- Looking after one horse (or possibly own horse and one other).

- Preparation for intended examination.

- Two daily lessons plus one lunge lesson.

- Teaching practice. When sufficiently experienced, taking class lessons or beginner lessons under supervision, or lessons suitable in standard as preparation for intended examinations.

MAINTENANCE PERSON

It makes for a better, tidier and safer yard if maintenance is done on a regular basis. Ideally there should be a Maintenance Book or File. This can contain information such as how much of what type of fertiliser is used on each field, when to apply specific weedkiller and in what quantity. Also, when vehicle MOTs and plating needs to be renewed and when servicing is due.

A maintenance person may be employed on a part-time basis depending on the type and size of the yard.

If a certain amount of time is allocated on a daily or even weekly basis much money can be saved and the yard will be safer and smarter.

Typical responsibilities:

- Liaising with stable manager regarding daily work.

- Stable repairs and yard maintenance. Field work and fence repairs.

- Grass cutting.

- Building and maintaining show jumps and cross-country fences.

- Care of car, horsebox and trailers.

- Maintaining tyre pressure in wheelbarrows. Lifting dropped hinges on doors and renewing washers on taps.

The maintenance person must receive relevant training and be qualified before using chemicals and machinery and must always wear appropriate safety equipment.

There should be a system for reporting the need for minor repairs and it is the yard manager's job to see they are done within an acceptable timescale.

Tasks such as washing out stables, cleaning windows and scrubbing down walls and doors can be weekly tasks for stable staff.

In small yards, the duties of chief instructor and stable manager can be amalgamated, and some of their duties can be reallocated to an Intermediate Instructor or senior BHSAI. Smaller yards are less likely to have paying students, or to do exam preparation, and tend to concentrate on providing instruction and hacking for the general rider.

CHILD AND ADULT HELPERS

The Children and Young Persons Act 1933–1963, the Education Acts 1944–1996, the Children Act 1989, the Children (Protection at Work) Regulations 1998, and the Health and Safety (Young Persons) Regulations 1997 lay out the basic legislation on the employment of children. This can be further amended by Local Authority by-laws, which may differ from Authority to Authority but mainly conform to guidance issued by the Department of Health and Safety. The Employment Act of 1989 should also be referred to. New legislation is frequently introduced from the European Union so it is important to keep up to date.

Traditionally, children, especially girls, have helped out during the holidays and at weekends at their local riding centre. This has been beneficial for both parties. The children have had something useful to do and have learned to care for and ride ponies which they otherwise might not be able to do and the riding school has had a useful pool of helpers at the times when the school has been busiest.

Points to consider:
- It is advisable ot contact your local authority for guidance.

- It is illegal to employ children under 13 years.

- No one under minimum school leaving age may be

employed before 7am or after 7pm.

- They may not be employed for more than two hours on any school day or Sunday.

- Most by-laws permit children under 15 years to work a maximum of five hours a day on Saturdays and school holidays, subject to a maximum of twenty-five hours a week.

- Children of 15 years and over may work a maximum of eight hours a day on Saturdays and school holidays, subject to a maximum of thirty-five hours a week.

- Most by-laws require employers to notify the Local Authority of the hours and conditions of the child's employment.

- Children who are not employed but receive remuneration in the form of rides etc. may not be covered by the yard's insurance policies.

- Children helping or working on the yard must have a suitable adult supervising them at all times.

- The children and the adult must have received suitable training in the tasks they perform.

- Parental permission must have been given.

- There should be written proof of the training given and the parent or guardian's permission.

- Forming an Affiliated Pony Club is an ideal way of providing the correct insurance cover.

- Appropriate risk assessments must have been done on all activities undertaken and appropriate training given.

- At all times the correct clothing must be worn for the task undertaken.

- Horse activities generally have a poor safety record and are recognised as fairly high risk. Care must be taken that the child is never put at risk and that the centre cannot be found negligent in the event of a claim being made against it.

The following training programme can easily be amended to suit the particular yard.

It is suggested that an appropriate fee is charged for the training and that a suitable certificate designed by the centre is awarded on satisfactory completion.

The training of helpers would be an ideal task for junior or trainee instructors.

Adult helpers

It is important that their role on the yard is clarified by some sort of written agreement signed by both parties.

- They must have personal and third party insurance.

- They must receive the appropriate training.

- They should be supervised in any new task undertaken.

- They should not be asked to supervise others unless suitably trained and experienced.

- They should always wear clothing suitable for the task.

- They should have an agreed personal mentor or supervisor.

Suggested Programme

Lesson 1	Safety on and around the stable yard. Handling horses.
Lesson 2	Stable routine.
Lesson 3	Grooming and tack cleaning.
Lesson 4	Tacking up and untacking.
Lesson 5	Care of the horse after exercise.
Lesson 6	Assisting with lessons.
Lesson 7	Watering and feeding.
Lesson 8	Revision, etc.
Lesson 9	Assessment.

DOMESTIC STAFF

A cook, a housekeeper and cleaners may be required. If staff and/or students and working pupils are to live in at the yard or in a staff house, arrangements have to be made for:

- Cleaning the house.

- Preparation of food.

- Mature staff living in separate accommodation may be expected to look after themselves, but young students and working pupils should not be required to do so. It is the responsibility of the school owner or manager to see that young members of staff are well looked after. They should have suitable accommodation, and should be encouraged to care for it and keep it clean and tidy.

Turnout of Staff, Students and Working Pupils

Some yards will have strict rules regarding dress and turnout. All yards should make sure that personnel are suitably dressed. It gives the yard a more professional appearance if staff are neatly and suitably turned out. They must also dress to conform with Health and Safety guidelines for the task they are undertaking.

If the public are being catered for, some sort of uniform such as a yard tee-shirt or sweatshirt will make it easier for staff members to be identified.

GENERAL STABLE DUTIES

Daily

1. Water.
2. Cleaning out water bowls.
3. Feeding.
4. Mucking out and sweeping yard.
5. Grooming.
6. Exercising.
7. Cleaning tack.
8. Washing feed bowls.
9. Tidying tack room and feed shed.
10. Washing sinks and floors.
11. Cleaning lavatories and basins.
12. Raking and harrowing school floor and track. (Raking done by hand; harrowing done by tractor.)
13. Washing stable tools, skips and wheelbarrows.

Weekly

1. Dusting down stables.
2. Checking salt licks.
3. Cleaning drains and traps.
4. Shaking and brushing rugs.
5. Disinfecting stable floors and drains – not deep-litter bedding.
6. Washing lavatory floors and checking supplies.
7. Washing grooming kit.
8. Cleaning headcollars and rollers.
9. Oiling tack if it is stiff.
10. Levelling school floor; salting and/or watering if necessary.
11. Preparing farrier list.
12. Dealing with saddlery repairs.
13. Washing down barn and stable passageways.

Monthly

1. Checking door bolts.
2. Checking string on tie-rings.
3. Checking drains.
4. Ordering feed supplies.
5. Checking other supplies: e.g. disinfectant, saddle soap, clipping blades, brooms, stable tools.
6. Checking bandages.
7. Checking saddlery for repairs.
8. Washing stable walls.
9. Checking first-aid box and veterinary cupboard.
10. Ensuring that horses are shod every 4–6 weeks.
11. Worming as needed.

Long term

1. Checking night and New Zealand rugs, washing and sending for repair.
2. Sending day rugs and blankets to be cleaned and repaired. Store away.
3. Painting wooden stabling and wood surfaces.
4. Painting block walls of stables.
5. Painting school walls.

6. Painting show jumps.
7. Repairing stabling. Repaint as necessary.
8. Checking roofs and yard surface. Repair as necessary.
9. Checking windows.
10. Buying hay, straw and other bedding.
11. Checking saddlery for replacement.
12. Checking fields, fencing and gates before turning out horses for spring.
13. Checking fire extinguishers.
14. Servicing clippers, groomers, corn mill, water heaters and other equipment.
15. Organising inoculations.
16. Checking teeth every six to twelve months.
17. Mucking out deep litter (twice a year minimum).

Allocate one hour a day for weekly tasks and half a day a week for monthly tasks. The horse's day off is an ideal time.

PLANNING THE WORKING DAY

In any professional yard it helps if there is a basic timetable. It is the task of the yard manager to produce one that is realistic and that suits the type of organisation.

Things that need to be considered are:

- Type of yard: e.g. some have many facets, e.g. livery, riding lessons, student training and evening clients. Hunting is still important in some areas.
- Identify the 'normal' working day.
- Identify any frequent 'abnormal' days. e.g. hunting or competition.
- Number of staff and/or trainees.
- Number of hours they work.
- The responsibilities of various staff members.
- Requirements of livery owners.
- Making best use of facilities.

- Making provision for staff training.
- Organising time off on a weekly basis and annual holidays.
- Ensuring best use of horses.

Task one is to decide whether the yard works a six-or a seven-day week. Traditionally yards gave all the horses the same day off each week.

Plus points are:

- Horse more relaxed without so much hustle and bustle.
- Good for organising staff time off.
- Opportunity for keeping up with maintenance etc.
- Opportunity to hire out facilities without major upheaval to routine.
- Cheapest way to utilise time when little demand for resources.

Minus points are:

- Wasting valuable resources.
- Wasting opportunity for staff training.

Task two is to divide the working day into blocks. Four is often a realistic number.

- Before breakfast or early stables.
- After breakfast or morning work.
- Afternoon work.
- Evening stables.
- Some yards may have evening work if they are in an urban area where clients wish to ride after work.
- There are also late-night checks to be considered.

Task three is to identify the tasks to be performed in each block.
Task four is to identify the staff and horses involved.

Task five is to identify staff time off.

Task six is to identify that all tasks have been covered.

It is important to plan the day's work because:

• People know what is happening.

• Horses work better to a routine.

• More can be achieved in a given time.

However, plans must be flexible to allow for changing circumstances such as:

• Extra clients.

• Sickness.

• Visitors.

• A change in the weather.

Certain basics are always present, depending on the type of yard. They might include:

• Mucking out.

• Feeding.

• Catching up.

• Exercise.

• Schooling.

• Lessons.

• Tack cleaning.

• Grooming.

Try to keep those that remain constant to the same times each day. For those that alter, try to allow sufficient time each day into which varying tasks can be fitted. For example 10.00 on Monday, staff lesson. On Tuesday, exercise and Wednesday lungeing.

Timetable a set time and a particular day for tasks that are done on a weekly basis. This might include cleaning windows, turning out the feed store or bringing up the weekly hay ration. In this way things are not forgotten or pushed into the background through lack of time.

Although parts of the day remain fairly rigid, e.g. feed times, try to ensure the timetable remains flexible. Then if something crops up, things can either be swapped around or reallocated to another day.

Don't plan too much for any one day. This ensures that what is done is done well.

Having planned the day as a whole, consider the tasks in particular and how they can be fitted together.

For example:

• Carrying all bedding and forage before sweeping yards.

• Tying all horses up before mucking out or quartering so time is not wasted opening and shutting doors.

• Picking out feet before sweeping floors.

• Washing buckets before feeds dry in them.

• Rinsing out skips and barrows straight after use.

• Brushing off horses before putting fresh water in the boxes.

• Doing all dirty, smelly jobs before changing into tidy clothes.

• Preparing all horses for exercise before exercising the first.

• Is it possible to save on tack without detriment to the horse, tack and rider?

• Is it possible to ride and lead?

• If horses are being turned out, do it as soon as possible. It saves on skipping out.

• If beds are free, set fair for the night with haynets etc.

• When cleaning tack, work in blocks. All washing done first, then bright work and finally soaping. The leather has more chance to dry and less soap gets rinsed into the bucket.

You will find many similar ways in which your yard can

Typical Daily Routine in a Riding School

Time	Work	Person responsible	Lessons, Teaching, Schooling	Person Responsible
0700	Check horses. Water and feed. Horses working at 0800 have small feeds and are fed after work.	Stable manager		
0800	Water. Muck out, bed down (or at 1215).	Staff	Private lesson	Chief Instructor
0900	Brush-off horses. Saddle-up for staff 1000 and 1100 lessons and for livery owners.Tidy muck heap and sweep yard.			
1000			Staff lesson	Chief I or II
1100			Client lesson	I or AI
1115	Small haynet all round. Groom horses.	Staff		
1215	Skip out. Water. Bed down.	Staff	Lungeing or schooling	Chief I or II
1230	Feed.	Stable manager		
1230	LUNCH BREAK			
1300			Private lesson	II
1345	Prepare horses for 1400 lesson.	Staff		
1400	Lectures for working pupils.	Stable manager	Lesson	AI or II
1430	Catch and prepare ponies for 1600 lesson. Groom horses.	AIs and working pupils		
1500			Lesson	AI or II
1600-1730	Feed. Skip out. Hay up.	Stable manager & staff	Children's lesson	AI and WP help
1730	Turn out ponies.	WPs		
1800	HOME			

Evening Rides

Time	Work	Person responsible	Lessons, Teaching, Schooling	Person Responsible
1700	Saddle up for 1800 lesson. Prepare hay and leave outside boxes of horses being worked.	Staff on evening rota	Lessons	Staff on evening rota
1800-2100	Prepare horses. Skip out boxes. Water. Check unsaddling and rugging-up. Put away tack. Give haynets.			
2100	Final check or after last lesson.	Stable manager		

work more efficiently. The main thing is to PLAN. Sit down and work out how best to do the work with the minimum of effort and the maximum efficiency. The time taken will be amply rewarded in the long term.

GENERAL DAILY ROUTINE

The following tasks are applicable to most stable yards:

1. Check the horse's general well-being:

• That he is moving comfortably round the box.

• That he is not pointing or resting a front foot – a sign of discomfort. If the opposite hind foot is also rested, it is a sign of relaxation after work.

• That there are no signs of injury such as those caused by getting cast.

• That the bed is in a satisfactory state and that the droppings are normal in appearance and number.

• That the feed and hay have been eaten.

2. If necessary, adjust rugs.
3. Water, feed and leave horse to eat in peace.
4. Muck out, pick out feet into a skip, bed down, sweep up. If there is time, tidy up the muck heap.
5. Brush off and saddle up. Horses should be tied up:

• If the groom is working in the stable.

• If they are saddled up ready for work, in case they try to roll.

6. Exercise.
7. On return from exercise, wash and pick out feet, unsaddle, give small feed of hay.
8. Groom.
9. Skip out box. Tidy muck heap (if not done earlier). Water, feed, lunch.
10. Finish grooming.
11. Clean tack.
12. Stable jobs.
13. Skip out. Set fair beds for the night.

14. Water and feed.
15. Sweep yard.
16. Give haynet.
17. Check:
    • Horse rugs.
    • Water.
    • Stable doors.
    • Feed shed.

18. Lock up tack rooms and close yard gate.
19. Later at night look round to ensure that all is well, but try not to disturb the horses.
20. Give water and late feeds if required.

Typical Routine for Competition Horses

This daily routine would be appropriate for a yard of three horses with one groom and help to ride.

0700	Check water. Feed and small haynet.
0730	Muck out. Bed down. Sweep up. Tidy up muck heap.
0830	Brush off.
0900	Schooling and/or exercise. Lunge one horse if one person responsible for all exercise. **NB:** Hay after work.
1200	Strap one horse. Set fair others.
1245	Feed.
1300	LUNCH
1400	Strap two horses.
1515	Stable jobs. Tack.
1600	Skip out. Water. Set fair beds for the night.
1630	Feed. Finish tack.
1730	Skip out. Water. Hay-up.
2030	Water. Fourth feed.

Typical Routine for Hunter Liveries

This daily routine would be appropriate for a yard of four horses. When getting the horses fit, extra help will be required if other duties are to be performed efficiently.

Example Weekly Timetable for a Yard with Multiple Interests

TIME	MONDAY	TUESDAY	WEDNESDAY	THURSDAY	FRIDAY	SATURDAY	SUNDAY
	Day off for horses	Hunting	Evening rides				
7.30-8.30	Morning stables	Morning stables	Morning stables	Morning stables	Morning stables	Morning stables	Morning stables
9.00-10.30	Turnout	Exercise 1	Load up	Staff time off	Exercise 1	Exercise 1	Exercise 1
or	or			or			
9.00-10.00	Deliveries	Lesson 1	Load up	Staff lesson	Lesson 1	Lesson 1	Lesson 1
10.30-12.00	or	Exercise 2			Exercise 2	Exercise 2	Exercise 2
	Staff lesson						
10.00-11.00	or	Lesson 2	Hunting	Staff theory	Lesson 2	Lesson 2	Lesson 2
11.00-12.00	Change turn out	Lesson 3	Lesson 3	Lesson 3	Lesson 3		
12.00-1.00	Long break	Lunch stables		Lunch stables	Lunch stables	Lunch stables	Lunch stables
1.00-2.00	Long break	Staff break	Staff break	Staff break	Staff break	Staff break	Staff break
2.00-3.00	Farrier	Lesson 4		Lesson 1	Lesson 4	Lesson 4	Lesson 4
or	or						
2.00-3.30	Maintenance	Exercise 3			Exercise 3	Exercise 3	Exercise 3
3.00-4.00	or	Lesson 5	Prepare for	Lesson 2	Lesson 5	Lesson 5	Lesson 5
	Staff lesson		return				
4.00-5.00	Evening stables	Evening stables	Evening stables	Lesson 3	Evening stables	Evening stables	Evening stables
5.00	Finish	Finish	Check horses	Lesson 4	Finish	Finish	Finish
6.00-7.00			Feed		Lesson 6		
7.00-8.00					Lesson 7		
8.00		Late feed	Check horses	Late feed	Late feed	Late feed	
10.00	Late checks	Late checks	Late checks	Late checks	Late checks	Late checks	Late checks

Obviously any day can be interchanged with any other, lessons can become hacks or treks and hunting might be competition. Staff would rotate days off; Monday being horses' rest day would require fewer staff as would Saturday and Sunday when clients would ride the horses. On late night teaching days, those teaching late could be off from 9.00 until 2.00.

0700	Check horses. Water. Feed. Hay	1245	Feed.
0730	Muck out.	1300	LUNCH
0830	Brush off. Saddle-up.	1400	Strap two horses.
0900	Ride and lead each pair for approximately one and a quarter hours.	1500	Clean tack.
		1545	Stable duties. Sweep yard.
1015	Return from exercise. Prepare second pair and take out.	1630	Feed.
		1700	Skip out. Check rugs. Water.
1130	Unsaddle. Haynet.	1730	Finish.
1145	Strap two horses. Skip out beds. Set fair. Sweep yard. Tidy muck heap.	2030	Check horses. Water.

General Considerations in a Hunter-livery Yard

• When the horse is fit and hunting twice a week, daily exercise can be reduced. In some cases three-quarters of an hour is sufficient.

• A warm mash may be given after hunting, but this is no longer thought to be so beneficial as in the past. See Chapter 23.

• The day after hunting, check legs, trot up, lead out for ten minutes. NB: One experienced (trained) groom should be able to do five horses if also not doing the exercising. A horse walker can be a great boon, and can save many hours spent exercising.

PREVENTION AND CONTROL OF FIRE

It is advisable to consult the local fire brigade headquarters about fire regulations relating to stables, and to seek their advice regarding a particular stable yard and its problem areas. For legal requirements, see Chapter 55.

Easy access for fire appliances needs to be maintained at all times. If the premises is secured at night, special keys can be used that allow the fire brigade access.

All gateways, archways and paths need to be wide enough to allow access. If water pressure is poor, cattle-type water troughs kept filled can provide a short-term supply of water whilst awaiting the fire brigade.

Recommended Procedures and Practices

• No smoking in stable and working areas. 'No Smoking' notices should be prominently displayed and no-smoking rules strictly adhered to.

• It is illegal to smoke in any public area or work place which is enclosed or which has a door opening to the outside.

• Fire notices should be displayed in all stable blocks and in all other ancillary buildings. Instructions for procedure in the event of fire must be clearly set out and legible.

• Fire drill should be held at regular intervals, particularly when there has been a new intake of staff or working pupils.

• Suitable fire appliances appropriate to the contents should be placed in all buildings, including covered school and gallery.

All personnel should be clearly instructed as to which appliances should be used on the following sources of fire:

Hay and straw.
Electrical faults.
Oil and petrol.

• A sufficient number of fire alarms should be available in accordance with the size of the yard. They should be tested regularly to ensure that they are in working order. They should be protected from frost.

• There should be an adequate number of hoses and water-points, so that the hoses reach all areas of stables, barns, and other buildings. Unfortunately, domestic water supplies seldom have sufficient pressure to be of much use but the fire officer will advise.

• Unless there is a risk of frost, the main fire hose should always be kept fitted to the water supply, and ready for use. In freezing weather, it should be drained and insulated.

Action to be Taken in the Event of Fire

These instructions should be given to all personnel:

1. Call the fire brigade, or make sure that someone else has called them.

2. Make sure they have the map reference.

3. Sound the fire alarm.

4. Assemble all staff and other personnel at designated assembly point and do a head count.

5. If the stables are on fire, or could catch fire, take or release the horses into a field or designated area. Begin with those nearest to the fire.

6. Ensure that the gate or door to the designated area is kept closed or has someone on it at all times. Horses will run back to their stables if they can.

7. Tackle the fire with appropriate fire appliances, without putting yourself at risk.

8. Leave headcollars on but remove ropes. If each animal has his own headcollar outside the stable and it is hung up by the noseband with the headpiece undone, it saves time when putting it on.

9. If possible, shut as many doors as possible to contain the fire and prevent accidents in a smoky environment.

Horses may be frightened and refuse to leave their stables. A coat or cloth put over the head and covering the eyes may make them more willing to move. If a stable rubber is kept handy it can be dunked in the water bucket and wrung out before covering the eyes and tucked into the headcollar. Being damp it is more likely to stay in place. In the case of a difficult horse, several people may be needed to move him. Inhaled smoke is very dangerous to horses, so make sure that they have access to fresh air. If they have inhaled smoke, it is advisable to seek veterinary advice.

It is a useful exercise to invite the local brigade down to the yard and give them a lesson in how to handle horses. They will also be able to familiarise themselves with the layout. Horses can be very frightened of fire officers in full protective gear.

The Most Common Causes of Fire

- See Appendix 8.

- Electrical fault in wiring or appliance. Installing a trip-switch, which cuts off the electricity supply in the event of a fault, should avert this.

- Electric or paraffin heaters.

- Clothing or rugs put too close to heaters when drying.

- Smoking. Careless use of matches and throwing away of cigarette ends.

- Children playing with matches.

- Self-combustion of hay in the stack.

- Bonfires placed too close to hay barns or other buildings.

- All electrical equipment should be checked by a qualified electrician on an annual basis and have a dated sticker attached to show when it was done.

55

THE LAW

Readers should be aware that any of the legal requirements quoted are subject to change. They should seek confirmation before assuming that they are accurate statements of the law currently in force. They are only outlines and are not a substitute for professional advice.

This chapter outlines the relevant contents of the Acts which cover horses and stables. The Acts most relevant to stable management are:

- Protection of Animals Act of 1911 amended 1988.

- Animals Act of 1971.

- Riding Establishments Acts of 1964 and 1970.

- Health and Safety at Work Act of 1974.

- Reporting of Injuries, Diseases and Dangerous Occurrences Regulations (RIDDOR) 1985.

- Control of Substances Hazardous to Health (COSHH) regulations.

- The Agricultural (Miscellaneous Provision) Act 1968.

- The Welfare of Farmed Animals (England) 2000 Regulations. There are similar Regulations in place for Scotland, Wales and Northern Ireland.

- The Farriers (Registration) Act 1975 and Amendments 1977.

There are also Regulations in place referring to:

- The slaughter of horses.

- The transport of horses.

- The tethering of horses.

Anyone with particular interest in any of the areas needs to consider the following:

- Getting hold of a full copy of the Act, which can be obtained from Her Majesty's Stationery Office (HMSO) London.

- Finding out if the Health & Safety Executive (H&SE) have issued guidelines on the subject.

- Getting professional advice to ensure full understanding of and compliance with the law.

The National Equine Welfare Council (NEWC) publishes excellent welfare guidelines for all equines.

The European Community (EC) issues European Legislation in a number of formats.

RIDING ESTABLISHMENTS ACTS 1964 AND 1970

The setting up, and to a large extent the running, of a riding establishment is governed by the combined effect of the Riding Establishments Acts 1964 and 1970. These are applicable in England, Scotland and Wales.

Northern Ireland has separate legislation entitled Riding Establishments Regulations 1980, and riding stables on the Isle of Man are governed by the Riding Establishment (Inspection) Act of 1968.

The Riding Establishment Acts 1964 and 1970 forbid the keeping of a riding establishment in England,

Scotland and Wales except under the authority of a licence issued by the local authority in whose area the premises (including land) are situated.

THE RIDING ESTABLISHMENT

The term Riding Establishment covers the carrying on of a business 'of keeping horses to let them out on hire for riding and/or for use in providing instruction in riding, for payment'.

Licences

A licence may be granted annually after application by an individual over the age of eighteen years, or by a company. The normal duration of a licence is twelve months. Licences are not renewable, and a new application and inspection of the premises is required on the expiry of the existing licence. Licences run from the date of issue, but some local authorities issue licences dated from 1 January.

As an alternative, if a local authority is not satisfied that a case has been made for a full licence it has the power to grant a provisional licence for a period of three months. This provisional licence can specify the conditions required, so that the licence holder has time to meet such conditions and will therefore eventually be granted a full licence. The local authority may extend the period for a further three months, but only on re-application by the licence holder. One of the purposes of such an extension is to give the licence holder the opportunity to complete work already begun in order to meet the specified conditions. The local authority may not issue provisional licences to any person or company for more than six months in any one case.

The cost of the licence, either full or provisional, is at the discretion of the local authority, and the total fee includes administrative and inspection charges. No provision is made for a charge to be levied for the three-months' extension to a provisional licence.

The Acts give the local authority complete discretion over the granting or refunding of a licence. However, an aggrieved applicant can appeal to a magistrates' court, in relation to both the refusal and to any conditions that the authority has imposed. The magistrates may then give such directions as they think proper in respect of the issuing of a licence or to the conditions.

There are no provisions within the Acts for third parties to appeal against the granting of a particular licence.

Planning Permission

Before consideration is given to the granting of a licence to a new applicant, the local authority should ascertain that under the Town and Country Planning Act of 1971 permission has been obtained either to erect new buildings, or for change of use of all or part of existing premises.

Qualification for a Licence

No one under eighteen is qualified to apply for a licence, nor is any person who for the time being is disqualified under any of the following:

- The Riding Establishment Acts.

- The Protection of Animals (Cruelty to Dogs) Act (1933) from keeping a dog.

- The Protection of Animals (Cruelty to Dogs) (Scotland) Act (1934) from keeping a dog.

- The Pet Animals Act (1951) from keeping a pet shop.

- The Protection of Animals (Amendment) Act of 1954 from having custody of animals.

- The Animal Boarding Establishments Act (1963) from keeping a boarding establishment for animals.

An applicant for a licence must be a qualified person within the above provisions, and must be able to satisfy the local authority that they are suitable, and qualified, either by practical experience in the management of horses or by being the holder of one of the following certificates:

- BHS Assistant Instructor.

- BHS Intermediate Instructor.

- BHS Instructor.

- BHS or ABRS Fellowship.

- Any other certificate prescribed by order of the Secretary of State.

An inspecting veterinary surgeon is required to consider the suitability of the applicant in accordance with the above conditions.

Inspections

Before granting a licence the local authority grants powers in writing to an officer from their own or from any other local authority; this person will be a veterinary surgeon or veterinary practitioner selected from the list specifically drawn up jointly by the Royal College of Veterinary Surgeons and the British Veterinary Association for this purpose. He should carry out a detailed inspection of the premises and submit a report to the local authority, who will consider whether the premises and the persons employed in the management of the riding establishment are suitable to be holders of a licence.

Inspectors are recommended to visit the riding establishment at any time within reason when all horses are likely to be at the stables: giving not more than 24 hours' notice of the visit. The inspection should be made at the time of year appropriate to the type of use of the animal, and to seasonal activities such as trekking or hunting. To determine the standard of care and management, the animals should be in full use.

Conditions of a Licence

Without prejudice to their discretion to withhold a licence on any grounds, the authority shall take particular regard to the following:

Accommodation

- Accommodation should be suitable for the animals in respect of size, construction, number of occupants, light, ventilation, drainage and cleanliness. Stalls should be wide enough and long enough to allow the animals to lie down and to get up easily and without risk of injury. Boxes should be large enough to allow the animal to turn round. Stalls and boxes should be free from fittings, projections or structural features which might cause injury. Doors should always open outwards. These and the following requirements apply to new constructions, and to buildings which have been converted for use as stabling.

The local authority considers the number of horses kept at an establishment (including animals at livery) in relation to the buildings and land available, and may impose a condition specifying the maximum number of horses of all categories (both for use in the riding establishment or otherwise) which should be kept at any time. Yards should provide sufficient space for every animal kept on the premises.

- Lighting should be good enough to preclude the use of artificial light during daytime. Switches, wires and other electrical equipment should be protected in such a way that horses cannot injure themselves.

- There should be adequate ventilation without draughts.

- Drainage must carry away any liquids voided, and be sufficient to keep the boxes and stalls dry. Provisions must be made for the storage and regular disposal of manure and waste bedding.

- Adequate and suitable food, water, and bedding, together with both rest and exercise where required, must be provided, as well as suitable facilities for the storage of reasonable reserves of food and bedding.

Grazing

- Where horses are kept at grass there must be adequate pasture, suitable shelter, and water at all times. When the animals are either in work, or during the winter period when the grass is not growing, the Acts require that adequate supplementary feed should be given. The veterinary surgeon takes into consideration the type of animal, together with the type and location of their pasture. Arabs, Thoroughbreds or hunter types require more protection from the weather than do native ponies.

- It is necessary within the Acts to maintain fences in a safe condition and to keep the grazing free from hazards and rubbish.

- A competent person who can recognise injuries or illness must visit the horses at grass daily.

Horses

- The term 'horse' within the Acts includes any mare, gelding, pony, foal, colt, filly, stallion, ass, mule or jennet. They are required to be kept in good health, physically fit, and suitable for the purpose for which they are being maintained.

- It is not permissible to use animals that are three years old or under, or mares heavily in foal or within three months of having foaled.

- Good, not thin, condition is required.

- It is not necessary for horses to be shod, but their feet must be kept well trimmed and in good condition. If they are shod, the fitting of the shoes must be correct.

- Animals must be free from illness, sores, galls, or injuries from the bit, saddle or other sources. Where injury or illness has occurred it is an offence not to provide curative care and treatments.

- On any inspection of the premises by an authorised officer of the local authority, a horse found to be in need of veterinary attention must be removed immediately from work on the verbal instruction of the officer. These instructions are generally confirmed in writing as soon as possible after the inspection. The horse cannot be returned to work until the licence holder has obtained at his/her own expense a certificate from a veterinary surgeon that the horse is fit for work, and has lodged the certificate with the local authority. This is a mandatory condition in the granting of a licence.

- A register of all horses three years old and under and in the possession of the licence holder must be maintained and must be available for inspection.

- Horses at part livery and partially used in the riding establishment are within the provisions of the Act and subject to inspection.

- Horses kept at full livery for private owners should be noted and can be inspected by the authorised officer who has powers under Section 1 (3) of the principal Act to inspect any horse found on the premises.

- It is very likely in the near future that all livery premises will require a similar licence. At the time of writing the word 'livery' has not been defined.

- It is an offence under the Acts to conceal, or cause to be concealed, any horse maintained on the premises, with the intention of avoiding an inspection of this horse.

- It is also an offence to allow a horse to be in such a condition that riding him would be likely to cause him suffering, as would letting him out for hire, or using him to provide, in return for payment, instruction in riding, or to demonstrate riding, whether for payment or not.

- When instruction in riding is given on a horse that is the property of the pupil receiving instruction, it is not usually considered that this requires a licence, regardless of where that instruction is given.

Saddlery

- All riding equipment must be maintained in good condition and, at the time when it is supplied to the rider, should not be subject to any defect which on inspection is considered to be likely to cause suffering to the horse or an accident to the rider. It also constitutes an offence to supply a saddle which is ill-fitting, causing a sore back; or bits, curbs, etc. which cause injury to the mouth; or bridles, girths, stirrup leathers and irons which might break due to faulty materials, manufacture, or stitching and thus place the rider in peril or render the horse liable to injury.

- The inspector examines the saddlery when fitted to the horse for which it is intended, and pays particular attention to the correct fitting of Western-type saddles and also to ex-army troop saddles, as many of these are not fitted with safety stirrup bars and might cause a falling rider to be dragged. This type of saddle should be used only with patent safety stirrup irons.

Infectious Diseases and First-aid Equipment

- All reasonable precautions must be taken against the spread of infectious diseases and, so far as it is possible, there should be provisions to isolate an infectious animal.

- Veterinary first-aid equipment and medicines must be kept on the premises in a suitable and clean place set aside for this purpose. It is recommended that before assembling this equipment, consultation as to its contents should be made by the licence holder with the establishment's veterinary surgeon. He will take into consideration the veterinary experience of the licence holder when advising on particular medicines etc., as well as on the standard contents, such as antiseptic solutions, powders, bandages, dressings, scissors and a clinical thermometer. It is also strongly recommended that the name, address and telephone numbers of the establishment's veterinary surgeon and doctor should be prominently displayed.

Fire Precautions

- Precautions must be taken for the protection of the horses in case of fire. Notices prohibiting smoking should be displayed.

- There must be clear access to all stalls and boxes, and where multiple numbers of stalls and boxes are housed within the same building, more than one exit is strongly recommended.

- Fire extinguishers must be regularly serviced, and an adequate supply of water should be available easily. The local fire-prevention officer should be consulted on the types of fire-fighting equipment most suitable for the premises.

- The 1970 Riding Establishments Act requires that there should be a notice on the outside of the premises, giving the name, address, and telephone number of the licence holder or other appointed responsible persons, together with directions as to the actions to be taken in case of fire. The directions should include particular advice on the removal of animals from the stables.

Management and Supervision

- A person under sixteen years of age must not be left in charge of the business. All horses let out on hire must be supervised by a person of sixteen years or over, unless the licence holder is satisfied that the hirer is competent to ride without supervision. Before he can be satisfied that the rider is competent to ride unsupervised, a licence holder must therefore have either previous knowledge, or have made an assessment of the capability of the rider and must then provide a horse 'suitable for the purpose' of that rider's requirements and ability. A licence holder who has failed to make the correct assessment might be unable to use this as a defence should litigation follow.

- The knowledge of the licence holder is an integral part of the granting of a licence, and should this knowledge be regarded as inadequate, the applicant can appoint a manager or other person to supervise the riding establishment on his/her behalf. The local authority can then issue a licence which will also carry the name of the person with the necessary knowledge or qualifications upon it. If this person leaves the establishment during the currency of the licence, it would appear that the licence becomes null and void.

- Similarly, it would appear that a riding establishment cannot be sold as a licensed business, because without the qualifications or experience of the licence holder the licence is ineffective. Any purchaser therefore has to make an application to the local authority for a licence before proceeding to operate the business, and to satisfy the authority that he/she has the necessary qualifications or experience.

- Provisions are made whereby, in the event of the death of a person holding a current licence, the licence passes to his/her personal representatives, and can be extended for one year (three months if a provisional licence) from the date of death. Such an extension can be made more than once if the local authority is satisfied that the extensions are necessary to wind up the estate.

Insurance

- The 1970 Riding Establishments Act clearly states that the licence holder shall hold a current Public Liability Insurance Policy which provides indemnity against liability at law to pay damages for accidental bodily injury sustained by the hirer of a horse, or those using the horse to receive instruction in riding. The licence holder must also insure the riders in respect of any liability which they might incur through injuries to any other person, caused or having arisen through the hire or use of the horse.

- The amount of indemnity is not specified, but licence holders are advised to make sure that the amount exceeds the highest awards the courts have made in respect of riding accidents.

- In addition, where the business employs staff, compulsory insurance is required under the following:

 – Employer's Liability (Compulsory Insurance) Act 1969.
 – Employer's Liability (Defective Equipment) Act 1969.

Rights of Local (Licensing) Authorities

- Powers of entry.

- The right to impose conditions upon a licence so as to secure all the objects specified within the Acts.

- The right to dispense with some conditions if they think that circumstances so warrant.

Five conditions in Section 2 of the 1970 Act are mandatory. They are:

1. The removal from work of horses which are in need of veterinary attention.
2. The supervision by responsible people aged sixteen years or over.
3. Leaving the premises in charge of a person over sixteen years.
4. The insurance policy requirements.
5. The register of horses three years old and under.

Any person who operates or has intentions of operating a riding establishment is advised to obtain copies of both the 1964 and 1970 Riding Establishment Acts in order to be fully conversant with their requirements.

THE HEALTH AND SAFETY AT WORK ACT 1974

The provisions of this Act apply to employers and employees engaged in the keeping and management of livestock. Riding schools, livery yards, etc. are not specified, but do come under the Act. Responsible employers should be aware of their duty, both to themselves and to their employees, to see that work conditions are as safe and as healthy as possible.

Any business employing more than five people,

including casual workers, must issue a Safety Policy Statement. Instructions to employees should be clearly set out. Assistance in drawing up this statement can be obtained from the BHS Riding Schools and Recreational Riding Office, The Deer Park, Stoneleigh, Warwickshire; or The Association of British Riding Schools, Old Brewery Yard, Penzance, Cornwall TR18 2SL; or the local Health and Safety Executive (address and telephone number in the local Yellow Pages Directory). The local office of ADAS also supplies leaflets and a poster on safety measures and safer working conditions.

In December 1986, HM Agricultural Inspectorate of Health and Safety published requirements extra to the 1974 Act. Many of the following directives are covered, but in addition there are strict regulations for health and safety in relation to food preparation, first aid, sanitation, etc. Responsibility for staff training, instruction, suitability of horses, dress, etc. are also covered. It is therefore essential for persons setting up – or running – a yard to obtain a copy of the *Horse Riding Establishments Guidance on Promoting Safe Working Conditions* by the Health and Safety Executive. They can thus ensure that they are able to comply with the necessary requirements of HM Agricultural Inspectorate.

General Obligations

- Employers must ensure the safety of their employees by maintaining safe systems of work, safe premises, and safe equipment.

- Employees and the self-employed must take reasonable care to avoid injury.

- Employers, the self-employed and employees must not endanger the health and safety of third parties.

- There should be a named person to whom any faults in equipment or other hazards can be reported.

- Employers must ensure that all employees and others on the premises are correctly instructed in any work

that they have to do and in any equipment that they have to use.

- It is advisable that written evidence of training given and received is kept on file.

- Employees should be encouraged to produce new ideas for improved safety measures and methods of working.

- Employers should ensure that their insurance policies cover the use of equipment and machinery by any member of staff, paid or unpaid.

- Employer's liability insurance is compulsory for all employers, and an up-to-date certificate of this must be displayed.

- The Health and Safety Executive issue and update directives from time to time to advise on such matters as the organisation of shows etc. The BHS also publishes guidelines on how to run a livery yard or format a working pupil contract, etc. It is always advisable to seek up-to-date information before embarking on a new venture and to check from time to time with an established business whether you are working within modern guidelines.

- Well-equipped first-aid facilities should be available on the premises and a responsible person should be always on call when required. Leaflets on first aid can be obtained from HMSO Publications Centre, PO Box 276, London SW8 5DT or the local Health and Safety Executive.

Risk Areas

- Employers should give these special attention.

- Employees should be instructed as to any special precautions which should be taken.

- Employees should be instructed in the correct and safe use of equipment and machinery.

Employees likely to be left in charge of the yard, in the absence of senior staff, should be fully briefed as to what to do should an emergency arise. A list of relevant telephone numbers – for doctor, veterinary surgeon, owner or manager, electrician – should be provided.

Employees should be instructed about:

• The working of the trip-switch and how it is re-set.

• The whereabouts of all water-main stop-cocks.

The main risk factors are:

COMBUSTIBLE MATERIALS – stables; hay barns; oil, diesel or petrol storage areas; electric, gas or oil heaters; bonfires.

ELECTRICAL EQUIPMENT AND MACHINERY such as clipping and grooming machines, corn mill, etc. All electrical wiring, fittings and equipment should be inspected regularly. Equipment should be regularly serviced. A circuit-breaker should be used with all electrical equipment. Electric cable should be inspected before using any equipment, to see that it has not been damaged by friction or by a horse treading on it. Plugs should be checked for faulty wiring and cracked casings. Personnel should be properly instructed in the equipment's use and care. Junior staff should be supervised when using electric clippers and groomers.

The corn mill and/or chaff cutter should be worked only by experienced staff. If it is not fitted with a dust extractor, face masks must be used. The dangers of inhaling dust should be explained.

CHAFF CUTTER If electrically powered, see previous paragraph. If either hand or electric powered, guards must be fitted to protect operator's hands. Warning notices should be fixed on the machine, and the risk of getting hands or clothing caught up should be explained. Hand-operated chaff cutters are very unlikely to pass H&S laws and are not recommended.

BARLEY BOILER If electrically powered, see Electrical Equipment, above. If gas powered, it should be well away from any combustible material, on a concrete floor and be worked only by experienced personnel.

TRACTORS, FIELD MACHINERY, HAY TRAILERS, ETC. Regulations and advice are published in a DEFRA pamphlet, which should be essential reading for all personnel.

• No extra persons should be allowed to travel on the tractor, hay trailer, or other farm vehicles.

• Personnel driving the tractor should have a current driving licence.

• Tractors must be suitably insured, and if driven on or across a road, the necessary road tax must be paid. The dangers of working on steep hills, close to deep ditches and boggy areas should be explained; also the risk of allowing children to play in the area where the tractor is kept or where it is working.

VEHICLE, VEHICLE AND TRAILER, HORSEBOX Drivers must check that children and animals are not near when drawing away or reversing.

HORSE WALKERS OR HORSE EXERCISERS These must be well maintained in a suitably fenced area. They should only be used by experienced personnel. Horses should not be attached to the machine by junior staff.

OUTSIDE STRUCTURES Buildings should be kept in sound order. In strong winds, loose tiles, slates or guttering can be dislodged and cause injury to anyone passing underneath.

STEPS AND STAIRS up to or down into working areas should be sound and with a level tread. It may be advisable to fit a hand-rail or rope.

LADDERS AND STEP-LADDERS must be strong enough for the work involved. Unsupervised junior personnel must not be allowed to use ladders. Two people should be responsible for putting up the ladder and for taking it down and putting it away. Ladders should never be left up against a stack or near a stack, as they can be knocked down, breaking the ladder and possibly causing injury. They may also be an invitation to children to climb up and play on top of the stack. This must never be allowed.

Unqualified persons should not work above 2.4m (8ft) off the ground unless suitably supervised.

LIFTING LOADS

- When collecting hay from a stack, employees must be instructed to take bales from the top of the stack and work down. Lower bales should not be pulled out, as this may cause the stack to fall, resulting in serious injury.

- When loading hay bales on to a trailer and taking them to the yard they must be stacked with care, so that the load is steady. If it is to be transported on a public road, the load should be roped for extra safety. Extra care should be taken on a steep or uneven surface.

- When lifting bales and sacks of feed, personnel must be instructed to lift weights in the proper manner. If in doubt, they should ask for help. Senior staff should check that the weights are not too heavy for the persons involved. They should not be allowed to risk straining their back.

Instructions for lifting sacks and other heavy weights:

- Estimate the weight and if necessary ask for help.

- Stand close to the sack.

- Square the sack up in front of you.

- Bend your knees; do not lean over and lift up.

- Take hold of the sack. Lift it by straightening the legs.

- Look where you are going. When putting the sack down, bend your knees. Try not to bend your back.

YARD AREA Stable tools must be carefully used and tidily replaced after use. If left about they are a hazard to staff and horses: they can fall down, be tripped over or stepped on, resulting in a cut foot and/or bruises to face and eyes. Rakes should always be left standing upright, with the head at the top.

BALING STRING When the bale is to be used, the string should be cut, tied up and placed in a suitable sack or bin. Left on the ground, uncut, it can cause a fall and injury should either a person or a horse get their feet caught in it.

WHEELBARROWS should never be left about. When in use, they should be placed parallel to the stable wall. Handles should never be left pointing outwards to the yard. When not in use, barrows should be parked tidily in the stable tool area.

YARD SURFACES should be swept clean. It may be necessary to hose them clean should a film of mud and manure form, as this can be very slippery. It is likely to happen in springtime when horses and ponies are brought in from the fields.

NARROW DOORS AND GATEWAYS should have warning notices. Internal swing doors for feed shed, tack rooms or office are dangerous and are not recommended.

COLD WEATHER CONDITIONS In freezing weather salt should be used if there is ice on the yard. (This should be obtained in the autumn.) In deep snow, working paths should be cleared and then kept clear with regular applications of salt. As an emergency measure, sand or coal ashes help to keep a slippery surface usable. In continuing freezing weather, straw or shavings manure tracks, 1.8m (6ft) wide, give a secure footing for horse and staff. This is more effective than using plain straw. Water buckets must be emptied carefully into a drain, and not spilt on the yard to create an icy surface.

FIELDS, FENCES AND GATES should be kept in good order. Heavy gates on broken hinges can cause a fractured leg for human or horse. Bog and deep ditch areas should be fenced off. If a field entrance on to a road is placed dangerously it should preferably be moved but, if this is not possible, warning notices should be fixed, and staff should be advised of the danger.

CAR PARK, YARD AND DRIVE ENTRANCES The following warning notices should be fixed:

- Speed restriction 5 mph.
- Children and horses.

Drives and access roads can be made safer by placing 'humps' at intervals to slow down traffic. Cars, horseboxes and trailers should be parked away from the stable yard, preferably in a car park. There should also be a special area set aside for bicycles.

TREES Tall old trees near the stable yard and car park area can be a hazard. They should be regularly inspected, and if necessary lopped or felled.

NEGLIGENCE

Claims for negligence are one of the most common forms of legal proceedings against equestrian businesses, especially riding schools.

The following notes are designed to give an overview and create an awareness of the areas in which proprietors and managers need to have policies and strategies in place. It is strongly recommended that advice is sought from your insurance company and the Health and Safety Authority.

Negligence has been defined as:

'The omission to do something which a reasonable person, guided upon those considerations, which ordinarily regulate the conduct of human affairs, would do, or, doing something which a prudent and reasonable person would not do.'

In cases of professional negligence, if someone has a special skill they are supposed to demonstrate it at the level of the average person in that profession. A qualified person working on a yard would be supposed to have a level of skill matching their qualification or experience.

To establish negligence it is necessary for the claimant to prove the following three elements:

- That there was a duty of care.
- That there was a breach of that duty of care.
- That as a result of that breach, damage or injury was caused.

Litigation is on the increase. Insurance premiums are increasing in cost. It can be weeks, months or years before it is apparent that a claim is being made. Therefore it is essential that all relevant information is collected as soon as possible after any incident or accident.

The burden of proof generally lies with the person making the claim, who must prove all three elements in order to be successful.

In all cases the claim is made against a named person within the establishment. That person may be the owner or manager of the establishment or a staff member deemed responsible at the time of the incident/injury.

If it is established that the incident/injury took place, the defendant needs to prove that all reasonable steps were taken in prevention.

With riding being recognised as a risk sport it is vital that those in responsible positions have all sensible strategies in place to minimise the risks involved. There is a duty of care towards staff, trainees, clients and visitors. It is not always easy to separate the responsibilities of the different staff members, especially on a small yard where one person may be fulfilling many roles. Initially, the ideal is to minimise the risk of a claim. This can be done in a number of ways that will be explained later.

Second, once a claim has been made, ensure that it can be defended in the most comprehensive and efficient way possible. Far too many equestrian establishments claim that there is not enough time to keep records. As a successful claim could well put a small establishment out of business, it is worthwhile making time. Once a system is in place and all relevant staff are trained in its use it is not so time-consuming. There are a number of excellent software packages on the market, one of which will suit most businesses.

Consider whether the following information is available weeks or months after a happening:

- Evidence of the claimant's level of experience.
- Were they correctly dressed?
- Were they provided with a suitable mount?
- Had they ridden that horse before?
- Had they been on a similar ride or lesson before?
- Were they riding with riders of a similar standard?
- Was the ride provided that they had requested?
- Who was in charge of the ride?
- Was the ride supervisor/teacher sufficiently qualified or experienced for the event?
- Was a record made of any accident or incident that took place?
- Did that record have the signatures and addresses of any witnesses?
- Did the claimant sign any description of the accident as a true and accurate account?
- If the accident occurred on the yard, was the claimant supposed to be in that area?
- Were they being properly supervised?
- Had they been given sufficient training for the activity engaged in?
- Had all reasonable steps been taken to prevent such an occurrence?
- Are there records of lessons given and ongoing schemes of work for regular pupils?
- Are there records of ongoing training for staff and trainees?
- Are there records of regular updates on H&S issues for all relative personnel?
- Are there records that all maintenance issues have been dealt with promptly?

It can be seen that fairly comprehensive records need to be kept but that, actually, in a well-run yard all this information is likely to be available at the time of the accident/incident.

If the answer to all the above questions is in the affirmative, it is likely that most preventative strategies are in place and the yard is well managed.

RISK ASSESSMENTS

Risk assessments are a fact of life! Any time someone considers crossing a road, they are making a risk assessment.

Formalising that action, having proof that the assessment has been made and that the appropriate action has been taken to minimise or remove the risk, is a vital part of running a yard.

How to make a risk assessment

Consider the following:

- Identify the risk.
- Is it valid?
- Who/what is at risk?
- Is it preventable?
- Can it be avoided?
- What action needs to be taken to minimise the risk?
- Who needs to be informed?
- What training needs to be provided?
- To whom?

Identifying the risk can be quite problematical.

People very quickly become familiar with their

Hazard Severity + Likelihood of Occurrence = Risk

5 Point Scale for Risk Severity		5 Point Scale for Likelihood of Occurrence	
5 VERY HIGH	Causing multiple deaths and widespread destruction.	**5 VERY LIKELY**	If the activity continues as it is, there is almost a 100% certainty that an accident will happen.
4 HIGH	Causing death or serious injury.	**4 LIKELY**	Outside sources or human carelessness could precipitate an accident, but this is unlikely to happen without such additional factors.
3 MODERATE	Causing injury or disease capable of keeping an individual off work for three days or more.	**3 QUITE POSSIBLE**	An accident may happen if additional factors precipitate an accident, but this is unlikely to happen without them.
2 SLIGHT	Causing minor injury which would allow the individual to continue work after first aid treatment on site or at a local surgery.	**2 POSSIBLE**	If other factors were present, this incident or illness might occur, but the probability is low and the risk minimal.
1 NIL	No perceived risk of injury or disease.	**1 NOT LIKELY**	There is really no obvious risk.

By using the formula above, a risk factor can be determined, ranging from 1 (no severity and unlikely to happen) to 10 (just waiting to happen).

surroundings and circumstances and adapt their behaviour accordingly.

When making a risk assessment consider from the point of view of a stranger or the least competent person likely to be involved.

Asking the opinions of others can be a useful exercise.

The validity of the risk is important. It is easy to become obsessed. Using the above table can help to keep the level of risk in perspective.

It is not only the **level of risk** but the **likelihood of it occurring** that needs to be taken into account.

• Decide on the level of risk.

• Decide on the likelihood of it occurring.

• Add the two figures together.

• Decide whether the activity is safe and valid.

Anything with a total of 5 or over would need very careful consideration, and should receive immediate action to rectify, be changed to lower the risk or abandoned as unsafe.

Who is at risk is an important factor. Fairly obviously the level of risk is likely to lessen given various circumstances. Consider the following:

• The level of knowledge and experience of those concerned.

• The age/size of those concerned.

• The amount of supervision available.

- The environment; facilities in which the activity is to take place.

Is it preventable? Can it be avoided?

Obviously if the answer to these questions is yes, once the risk has been identified, it can be removed.

What action needs to be taken? Things to consider are:

- The timescale, how soon can the risk be removed or lessened?

- By whom?

- How?

- Is training involved?

- Who will receive it?

- Who needs to be informed?

- Update the records.

If it is a question of maintenance, the sooner the problem is rectified the better. For instance, filling one small pothole in the car park as soon as it appears not only prevents accidents but also is a much cheaper option than dealing with a claim if an accident occurs, and is good customer relations.

As soon as a fault is noticed or reported, it should be entered in the maintenance book with the date. Who made the repair, when and at what cost is entered as soon as the repair is complete.

When training is involved, it should be put in place as soon as possible. All those who received it should be noted and in future, any others should be added as soon as possible.

It may be that temporary measures have to be put in place initially while a permanent solution is arranged. This is perfectly acceptable as long as all those who need to know are informed.

The yard manager needs to make risk assessments of all areas of their responsibility. They should use a format that is user-friendly, sufficiently detailed for their enterprise and that can be easily updated and referred to.

The list of what should be risk-assessed is too exhaustive to be detailed here, see page 454 for some suggestions. It will obviously vary with the type of yard being run. It will start with such mundane activities as mucking out and the safe storage of tools, may progress through the safe turning out and bringing in of the animals, cover such activities as safe lifting procedures, safe stacking and removing of bales and continue with more specialist activities such as clipping, using horse walkers and the handling of stallions.

It should be stored alongside the safety policy which has been put in place for that activity.

Proof of who has received relevant training can be stored in the personal records of those concerned.

All assessments should be reviewed regularly, at least annually. Any new intake of staff, students or clients should be made aware of or trained in areas relevant to them on induction. **They should not be allowed to perform tasks until the person responsible is satisfied that they are safe and competent.**

THE ANIMALS ACT 1971

This Act is not applicable in Scotland or Northern Ireland. It is based on strict liability and deals with the injury that horses and various other animals may cause, and with damage arising from their straying. Strict liability means that there is liability without proof that the person claimed against was negligent, if he was responsible for the animal, and the animal has caused injury or damage.

Animals

These are divided into animals belonging to a dangerous species, and those which do not. Bulls and wild and unbroken stallions may come within the former category. Liability for injury caused by animals of a dangerous species will be placed on the 'keeper' unless he can bring himself within one or more of the exceptions of the Act. Liability for damages caused by an animal which is not of a dangerous species (such as a horse or pony) also rests with the 'keepers' in the following circumstances.

The damage is of a kind likely to be caused, and when caused is likely to be severe, unless the animal is restrained; and the likelihood of the damage, or of its being severe, must be due to the characteristics of that particular animal which are not normal in animals of this species except at particular times or circumstances: e.g. mares in season, etc., and those characteristics were known to the keeper or known to any other person who had charge of the animal as the keeper's servant, or where that keeper is the head of a household, or were known to another keeper of the animals, who is a member of that household and under sixteen years old.

Who is a Keeper?

A person will be treated as a keeper if:

• he owns the animal, or has it in his possession,

or

• he is the head of the household of which a member under sixteen years of age owns the animal or has it in his possession.

The keeper must be an individual. The person who has control over company-owned horses would be regarded as the keeper. Liability for damage rests on the person who at the time has possession; he need not be the owner. Anyone who takes possession of and keeps horses to prevent them from causing damage or to restore them to their owner is **NOT** a keeper.

Damage by Trespassing Stock

In broad terms an animal is said to trespass in the same way as humans: that is, where it is on land on which it has no right to be, or where its owner has no right to put it. This includes animals straying on to a highway or from a highway on to private land. Exceptions exist with regard to animals straying from unfenced common

land on to highways.

The only lawful use of the highway (unless they have grazing rights on the verges) is to pass and repass on it. The highway need not adjoin the land; the stock may have wandered through other land to the highway. Bridlepaths are highways.

Section 8 of this Act imposes a duty on the person placing horses on the land to take care to prevent them from straying on to the highway: the only exception being if they stray from unfenced land, and providing the person who placed them on the land had a 'right' to do so. Unfenced land is regarded as land in an area where fencing is not customary; this is common land, town or village greens or some moorlands.

Claims under Section 2 for Injuries and Damage Done by Animals

1. Where a horse strays on to land owned or occupied by another person, the owner of the horse is strictly liable for the following damage and expenses:

(a) Damage done to the land or to any property on the land which is owned or in possession of another person.

(b) Expenses which are reasonably incurred by the other person in keeping the horse until it can be returned to the owner.

(c) The expense of finding out to whom the horse belongs.

(d) Expenses incurred by the occupier of the land in exercising his right to detain the horse.

Injuries caused by the straying horse, death of, or injury to, a person is included in the word 'damage'.

2. There would be NO responsibility for straying livestock if:

(a) The damage is due wholly to the fault of the person suffering it, but that person cannot be regarded as at fault just because he could have prevented it by fencing, or

(b) It is proved that the straying would not have occurred but for a breach of duty imposed on another person who has interests in the land to fence it, or

(c) The person suffering the damage has voluntarily accepted the risk. But where a person employed by a keeper incurs a risk as a result of his employment he shall not be treated as accepting it voluntarily.

3. The occupier of the land on to which the animal strays without being under the control of any person has the right to detain it, unless ordered by a court to return it. The right ceases, however:

(a) At the end of 48 hours unless the occupier notifies a police officer and also the person to whom the horse belongs, if that person is known.

(b) If the person claiming the horse offers the occupier sufficient money to cover any proper claim for damage and expenses.

(c) If the occupier has no proper claim, when the horse is reclaimed by someone entitled to its possession.

4. If a horse has been detained for at least 14 days the occupier may sell it at market or by auction, unless any court proceedings are pending. The occupier is entitled to the proceeds of the sale, but any excess over his claim has to be paid to the person who but for the sale would have been entitled to possession.

5. Occupiers are liable for any damage caused to the horse that they have detained, by failing to treat it with care, or by failing to supply it with food and water.

6. Occupiers who sell the animal have no right to sue for damages. They must choose one remedy or the other.

Fencing

The Act does not define a 'duty to fence', so common-law rules have to be considered. These show that the law has never imposed any obligation on a person to fence his land, but obligations may have been created by formal agreements or may have become established through long usage or custom.

For example, if a person has maintained a fence for, say, forty years and upwards this would indicate that he thought he had a duty to do so. He cannot then deny the obligation, and his actions have created a liability on him and his successors in title.

Where horses stray from common land where they had a 'right' to graze, the position might differ if it can be established that it was the responsibility of the land owner to fence against animals straying from it. Any fences erected must be kept in a proper state of repair so as not to constitute a danger to adjoining occupiers or to people on a highway.

Dogs

This Act also gives protection against dogs either killing or causing injury to livestock. For proceedings and defences, reference should be made to Section 9 of the Act.

PROTECTION OF ANIMALS ACT 1911 – ENGLAND AND WALES, AND PROTECTION OF ANIMALS ACT 1912 – SCOTLAND

These two Acts are perhaps the most widely used of the many Welfare of Animals Acts currently on the statute book. Both Acts are similar in content. Any reference to magistrates in the Protection of Animals Act 1911 should be read as a reference to the sheriff in the Protection of Animals Act (Scotland) 1912. As the powers of courts in regard to penalties are subject to changes under the Criminal Justices Act, these have not been included.

The Acts consolidate the laws relating to cruelty to domestic and captive animals. The expression 'domestic animal' covers any animal of whatever species which is tame, or which has been, or is being sufficiently tamed to serve some purpose for the use of man. 'Captive animal' means any animal which is in captivity or confinement.

The 1911 Act has 15 sections but this chapter only deals with those sections which are relevant to horses. The expression 'horse' includes mare, gelding, pony, foal, colt, filly, stallion, ass, mule or jennet.

The Offences of Cruelty in Section 1 read that if any person:

(a) 'Shall cruelly beat, kick, ill-treat, over-ride, over drive, over-load, torture, infuriate, or terrify any animal, or shall cause or procure, or, being the owner, permit any animal to be so used, or shall, by wantonly or unreasonably doing or omitting to do any Act, or by causing or procuring the commission or omission of any Act, cause any unnecessary suffering, or being the owner permit any unnecessary suffering to be so caused to any animal, shall be guilty of an offence.'

This long paragraph indicates, among many other things, that if a person carries out any of the above offences, or hires or permits any other person to commit them, it will be an offence. It also means that by unreasonably preventing any of the following from taking place, the owner and/or offender will be guilty within the meaning of the Act. Failure to feed, failure to provide veterinary treatment, or failure to slaughter an animal which is incurably diseased and thereby causing unnecessary suffering may well be offences of omission. The abandonment of animals was not an offence under this Act as it was originally passed, so the Abandonment of Animals Act 1960 was passed to rectify the omission. It is now an offence to abandon an animal (whether permanently or not) in circumstances likely to cause that animal any unnecessary suffering. This would appear to include both liberating animals in order to get rid of them, and leaving animals shut up unattended.

The clause of causing or procuring the commission of certain acts by others, could be interpreted so that the parents of children who, acting on the instructions of their parents, perform acts of cruelty, could be guilty. In such a case it would be irrelevant if the child is below the age of criminal responsibility. There is no reason why one person should not be charged with 'causing' or presumably 'permitting' and another with ill-treating in respect of the same act. This would be the case where a horse is ridden in an unfit state (e.g. lame), the stable manager (or the owner) knowing/causing (or permitting) it to be ridden, and the rider for knowingly riding it.

Cruelty and Unnecessary Suffering

The mere infliction of pain is not sufficient to constitute any offences given in the Act. It has been ruled that cruelty is defined as: 'causing unnecessary suffering', and courts have to examine whether the defendant is doing something which it was not reasonably necessary to do. If the reason was of sufficient importance to justify the act done then no offence has been committed. Suffering must not only be disproportionate to the alleged reason for which it was inflicted, but must also be substantial. What is clear from judgments given is that 'cruelly' and 'so as to cause unnecessary suffering' mean exactly the same thing. The inflicting of mental suffering by the defendant's own positive act could be within the category of cruelly infuriating and terrifying animals; it may also be included in the category of torturing animals.

(b) 'Shall convey or carry or cause or procure, or, being the owner permit to be conveyed or carried, any animal in such a manner or position as to cause that animal any unnecessary suffering'. This sub-paragraph refers to all kinds of animals carried, and in regard to horses it is generally assumed to be by mechanical methods. Other legislation exists where offences of carrying can occur both by air or sea, but perhaps the most relevant legislation is the Transit of Animals (Road and Rail) Order of 1975 and amendments 1979.

(c) 'Shall wilfully, without any reasonable cause or excuse, administer, or cause or procure or being the owner permit such administration of, any poisonous or injurious drug or substances to any animal, or shall wilfully without any reason cause or excuse, cause such substances to be taken by any animals'.

This means that the administration of any injurious drug which causes unnecessary suffering, or the owner attempting or permitting an attempt by another person, to poison an animal is regarded as an offence.

(d) 'Shall subject or cause or procure, or being the owner permit, to be subjected, any animal to any operation which is performed without due care and humanity'.

Treatments and operations to agricultural animals (as defined in the Agriculture Act 1947) which are permitted to be carried out by unqualified persons are specified in Schedule III of the Veterinary Surgeons Act 1966.

The Powers of a Court to Order Destruction of Animals in Section 2

Where the owner of an animal is convicted of an offence of cruelty within the meaning of this Act, the court has powers, providing they are satisfied that it would be cruel to keep the animal alive, to direct that:

(a) the animal should be destroyed, and
(b) the animal should be assigned to any suitable person for destruction, and the person to whom it is assigned shall as soon as it is possible destroy that animal or arrange for its destruction in his/her presence without unnecessary suffering.

The court may order that any reasonable expenses incurred in the destruction shall be paid by the owner of the animal or be recoverable by a summons as a civil debt. It should be noted that unless the owner agrees to the destruction, a veterinary surgeon must give evidence to the court to the effect that it would be cruel to keep the animal alive. If no such consent, or evidence, is given, courts cannot make an order for destruction.

There can be no appeal against an order for the destruction of an animal. However, the magistrates may themselves suspend or rescind an order on complaint.

The Powers of Confiscation in Section 3

If the owner of any animal shall be guilty of cruelty within the meaning of this Act, the courts, upon conviction of the owner, may if they think fit, in addition to any other punishment, deprive such a person of the ownership of the animal, and they may also make an order as to the disposal of the animal as they think fit under the circumstances. They are not permitted to make such an order, unless it is shown by evidence of a previous conviction, or as to the character of the owner, or otherwise, that if the animal is left with the owner, it is likely to be exposed to further cruelty.

The Regulations for Knackers in Section 5

Any police constable has a right of entry to a knacker's yard during hours when business is usually being carried out, for the purpose of examining whether there has been any contravention of or non-compliance with the provisions of this Act. For the purposes of Section 1 of this Act relating to offences of cruelty the knacker shall be regarded as the owner of any animal delivered to him. The expression 'knacker' means a person whose trade or business is to kill any cattle including horses for the purpose of the flesh not being used as butchers' meat.

Animal Pounds in Section 7

If anyone impounds, or causes to be impounded or confined in any pound, any animal, they shall while the animal is so impounded or confined, be responsible for supplying a sufficient quantity of wholesome and suitable food and water to that animal, and if they fail to do so will be liable upon conviction to a fine.

The person taking the animal to the pound is therefore responsible for it under this Section, not the pound keeper. The pound keeper may be guilty of an offence under sections of this Act if it can be shown that he was legally responsible for performing that act.

If any animal impounded or confined is without sufficient suitable food or water for six successive hours, or longer, any person may enter the pound for the purpose of supplying the animal. The reasonable cost of the food and water supply shall be recoverable from the owner of the animal as a civil debt.

Poisoned Animal Food in Section 8

It is an offence to offer for sale, to give away or to cause or procure any other person to do so any grain or seed which has been rendered poisonous, except for bona-fide use in agriculture. It is also an offence to place, cause some other party to place, or knowingly be a party to the placing in or upon any land or building any poison or fluid or edible matter (which is not sown seed or grain) that has been rendered poisonous.

The defence can be used that the poison was placed by the accused for the purpose of destroying insects or small ground-vermin where such is necessary in the interest of public health, agriculture or the preservation of other animals, or for the purpose of manuring the land, providing that all reasonable precautions to prevent injury to all domestic animals and wild birds were taken.

Diseased and Injured Animals in Section 11

(i) If a police constable finds any animal so distressed or so severely injured, or in such a physical condition that in his opinion, there is no possibility of removing it without cruelty, he shall in the absence of the owner, or if the owner refuses to consent to the animal being destroyed, summon a veterinary surgeon if any reside within a reasonable distance and providing it appears by the certificate of that veterinary surgeon that the animal is mortally injured, or so severely injured, or so diseased, or in such a physical condition that it is cruel to keep it alive, it is lawful for the police constable, without the owner's consent, to slaughter or arrange for the slaughter, with such instruments or appliances, and with such precautions, and in such a manner as to inflict as little suffering as is possible. The constable also has powers to arrange for the removal of the carcase if the slaughter of the animal takes place on a public highway.

(ii) If a veterinary surgeon certifies that the animal can be removed without cruelty, it is the responsibility of the person in charge to arrange for the removal with as little suffering as possible, and if the person in charge fails to do this, the police constable may without the consent of the person in charge cause the animal to be removed.

(iii) Any reasonable expenses incurred including those of the veterinary surgeon and regardless of whether the animal is slaughtered or not may be recovered from the owner as a civil debt.

(iv) 'Animal' in this section applies only to horses (as already defined), and to bulls, sheep, goats or pigs.

The Summons in Section 13

Frequently, the most valuable piece of evidence is the animal itself. If the owner refuses to produce the animal, or to have it examined by a vet, a summons may be applied for ordering the production of the animal in the same way as a summons to an accused person.

Rights of Appeal in Section 14

(i) Any appeal from conviction or order (other than appeal against destruction in Section 2) made by a summary court, shall be made to a Crown Court.

(ii) Where there is an appeal against a summary court conviction or order, the court may order the owner not to sell or part with the animal until the appeal is determined or abandoned, the court may order that the animal be produced on the hearing of the appeal providing such production is possible without cruelty being incurred.

PROTECTION OF ANIMALS (AMENDMENT) ACT 1954

This Act, which applies to Scotland but not to N. Ireland, extends the powers of the court to disqualify from having custody of animals a person previously convicted of an offence of cruelty to an animal.

Powers of Disqualification in Section 1

(i) Where a person has been convicted under the Protection of Animals Act 1911 or the Protection of Animals (Scotland) Act (1912), and is subsequently convicted under either of these Acts of an offence, the court by which the subsequent conviction is made may if it thinks fit either in addition to, or in substitution for, any other punishment, order the person to be disqualified, for a such period as it thinks fit, from having custody of any animals or any animal of a kind specified.

(ii) A court which has made such a disqualification order may if it thinks fit suspend the order:
  (a) For a period of time as the court thinks necessary to enable arrangements to be made for the custody of any animals to which the order relates; or
  (b) Pending an appeal.

(iii) Any disqualified person may after twelve months from the date of the order and subsequently from time to time, apply to the court by which the order was made for removal of the disqualification, and

the court will consider the character of the applicant, the conduct following the order, the nature of the offence of which he was convicted, and any other circumstances of the case; and either:
  (a) Direct the removal of the disqualification from such a date as they specify, or shall vary the order to apply only to animals of a kind specified; or
  (b) Refuse the application.

Further applications for variations cannot be made within 12 months after the date of the direction or refusal.

ADDITIONAL EFFECTS OF DISQUALIFICATION. Any person disqualified under this Act from having custody of an animal may not be granted a licence to keep either an animal-boarding establishment or a riding establishment, a pet shop, or dog-breeding kennels.

Further penalties can be imposed for breaches of any disqualification order.

PROTECTION OF ANIMALS (AMENDMENT) ACT 1988

Gives power to the court to disqualify a person convicted of cruelty to animals from having custody of animals.

PROTECTION AGAINST CRUEL TETHERING ACT 1988

It shall be an offence to tether any horses, asses or mules under such conditions or in such a manner as to cause that animal unnecessary suffering.

RIDDOR

RIDDOR (Reporting of Injuries, Diseases and Dangerous Occurrences Regulations) 1995

It is a legal requirement to report accidents and ill health at work to the Health and Safety Executive. This enables them and the local authorities to identify where and how risks arise and to investigate serious accidents. A report needs to be made when:

- Someone connected with your work or premises is killed.

- Someone suffers serious injury.

- Someone is taken to hospital following an incident at work.

- A doctor reports to you that a person is suffering from a work-related disease.

- A person is not seriously injured but is away from work for more than three days.

- There is a dangerous occurrence.

- Fatalities and serious accidents must be reported by phone immediately, followed with a written report within seven days.

A dangerous occurrence is one where, if something happens, no one is injured but they might have been. There are appropriate forms available from the HSE. All records must be kept for at least three years.

The report must include the following information:

- Date and time of the accident.

- Name, address and occupation of the person involved.

- Where the accident occurred, the nature of it and a description of the circumstances.

- Any additional information that might be useful, such as witness statements or photographs.

Some of the diseases that might occur in a stable environment are:

- Leptospirosis, also known as Weil's disease. This is spread to humans through water contaminated by infected animals, especially rats. Anywhere where rats habitually urinate may be infected.

- Occupational asthma, which may follow exposure to the handling of cereals and their derivatives.

- Extrinsic alveolitis, commonly known as farmer's lung. This is caused by exposure to moulds or fungal spores such as may be found in forage and bedding.

- Anthrax, a disease of farm animals that can be passed on to humans. It is extremely rare and is a notifiable disease and as such subject to strict controls.

COSHH (CONTROL OF SUBSTANCES HAZARDOUS TO HEALTH) 1989

Every employer has a responsibility to assess the risks associated with hazardous substances in the workplace and to take steps to eliminate or control those risks.

Every employee has a responsibility to:

- Ensure their own safety and that of others.

- To abide by such rules and regulations as are in place.

- To wear appropriate clothing and to ensure they have received the appropriate training.

Hazard

The hazard presented by a substance is its potential to cause harm. It may be able to make you cough, damage your liver or even kill! Some substances harm in several different ways, e.g. they can be breathed in, swallowed or absorbed by the skin.

Risk

The risk from a substance is the likelihood that it will

cause harm in the actual circumstances of use. This will depend on:

- The hazard presented by the substance.

- How it is used.

- How it is controlled.

- Who is exposed to it, how much, for how long.

- What are they doing?

Poor control can lead to a substantial risk even from a substance with low hazard. With proper precautions even the most hazardous substance can be adequately controlled.

The COSHH regulations require employers to assess the risks created by the work in which a hazardous substance is used.

- First, the hazardous substance has to be identified.

- Second, it has to be controlled.

- Some, such as dust and fungal spores, are produced naturally.

- Others such as disinfectants, paints, liniments and medicines are bought in.

- With natural substances it is important that exposure is limited to safe levels, that protective apparel is worn as appropriate and that the amount of dust etc. is kept as low as possible.

With substances in containers: always ensure correct and secure storage; always ensure the substance is correctly labelled according to law and that it has the correct warning symbols and guidance phrases.

- Assess the risk to people's health from the way it is used in the specific establishment.

- Prevent all but essential people from exposure to the substance.

- Decide how to control exposure to reduce risk.

- Establish effective controls.

- Ensure that appropriate safety clothing is available and is used.

- Train and inform the work force.

- Monitor employees' exposure as necessary.

- Keep records of all risk assessments, control measures and training given.

APPENDICES

MEASUREMENTS

Land-based industries in Britain went metric in 1976 and ever since the feed room has been a muddle of metric and imperial measurements. Now, with our closer ties to mainland Europe, it is important that everyone in Britain should try to use metric measures.

Weight

If in doubt remember: 'two and a quarter pounds of jam weigh about a kilogram.'

pounds (lbs)	kilograms/pounds (kg/lbs)	kilograms (kg)
2.2	1	0.45
4.4	2	0.9
6.6	3	1.36
8.8	4	1.81
11.0	5	2.27
13.2	6	2.72
15.4	7	3.18
17.6	8	3.63
19.8	9	4.00

• Note the weight on sacks and containers.

• Resolve to make every feed board metric.

Typically:

• Horse cubes come in 25kg bags but some straight feeds come in 40kg sacks.

• Fertiliser comes in 50kg bags (used to be supplied in 1cwt bags).

• Hay bales weigh about 25kg (40 to the tonne).

• Straw bales weigh about 16.5kg (60 to the tonne).

• Stacked hay takes up about 7 cubic metres per tonne.

• Stacked staw takes up 10.5 cubic metres per tonne.

• A hay crop of 10 tonnes per hectare used to be reckoned as 4 tons per acre. (A hectare is about 2.5 acres, which is about the size of a professional football pitch).

• A ton and a tonne (metric) are nearly the same.

• Hay and straw will lose weight as the bales dry out.

Volume

• A litre is about 1¾ pints, or remember the phrase: 'A litre of water's a pint and three-quarters'.

• We know from filling up with petrol at a garage that whereas we used to take 10 gallons we now take 45 litres.

• A 5-litre container holds just over 1 gallon.

THE BRITISH HORSE SOCIETY

WHAT IS THE BRITISH HORSE SOCIETY?

The British Horse Society is a charity to promote the welfare, care and use of the horse and pony; to encourage horsemastership and the improvement of horse management and breeding; and to represent all equine interests.

The Society is internationally recognised as the premier equestrian riding, training and examination organisation in the United Kingdom, and operates an Approvals scheme for all types of equestrian establishment. It incorporates some 420 Riding Clubs and works closely with the Pony Club. The Society is also the national governing body for recreational riding and fully supports the independent sporting disciplines within the British Equestrian Federation.

The BHS plays a major role in equine welfare, safety, provision of access to the countryside, and protection of riding and driving Rights of Way. It represents riders to Government and to the EU in Brussels in all matters, especially those concerning taxation, rates, planning and the law.

Gold membership benefits include £10 million public liability insurance, personal accident insurance (terms, conditions and territorial limits apply), a yearbook, magazines, special facilities and discounts at BHS functions, and access to BHS advice and support.

With membership approaching 70,000 and approximately 38,000 riding members, it is the largest organisation within the British Equestrian Federation.

By joining the Society you are supporting the UK's largest equestrian charity working on behalf of every horse and rider. For further information and membership details write to: The British Horse Society, Stoneleigh Deer Park, Kenilworth, Warwickshire, CV8 2XZ • tel: 01926 707700 • email: enquiry@bhs.org.uk • website: www.bhs.org.uk

WHY CHOOSE A BHS-APPROVED ESTABLISHMENT?

Whatever your reason for seeking out a riding centre – be it for a pleasant hour's hacking, or training up to advanced level – you will want to choose an establishment that is both reputable and well run.

By selecting one of the establishments listed in **The BHS Directory of Where to Ride, Train and Stable Your Horse,** or on the BHS website (see above), you will not only be able to satisfy yourself on that point, but you will also be able to discover a good deal about the centre before you pick up the telephone to discuss your ride.

Each of the establishments listed in the directory has been inspected by a fully qualified representative of the British Horse Society, who will have looked carefully at the level of instruction available to clients, the on-site facilities and equipment, and the standards of safety, horse care and management.

A riding centre will not be approved by the BHS unless it has a Local Authority Licence. Every riding establishment is supposed to have a Local Authority Licence; without this licence it will not have proper third-party insurance cover. To hold such a licence, granted annually, the establishment will have been inspected by a council representative and a council-appointed veterinary surgeon, who will have been concerned primarily with riders' safety and the welfare of the animals being used. Unlike the BHS inspector, the council inspector will not have assessed the standard of the instructors or whether the horses are well-schooled and forward-going.

It is also reassuring to know that at an Approved establishment you will not be allowed to ride without the correct protective headgear. An Approved centre may be able to supply you with an appropriate hard hat if you do not already possess one of the correct standard. Newcomers to riding can expect to be offered helpful advice on what to wear so that their first lessons are safe and enjoyable.

Another advantage is that many BHS-Approved establishments run the BHS Progressive Riding Tests, a scheme of instruction and assessment designed for riders of all ages and abilities. Further details of these tests – which can be administered only by an Approved centre – will be available from your chosen BHS-Approved centre.

The staff at the **Approvals Office** are available to answer any queries during normal working hours, whether you want to know more about the Society's system of approving riding establishments, about an individual Approved Establishment or just have a general enquiry about finding your nearest Approved Centre. The phone number is 01926 707700, and they are always pleased to deal with any enquiries. Please do not hesitate to contact them.

BHS EXAMINATIONS AND PROFESSIONAL QUALIFICATIONS

The British Horse Society has developed an examination system designed to meet the requirements of the riding instructor, yard management, riding holiday sector, and those who wish to further their knowledge in riding, stable management and horse care. It holds these examinations – aimed primarily at career students – at BHS-Approved centres throughout the British Isles and overseas.

Before embarking on a career with horses it is important to select the place of training carefully. Whilst it is not obligatory for candidates to receive their training at a BHS-Approved centre, it is certainly advisable to do so. Details of approved BHS Training Centres can be found in the publication **The BHS Directory of Where to Ride, Train and Stable Your Horse,** available from the British Horse Society Bookshop, Stoneleigh Deer Park, Kenilworth, Warwickshire, CV8 2XZ, tel: 01926 707762 (or from Kenilworth Press).

Examinations are taken at officially appointed BHS-Approved centres throughout the UK and overseas.

Candidates for all examinations must be members of the BHS at time of application and on the day of their examination.

Stage 1

The minimum age for entry is 14 years. The candidate must understand the basic principles of horse care and, working under supervision, must show some knowledge and practice of looking after a well-mannered horse in the stable or at grass. He/she must be capable of riding a quiet, experienced horse or pony in an enclosed space.

Many BHS-Approved riding establishments run the Society's Progressive Riding Tests 1–6, which give weekly riders an aim and standard to work for. Achievement of all six Progressive Riding Tests gives exemption from the BHS Stage 1 exam and enables the holder to begin to study for Stage 2.

Stage 2

The minimum age for entry is 16 years. Before entering the riding section of this examination the candidate must have passed the BHS Riding and Road Safety test. The candidate must understand the general management and requirements of horses for their health and well-being. Working under regular but not constant supervision, the candidates should be able to carry out the care of a stabled and grass-kept horse during all seasons of the year. The candidate must be capable of riding a quiet, experienced horse or pony in the countryside and on the public highway, as well as in a manege.

Prerequisites: Stage 1 Care (for Care section); Stage 1 Riding(for Riding section); S/NVQ Level 2 (riding/schooling horses) or PRTs 1–6.

Stage 3

The minimum age for entry is 17 years. The candidate must show an ability to look after up to four horses under a variety of circumstances. He/she should be tactful, yet effective, understanding the reasons for his/her actions, both in horse care and while riding. At this level there is an increase in responsibility. The Stage 3 Care Groom's Certificate requires candidates to look after up to four horses or ponies with minimum supervision.

Prerequisites: Horse Knowledge, Care and Riding Stage 2; S/NVQ 2 or 3 (riding/schooling horses). Direct entry with APL – contact Exams Office for details.

BHS PRELIMINARY TEACHING TEST (PTT): The minimum age for entry is 18 years of age. Candidates must show that they have the required qualities and can apply the basic principles of coaching. They should have the ability to improve their rider's horsemastership using a progressive plan. They must know the safety procedures and principles involved in the organisation of a lesson or hack. All coaching should be relevant to the rider in front of them and they should be experienced enough to modify sessions to facilitate this. They should evaluate their own performance and show ability to assess progress in their pupils. Holders of this qualification will have the opportunity to gain the UKCC endorsed Level 2 Certificate in Coaching.

Prerequisite: Stage 2 Care and Riding. Direct entry with APL – contact Exams Office for details.

BHS ASSISTANT INSTRUCTOR'S CERTIFICATE (BHSAI): This certificate is awarded to holders of the Preliminary Teaching Test and Horse Knowledge, Care and Riding Stage 3 certificate. Completion of a portfolio of evidence is also required plus a current equine-specific first-aid certificate or Health & Safety Executive First Aid at Work certificate.

Stage 4

The minimum age for entry is 18 years for Stage 4 Riding, and 19 years for Stage 4 Care. The candidate must be capable of taking sole charge of a group of horses of various types in stables and at grass. He/she must be an educated rider capable of training and improving horses in their work on the flat and over fences. Candidates passing the Horse Knowledge and Care section will be awarded the Intermediate Stable Manager's Certificate.

Prerequisite: Stage 3 Riding (for Riding); Stage 3 Care (for Care); S/NVQ Level 3. Direct entry with APL – apply to the Exams Office for details.

BHS INTERMEDIATE TEACHING EXAMINATION (BHSIT): The minimum age for entry is 20 years. For candidates who hold the Preliminary Teaching Test and have completed a portfolio of evidence (post 1 January 2007) or 500 hours of logged teaching (pre 1 January 2007) and a current equine-specific first-aid certificate or Health & Safety Executive First Aid at Work certificate. Candidates should demonstrate their ability to give safe and competent lessons from beginner to elementary standards, without supervision. The candidate will be able to show genuine improvement of the horse and rider. They will demonstrate practical business knowledge and be conversant with the running of a commercial yard. Holders of this qualification will have the opportunity to the gain the UKCC endorsed Level 3 Certificate in Coaching.

The British Horse Society Examination System

Outline of progression route through BHS examinations

International Expert

FELLOW FBHS

BHS Stable Manager + Equitation and Teaching = **INTERNATIONAL INSTRUCTOR LEVEL 3 BHSI**

Intermediate Stable Manager
Horse Knowledge and Care Stage 4
+ Riding Stage 4 + Intermediate Teaching Test = **INTERNATIONAL INSTRUCTOR LEVEL 2 BHSII**

= **INTERNATIONAL INSTRUCTOR LEVEL I BHSAI**

Groom's Certificate
Horse Knowledge and Care Stage 3
+ Riding Stage 3

Horse Knowledge and Care Stage 2
+ Riding Stage 2 + Preliminary Teaching Test + Riding and Road Safety Test = **PRELIMINARY TEACHER BHSPTC** + Portfolio of evidence. H & S at Work or ESFAC plus safeguarding children course attended

Horse Knowledge and Care Stage I
+ Riding Stage I

KEY
– – – Stable Management only
——— Instructors Qualifications
— · — Levels of the International Group for Training Horse and Rider

BHS INTERMEDIATE INSTRUCTOR CERTIFICATE (BHSII): This is achieved by passing the Intermediate Teaching Examination and the complete Horse Knowledge and Riding Stage 4 examination. Candidates are also required to hold a full Health & Safety Executive First Aid at Work certificate or equine-specific first-aid certificate.

(a) **BHS Stable Manager's Examination:** This is also an examination in its own right and candidates need not necessarily go on to complete the full Instructor's Examination by taking (b) below. The entry requirement for this examination is the Intermediate Stable Manager's Certificate (HK & C Stage 4). The minimum age for entry is 22 years.

(b) **BHS Equitation and Teaching Examination:** On passing this examination and the Stable Manager's exam, the candidate completes the full BHS Instructor (BHSI) Certificate. The entry requirements are the Intermediate Instructor (BHSII) Certificate. Direct entry with APL – apply to the Exams Office for details.

BHS FELLOWSHIP EXAMINATION (FBHS): The BHS Fellowship Certificate is the senior qualification. The minimum age for entry is 25 years. The candidate must show a depth of knowledge and effectiveness in all aspects of equitation and horsemastership; proving themselves to be persons to whom others can turn for advice in the various spheres of equestrian activities. The Fellowship is available in four formats – General Fellowship, Show Jumping Specialist, Dressage Specialist, and Eventing Specialist – to assist those who have followed specific disciplines.

Equestrian Qualifications GB Ltd (EQL) awards qualifications on behalf of the BHS. In addition, EQL is an awarding body for Scottish and National Vocational Qualifications (S/NVQs) in the horse industry. Full details on request from EQL at Stoneleigh Deer Park, Kenilworth, Warwickshire, CV8 2XZ. It also awards the new UKCC Coaching Certificates on behalf of the British Equestrian Federation.

The present structure of the BHS examination system is shown on the previous page. If you wish to find out more about the syllabi and requirements of the different exams, contact the Training & Education Office, The British Horse Society, Stoneleigh Deer Park, Kenilworth, Warwickshire, CV8 2XZ. Tel: 01926 707700.

3 EQUINE PASSPORTS

Since 2003 all equines have been required to have a valid passport, with the exception of some ponies living wild on moorland who are exempt whilst they stay on the moor.

No animal should be bought or sold or be sent to slaughter without the passport being produced.

No animal is allowed more than one passport, and owners of those who already have one may need to send them to the issuing body to have them updated.

The Department of Environment, Food and Rural Affairs (DEFRA) have approved a number of Passport Issuing Offices (PIOs).

If the horse already has a passport or his breeding is known, deal with the relevant breed society. Refer to the flow chart on the following page.

Once the passport has been obtained it is important to keep it updated. It should accompany the horse on his travels and to competition. However, care must be taken to prevent theft.

Where to Obtain a Passport

Do you have a passport for your equine? All horses, ponies, donkeys and mules **MUST** have a passport with effect from December 2003.

Yes

No

Is it from a recognised passport issuing organisation (PIO)? Are they still operating?

No

Yes

What type of equine do you have and what are the aims? It is important to think about your equine's future when getting a passport. Is it eligible for one of the below?

Equines can only hold one passport. The passport may be accepted by certain PIOs for over-stamping.

Your passport will still be valid and may not need any additional paperwork. Check with your PIO.

Pure bred/part bred

It is important to register with the breed society if your equine has any known breeding, which may result in it competing in breed or show classes, or, if you have plans to breed from it in the future. Even if *you* don't intend to do this, should you sell the equine, future owners may – and it could be a selling point. Contact the relevant breed society.

Colour

Is your equine of any specific colour, e.g. piebald, spotted, palomino, skewbald? If so, you may wish to register with one of the relevant societies.

Affiliated competition

Are you likely to compete in any discipline – jumping or showing for instance? If so, registering with perhaps the BEF, BD, BHRC, POLO, NPS or SHB (GB) to build up a competition record may be useful. Contact the relevant organisation.

None of these

If your equine is of unknown origin and not eligible to be registered with a recognised breed society or any of the above, then you can obtain the necessary passport for your horse from SHB, NPS, or The British Horse Society. Contact the BHS on 08701 299992.

4 VACCINATIONS

In Britain horses are routinely vaccinated against two common ailments: tetanus, also known as lockjaw, and influenza, usually called flu.

Tetanus

The horse is most susceptible to tetanus. The causal organism, the bacterium *Clostridium tetani*, is commonly found in the soil and sometimes in horses' faeces. It usually enters the body via a wound. This may be a deep and penetrating wound but is just as likely to be a scratch or thorn prick that goes unnoticed.

The tetanus organism thrives in an environment deprived of oxygen, which is one reason why puncture wounds need to be treated with care.

All horses should be vaccinated against tetanus. This is quick, simple and highly effective and is the only practical means of long-term protection. Horses can begin the vaccination course from the age of three months.

Once the horse has contracted tetanus it is unlikely that it can be saved, as the disease has a 90% mortality rate. If the horse suffers an obvious wound and is not known to be vaccinated, the veterinary surgeon can administer tetanus antitoxin within 24 hours of the wound being inflicted.

The permanent vaccination course with tetanus toxoid consists of two primary injections given about four weeks apart, followed by a booster a year later and thereafter at 2–5-yearly intervals.

Equine Influenza

Flu is a highly contagious viral disease of the respiratory tract. It debilitates the horse leaving it open to secondary infections, and if it is worked hard whilst incubating the disease the horse can suffer permanent and serious respiratory damage. An infected horse can infect others before there are any clinical signs and will remain infectious for at least another 6–10 days. This means it is easy for the infection to spread rapidly.

Because flu is a viral disease it is liable to change and there are different strains and sub-types. However, the various vaccines available are designed to cope with the most generally occurring strains. Veterinary advice must always be sought and will be required to administer injections.

For many competition horses vaccination is mandatory within their discipline and many yards, stables and competition venues will not allow unvaccinated animals on their premises. It is mandatory for all animals visiting racecourses, for whatever reason, to be vaccinated. The vaccination requirements are VERY strictly adhered to, and being even one day out of date will invalidate the whole programme.

Each horse must have a valid vaccination certificate, usually part of his passport, so that it undeniably belongs to him. It must be completed, signed and date stamped on each line by a veterinary surgeon who is not the owner of the animal. There must be no sign that the record has been tampered with or altered.

- The record should show that the horse has received two injections for primary vaccination not less than 21 days apart and not more than 92 days apart. After this a horse may be allowed to compete.

- In addition a first booster must be given not less than 150 days and not more that 215 days after the second primary injection.

- Subsequently, booster injections must be given at intervals of not more than one year apart, commencing after the first booster injection. Some organisations recommend six-monthly intervals.

- None of these injections may be given within the preceding 7 days, including the day of entry to the stables or competition.

It is possible to give a joint tetanus and flu vaccine in the years when this is required.

Some horses react quite severely to the flu vaccine and may need a quiet few days after being injected.

Pregnant mares are often given a tetanus booster in the late stages of pregnancy. This increases the antibodies available to the foal through the colostrum.

GOVERNMENT PUBLICATIONS AND CODES OF PRACTICE

ANNEX A

- **Summary of the Law Relating to Farm Animal Welfare (DEFRA 1996)** This guide provides a summary of the legislation relating to the welfare of animals on the farm, with reference to horses, ponies, asses and mules. It also shows in summary form for each species, including horses, what operations are permitted, at what age, by whom and whether an anaesthetic is needed.

- **Export of Horses and Ponies from Great Britain – Welfare Arrangements – Guidance Notes for Exporters (DEFRA, SEERAD, NAWAD 2000)**

  The notes provide guidance to exporters on the requirements of the law in relation to the export of horses from Great Britain including: export licences, animal health requirements, minimum values and Customs and Excise requirements.

- **Guidance Notes on the Welfare of Animals (Transport) Order 1997 (DEFRA)**

  The guidance is issued to aid consistency of understanding and enforcement of the Order. It is a useful reference document for anyone engaged in the transport of animals, including horses, to ensure that they are familiar with the regulatory provisions and comply with the law.

- **Horse Passports (England) Regulations 2004: Guide to the Horse Passport (England) Regulations 2004**

  Guidance on the application of the regulations in England.

- **Code of Practice – The Welfare of Horses, Ponies & Donkeys at Markets, Sales and Fairs Order 1990**

  The Code of Practice supplements the Welfare of Horses at Markets (and other places of sale) Order 1990, with practical guidance on transport, control and handling, penning, feeding and watering, sale rings, facilities, wild ponies and general conduct.

- **Code of Practice on how to prevent the spread of Ragwort (DEFRA 2004)**

  The Code aims to define the situations in which there is a likelihood of ragwort spreading to neighbouring land where it will then present an identifiable risk of ingestion by vulnerable animals, and to provide guidance on the most appropriate means of control, taking into account both animal welfare and environmental considerations.

Copies of the above publications can be obtained, free of charge, from DEFRA Publications, Admail 6000, London SW1A 2XX. Telephone orders 0845 955 6000, email: defra@sr-comms.co.uk
website: http//www.defra.gov.uk

ANNEX B

CODES OF PRACTICE

For the purpose of this Compendium Codes of Practice are defined as 'guidelines to best practice produced by a group of experts in consultation with industry and validated through the consultation process by that industry'.

Conservation Grazing

- A Guide to Animal Welfare in Nature Conservation Grazing (GAP 2001)

Disease Control

- Codes of Practice on Contagious Equine Metritis (CEM), Klebsiella pneumoniae, Pseudomonas aeruginosa, Equine Viral Arteritis (EVA), Equid Herpesvirus-1 (EHV-1) and Guidelines on Strangles (HRBLB 2005)

- Rules of Racing (The Jockey Club 2005 – revised annually)

- Code of Practice for Respiratory Diseases (National Trainers Federation 2005)

Donkeys

- Donkey Derbies a Code of Practice (The Donkey Sanctuary 2004)

- Beach Donkeys a Code of Practice (The Donkey Sanctuary 2005)

Farriery

- A Farrier's Guide to Professional Conduct (Farriers Registration Council)

General Welfare

- Horses in the Countryside A Code of Practice for Owners and Riders (Countryside Commission Revised 1997, now Countryside Agency)

- The FEI Code of Conduct for the Welfare of the Horse (FEI 2005)

Grazing

- Horse Pasture Management (Countryside Agency 2001)

Markets, Sales and Fairs

- The Welfare of Horses, Ponies & Donkeys at Markets, Sales & Fairs (DEFRA 1990)

- Code of Practice for Markets and Sales Involved with the selling of Horses, Ponies & Donkeys (NEWC 2003)

Riding Schools, Livery Yards & Trekking Centres

- Code of Practice for Livery Yards (BEVA/BHS/RSPCA/ILPH on behalf of the Horse Industry 2001)

Tethering

- Code of Practice to Tethering Horses and Ponies (NEWC, 2005)

Welfare Charities

- Code of Practice for Welfare Organisations involved in the keeping of Horses, Ponies and Donkeys (NEWC 2000)

ANNEX E

CODES OF RECOMMENDATION AND ADVISORY PUBLICATIONS

For the purpose of this Compendium, Codes of Recommendation are defined as 'guidelines to best practice produced by individuals or organisations but not validated by the consultation process'.

The National Equine Welfare Council (NEWC) maintains information on current advisory publications on horse, pony and donkey welfare, management and related topics.

This can be accessed at www.newc.co.uk or by contacting NEWC on 01295 810 060.

ANNEX F

ORDERS AND STATUTORY INSTRUMENTS

AGRICULTURE (relates to Agricultural Livestock only)

- Weeds Act 1959
- The Agriculture (Miscellaneous Provisions) Act 1968
- The Welfare of Farmed Animals (England) Regulations 2000 (SI 2000/1870)
- The Welfare of Farmed Animals (Wales) Regulations 2001 (SI 2001/2682)
- The Welfare of Farmed Animals (Scotland) Regulations 2000 (SI 2000/442)
- The Welfare of Farmed Animals (Northern Ireland) Regulations 2000 (SI 2000/270)

CRUELTY

- The Animals Act 1907
- The Protection of Animals Acts 1911 to 1988
- The Protection of Animals (Scotland) Acts 1912 to 1988
- The Protection of Animals (Scotland) Act 1993
- The Abandonment of Animals Act 1960
- The Animals Act 1971
- The Protection of Animals (Penalties) Act 1987
- The Protection of Animals (Amendment) Act 1988
- The Protection of Animals (Amendment) Act 2000

DISQUALIFICATION

- Protection of Animals (Amendment) Act 1954 (as amended by the Protection of Animals (Amendment) Act 1988

EXHIBITION OF EQUINES

- Performing of Animals (Regulations) Act 1925
- Protection of Animals Act 1934

FALLEN STOCK

- Animal By-Products Regulation 2003

FARRIERY

- Farriers (Registration) Act 1975 as Amended by the Farriers (Registration) (Amendment) Act 1977 as Amended by Statutory Instrument No 1597 (effective from 16th July 2002)

HEALTH, DISEASE CONTROL

- The Infectious Diseases of Horses Order 1975 (SI 1975/888)
- The Animal Health Act 1981 and 2002
- The Infectious Diseases of Horses Order 1987 (SI 1987/790)

- Equine Viral Arteritis Order 1995 (SI 1995/1755)

HORSE PASSPORTS

- Horse Passports (England) Regulations 2004
- Horse Passports (Scotland) Regulations 2005
- Horse Passports (Wales) Regulations 2005

HORSE WASTE MANAGEMENT

- The Waste Management Licensing Regulations 1994
- The Waste Management Licensing (England and Wales) (Amendment & Related Provisions Regulations 2005)

IMPORT AND EXPORT OF EQUINES

- The Export of Horses (Veterinary Examination) Order 1966 (SI 1966/507)
- The Export of Horses (Excepted Cases) Order 1969 (SI 1969/1742)
- The Export of Horses (Protection) Order 1969 (SI 1969/1784)
- The Equine Animals (Importation) (Amendment) Order 1972 (SI 1972/761)
- The Equine Animals (Importation) Order 1973 (SI 1973/470)
- Importation of Animals Order 1977 (SI 1979/1701)
- Importation of Equine Animals Order, 1979 (SI 1979/1701)
- Export of Animals (Protection) Order 1981
- The Animal Health Act 1981 and 2002 (Sections 40–48)

MARKETS, SALES AND FAIRS

- Markets, Sales and Fairs Order 1995
- Welfare of Horses at Markets (and other Places of sale) Order 1990 (SI 1990/2627)
- Welfare of Animals at Markets Order 1990 (as amended by the Welfare of Animals at Markets (Amendment) Order 1993)

OPERATIONS ON EQUINES

- Docking and Nicking of Horses Act 1949
- The Protection of Animals (Anaesthetics) Act 1954, and as amended
- The Veterinary Surgeons Act 1966
- Farriers (Registration) Act 1975
- The Veterinary Surgery (Artificial Insemination of Mares) Order 2004
- Farriers Registration (Amendment) Act 1977
- The Animals (Scientific Procedures) Act 1986

RAGWORT

- The Ragwort Control Act 2003

RIDING ESTABLISHMENTS

- Riding Establishments Act 1964
- Riding Establishments Act 1970

SLAUGHTER OF EQUINES

- Slaughterhouses Act 1974
- Slaughterhouses (Hygiene) Regulations 1977
- Slaughter of Animals (Humane Conditions) Regulations 1990

- The Welfare of Animals (Slaughter or Killing) Regulations 1995, as amended 1999

TETHERING

- The Protection Against Cruel Tethering Act 1988

TRANSPORT OF EQUINES

- The Transport of Animals (Road and Rail) Order 1975 (as amended) (SI 1975/ 1024)

- The Welfare of Animals (Transport) Order 1997 (SI 1997/1480)

- The Welfare of Animals (Staging Points) Order 1998 (SI 1998/2537)

- The Welfare of Animals (Transport) (Amendment) Order 1999 (SI 1999/1622)

- The Transport of Animals (Cleansing and Disinfection) (England) (No 2) Order 2000 (SI 2000/ 1618)

VETERINARY SURGEONS

- The Veterinary Surgeons Act 1966

YOUNG RIDERS

- The Horses (Protective Headgear for Young Riders) Act 1990

- The Horses (Protective Headgear for Young Riders) Act 1990 (Commencement) Order 1992 (SI 1992/1200)

- The Horses (Protective Headgear for Young Riders) Regulations 1992 (SI 1992/1201)

THE NATIONAL EQUINE DATABASE

This is a Government sponsored DEFRA initiative. All Passport Issuing Offices (PIOs) are required to send passport data to the National Equine Database (NED). They are also asked to volunteer breeding and competition data on all British-bred horses, the idea being that would-be buyers or breeders would be able to access this information for a fee which would help pay for the service.

This initiative has been subject to many delays, and at the time of going to press the date for its inception is still open to change.

ANIMAL TRANSPORT CERTIFICATE AND ROUTE PLAN

In January 2007 new EU regulations for the transporting of horses came into effect. Under these new regulations anyone transporting animals must ensure:

• Journey times are kept to a minimum.

• The animals are fit to travel.

• Those handling the animals are trained and competent.

• The vehicle and its loading and unloading facilities are designed, constructed and maintained to avoid injury and suffering.

• Water, feed and rest are given to the animals as needed and sufficient floor space and height is allowed.

If you transport horses in connection with an economic activity over 65km (approx. 40 miles) you will need to apply for a transporter authorisation. This will be valid for 5 years. Any previously granted authorisation issued under the Welfare of Animals (Transport) Order 1997 is invalid from January 2007.

The Animal Transport Certificate (ATC) and the Route Plan are two forms which need to be filled out by anyone travelling horses for gain. They will certainly be required by any licensed haulier. It is unclear under what circumstances private people transporting horses may be required to fill them out.

Anyone transporting their own animals for pleasure riding, veterinary treatment or competition does not need one.

Someone giving a friend's horse a lift under such circumstances and receiving petrol money in return, is not intended to need one.

Anyone transporting a friend's pet horse which is accompanied by the owner should not need one.

A livery yard owner, transporting clients' horses for them might well. There are a number of grey areas open to interpretation.

The two example forms shown overleaf need to be filled out whilst referring to the notes published with them. These can be downloaded from the Department for Environment, Food and Rural Affairs (DEFRA) Welfare in Transport Implementation Team.

When you have decided to use the forms, they should travel with the animals in the vehicle and be available for inspection on demand.

Department for Environment, Food & Rural Affairs
Scottish Executive Environment Rural Affairs Department
National Assembly for Wales Agriculture Department
The Welfare of Animals (Transport) Order 1997 (Article 13)

Route Plan (please complete in BLOCK LETTERS)

During the journey the consignment MUST be accompanied by the Route Plan.

Section 1 : To be completed BEFORE the journey by the Transporter responsible for the whole journey

1. Transporter's name and full postal address:

   Business name   Postcode

   Telephone No. (incl. STD code):

   Fax No. (incl. STD code):

2. Full postal address of place of departure:

   Postcode

   Planned **date** of departure:

   Planned **time** of departure:

3. Animal species: No. of animals:

4. No. of registration plate(s) and trailer(s):   Transporter's authorisation reference

5. Air or sea stage:

Name of Shipping Company/Airline	Port/Airport of departure	Estimated time of departure	Port/Airport of arrival	Estimated time of arrival

6. Rest period, staging point or transfer point: (please see notes at paragraph D, bullet point 9, page 3)

Full address	Planned date of arrival		Planned length of stop	Reason
	Date	Time		

7. Full postal address of place of destination:

   Planned **date** of arrival: Planned **time** of arrival:

   Please refer to paragraph A on page 2 of this form for information on the Data Protection Act 1998

   Transporter's signature

   Please now submit this form to the DVM

   DVM stamp, signature and date of area of the place of departure

   This route plan is valid for journeys starting within 10 days from date of stamp

   Number(s) of Health Certificate(s) or accompanying document(s)

Animal Transport Certificate

The Welfare of Animals (Transport) Order 1997

> **Please read the notes overleaf before starting to complete this form.**

1. Name and address of transporter	2. Name and address of owner of animals
Telephone no. Fax no.	Telephone no. Fax no.

3. Registration number of vehicle(s) and trailer(s)

4. Species of animals	5. Number of animals

6. Status of animals *(Please circle appropriate entry)*

Slaughter   Fattening   Breeding   Other (specify)

7. Address of place animals loaded	8. Address of final destination

9. Date of loading	10. Time first animal loaded

11. Date of departure	12. Time of departure

13. Time(s) and place(s) where rest stops undertaken, including if the animals were watered and/or fed

14. Date last animal unloaded	15. Time last animal unloaded

STABLE FIRES

Fire is possibly one of the most horrific dangers facing stabled horses. Prompt action, coolly undertaken, by owners and staff is an essential requirement.

1. Dial 999 (in UK) ask for fire services, give name, address (map grid reference if known) of fire and telephone number you are speaking from.

2. Extricate firstly those horses nearest the fire, to the closest paddock or enclosure not likely to be affected by the fire.

   Secure control of the frightened animals is essential; always have a headcollar conveniently placed if the horses are in loose boxes, or a spare shank if they permanently wear headcollars or are tied in stalls.

   A coat, sack or saddle blanket placed over the horse's head as a blind-fold may help, but time in fitting could be wasted if panic has commenced.

3. Remove all horses, working progressively away from the fire area.

4. If working single-handed in a large yard **do not** attempt to fight an established fire until all horses are safely removed.

5. **Small** outbreaks of fire, if you are present at the onset, and they can be immediately contained, should be fought if equipment is to hand.

6. If the fire is confined to one stable or building from which the occupants have been removed, or it is unoccupied, close all doors and windows (providing this can be achieved without danger to persons). This will help to contain the fire.

7. **Never** turn horses out loose into the yard unless there is no alternative exit. Close all loose-box doors after removing horses, as they regard their stables as places of refuge and might attempt to re-enter the burning building.

   A yard full of loose horses will cause great difficulties for the fire service on their arrival, and the horses might escape into the highway. Designate an alternative site and keep the gate closed.

PREVENTION

Consult your Fire Prevention Officer for advice.

1. **ALWAYS** equip stable yards with the following:
   a) An alarm signal, regularly tested.
   b) Extinguishers, regularly tested.
   c) A hose-pipe permanently attached to the mains supply, and of sufficient length to reach all the buildings. The pipe should be maintained in a reel, and regularly extended and tested for leaks. There needs to be sufficient water pressure for this to be useful.
   d) **NO SMOKING** notices should be displayed.
   No inflammable materials such as petrol, paraffin or

paints should be stored in the stable vicinity.

e) If staff are employed, ensure that they have received instruction in fire drill, and that drill practices are carried out.

f) Where several horses are stabled in the same building, always try to have more than one **EXIT** to the building.

g) **NEVER** construct cage boxes in a building unless the passageway is a minimum of 6ft (1.18m) wide and all box doors, which should open outwards, are designed to fold back flat, to the front of the box, or are of the sliding design.

h) **NEVER** leave inflammable material in the passageways or adjoining stables, to reduce the risks of spontaneous combustion.

i) **NEVER** allow bonfires or fireworks to be lit near to stables.

j) Display a notice which informs of the location of a second telephone, should the stable telephone become unusable.

k) Consider the installation of a fire hydrant if one is not in proximity.

l) Remove cobwebs from lights regularly. Hot cobwebs falling onto bedding cause fires.

2. KEYS

If the stable owner or staff do not live on the premises (lock-up stables), make arrangements for one or two key holders nearby. Inform the fire service and police of your home address and also the name and address of the key holders in advance.

3. ELECTRICAL FITTINGS

All cabling should be away from areas within easy reach of the horses; all cabling should be PVC covered and waterproof.

Switches to be located outside the stable and away from the reach of the occupants; switches to be of an approved water-tight design.

Master switch panels, transformers, meters and trip switches should be located in a separate building, or secured in a horse- and water-proof cabinet.

Many fires are started through electrical faults. Make it a weekly routine to check for:

- Visible signs of loose wires in plug tops.

- Visible signs of cracked plugs.

- Visible signs of frayed, cracked or gnawed leads.

- Signs of over-heating on plug tops and socket outlets.

All installations should comply with present legislation, and be fitted by an approved contractor.

Check all electrical equipment which is only in seasonal use, such as clippers, for the above signs **before** using.

Extension cables should not be left in hay or straw. There is a real chance of a fire through a shorting of the circuit. All coiled cables when in use generate a lot of heat.

Even the quietest horse can be startled, and no horse should ever be left unsupervised near electrical equipment such as clippers or unprotected infra-red light banks. Even though the last mentioned hang suspended from the ceiling, a wrong movement by the horse could cause a fire. Because of the heat created by these particular lamps it is important that they are dusted regularly so no heavy deposits are formed on top.

Keep stables free from cobwebs which, when dust-laden, make the flash-point more acute.

At no time should personnel be put at risk in order to save horses.

FURTHER READING

The following books and booklets can all be obtained from the BHS Bookshop.

The BHS Veterinary
Manual

The BHS Manual for
Coaching and Teaching
Riding

The BHS Complete
Manual of Equitation

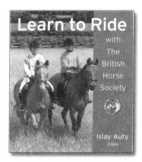

Learn to Ride
with the BHS

The BHS Training
Manual for the PTT
Incorporating the
UKCC Level 2

The BHS Training
Manual for Progressive
Riding Tests 1-6

The BHS Complete
Training Manual for
Stage 1

The BHS Complete
Training Manual for
Stage 2

The BHS Complete
Training Manual for
Stage 3

The BHS Stage 1
Workbook

The BHS Stage 2
Workbook

The BHS Riding and
Road Safety Manual
12th Edition

BHS TREC

The BHS Directory of
where to Ride, Train
and Stable Your Horse

Guide to BHS
Examinations

Examinations
Handbook 5th Edition

BHS Guide to
Careers with Horses

BHS Duty of Care

INDEX

access road 384, 385
accident book 426
accident forms 426
accountant 427
accounts 423, 424
acorns 360
action
    assessment 31, 79
    defective 29–30
afterbirth (foetal membranes) 48
ageing of horse 35–8
Agricultural Development and
        Advisory Service (ADAS)
        346–7, 353
air bricks 397
air extractors 397
air travel 344
alarms, stable yard 382
alfalfa (lucerne) 171, 175, 176, 197
allergies 64
alveoli 135
American barn 385, 387–8, 390, 393
amino acids, essential 169
anaemia 171
Animal Transport Certificate (ATC)
        487, 489
Animalintex poultice 129
Animals Act (1971) 460–2
anti-cast ridge 395
anti-cast roller 150, 267–8
anti-crib biting strap 146
anti-weaving grid 145
antibiotics 185
anus 162–3
aorta 136, 137
Appaloosa 58
appetite, loss 126, 200, 201
apples 179
Arab horse 40, 44
arenas, see indoor school; outdoor
        school
Army reversible bit 253

arteries 136
artificial insemination 54
Association of British Riding Schools
        454
Atherstone girth 220
auction sales 63
    codes of practice 482
Australian noseband 230, 253
azoturia (set fast, tying up) 203

back
    conformation 21, 22
    sore/inflamed 130, 378
'bad doers' 200–1
balance, spring-loaded 211
balancer cubes 181
balancing rein 242
Balding girth 220
baling string 456
bandages
    pressure 131
    stable 259, 260–1
    support 261
    tearing 148
    under-bandage protection 260
bandages, leg 259–63
    causes of damage 259
    cold 132
    dressage horse 299
    event horse 294
    exercise 259, 262–3
    fastenings 260
    removal 262–3
bandages, tail 260, 263–4
bandaging
    foot 130, 131
    knee and hock 130–1
banks (fences) 362
barbed wire 363
barley 178
    boiled 183

nutritive value 191
barley boiler 455
barley grass 167
barley straw 176
barn, hay storage 381, 418–19
barn-type stabling 385, 387–8, 390,
        393
bars (foot) 102
bars (mouth) 243
bathing horse 85
beans 178, 191
bedding 116–18
    buying 417, 418, 420, 428–9
    choice of 116–17
    deep litter 122
    depth 121
    disposal 117
    eating 148
    mucking out 119–22
    semi-deep litter 120–1
    setting fair 122
    sick horse 125
    storage 118, 418
beet, whole 179
behaviour
    grazing 164
    natural instincts 32, 33, 163, 367
behavioural problems 33, 144–9
    causes 32–3
    clipping 91, 94
    loading 33
    restraining horse 73–6
benzimidazole 141, 142
BHS qualifications, levels and
        responsibility 70
bib 76
bib martingale 232
billet studs 276–7
biotin 106, 173
bishoping 38
bit
    actions 243

bridoon 228, 249, 250, 276
    checking for soundness 278–9
    cleaning 275, 277
    construction 244–5
    fitting problems 244
    key-ring mouthing 249
    materials 245
    measuring 245
    stallion 249
    types 245–6
    see also snaffle bits
bit attachments 253
bit guards 253
biting 33, 73, 148
bitless bridle 253
blanket clip 89, 90, 93
blankets, under-rug 265
blood cells 136
blood testing
    competition horse 194, 289
    pregnancy 54
    prior to purchase of horse 64
body
    depth 20–1
    markings 59
body brush 81, 83
body weight, see condition; weight
bolts, stable door 80, 398
'bone' 20
bookkeeper 427
boot, poultice 258
boots 256–9
    application 256
    brushing 256
    dressage horse 299
    event horse 294
    exercise 255
    fastenings 255–6
    materials 255
    medicine 257
    point-to-pointer 318
    polo 257, 327

boots *cont.*
poultice 129–30
purpose of 254, 255
tendon 255
travelling 258–9, 261
turnout 255
boredom, stabled horse 144, 147, 388
bots (gadfly/*Gasterophilus* spp.) 140, 369
botulism 175, 356
box rest 127–8, 201
bran 171, 178, 191
bran mash 182–3, 196
bran poultice 129
brand marks 55
'breaking out' 83, 312
breastgirth, 'Aintree' 233
breastplates 233, 294
fitting 280–1
lungeing 239
breed societies 39
breeding
facilities 45
selection of stock 28, 45
see also broodmare; foaling; stallion
bridles
bitless/hackamore 253
checking for soundness 278
cleaning 275–6
endurance 304
event horse 293
leading horse in 74, 78
Pelham 227, 229, 252
polo pony 327
putting on 281–2
putting up 276
removing 282
show horse/pony 321–2
stallion 76, 323
storage 405, 431
see also double bridle; snaffle bridle
bridoon bit 228, 249, 250, 276
bridoon rein 228–9
British Horse Society (BHS) 454, 472
approved establishments 472–3
examinations and qualifications 473–6
Instructors' Register 426
membership 426, 472
Progressive Riding Tests 473
roles of 472
British Sport Horse 39–40
British Warmblood 40, 45

bronchi 135
bronchioles 135
broodmare
covering 54
feeding 50, 51, 53, 188, 191, 198
foaling 47–9
general management 45–7, 49–50
lactation 50–1, 153, 191
selection 28, 45
showing 322
vaccinations 480
brooms, stable 119
browband 227
brushes
grooming 82, 83–4
stable 119
brushing boots 256
brushing injury 254
buckets
feed 69, 168, 209–10
water 155
buckles 277
buffalo hide 215, 221
buffer 108
buying a horse 61–4

caecum 162
calcium 171
cane, showing 323
cannon bones 20
canter work 135, 288, 315
capillaries 136, 137
car park, safety regulations 457
carbohydrates 161, 169
carbon dioxide 136
carrots 167, 179
cash
handling 422
petty 423
cash book 424
cast horse 149–50
cat hairs 95
catching 372
difficult horse/pony 33, 373–4
foal 51
catering 430
cattle, grazing 351, 352, 362
cattle lorry 332
cavesson, lunge 74, 238
ceilings, stable 396
cereals, *see* grain
certificate of identification 59–60
cess pit 391
chaff 176, 192
chaff cutter 455

Chambon 241, 242
changing rooms 385, 407–8
chaser clip 89, 90
cherry roller snaffle 248
chest, conformation 19
chestnuts 59
chewing, stable 80
chewing (mastication) 163
chief instructor 436
Chifney bit 74, 249
child helpers 438–9
chlorine 171
choke 149, 164
chop 176, 192
chrome-tanned leather 215
chronic obstructive pulmonary disease (COPD), feeding 204, 206
circulatory system 136, 137
Cleveland Bay 40
client rest room 407
clients
duty of care 383
payments 422–3
personal accident insurance 426
recommended dress 429–30
clipper blades 92
clippers 91–2, 401, 455
clipping
competition horse 89
difficult horses 91, 94
dressage horse 298
grass-kept horse/pony 88
mane 95
methods 92–4
polo pony 329
preparation 90–1
reasons for 88
safety 91, 455
show horse/pony 88–9, 319
show jumper 300–1
utility box 401
clips
shoe 107
types and uses 89–90
clothing
for clipping 91
in-hand showing 323
riding clients 429–30
staff and student turnout 440
for working with horses 68, 73
clothing shop 408–9
coarse mixes 181, 189
cob, definition 44
cobalt 171

cod liver oil 172
codes of practice 481–3
cold bandages 132
cold hosing 132
cold packs 132
cold weather conditions 367
cold-blood, definition 44
colic 50, 202–3
colon 162
colostrum 47, 51, 480
coloured horse/pony 44, 58
colours, correct description 57–8
combined management system 371–2
combs
mane 84
mane-thinning 96
plaiting 84
comfrey 179
communication 70
competition horse
blood tests 289
checks during training 288–9
clipping 89
daily routines 445
dressage 195, 298–9
driving horse/pony 307–8
feeding 166, 170, 194–6, 289
fitness programmes 287–8
passport 287
point-to-pointer 314–18
polo pony 326–9
show horse/pony 319–25
show jumper 300–1
vaccinations 287, 479–80
worming 287
see also endurance horse; event horse
competitions, overnight stays 289–90
compound feeds 180–1, 189
bulk buying 421
racehorse 317
computer systems 427
concentrates 176–7
compound feeds 180–1, 189
definition 163
for grass-kept horse/pony 367
purchase and storage 209–10, 420–1
roughage:concentrate ratio 193, 195
straight cereals 177–9
concrete
stable floor 393
yard surfaces 384–5
condition 187

condition *cont.*
    broodmare 50, 51
    and conformation 13
    and feed ration 188
    fit horse 28
    grass-kept horse/pony 369
    polo pony 326
    poor/loss of 13, 200–1
    show horse/pony 319
condition scoring 26–8
confidentiality 383, 427
conformation 13, 18–24
    and action 29
    assessment 24–6
    breeding stock 28
    foot 13, 18, 103–6
    and saddle fitting 224
Connemara pony 42
contagious disease 125, 127
Contract of Sale Conditions 63
control halters 74, 237
convalescence 127–8
cooling of horse 296–7, 304, 306
copper 171–2
copper bits 244, 245
corn oil 170
coronary band 101, 102
coronet boot 257
corrugated iron roofing 395
COSHH (Control of Substances
    Hazardous to Health) (1989)
    467–8
covering 54
covering fees 54
cowls, ventilation 397
crab apples 360
cracked heels 369–70
cradle 76
creoline derivatives 128
crest 18, 26, 369
crib biting 38, 145–6
cruelty, legislation 483
cruelty offences 463–4
crupper 236, 240
cubes 180–1, 189
    bulk buying 421
    horse and pony 191, 197
    nutritive value 191
curb chain 252
    double bridle 228, 250, 276
    fitting 228–9
    Kimblewick 253
    leather-covered 228
    Pelham bridle 229, 252
curry comb 84

plastic 84
rubber 81, 84, 86
Cytek shoe 115

Dales pony 43
damp course 394
dandelions 179, 360
dandy brush 83, 86
Dartmoor pony 43
de Gogue 241
deadly nightshade 360
deep litter 122, 392
DEFRA 347, 477
dehydration 153, 156, 203
    causes 156–7
    signs of 156
deliveries 429
dental care 34, 38, 76, 165, 287
description of horse, colours 56–60
diaphragmatic flutter, synchronous
    (thumps) 156
diarrhoea 157, 203
diary 423
    daily 427
Dick Christian bit 247
diesel tank 381
diet
    associated problems and ailments
        202–4
    changes to 163, 167
    horses' natural 159–60, 163
    see also feeding
digestible energy (DE) 190–1
digestive problems
    causes 180–1
    signs of 164
digestive system 161–3, 167
digital cushion 101, 102
disease control
    codes of practice 482
    legislation 483–4
dishing 29, 30
disinfectants 128
dock (tail) 22
docks 360
doeskin, cleaning 273
dogs, stable yard 404
domestication of horse 160
donkeys
    codes of practice 482
    worming 141
doors
    barn stabling 393, 398
    indoor school 411

safety 456
    see also stable door
dorsal stripe 59
double bridle 249–52
    action 249–50
    cleaning 275–6
    curb chain fitting 250, 251
    fitting 228–9
    parts 226
    putting on 282
    showing 321, 322
    types of bit 251
Dr Bristol bit 247
drainage
    grassland 348
    indoor school 411–12
    outdoor school 414
    stable yard 384
    stabling 116, 121, 391–3
    traps and gullies 392
draw reins 240
drawing knife 109
drenching 77
dressage horse 195, 298,
    298–9
dressage saddle 218, 219
drinking, *see* watering
driver, horse transport 334–5
driving harness 308
driving horse/pony 307–8
drop noseband 229–30
droppings 123–4
    consistency 164
    healthy 123
    horse eating 147–8
    number/frequency of 164
    picking up from pastures 141–2,
        351
drying horse, after hunting 313
dumping 112
duodenum 162
dust 69, 117
dust control
    indoor school 413
    outdoor school 415
    stables 121, 388
Dutch gag (bubble bit) 248
duties
    general stable 440–1
    staff members 436–8
duty of care, clients 383

ears 18
    trimming 95

Easy-Glu shoe 115
electric fencing 363
electrical equipment
    clippers 91–2
    grooming machines 87, 90
    safety 455, 491
electricity supply 402–3
electrolytes 155, 158, 195, 202, 295,
    296, 304
electuary 77
Elevator bridles 251–2, 276
embryo transplantation 54
employers liability, insurance 425,
    454
Employment Act (1989) 438
endurance competitions
    compulsory halt (vet gate) 306
    preparation 304–5
    types 302–3
Endurance GB 302, 306
endurance horse 302–6
    care during competition 305–6
    equipment 305
    feeding 195, 303–4
    fittening 303
    general management 304
    saddlery 222, 304
    veterinary inspection 305–6
    watering 155
endurance saddle 219
energy 159
epiglottis 135
epiphysitis 198
Epsom salts 129, 131
Equi-Boot 129, 130, 257–8
equine influenza vaccinations 479–80
equine rhabdomyolysis, *see* azoturia
ermine markings 59
event horse
    care during competition 294–7
    condition 187
    feeding 194–5, 294
    fitness 28
    fitness programme 291–3
    tack and equipment 293–4
    two/three day competitions 292
    veterinary inspection 297
    watering 155, 295
exercise bandages 259, 262–3
Exmoor pony 42
export of equines, regulations 484
extractors, stabling 397
'eye' for a horse 24–6
eyes 18
    irritation from flies 369

faeces, *see* droppings
farm buildings, conversion 388
farmyard manure (FYM) 350
farrier 18, 101, 106
    forge 402
    owner's responsibility 101
    shoeing process 109–11
Farriers (Registration) Act (1975)
    101
farrier's tools 108–9
farriery
    codes of practice 482
    legislation 101, 483
    qualification and registration 101
fast work 288
    event horse 291
    point-to-pointer 315
fats, dietary 170, 178–9
fear, horse 32
feather, trimming 95
feed balancers 185
feed bins 208
feed blocks 367
feed bowls/bucket 69, 168, 209–10,
    400, 431, 432
feed chart 211, 432
feed merchant 208–9, 417, 428
feed ration, *see* ration
feed scoop 168
feed shed 404
    equipment 209–12
    hygiene 69
    layout 208–9
    organisation 431–2
    security 209, 431
    siting 209, 382, 385
feed trolley 212, 432
feed trough/manger 399–400
feeding
    aims of 159
    art versus science 186
    'bad doer' 200–1
    broodmare 46, 48, 49, 50–1, 53
    children's ponies 197–8, 319
    competition horses 170, 289
    cost-effectiveness 189
    dressage horse 195, 298
    driving horse/pony 307
    during fittening programme 134
    endurance horse 195, 303–4
    event horse 194–5, 294
    grass-kept horse/pony 193–4, 207,
        366–7
    horse brought up from grass 376
    hunter 309–10, 312

modern methods 160
non-competitive horse 197
point-to-pointer 196, 316–17
polo pony 328
prior to competition 294, 300
riding school horse/pony 197, 198
routines 167
rules of 166–8
show horse/pony 319–20
show jumper 300
sick horse 126, 201
stallion 199
succulents 167
supplements 158, 179, 183–5
and temperament 188–9
theoretical knowledge 159
travelling 157, 201–2, 206, 343
wind problems/COPD 204, 206
and work 167–8, 186, 188, 191–2
youngstock 51, 188, 191, 198–9
feeds
    packing for journey 290
    size of 164, 167, 192
feedstuffs
    buying and storage 417–21, 428–9
    contamination 194
    lifting 456
    nutritive value 190, 191
    processing 181–2
    quality of 166
    supply and quality 189
fees 434–5
feet
    balance 104–5, 110
    conformation 13, 18, 26, 103–6
    external structure 102–3
    internal structure 15, 101–2
    measurement for shoeing 110–11
    picking up 69, 71–3, 82–3
    poulticing 129–30
    tubbing 131
    see also shoeing
Fell pony 43
felt numnah 274
fences, stable yard 382, 385
fencing 361–5
    Animals Act obligations 462
    erection 364–5
    outdoor school 414
    types 361–4
    unsuitable 365
fertilisers 349–50
fetlock boot 256
fetlocks
    conformation 20

trimming 95
fibre, dietary 166, 169, 304
field
    choice for grazing 357–8
    saddling horse in 282
    see also grassland management;
        grazing
field shelter 361
filled legs 203–4, 261
finances 67
fire
    action in event of 490
    barn-type stabling 387–8
    common causes 447
    compulsory measures 452
    prevention 446–7, 490–1
fire alarms 446
fire drill 446
fire extinguishers 452
fire hose 446
first aid box, human 424
fitness
    categories 28
    definition 133, 287
fittening programme 133–5, 287, 288
    dressage horse 298
    driving horse/pony 307
    endurance horse 303, 378
    event horse 291–3, 378
    feeding during 192–3
    hunter 309, 378
    point-to-pointer 314–15
    polo pony 326–7
    show jumper 300
    timetables 378
    unfit horse up from grass 377–8
flash noseband 230
flesh marks 59
flies 369
flight instinct 32
floors
    horse transport 330, 334
    stable 393
flu vaccinations 479–80
flute bit 146
fly repellents 325, 369
foal slip 51–2, 73, 76, 236, 237
foaling 47–9
foals
    feeding 51, 191, 198–9
    handling 51–2, 76
    weaning 52–3
    worming 50, 140, 141
foetal fluids 48
folic acid 173

fomenting 131–2
food
    categories 168
    necessity of 159
    refusal of 200
    see also feedstuffs *and types of foods*
foot balance 104–5, 110
foot care 106–7
    grass-kept horse/pony 107
    roughed-off horse 375
    youngstock 52, 107
    see also shoeing
footwear
    riding clients 429
    yard work 68
forage 163–4
    buying 416–18
    feeding methods 205–7, 400
    feeding rations 192
    for sick horse 126
    storage 209
    vacuum-packed 209
    weighing 211
    see also grass; hay; haylage;
        roughage
fore legs
    action 29–30
    conformation 19–20
    holding to restrain horse 75
foregirth 233–4
forge, farrier's 402
forge tools 108–9
forging 30
fork, stable 119
freelance instructors, insurance
    426
freeze-marking 55, 382
French bridoon 247
French drains 384
frog 102, 103
fuel storage 381
Fulmer snaffle 246, 247
Fybagee pads 260

'gadgets' (training aids) 240–2
gag, mouth examination 76
gag snaffles 248
gallery, indoor school 412
Galvayne's groove 38
Gamgee 130, 132, 260, 261
garden waste 360
garlic 179
gates
    field 365–6, 456

gates *cont.*
  stable yard 80, 385, 456
gateways 366, 456
General Stud Book 39
girth galls, prevention 378
girth (horse's), measurement 187
girth straps 218
girths 220
  checking for soundness 278
  cleaning 274
  fastening 280
  foregirth 233–4
  overgirth/surcingle 233, 294
globe cheek snaffle 253
gloves, yard work 68, 69, 119
glucose 158
glycerine and epsom salts poultice
  129
good practice 67–8
'goose-rumped' horse 22
grain
  boiled 183
  buying and storage 208, 420–1
  nutritive value 191
  processed 182
  'straights' 177–9
Grakle noseband 230
grass
  bringing horse up from 376–8
  dried cubes 176
  nutritive value 191
  vacuum-packed (haylage) 175–6,
  356
  see also grazing
grass meal 191
grass reins 236
grass-kept horse/pony
  clipping 88
  company 367
  daily care 367–8
  feeding 193–4, 207, 366–7
  field choice 357–8
  foot care and shoeing 107
  grooming 86–7
  groups of 366, 367
  health 368–70
  water supply 358–9
  working 371
grasses 354
grassland management 347
  alternative grazers 351, 352, 353
  codes of practice 482
  drainage 348
  harrowing 348
  haymaking 354–6

rolling 348–9
rotational 350–1
soil analysis 346–7
soil fertility 349–50
weed control 352–3
winter 351–2
worm control 141–2, 349, 351
grazing 163
  for breeding stock 45, 46, 49
  feeding value 163, 173, 190
  gates and security 365–6
  horses effects on 347, 351
  improving 352–4
  litter 361
  nutritive value 167, 192–3
  requirements for local authority
    licence 450
  restriction 357
  rotational 351–2
  shelter 361
  stocking rates 352
  turning out horse/pony 374
  valuable grasses and herbs 354
  winter months 351–2, 359
  see also grassland management
grazing behaviour 164
grease, legs 295, 297
grooming
  brushing off 83
  endurance horse 304
  grass-kept horse/pony 86–7
  methods 81–3
  objectives 81
  polo pony 329
  quartering 83
  racing/point-to-point yards 87, 317
  restraint of horse 73
  show horse/pony 320, 325
  sick horse 125
grooming machines 87, 90
  safety 87, 455
grooming tools 83–4
gruel 182, 196–7, 312
guard dog 404
gully traps 392
guttering 393

hack 44
hackamore 253
hacking 288, 300, 327, 377
Hackney horse 40–1
Halamide 128
halters 237
  control 74, 237

slipping 149
'Yorkshire' webbing 237
hammer, shoeing 108
handling 68, 69
  anxious horse 68
  control/restraint methods 73–6
  foal 51–2
  legs and feet 69, 71–3, 82–3
  rough 73
  safety precautions 69, 80
  stallion 53–4, 76
  use of voice 69, 77–8
  see also leading
'Happy Mouth' bits 245
harness, driving 308
harrowing 348
hay 174–5
hay:concentrate ratio 193
hay
  buying 418, 420
  clover 175
  feeding 163–4, 192, 197, 205–7,
  400
  feeding to grass-kept horse 366–7
  judging value of 174
  making 354–6
  meadow 175, 320, 355
  new 174
  nutritive value 191
  poisonous plants 174, 360
  seed 174–5, 355
  for sick horse 126
  soaking 206
  storage 209, 418–19
  weight 211, 420, 471
hay bales
  lifting 456
  weight 420
hay barn 381, 385–6, 418, 419
hay mangers 205–6, 400
hay racks 206, 400
hay stack 418–20
haylage 175–6
  big bale 197, 419
  buying 418
  feeding 176, 192, 197, 207
  making 356
  nutritive value 191
  storage 176, 356, 419
haynets 205, 206, 207, 400
  horsebox/trailer 337
head
  conformation 18
  trimming 95, 320
  white markings 58–9

head shaking 64
headcollar 71, 73
  control 74, 237
  field/turnout 373
  fitting 236
  foal 51–2
  leading horse 78
  slipping 149
  types and materials 236
  yearling 73, 236
headgear, protective 68, 429
  legislation 485
health, signs of 123, 367–8
Health and Safety at Work Act
  (1974) 407, 429, 453–7
heart 136, 137, 160
heart rate, *see* pulse
heat, extreme 296–7
heating
  staff room/lecture room 407
  tack room 405
heavy horse breeds 41
hedges 362
heels 103, 105
  bandaging 131
  over-lowering 112
  trimming feather/hair 95
height
  certification 61
  measurement 56
helpers, child and adult 438–9
helvetia leather 215
herbicides 352–3, 360
herbs
  feeding 179–80
  grassland 354
herd instinct 33, 367
'herring-gutted' 21
Highland pony 43
hill work 134, 188, 291, 377
hind legs
  action 29, 30
  conformation 23–4
  handling 72–3
hindquarters, conformation 22–3, 26
hinges 398
hinny 44
'hip down' 22
hock boots 258–9
hocks
  bandaging 130–1
  conformation 23–4
hogging 95
hoods 266
hoof 102–3

hoof *cont.*
   brittle 106
   rings/ridges 18, 102, 106
   texture 18
   see also feet
hoof boots 257–8
hoof dressings 106, 325
hoof pick 84
hoof/pastern axis 20, 103–4, 105
horse, definition 44
Horse Riding Establishments Guidance
   on Promoting Safe Working
   Conditions 454
horse 'toys' 144
horse walker 315, 455
horsebox 331–2
   construction 330–1
   driver 334–5
   loading 335–7
   loading equipment 342
   loading problems 337–9
   packing 290
   unladen weight 331
   unloading 339–40
horses, requirements for local
   authority licence 451
hose, fire 446
hosing, cold 86, 132
hot weather conditions 295, 297
hot-blood 44
hunter clip 89
hunter liveries, routines 444–6
hunter shoe 108
hunters 44
   breeding show classes 322–3
   bringing up from grass 377–8
   feeding 196–7, 309–10
   fittening 309
   travelling 311
   watering 155–6
hunting 288, 309, 314
hygiene
   human food handling 430
   stable yard 69, 125

Iberian plait 98
ice, application of 132, 297
identification
   brand marks 55
   description of horse 56–60
   freeze-marking 55
   micro-chipping 55
   tack 404, 430–1
identity, certification 59–60

ileum 162
ill-health, signs of 123–4, 164
import of equines, regulations
   484
incident (accident) book 426
indoor school 410–13
indoor shows 410
infectious disease 125, 127
infra-red lamp 125
injections, administration 77
injuries
   event horse 296
   hunter 311–12
   legs (self-inflicted) 254–5
   polo pony 196, 255, 329
instincts 32, 33, 163, 367
instructors
   assistant 437
   chief 436
   freelance 426
   intermediate 437
insulation, stabling 394
insurance 425–6
   compulsory 425, 453, 454
internal organs 160–1
interval training 292, 303
inventory 429
Irish Draught 40
Irish martingale 232–3
iron 171
isolation box 401–2
ivermectin 140, 141, 142

jaw
   malformations 38
   trimming 95
jejunum 162
jewellery 68
jockey wheel 333
'jockeys' 273
Joint Measurement Scheme 56, 61
jump studs 113–14
jumps, storage 412, 416

kaolin poultice 129, 130
kicking
   stable door 147
   stable walls 146
   when groomed/handled 33
kicks, minimising danger of 69
Kimblewick 229, 252–3
Kineton noseband 230
knee caps 76, 258

knees
   bandaging 130–1
   conformation 20
knife
   drawing 109
   stable 80
knot
   figure-of-eight 72
   quick-release 71
Kournakoff irons 221

lacing 29
lactation 50–1, 153, 191
lactic acid 295
ladders 455–6
lameness, caused by incorrect
   feeding 204
laminae, sensitive 101–2
laminitis 64, 368
large intestine 162
larynx (voice box) 135
lateral cartilages 101, 102
laurel 360
lavatories 385, 407
leading 73–4, 77–80
   in bridle/saddle 78
   for exercise 79
   foal 52, 76
   handler clothing 73
   for inspection/assessment
      79
   in and out of stable 79
   on road 79
   stallion 54, 76
   to and from grazing 78–9
leather 215–16
   care and cleaning 272–3
   colours 215
   quality 216
   saddle lining 218
   stirrup leathers 221–2
   storage 272
   tanning 215
   texture 215
   types 215–16
leather dressings 272
lecture room 407
leg wraps 260
legislation 448, 483–5
   agricultural 483
   animal welfare 460–6, 483
   buying of horse 63
   children 438
   COSHH 467–8

Health and Safety at Work Act
   407, 429, 453–7
   import/export of equines 484
   Riding Establishments Acts
      (1964/1970) 448–9
   transport of equines 485
legs
   filled 203–4, 261
   handling 69
   trimming 95
   washing 85
   white markings 59
lice 370
licence, local authority 449–53
lifting, guidelines 456
lighting
   indoor school 412
   stable yard 382, 403, 404
   stabling 391, 402, 450
lime, grassland dressings 349
linseed 179, 191
   boiled 183
lip strap 228, 276
liver 160
liveries
   DIY 435
   fees 434–5
   tack room 431
   working 435
loading 335–9
   problems 33, 337–9
   training of horse 336
local authority
   licensing of riding establishments
      449–53
   planning permission 410, 449
   rights of 453
lockers, personal 407
loins 22
long reining 240
loosebox, mare and foal 45
looseboxes 387
   drainage 392
   size 389
   wooden sectional 390
lucerne, *see* alfalfa
lunge cavesson 74, 238
lunge rein 74, 78, 239–40
lunge whip 240
lungs 135–6, 160, 161
lungworm (*Dictyocaulus arnfeldi*)
   141
lying down, refusal 148
lymphangitis 203–4
lymphatic system 137

lysine 169

Magenis snaffle 248
magnesium 171
maintenance person 438
maize 178, 191
management methods, factors in
    choice 67
mane
    clipping 93, 95
    grooming 82
    plaiting 96–8
    pulling/thinning 96
    washing 84
mane comb 84
mangers 210, 399–400
    hay 205–6, 400
manures 350
mare, *see* broodmare
Market Harborough 242
markings 58–9
martingales 231–2, 277
    bib 232
    combined 232
    fitting 280–1
    Irish 232–3
    leading horse in 78
    running 231–2
    standing 232
mastication (chewing) 163
mastitis 53
Matthew Harvey Grinder bit
    146
mebendazole 141
medicine boots 257
medicine cabinet 432–4
medicines 433
    administration 77, 126
    requirements of local authority
        licence 452
    storage 211
micro-chipping 55
micro-organisms, gut 162, 163, 167
milk, mare's 50–1
milk pellets 179
minerals 170–2
mirrors, indoor school 412
mobile phone 422
molars 34
'Monday Morning Disease'
    (lymphangitis) 203–4
mould spores 206
mountain and moorland pony, *see*
    native ponies

mouth
    conformation 18, 38
    inspection 38, 76
    measurement for bit fitting 245
    opening 281
    polo pony 196, 329
    problems 243–4
    structure 243
mouthing bit 249
muck heap 117, 118, 385
muck sacks 119
mucking out
    equipment 118–19
    procedure 119–22
    sick horse 125
mud, removal 86, 312, 313
mud fever 369
mule 44
muscle bulk 187
muscles, superficial 16, 17

nail bind 112–13
nail prick 113
nails, horseshoe 107, 110
nasal passages 135
Nathe bits 245
National Equine Database (NED) 61,
    486
National Equine Welfare Council
    (NEWC) 483
native ponies
    branding 55
    breeds 41–4
    showing 319, 320, 321–2
    summer feeding 193
    winter feeding 194
neatsfoot oil 272
neck, conformation 18, 26
neck cover 266
neck strap 236
negligence 457–8
neoprene 255
nettles 180, 360
New Forest pony 42
New Zealand (turnout) rug 267, 368,
    375
nitrogen, soil 349
non-Thoroughbred Register 39
nosebands 229–30, 244
    Australian cheeker 230, 253
    cavesson 228
    double bridle 252
    drop 229–30
    flash 230

grakle 230
    sheepskin 230
nostrils 135
note pad 70
noticeboard 406
numnahs 234–5, 378
    care of 235, 274
    dressage horse 299
    fitting 280
nursing 124–6

oat straw 176
oats 177–8, 183
    nutritive value 191
oesophagus 161
office
    inside requirements 408
    organisation 422–4
    outside requirements 408
    siting 385
office person 422
oils, dietary 170, 178–9
older horse, feeding 188
olfactory nerve endings 135
onduline sheeting 395
outdoor school 413–16
over-feeding 202
over-grazing 347, 351
over-reach boot 257
over-reach injury 30, 131, 254
overgirth 233
oxygen 136

paddock-sheet 316
padlocks, grazing fields 365–6
pads, shoe/foot 114
pancreas 160–1
panels, saddle 217–18, 219
passports, equine 59–60, 61, 287,
    318, 477
    guidance and regulations 481, 484
    vaccination records 479–80
    where to obtain 478
pastern 20, 105
    hoof/pastern axis 20, 103–4, 105
pawing ground 148
payments 422–3
peacock irons 221, 278
peas 178
pecking order 32, 33
Pelham, Rugby 321–2
Pelham bridle 227, 229, 252, 321
perfume (scent) 68

periople 102
peristalsis 161
personal accident insurance 426
petrol tanks 381
petty cash 423
petty cash book 425
pH, soil 349
pharynx 135, 161
phosphorus
    diet 171
    soil 349
piebald 58
pigeon-toed 30
pincers 109
pinch test 156
pin worms (*Oxyuris equi*) 140
plaiting
    dressage horse 298
    hunter 310
    mane 96–8
    show horse/pony 324
    show jumper 301
    tail 100
plaiting (defective action) 29, 30
planners, yearly 424
planning permission 410, 449
planning regulations 384
plants
    beneficial grassland 354
    poisonous 353, 359–60
plasma 136
plastic granules 415
platelets 136
'plates', racing 108
pleura 136
poaching, grassland 351–2, 353
point-to-point season 314
point-to-pointer 196, 314–18,
    316–17
points of the horse 14
poisonous plants 353, 359–60, 362
poles, storage 416
poll piece, clipping 93, 95
polo boots 257, 327
polo match 327
polo pony 44, 197, 326–9
    injuries 196, 255, 329
polo wraps 260
polyuria 157
pony, definition 44
Pony Club, affiliated 439
post and rail fencing 362–3
potassium
    dietary 171
    soil 349

poultice boot 129–30, 258
poultices 128–30
    foot 129–30
    leg 129, 261
powders, administration 77
power lines 386
power points
    feed room 210
    stable yard 403
pregnancy 50
pregnancy testing 54
pressure bandage 131
privet 360
probiotics 185
prohibited substances 194
prolite, leg pads 260
property insurance 425
prophet's thumb mark 59
Protection Against Cruel Tethering
    Act (1988) 466
Protection of Animals Acts 462–6
Protection of Animals (Amendment)
    Act (1954) 466
Protection of Animals (Amendment)
    Act (1988) 466
protective equipment 68, 429, 485
protein, dietary 169–70, 191
psychology of horse 32–3
public liability insurance 425, 453
pulling back, when tied up 33, 149
pulmonary vein 136, 137
pulse (heart rate) 123, 126
    endurance horse 302, 303
    recording 126–7
pyloric sphincter 162
pyrantel 141, 142

quarter marks 325
quartering 83
quarters, conformation 22–3, 26
quick-release knot 71

rabbit holes 361
racehorse
    fitness and condition 28
    grooming 87, 317
    see also point-to-pointer
racehorse cubes, nutritive value 191
racing plates 108, 317
racing tack 218, 219, 222, 317
ragwort 174, 360
    laws and code of practice 481, 484
rain jackets 429–30

rain scald 369
Rare Breeds Survival Trust 39
rasp 108–9
ration
    calculation 187–90, 193
    competition horses 194, 289
    factors determining 166
    finalising 192–3
    grass-kept horse 193
    maintenance 186
    spring/summer maintenance 193
    winter maintenance 194
    and work 186, 188
rawhide 215, 221
record keeping 427–8
records, confidentiality 383, 427
rectum 162
red blood cells 136
redworm
    large (*Strongylus vulgaris*) 139
    small (*Cyathostomes*) 139
reins 227
    bridoon 228–9
    cleaning 275, 277
    cross-country 294
    grass 236
    length 227, 228
    martingale stops 232
    types and materials 227
respiration rate 123, 127
respiratory system 135–6
responsibility
    levels of 70
    staff members 435–8
restraint of horse 73–6, 91
rhododendron 360
ribs 21
RIDDOR (Reporting of Injuries,
    diseases and Dangerous
    Occurrences Regulations) 467
rider, crookedness 225
riding establishment
    definition 449
    licensing 449–53
Riding Establishments Acts 448–9,
    452
riding and leading 79
riding school horse/pony, feeding
    197, 198
rig 56
ring-fence 382
ringworm 127, 370
riser pads 235
risk assessments 458–60
river, water supply 359

roach back 21, 22
road studs 113
roads, leading horse 79
roadwork 300
roan 58–9
rock phosphate 349
rock salt 184
Rockwell snaffle 248
roller
    anti-cast 150, 267–8
    lungeing 238
    stable rugs 267, 271
rolling, grassland 348–9
roofs, stable 395
    flat 394
    height 389, 394
    materials 395
    overhang 395
    pitch 394
    ridge 394
ropes 71, 237
rotational grazing 351–2
roughage 163, 166, 173–6
roughage:concentrate ratio 193, 195
roughage
    definition 163
    see also fibre; forage; hay; haylage
roughing off 328, 374–5
'roughs and lawns' 347, 353
roundworm (*Parascaris equorum*) 140
routines
    feeding 167
    riding school 441–4
    stable yard 444–6
rubber, arena surface 415
rubber bits 245
rubber curry comb 81, 84, 86
rubber matting 117, 148, 393
rubber ring boot 257
rug room 406
rugs
    belly straps 268
    day 266
    fittings/straps 268, 271
    hanging outside stable 402
    hunter 311, 312, 313
    measuring for 268
    New Zealand/turnout 267, 368,
        375
    point-to-pointer 318
    putting on 268–9
    removing 269–70
    sick horse 125
    stable 265
    storage 272

sweat 265–6, 341
tearing 146–7
travel 341–2, 343
washing 271–2
waterproof 266
run-off 384
running martingale 231–2
running reins 240
Russian trellis 97–8

saddle
    buying 222
    cleaning 273–4, 276
    close-contact 219
    competition 219–20
    dressage 218, 219
    endurance 219, 304
    eventing 293–4
    examining for damage 223–4,
        277–8
    general purpose 217, 219
    jumping 218–19
    linings 218, 273, 277
    modern designs 220
    panels 217–18, 219
    polo 219, 327
    putting on/removing 280–3
    putting up 274–5
    racing 218, 219, 317
    seat 217
    showing 219, 321
    synthetic materials 220, 273–4
    treeless 216, 224
saddle cloths 234
saddle fitting 222–4, 378
    poor 224–5
saddle pads 235, 274
saddle patch, clipping 89, 93
saddle racks 405, 431
saddle soap 272
saddle sores, prevention 378
saddle tree 216
    carbon fibre 220
    damage 223–4, 277
    rigid 216, 223
    spring 216, 223
saddled horse
    leading 78
    leaving in stable 282
saddler 222
saddlery
    checking for soundness 277–9
    cleaning 272–7, 323
    identification 404, 430–1

saddlery *cont.*
   requirements for local authority
      licence 451–2
   see also bridles, saddle and other items
      of saddlery
saddling/unsaddling 280–3
safety
   clipping 91
   clothing 68
   electrical equipment 87, 91, 455,
      491
   fire prevention 446–7, 490–1
   handling horses 69, 80
   regulations 453–7
Safety Policy Statement 454
safety stirrup irons 221, 278
Sale of Goods Act 63
sale of horse 63
sales 63
   codes of practice 482, 484
saline solution 434
saliva 161
salivation 165
salmon marks 59
salt 171, 179, 183
   feeding 184–5, 195, 303
   storage 209
   see also electrolytes
salt lick 184
salt-lick holders 401
sand colic 359
sand surfaces 415
sausage boot 257
sawdust 118, 420
scales 211
Schoolmasta 241
Scorrier snaffle 248
scouring (foal) 49–50
sea travel 344
searcher knife 109
seasonal allergic disorders 64
'seat of corn' 102
seaweed, calcified 349
secretary 437
security 381–3
   feed room 209, 431
   grazing fields 365–6
   horses 55, 382
   office 424
   tack room 404, 431
sedation of horse 94
seed mixes 354
selenium 171
semen, collection 54
septic tank 391

shampoos 83, 85
sheath, washing 86
sheep, grazing 351, 353, 362
sheets
   exercise/paddock 266
   summer 266
shelter
   field/grazing 361
   outdoor school 414
Shetland pony 43–4
shins, bruised 255
shoe (horseshoe)
   aluminium 108
   parts of 107
   plastic glue-on 115
   removal 109–10
   types 107–8
shoeing 109
   alternative methods 114–15
   appearance of newly-shod foot 111
   behavioural problems 33
   cold 110
   dressage horse 298–9
   driving horse/pony 308
   faults 112–13
   frequency 109
   grass-kept horse 107
   hot 110, 112
   pads 114
   point-to-pointer 317
   polo pony 329
   process 109
   show horse/pony 320
   show jumper 301
shoeing tools 108–9
shoulders, conformation 18, 19, 29,
      224
shovel 119
show horse/pony
   child's pony 319
   clipping 88–9, 319
   equipment 323–4
   feeding and condition 319–20
   in-hand classes 322–3
   ridden classes 321–2
   show day 324–5
show jumper 196, 300–1
sick horse 125–7, 201
sickle hocks 23
side reins 239
silage 175, 176, 356, 419
skeleton 15
skewbald 58
skip 119
slaughter, regulations 484–5

sliphead 228, 252
slipping up 80
slosh bottles 304, 306
slot seeding 353
small intestine 162
snaffle bits 246–9
   action 246
   fitting 227–8, 249
   new designs/materials 247–8
snaffle bridle
   fitting 227–8
   parts 226
soak-away 384, 391
sodium 171
soil analysis 347–8
soil nutrients 349–50
sole, dropped 106
sole (foot) 102–3
soundness, assessment 31, 79
soya meal 171, 191
soya oil 178
speedicut injury 254
sponges 84
sponging down 85–6
Sport Horse Breeders of Great Britain
      (SHB) 39
spotted horse 58
stable door 397–9
   banging/kicking 147
   bolts 80, 398
   construction 398–9
   fitting 398
   grille 145
   hinged 397–8
   iron bar 399
   size 397
   sliding 393, 398
   ventilation 396
   webbing 'gate' 396
stable fittings 399–400
stable manners 68
stable rubber 84
stable stains 82
stable 'vices' 144–9
stable yard
   access road 384, 385
   drainage 384, 392–3
   foundations 384
   layout 381
   maintenance 403
   security 381–3
   site and shelter 381, 385
   surface 384–5, 386
stables
   aspect and shelter 385, 396

barn-type 117, 387–8, 390
ceilings 396
cleaning and disinfection 121, 128
construction materials 389–90
doors 397–8
drainage 116, 121, 391–3, 450
electricity 402
floors 393
guttering 393
isolation box 401–2
looseboxes 387
requirements for local authority
      licence 450
roof height 389
roof materials 395
roof overhang 395
sick horse 124–5
size of individual 389
ventilation 385, 388, 396–7
walls, external 394–5
walls, internal 390–1
wooden sectional 390, 395
staff
   accommodation 382, 385, 407–8,
      430
   catering 430
   contracts 435–6
   domestic 439–40
   duties and responsibilities 436–8
   turnout 440
stallion
   feeding 199
   handling 53–4, 76
   selection 45
   stud fees 54
stallion bridle 76, 323
stalls 71–2, 388–9, 392
stamping 148
standing horse up 80
standing martingale 232
stethoscope 303
stirrup bars 216–17
stirrup control system 221
stirrup irons 221–2, 278
   bent leg 221
   bent top/polo 221
   cleaning 273
   Kournakoff 221
   nickel 278
   safety 221, 278
   stainless-steel 278
   treads 222
stirrup leathers 220–1, 273, 278
stock, ordering and monitoring
      428–9

stolen horse, description 60
stomach 161–2, 167
stomach tube 77
store room 406
strapping (wisping) 82–3
straw
  bedding 117, 118, 148
  buying 418
  feeding 176
straying horses 461–2
streams, water supply 359
stress 201, 289
stud fees 54
stud rails 363
students
  paying 437–8
  turnout 440
  working 437
studs 107, 113–14
  dressage horse 299
  driving horse/pony 308
  fitting 114
  show jumper 301
succulents, feeding 167, 179
suede, cleaning 273
sugar beet 171, 178, 197, 198
  nutritive value 191
summer, health problems 64, 368
sun blister 369
sunlight 172
supplements 158, 179, 183–5
surcingle
  rugs 268, 271
  saddle (overgirth) 233, 294
surfaces
  indoor school 412–13
  outdoor school 414–15
  yard and access road 384–5, 456
Swales three-in-one bit 253
sweat, removal 85–6, 312
sweat rugs 265–6, 341
sweat scraper 83, 84
sweating 157
  'breaking out' 83, 312
sweet iron bits 245
sweet itch 64, 368–9
synthetic materials
  bridles 226
  cleaning 273–4
  girths 220
  leathers 221
  saddles 220

tack cleaning 272–7, 323

tack room 404–6
  liveries 431
  organisation 405–6, 430–1
  security 404, 431
  siting 382, 385
tack shop 408–9
tail 22
  bandaging 260, 263–4
  grooming 82, 86
  plaiting 100
  pulling and trimming 98–9
  putting up 99
  rubbing 148
  washing 84–5
tapeworms 141
tarmac
  arena base 416
  yard and road surfaces 384–5
Tattersall yearling bit 249, 323
teeth 161
  ageing horse 35–8
  'bishoping' 38
  examination and care 34, 38, 76,
    165, 287
  hooks 38
  milk (deciduous) 36, 37, 38
  parts of 35
  types and number 34–5
  wolf 35, 243
teething 35
telephones 70, 382, 422
temperament
  assessment 28
  and feeding 189–90
temperature
  in extreme heat 296–7
  normal 126
  recording 126
tendon boot 257
tendons, foot 101, 102
tetanus vaccinations 287, 479
tethering, laws and codes 466, 482,
    485
thatching 313
theft, prevention 382–3
thermometer 126
thiabendazole 140
thiamine 173
thistles 360
thorn injuries 311–12
Thoroughbred (TB) 39
threadworm (*Strongyloides westeri*)
    140
throatlash 228
thrush 370

'thumps' 156
timetables, working day 441–4
toeing knife 109
tongue 161
  holding 76
  over the bit 244
tongue grid 253
tongue guards 253
tools, yard 68–9
'top line' 13, 18
top-cutting, grassland 351
towing attachment 333
towing vehicle 332, 333–4
trace clip 89, 90, 93
trace elements 170, 171–2
trachea (windpipe) 135
tractor, regulations 455
tractor shed 381
Trades Description Act 63
trailer 332–3
  care of horse during travel 341–2
  driver 334–5
  loading 335–6
  loading problems 337–9
  reversing 335
  towing vehicle 332
  unloading 339
training devices ('gadgets') 240–2
Transit of Animals (Road and Rail)
    330
transportation
  abroad/long distances 202, 342–4
  air 344
  avoiding stress 144
  boots and bandages 258–9, 261
  care of horse 340–2
  construction 330–1
  driver 334–5
  equipment 342
  EU regulations 487–9
  feeding and watering 157, 201–2,
    206, 343
  floor 330–1, 334
  hired 334
  hunter 310–11
  legislation and guidance 330, 481,
    485, 487–9
  loading equipment 342
  loading horse 33, 335–9
  overnight stay 289–90
  procedure after travelling 335
  procedure before travelling 333–5
  sea 344
  show horse 324
  tacked up horse/pony 341–2

tail bandaging 263–4
  types 331–3
  unloading 339–40
tread injury 255–6
trees, safety 457
trespassing stock 461
trimming 94–5
  head 95, 320
  legs 95
  tail 98–9
trot up
  assessment of soundness/action 31,
    79
  showing classes 321
trot work, fittening 135
tubbing 131
turning out (field) 374–5
turnout
  hunting 310
  point-to-pointer 317–18
  polo pony 327
  staff and students 440
turnout boots 255
tushes 34–5, 243
twitch
  clipping horse 94
  humane 75
  rope 75
'tying up', *see* azoturia
tying up horse 69, 71–2
  horsebox/trailer 335
  outside box 80
  pulling back 33, 149
  safety precautions 71, 80, 399
  stable or stall 71–2, 399
  training young horse 80

ultrasound scanning, broodmare
    54
umbilical (navel) cord 48
under-feeding 202
underweight horse 13, 188, 200–1
unsaddling 282–3
unshod horse/pony 106–7
urination, excessive (polyuria) 157
urine testing, pregnancy 54
utility box 401

vaccinations 479–80
  competition horse 287, 479–80
  endurance horse 304
vandalism, prevention 382–3
vehicle insurance 425

Vehicle and Operators Service Agency (VOSA) 332
veins 136
Velcro fastenings 255, 256
vena cava 136, 137
ventilation, stables 385, 388, 396–7
vermin, stable yard 69
'vest' 266
veterinary examinations
  endurance horse 305–6
  event horse 297
  pre-purchase 61, 64
veterinary inspections, riding establishment 450
veterinary surgeon
  foaling 48, 49
  when to call 124
veterinary surgeons, legislation and codes 484, 485
'Vetrap' 130, 131, 132, 260
vitamins 161, 167, 172–3
  B group 171, 173
  vitamin A (retinol) 172
  vitamin D (calciferol) 172
  vitamin E (tocopherol) 171, 173
  vitamin K 173
voice, use of 69, 77–8
volumes 471
vulcanite bits 245
vulva 28

walk, fittening programme 135, 377
wall eye 58, 59
walls
  field boundary 362
  stable 390–1, 394–5
warble fly 369
warm-up
  event horse 295
  show jumper 301
warmbloods 40, 41, 44
warmth, sick horse 125
wash room 406
washing horse 83, 84–5, 312
waste management, regulations 484
water 168
  digestive system 164

purity of 154
roles in body 153
stabled horse requirement 153
see also watering
water bowls, automatic 154
water brush 83
water buckets 155
water dropwort 360
water main 384
water supply, feed room 210
water trough 358–9
watering 154–5
  competition horses 155–6, 295, 296, 297, 304, 306, 328
  grass-kept horse 358–9
  hunter 311
  principles 154
  rivers and streams 359
  sick horse 125–6
  travelling 157, 201–2, 343
watering systems, indoor school 413
weaning 52–3
weather conditions
  and feeding 189
  freezing/cold 367, 456
  hot 295, 297
Weatherbys 39, 318
weaving 144–5
weed control 352–3, 360
  code of practice 481
weight
  calculating 187
  and dry food requirement 188, 189
  excessive 187, 377
  loss 200–1
  see also condition
weight cloth 234
weights and measures 471
welfare
  code of practice 481
  legislation 460–6, 483
Welfare of Animals (Transport) Order (1997) 337, 340, 487–9
Welfare Bill 124
Welsh ponies 41–2
  Section A (Welsh Mountain) 42
  Section B 42
  Section C 42

Section D (Welsh Cob) 42
Weymouth, sliding mouthpiece 251
wheat bran 171, 178, 191
wheelbarrows 119, 456
whips, lungeing 240
whiskers, trimming 95, 320
white blood cells 136
white line 102
white markings
  description 58–9
  grooming 325
whorls 59
Wilson snaffle 248
wind problems, feeding 204, 206
windows, stable 396
windpipe (trachea) 135
windsucking 145–6
winter
  grass-kept horse/pony 366–7, 369–70
  grassland management 351–2, 358–9
  health problems 369–70
  maintenance feeding 194
  water supply 359
  yarding of ponies 372
wire fencing 363
wire mesh fencing 363
wisp 82
wisping (strapping) 82–3
wither pads 235–6, 274
withers, conformation 19, 224
wood chewing 147
wood shavings 118, 420
wood-based surfaces 413, 415
work
  categories 192
  feed requirement 167–8, 186, 188, 191–2
working pupils 437
wormers 142–3, 434
  administration 77, 142
  drug groups 142
  parasite resistance 141
worming
  competition horse 287
  foals 50
  frequency 142–3

worms (internal parasites) 138
  bots 140, 369
  control 141–3
  faecal egg counts 138–9, 142–3
  large redworm (*Strongylus vulgaris*) 139
  life cycle 139
  lungworm (*Dictyocaulus arnfeldi*) 141
  pinworms (*Oxyuris*) 140–1
  roundworm (*Parascaris equorum*) 140
  small redworm (*Cyathostomes*) 139–40
  symptoms of infestation 138
  tapeworm 141
  threadworms 140
Worshipful Company of Farriers 101
wound dressings 433, 434
  prevention of chewing 76

X-rays, prior to buying horse 64

'Y-mouth snaffle 248
yard equipment 68–9
yard management, flow chart 423
yard manager, responsibilities 436, 460
yarding of ponies 372
yew 360, 362
Yorkshire boarding 397
Yorkshire boot 256–7
young horses
  action 29
  conformation 21
  feeding 51, 188, 191, 199
  foot care 107
  picking up feet 82–3
  showing 322–3
  teeth 35, 36, 37, 38
  training to tie up 80
young riders, legislation 485

zebra marks 59

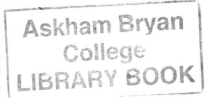